Human Brain Dynamics

Human Brain Dynamics

Editor: Latia Smothers

AMERICAN
MEDICAL PUBLISHERS
www.americanmedicalpublishers.com

AMERICAN
MEDICAL PUBLISHERS
www.americanmedicalpublishers.com

Cataloging-in-Publication Data

Human brain dynamics / edited by Latia Smothers.
p. cm.
Includes bibliographical references and index.
ISBN 979-8-88740-187-4
1. Brain. 2. Brain--Metabolism. 3. Central nervous system.
4. Neurophysiology. I. Smothers, Latia.
QP376 .H86 2023
612.82--dc23

American Medical Publishers,
41 Flatbush Avenue,
1st Floor, New York,
NY 11217, USA

ISBN 979-8-88740-187-4 (Hardback)

Contents

Preface

Brain dynamics characterize expert cognitive-motor performance based on neural and psychomotor efficiency. It is relevant to consider the dynamics for all aspects of mental activity—perception, cognition, and emotion because brain activity keeps on changing rapidly even in a stable environment. Several measuring tools and techniques like electroencephalogram (EEG), event-related potential (ERP), functional magnetic resonanceimaging (fMRI), and EEG coherence are used to obtain the details of brain activity. The study of brain dynamics majorly focuses on evaluating the internal states of the human brain and its dynamics. This book includes some of the vital pieces of work being conducted worldwide on various topics related to human brain dynamics. From theories to research to practical applications, case studies related to all contemporary topics of relevance to this field have been included herein. Students, researchers, experts, and all associated with human brain dynamics will benefit alike from this book.

The information contained in this book is the result of intensive hard work done by researchers in this field. All due efforts have been made to make this book serve as a complete guiding source for students and researchers. The topics in this book have been comprehensively explained to help readers understand the growing trends in the field.

I would like to thank the entire group of writers who made sincere efforts in this book and my family who supported me in my efforts of working on this book. I take this opportunity to thank all those who have been a guiding force throughout my life.

Editor

1

Long-range neural activity evoked by premotor cortex stimulation: a TMS/EEG co-registration study

Marco Zanon[1], Piero P. Battaglini[2], Joanna Jarnolowska[2], Gilberto Pizzolato[3†] and Pierpaolo Busan[2*]

[1] Cognitive Neuroscience Sector, International School for Advanced Studies, SISSA, Trieste, Italy
[2] Department of Life Sciences, BRAIN Center for Neuroscience, University of Trieste, Trieste, Italy
[3] Department of Medical, Surgical and Health Sciences, University of Trieste, Trieste, Italy

Correspondence:
Pierpaolo Busan, Department of Life Sciences, BRAIN Center for Neuroscience, University of Trieste, via Fleming 22, Trieste 34127, Italy
e-mail: pbusan@units.it

† The present manuscript wishes to be the authors' personal honor to the memory of Prof. Gilberto Pizzolato, as a tribute to his scientific competence, and the contribution that he gave to our research projects in these years of proficient collaboration.

The premotor cortex is one of the fundamental structures composing the neural networks of the human brain. It is implicated in many behaviors and cognitive tasks, ranging from movement to attention and eye-related activity. Therefore, neural circuits that are related to premotor cortex have been studied to clarify their connectivity and/or role in different tasks. In the present work, we aimed to investigate the propagation of the neural activity evoked in the dorsal premotor cortex using transcranial magnetic stimulation/electroencephalography (TMS/EEG). Toward this end, interest was focused on the neural dynamics elicited in long-ranging temporal and spatial networks. Twelve healthy volunteers underwent a single-pulse TMS protocol in a resting condition with eyes closed, and the evoked activity, measured by EEG, was compared to a sham condition in a time window ranging from 45 ms to about 200 ms after TMS. Spatial and temporal investigations were carried out with sLORETA. TMS was found to induce propagation of neural activity mainly in the contralateral sensorimotor and frontal cortices, at about 130 ms after delivery of the stimulus. Different types of analyses showed propagated activity also in posterior, mainly visual, regions, in a time window between 70 and 130 ms. Finally, a likely "rebounding" activation of the sensorimotor and frontal regions, was observed in various time ranges. Taken together, the present findings further characterize the neural circuits that are driven by dorsal premotor cortex activation in healthy humans.

Keywords: premotor cortex, propagated activity, TMS/EEG co-registration, sLORETA, TMS-evoked potentials

INTRODUCTION

In the last decades, many studies have contributed to disentangle the anatomical and functional organization of the cortical circuitries characterizing motor structures. Most have focused on control of motor behavior (see for a brief review Rizzolatti and Luppino, 2001), and/or on goal-directed movements under visual guidance (Naranjo et al., 2007). The dorsal premotor cortex (PMd) plays a key role in these motor networks (Davare et al., 2006). It is actively involved in several functions ranging from the planning of a proper motor response to the correct allocation of attentive resources (Rushworth et al., 2003) and/or eye-related activity (Luppino and Rizzolatti, 2000; Amiez and Petrides, 2009). As a consequence, the PMd is directly or indirectly linked with a series of structures in the brain (Hagmann et al., 2008), ranging from the primary motor cortex (Matsumoto et al., 2007; Huang et al., 2009) and the supplementary motor area (Matsumoto et al., 2007) to the superior parietal cortex (Kurata, 1991; Massimini et al., 2005; Rottschy et al., 2012), parieto-occipital regions (Shipp et al., 1998; Caminiti et al., 1999), and the prefrontal cortex (Barbas and Pandya, 1987; Lu et al., 1994), in order to allow effective exchange and elaboration of information.

Taking into consideration the goal-directed movements under visual guidance, Milner and Goodale (2006) suggested the existence of different streams mediating the sensory-motor transformations necessary for visually guided movements. Signals elaborated in the primary visual cortex are sent to areas for integration with other sensory information to organize a representation of the action to be performed. The information is then transmitted to the frontal cortex, such as Brodmann area 6, which constitutes the premotor cortex in humans and successively sends motor programs to the primary motor cortex (see for a brief review Luppino and Rizzolatti, 2000; Rizzolatti and Luppino, 2001). Furthermore, the PMd can be functionally subdivided in subregions, according to the specific computation it is mainly involved in. For example, neurons involved in reaching movements have been identified in the dorsal part of the lateral premotor cortex, whereas its ventral part is likely involved in grasping movements (Rizzolatti et al., 1998; Rizzolatti and Luppino, 2001; Matsumoto et al., 2007).

Most of the knowledge about the functional and anatomical organization of PMd derives from studies on animals, and in particular on non-human primates (Rizzolatti et al., 1998), but also on electrophysiological recordings during neurosurgery, as in the case of epileptic patients (Matsumoto et al., 2003, 2007). However, the development of non-invasive neuroimaging techniques extended knowledge of PMd connectivity and functions even in humans (Picard and Strick, 2001; Massimini et al., 2005; Rottschy et al., 2012). Early electrophysiological studies on monkeys have shown that PMd neurons respond, for example, to the appearance of visual signals and discharge during the preparation and execution of movements under visual guidance (Hoshi and Tanji, 2006). The PMd is also activated by viewing an object that has motor valence, even in the absence of a subsequent movement (Grafton et al., 1997). Moreover, it is also involved in motor attention and motor selection (Rushworth et al., 2003). Some of these findings have also been observed in humans (Davare et al., 2006) and it is now clear that the PMd is part of a fronto-parietal circuit for goal-directed movements, where it plays a key role in the planning aspects of motor commands (Luppino and Rizzolatti, 2000; Rizzolatti and Luppino, 2001; Davare et al., 2006; Milner and Goodale, 2006; Naranjo et al., 2007; Busan et al., 2009a).

The PMd organizes and selects appropriate and effective motor commands, on the basis of representations, provided by the parietal regions, and intentions, elaborated in the prefrontal areas (Tanne et al., 1995; Matelli and Luppino, 2001; Galletti et al., 2003). The role of the PMd as an integration center is also supported by studies that have shown a functional gradient of neuronal projections with its rostral part mainly connected to prefrontal regions, and caudal portions sending projections mainly to the primary motor cortex and spinal cord. This organization has led to the hypothesis that the former are more likely involved in higher-level, cognitive aspects of behavior preparation, whereas the latter are probably involved in less complex functions that are more related to motor execution (Picard and Strick, 2001; Matsumoto et al., 2003). The PMd seems to be involved in the control of eye movements and in the control of eye-related neural activity or in specific tasks that require eye-hand coordination (Luppino and Rizzolatti, 2000; Amiez and Petrides, 2009).

Due to the functional relationship between the parietal and frontal areas, it has been suggested that the flow of information is not unidirectional from the former to the latter, but that it can re-enter the parietal cortex through fronto-parietal connections. This reciprocity of cortico-cortical connections implies that coding of information cannot be regarded as a serial sequence of transformations, each performed by a given cortical area, but rather as a recursive process that can also involve relatively remote regions (Paus et al., 1997; Battaglia-Mayer et al., 1998; Massimini et al., 2005). In spite of all this information, effective and functional connections of PMd in humans are still far from being fully understood.

Different techniques to investigate brain connectivity have been developed during recent years, and among these, the combination of transcranial magnetic stimulation (TMS) with electroencephalography (EEG) acquisition (TMS/EEG) has been demonstrated to be a useful approach. It allows the study of the propagation of neural activity from the stimulated cerebral area to other brain regions, providing a new way to look for their connections (e.g., Ilmoniemi et al., 1997). In fact, thanks to the optimal temporal resolution offered by EEG and the reconstruction of the EEG neural sources (Michel et al., 2004), it is possible to successfully characterize the neural temporal dynamics of events evoked by TMS (TMS-evoked potentials, TEPs; e.g., Paus et al., 2001; Bonato et al., 2006).

Although the mechanisms underlying TEPs are not completely understood, they might provide useful information with respect to brain functions and networks (Massimini et al., 2005; Komssi and Kahkonen, 2006; Miniussi and Thut, 2010; Frantseva et al., 2012; Manganotti and Del Felice, 2013). Furthermore, the development of improved methods to obtain a reliable EEG source estimation allows adding spatial information on the evoked neural activity (e.g., Ilmoniemi et al., 1997; Pascual-Marqui, 2002).

TMS/EEG is usually performed by using an "inductive" approach (Miniussi and Thut, 2010), and a long-scale network of neuronal connections has been shown to be engaged when TMS-related activation spreads from the stimulation site toward different brain regions, an activity that can last even hundreds of milliseconds (e.g., Ilmoniemi and Karhu, 2008). The properties of the TMS-evoked responses have been shown to depend on a series of parameters, such as the stimulus intensity (Casarotto et al., 2010). In this regard, while the initial part of the TEP can reflect the "reactivity" of the stimulated cortex, the later spatio-temporal propagation of the electrical activity toward different brain regions might unravel the presence of intra- and/or inter-hemispheric cortico-cortical connections as well as intermediate links, such as subcortical structures.

In an effort to better characterize PMd connectivity, we used TMS/EEG co-registration to investigate the cortico-cortical long range connections and activity propagation pathways. We focused on the stimulation of the left hemisphere, usually viewed as the dominant one in right-handed people (e.g., Iacoboni, 2006; Vingerhoets et al., 2013). In this sense, the left hemisphere seems to play a special role also in organizing movements during visually-guided praxis (e.g., Goodale, 1988; Janssen et al., 2011).

MATERIALS AND METHODS

SUBJECTS AND TRANSCRANIAL MAGNETIC STIMULATION

Twelve healthy subjects (7 males and 5 females, age range 22–26 years, mean age 23.4 years, $SD = 1.2$) underwent single-pulse TMS (Medtronic MagPro R30) applied on a scalp position that putatively allowed the stimulation of the dorsal premotor cortex (see **Figure 1**). All subjects were right-handed as confirmed

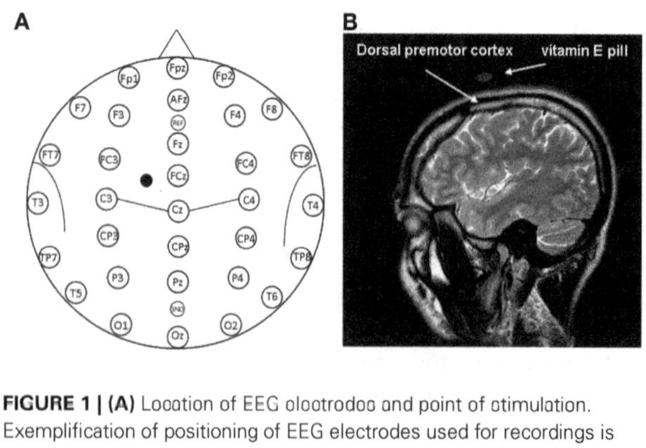

FIGURE 1 | (A) Location of EEG electrodes and point of stimulation. Exemplification of positioning of EEG electrodes used for recordings is reported on a model also indicating some of the main brain sulci. The point on the scalp where TMS was applied is indicated by a mark. **(B)** Structural magnetic resonance indicating the point of stimulation. Anatomical magnetic resonance acquisition performed in a prototypical subject. The point of stimulation is indicated by the positioning of the vitamin E pill. The positioning of the dorsal premotor cortex is also indicated on the basis of Duvernoy (1999).

by a dedicated questionnaire (Edinburgh Inventory; Oldfield, 1971). Participants gave written informed consent after receiving exhaustive information about all procedures, in compliance with the Declaration of Helsinki. Favorable judgment of the Ethics Committee of the University of Trieste was obtained. Participants could leave the study at any time, although all completed the experiments.

The stimulated scalp position was determined using an adapted EEG coordinate system (see Herwig et al., 2003; Okamoto et al., 2004; Jurcak et al., 2007) and a probabilistic method (Steinsträter et al., 2002; http://wwwneuro03.uni-muenster.de/ger/t2tconv/). TMS was delivered on a scalp location that corresponded to a position situated 10% of the biauricolar distance to the left of the vertex and 7.5% ahead the nasion-inion distance (see **Figure 1A**). A very rough estimation, in MNI (Montreal Neurological Institute) coordinates, of the center of the stimulated region was: $x = -30$, $y = 10$, $z = 65$ (best match: Brodmann Area—BA—6). The resulting point of stimulation was marked on the EEG cap.

For each participant, TMS was delivered through a figure-of-eight coil (diameter of each wing about 7 cm), oriented tangentially to the scalp (single pulse stimulation; biphasic waves; pulse duration: 280 μsec). The coil was secured on the scalp by hand and its position was continuously visually checked and readjusted if necessary. The coil was maintained with a 45° orientation with respect to the inter-hemispheric fissure with the handle pointing downward and backward. The subject's head was not restrained, although participants were asked to maintain a stable position for the entire experiment with their chin backed on a metal structure. The stimulation coil was also maintained in the same position when sham TMS was delivered.

PRE-EXPERIMENTAL PROCEDURES

Before each experiment, the optimal cortical point for activating the first dorsal interosseous muscle (FDI) of the right hand was individuated and, successively, resting motor threshold (RMT) was measured as the stimulus intensity triggering at least a 50 μV response on electromyography traces (EMG; band pass filtering 20–2000 Hz) in half of the stimulations (Rossini et al., 1994). A tendon belly montage was used by applying surface Ag/AgCl electrodes. During experimental sessions, the intensity of TMS was set at 110% RMT to limit current diffusion to neighboring areas, such as the primary motor cortex. To check for unintended current diffusion, the selected stimulation point on PMd was stimulated immediately after the evaluation of RMT, before the beginning of the experiment. Specifically, muscular responses on different right hand and right arm muscles, detected by EMG (band pass filtering 5–2000 Hz), were considered as unwanted activation of the primary motor cortex at the individuated experimental intensity. On the same line, it was verified that stimulation of the premotor cortex did not evoke evident facial muscular artifacts (e.g., Julkunen et al., 2008; Mütanen et al., 2013). When a muscular response was highlighted, one of the following operations or combination was used to reduce these muscular activations until no response was evident: a) the stimulation intensity was slightly dampened; b) the coil position was slightly moved anteriorly; c) the coil was slightly rotated from its original position. Some of these suggestions have been already shown to be effective in reducing muscular artifacts (Ilmoniemi and Karhu, 2008; Ilmoniemi and Kicic, 2010). As a consequence, for each subject we found the methodological solution that minimized variability with respect to the original setting in terms of stimulation intensity, stimulated scalp position, and coil position. It is evident that the application of these procedures could make individuation of the premotor cortex a little bit more uncertain, but they also allowed minimizing possible contamination from neighboring neural regions, especially the primary motor cortex, reducing, for example, artifacts related to sensory feedbacks obtained after distal muscular activations.

TMS/EEG EXPERIMENTAL SETTING

Subjects were asked to sit with eyes closed for the entire duration of stimulation blocks (real and sham TMS sessions) to reduce ocular artifacts.

The experiment consisted of three blocks of 65 real magnetic stimuli (real TMS) and three blocks of 65 sham stimuli (sham TMS), interleaving one real TMS block and one sham TMS block. The starting block (real or sham TMS) was randomly defined. During stimulations, EMG was constantly checked to verify that the stimuli did not evoke any muscular response that could interfere with EEG recorded potentials, such as that evoked by direct motor activation or somatosensory feedbacks successive to distal muscular activations. For this purpose, right hand muscles (first dorsal interosseous muscle, abductor digiti minimi muscle and opponens pollicis brevis muscle) were routinely monitored as well as right arm biceps brachii muscle, right arm deltoid muscle and/or right arm flexor and extensor muscles. Monitoring was performed by applying surface Ag/AgCl electrodes on the targeted muscles and using a band-pass filtering of 5–2000 Hz. Trials showing an evident motor response were discarded from successive analyses.

Sham TMS was performed by applying the coil on the scalp in the same manner as real TMS condition, and using the same intensity of stimulation. In this condition, however, a 3-cm-thick block of wood was placed between the coil and scalp to reduce the intensity of the magnetic field that reached the scalp. Both in real and sham conditions, about 0.5 cm of foam was applied between the scalp and coil to limit the somatic sensation specifically related to TMS stimulation; subjects wore earplugs to reduce acoustic stimulation. In this way, sham TMS allowed to control for the acoustic activation related to magnetic stimulation (Nikouline et al., 1999), while a reliable control for the somatic sensation of TMS is not so simple to obtain. Safety guidelines for TMS were always taken into consideration (e.g., Wassermann, 1998; Rossi et al., 2009).

EEG DATA

EEG traces were acquired by using a commercially-available system (MIZAR-SIRIUS system, acquisition software Galileo NT, EBNeuro, Italy). Specifically, an amplifier compatible with magnetic resonance acquisition (BASIS BE, EBNeuro, Italy) was used. Subjects wore an EEG elastic cap with 32 flat electrodes (Bionen sas, Italy). Electrode positions corresponded to classical positions and are reported in **Figure 1A**. More specifically, the following sensor positions were placed on the scalp: Fp1, Fp2, Fpz, AFz, F7, F3, Fz, F4, F8, FT7, FC3, FCz, FC4, FT8, T3, C3, Cz, C4, T4, TP7, CP3, CPz, CP4, TP8, T5, P3, Pz, P4, T6, O1, Oz, O2. The reference electrode was positioned between the AFz and Fz electrode, while the ground electrode was placed between the Pz and Oz electrode. EEG impedances were maintained under 10 KΩ. An electro-oculogram (EOG) was also acquired to allow accurate selection and rejection of noisy epochs. For this purpose, surface Ag/AgCl electrodes were placed above (near the external canthi) and below the right eye. Specific hardware and software settings were used to limit the impact of the TMS artifact on EEG traces. In particular, the sampling rate was set at 4096 Hz, with an analog band-pass filtering of 0.01–1843.2 Hz. The acquisition range was adjusted at $\pm$ 65500 μV to limit amplifier saturation. Moreover, electrode wires were carefully placed to limit the influence of TMS pulses on the EEG signal (Sekiguchi et al., 2011). Raw data were subsequently marked (real or sham TMS trials) and digitally filtered (band pass infinite impulse response filter 0.01–1000 Hz) using Neuroscan software (Compumedics Neuroscan Inc., El Paso, USA). EOG data were further elaborated by using a similar low pass filter at 50 Hz. Data were then segmented in epochs, considering a time window between −100 and 500 ms with respect to the delivery of TMS (0 ms) and corrected for baseline (from −100 to −10 ms before the delivery of the TMS pulse). Epochs were subsequently subdivided according to the considered condition (real or sham TMS) and visually inspected to discard those that presented excessive noise. In this sense, epochs that presented, for example, blink artifacts or that showed the presence of a drift that did not allow a reliable alignment of the trace (even if a baseline correction was performed) were not considered for further analyses. An average of 137.3 ($SD = 21.3$) epochs per subject was accepted for the real TMS condition, while 144.7 ($SD = 25.8$) epochs per subject were considered for the sham TMS condition. These epochs, grouped by conditions (real and sham TMS), were further analyzed with EEGLAB (Delorme and Makeig, 2004). An independent component analysis (Jung et al., 2000) was conducted to reduce the TMS-induced electric artifact and increase the quality of recorded data (e.g., Hamidi et al., 2011). Because of the large TMS artifact, which would highly impair the decomposition in independent components, ICA was performed considering a time range between 45 and 250 ms after delivery of the magnetic pulse. This approach allowed excluding most of the TMS artifacts that appeared immediately after TMS delivery (fast rising/decaying peak of signal, recharging artifacts, etc.) and, as much as possible, the residual part of the TMS artifact, and specifically the slow recovery of the signal after the delivery of the pulses (see **Figures 2D,E**).

It has been decided to reduce the considered time window of analysis until 250 ms after the delivery of the magnetic pulse in order to have a more direct comparison with previous works (Zanon et al., 2010; Busan et al., 2012). In fact, in these previous studies (Zanon et al., 2010; Busan et al., 2012) the more interesting results were mainly comprised in similar time ranges. A longer time window (see above) was initially considered only to allow a more reliable epochs selection for subsequent analyses even if, generally, it was noted the presence of further components (see **Figures 2F,H**), preferably stronger in the real TMS condition. For example, the component appearing after about 250–300 ms from TMS delivery, could be ascribed as an evidence arising from the stimulation of motor networks (e.g., Massimini et al., 2005; Ferreri et al., 2011), even if the possibility remains that it also arises from acoustic stimulation (e.g., Nikouline et al., 1999).

A further step was implemented for eliminating as much as possible the remaining TMS artifact: after averaging the epochs and obtaining real and sham TMS-evoked potentials, a "linear detrend" function was applied when needed (e.g., Van Der Werf and Paus, 2006). Averaged real and sham TEPs were re-referenced to a common average reference based on all the recorded 32 electrodes. Finally, grand-averaged TEPs were visually inspected by means of a butterfly-plot representation: this allowed to highlight the more evident time windows of analysis in a time range comprised between 45 and 250 ms (see below the sLORETA analysis section). In every time window, the relative local maxima peak of amplitude (and its latency) was highlighted in a series of representative electrodes: F3, Fz, F4, FC3, FCz, FC4, C3, Cz, C4, CP3, CPz, CP4, P3, Pz, and P4. Amplitudes (in μV; with respect to the zero value), as well as latencies (in ms; with respect to the delivery of TMS), were averaged among electrodes and considered as dependent variables. Data were successively analyzed by means of repeated measures ANOVA by considering main effects and interactions between time windows and stimulation condition (TMS vs. sham) for every dependent variable. *Post-hoc* analyses were conducted by using T-test. Significance was set at $p < 0.05$. Data were checked for their normality by means of the Shapiro–Wilk test and corrections were used in order to manage data that did not respect the assumption of sphericity and in order to correct for multiple comparisons.

Characterization of the TMS-induced artifact on the EEG signal was also performed on a watermelon, using the highest TMS intensity used in the present experiments and following the suggestions of Veniero et al. (2009). In this case, all EEG settings were similar to those used for real and sham TMS experiments.

sLORETA ANALYSIS

Although scalp topography of electric potentials can provide some information about underlying neuronal dynamics, the distribution of EEG signal sources better allows investigation about the spatial localization of activated areas (Michel et al., 2004; He et al., 2011). Therefore, EEG source imaging was applied to both real and sham TMS evoked-potentials and a statistical comparison was performed between these conditions.

Standardized low resolution brain electromagnetic tomography (sLORETA; Pascual-Marqui, 2002) implemented in sLORETA-Key software (http://www.uzh.ch/keyinst/loreta.htm) was used to reconstruct the cortical three-dimensional distribution of the neuronal activity underlying real and sham TEPs. The sLORETA algorithm is a standardized discrete, three-dimensional distributed, linear, minimum norm inverse solution (Pascual-Marqui, 2002). Computations were realized in a realistic head model (Fuchs et al., 2002) based on the MNI152 template (Mazziotta et al., 2001), with three-dimensional space solution restricted to cortical gray matter, as determined by using the probabilistic Talairach atlas (Lancaster et al., 2000). Therefore, the intracerebral volume considered for the analysis comprised

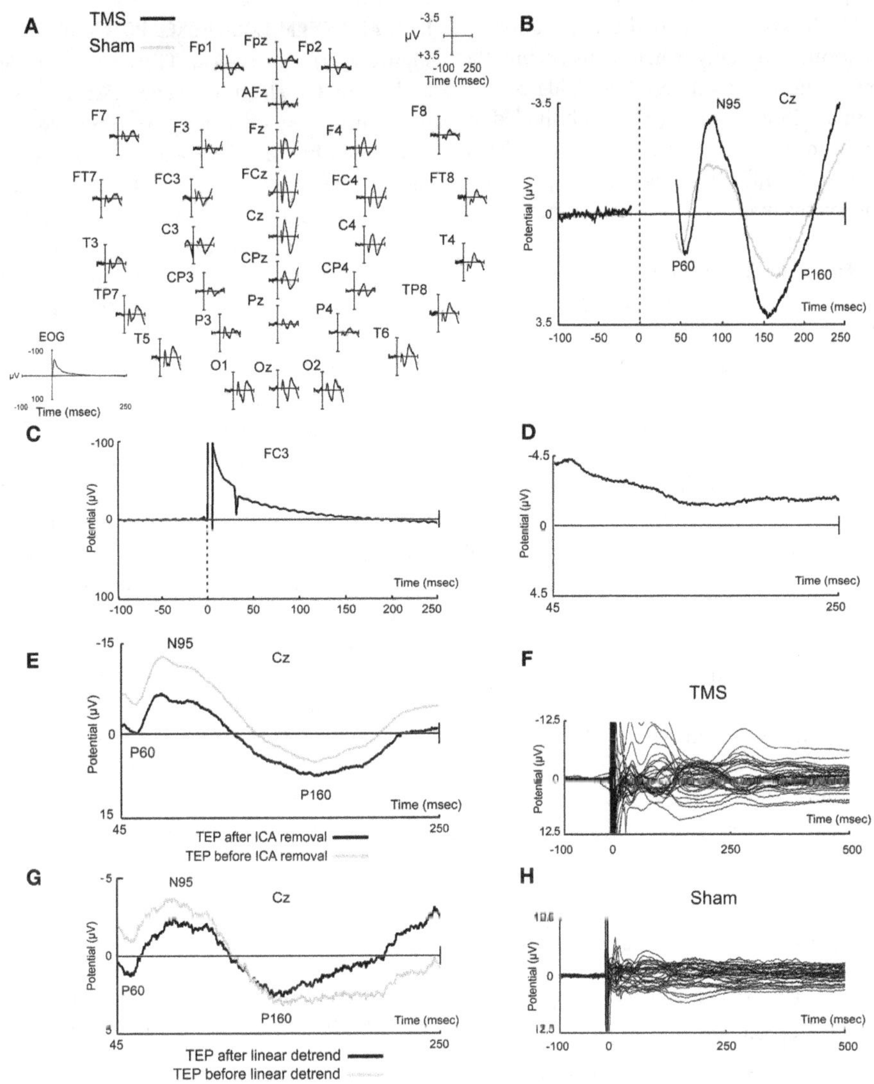

FIGURE 2 | Real and sham TMS-evoked potentials. Evoked potentials obtained in real and sham TMS conditions as recorded in all electrodes **(A)** and in the representative Cz electrode **(B)**. In EOG data, TMS artifact is fully reported and appears longer likely due to filtering settings **(A)**. Potential that has been obtained in a prototypical electrode after the stimulation of the watermelon is also shown **(C)**, as well as a prototypical independent component, evidently related to TMS artifacts, that has been removed from data **(D)**. A TMS-evoked potential of a prototypical subject before and after ICA removal is also represented **(E)**. Finally, the butterfly plots of the grand-averaged TMS and sham raw data (before ICA decomposition and removal, and before linear detrend) are shown **(F,H)** in order to highlight that data tend to the baseline after the last components that appeared at about 250–300 ms after the delivery of the magnetic stimuli. An example of data before and after linear detrend is also shown **(G)**.

6239 voxels at a 5-mm spatial resolution. Finally, electrode positions were superimposed on the MNI152 scalp (Oostenveld and Praamstra, 2001; Jurcak et al., 2007) and localization error was reduced by applying a regularization factor in all source reconstructions. Specifically, the mean signal-to-noise ratio in ERPs for each subject and condition was computed using the method of the 20th percentile, in a time window between 45 and 250 ms after stimulus onset. Anatomical labels and Brodmann areas were reported in the MNI space, with the possibility to correct to the Talairach space (Brett et al., 2002).

A voxel-by-voxel within-subject comparison of EEG sources was performed, and significant differences in real and sham TMS conditions were assessed with non-parametric statistical analysis based on a permutation test (Statistical non Parametric Mapping: SnPM; Nichols and Holmes, 2002), implemented in sLORETA-Key software. Both *t*-statistic and log of F-ratio were computed, to obtain a more comprehensive evaluation of the possible activations elicited by the present protocol.

Furthermore, statistical analyses were conducted comparing real and sham TMS signals in each time-frame (time-frame by time-frame analysis) and the mean source signal in selected time intervals of interest (mean signal analysis). In both cases, analyses were restricted to time windows ranging from 45 to 213 ms after stimulation, chosen after visual inspection of the grand-average butterfly plot of real TMS and sham TEPs and in order to limit possible biases related to the application of the linear detrend function, especially when considering the end of the original time window of interest (i.e., 250 ms after TMS delivery). Thus, this window was further subdivided in 3 windows of interest: from 45 to 70 ms, from 70 to 130 ms, and from 130 to 213 ms. Significance was set at $p < 0.05$; this threshold was conservatively corrected with respect to the number of time windows that were considered in each analysis. Importantly, SnPM in sLORETA automatically allowed for correction of multiple comparisons in each computed analysis even with respect to all examined voxels and time samples. When considering time-frame by time-frame analyses, in order to assure a greater confidence in results obtained from the main statistical analyses, we also reported the number of time-frames that resulted in a consecutive activation, at a trend level ($p < 0.1$; see **Tables 1, 2**), of every maximal peak of activation obtained from main analyses. This has been done considering that reliable and meaningful brain activations should occur in microstates.

ANATOMICAL LOCALIZATION

In order to verify the cortical areas beneath the selected stimulation site, TMS coil position on the scalp of a prototypical subject was marked with a vitamin E pill. Immediately after, magnetic resonance imaging (MRI) anatomical acquisition was performed (T2-weighted, slide thickness 4 mm, TR = 3833.13 ms, TE = 100 ms, fov 230 × 230, acquisition matrix 256 × 256 pixels, pixel spacing 0.4 × 0.4).

RESULTS

REAL AND SHAM TMS-EVOKED POTENTIALS

Figure 2 reports typical TEPs from all electrodes (**Figure 2A**) and from Cz electrode (**Figure 2B**), to show, in more detail, the main peaks of activity we observed. On this representative electrode, after real TMS, a first positive component (mean amplitude 2.29 μV; SD 2.34), named P60, appeared at a mean latency of 57.1 ms (SD 3.9), followed by a negative component (mean amplitude −4.42 μV; SD 3.43), named N95, with a mean peak latency of 95.2 ms (SD 23.6), and by a second positive component (P160) at 158.7 ms (SD 20.5), with a mean amplitude of 4.87 μV (SD 2.75).

Sham evoked potentials showed similar deflections, but with reduced amplitudes compared to real TMS (**Figures 2A,B**). A positive component was observed at 54.6 ms (SD 5.7), with a mean amplitude of 1.61 μV (SD 1.10); a negative component appeared at a mean latency of 92.0 ms (SD 16.8) with a mean amplitude of −2.23 μV (SD 0.81); the third, positive component was detected at 169.3 ms (SD 17.3) with a mean amplitude of 2.75 μV (SD 1.28). The strict similarity of waves can be ascribed to acoustic contamination (Nikouline et al., 1999).

Mean real TMS amplitudes obtained for every time window of interest on a series of representative electrodes (see Materials and Methods section) were 1.18 μV (SD 0.92), −2.18 μV (SD 1.41), and 2.17 μV (SD 1.24), respectively. On the other hand, mean sham amplitudes resulted 0.91 μV (SD 0.72), −1.11 μV (SD 0.42), and 1.31 μV (SD 0.55), respectively. Statistical analyses showed that amplitudes were different with respect to the different time windows considered [$F_{(1.149,\ 12.640)} = 46.252$, $p <$

Table 1 | Results from time-frame by time-frame sLORETA analysis (t-statistic).

Time of activation (ms)	Maximal peak of activation (MPA)			Other significant voxels (BA)	Number of activated voxels (mean and *SD*)	Number of MPA time-frames (~ms) at $p < 0.1$
	X, Y, Z (MNI coordinates)	*BA*	Anatomical landmark			
59–60	−65, −15, −5	21	Left middle temporal gyrus	/	3 (1.4)	8 (~2)
132–133	45, −20, 40 40, −20, 40	4	Right pre-central gyrus	/	1 (0)	22 (~5.5) 19 (~5)
134–137	45, −20, 40 40, 35, 35 45, 40, 30 35, 30, 35 35, 25, 35 45, 30, 25 35, 20, 35 35, 5, 30 30, 35, 30	4, 9, 46	Right pre-central gyrus, Right superior frontal gyrus, Right middle frontal gyrus, Right inferior frontal gyrus	2 R, 3 R, 6 R, 8 R, 10 R, 24 R, 32 R, 40 R, 46 R	14.8 (13.8)	22 (~5.5) 18 (~4.5) 22 (~5.5) 24 (~6) 26 (~6.5) 21 (~5) 25 (~6) 19 (~5) 19 (~5)
138–139	35, 40, 25 40, 45, 30	10	Right middle frontal gyrus	9 R	4 (1)	18 (~4.5) 17 (~4.5)
140	30, 20, 15	13	Right insula	46 R	4 (–)	9 (~2)

Time of activation and location of maximal peaks that were significant with analysis made on discrete time windows of interest. The remaining significant voxels are also reported by indicating BA. BA, Brodmann Area; L, left; R, right.

Table 2 | Results from time-frame by time-frame sLORETA analysis (log of F-ratio).

Time of activation (ms)	Maximal peak of activation (MPA)			Other significant voxels (BA)	Number of activated voxels (mean and SD)	Number of MPA time-frames (~ms) at $p < 0.1$
	X, Y, Z (MNI coordinates)	BA	Anatomical landmark			
61–65	−45, 10, 55 −45, 30, 40	6, 9	Left middle frontal gyrus	8 L	10.1 (8.9)	29 (~7) 27 (~7)
88–89	−35, 50, 30 −35, 55, 20	10	Left superior frontal gyrus	46 L	2.3 (0.58)	40 (~10) 34 (~8)
90	−35, 55, 20 −35, 50, 30	10	Left superior frontal gyrus	46 L	3 (3.5)	34 (~8.5) 40 (~10)
199	−45, 10, 55	6	Left middle frontal gyrus	1 L, 2 L, 3 L, 8 L, 40 L	20 (–)	21 (~5)

Time of activation and location of maximal peaks that were significant with analysis made on discrete time windows of interest. The remaining significant voxels are also reported by indicating BA. BA, Brodmann Area; L, left; R, right.

0.0009] and also an interaction between stimulation condition (TMS vs. sham) and time window of interest was present [$F_{(2, 22)} = 7.183$, $p = 0.004$]. *Post-hoc* analyses showed that real TMS amplitudes were significantly higher with respect to sham amplitudes when considering the second and the third time window of interest [$t_{(11)} = 3.26$, $p = 0.008$; $t_{(11)} = 2.92$, $p = 0.014$, respectively].

Mean real TMS latencies on a series of representative electrodes, for every time window of interest (see Materials and Methods section), were 60.6 ms ($SD = 4.3$), 101.6 ms ($SD = 13.4$), and 164.5 ms ($SD = 14.2$), respectively. On the same line, mean sham latencies resulted 55.5 ms ($SD = 1.5$), 99.8 ms ($SD = 13.2$), and 166.2 ms ($SD = 12.5$), for every time window of interest. Statistical analyses showed that latencies were different with respect to the different time windows of interest [$F_{(2, 22)} = 635.013$, $p < 0.0009$], but the interaction between stimulation condition and time window of interest resulted only in a trend toward significance [$F_{(2, 22)} = 2.865$, $p = 0.078$]. Scalp topographies, with respect to the different conditions, are also shown in **Figure 3**.

Stimulation of the watermelon, carried out according to Veniero et al. (2009), showed that a slower artifact was evident, after the initial and greater fast-rising and fast-decaying TMS-related artifact, which lasted several ms after TMS administration. Unfortunately, we found it difficult to properly reduce the impedances, which were generally worse than those obtained from the subject's scalp. Therefore, whereas proper conclusions cannot be achieved, we believe that impedance might influence the size and the duration of the TMS-related artifacts (for a discussion see Julkunen et al., 2008; Veniero et al., 2009). Finally, a further artifact was evident that was related to the TMS recharge after delivery of the stimulus. A prototypical characterization of the artifacts related to the delivery of TMS on watermelon is showed in **Figure 2C**.

sLORETA: TIME-FRAME BY TIME-FRAME ANALYSIS

Non-parametric time-frame by time-frame statistical tests showed significantly different cortical activations between real and sham TMS conditions, in a time window between 45 and 213 ms.

Tests based on *t*-statistic (**Table 1** and **Figure 4**) revealed significant neuronal activity induced by real TMS (minus sham TMS) at about 60 ms after stimulus delivery and in an interval roughly between 132 and 140 ms. The left temporal cortex (middle temporal gyrus; BA 21) was more active in real TMS (minus sham TMS) at early time points, whereas at later time intervals differences were observed in the sensorimotor regions of the right hemisphere, contralateral to the side of stimulation. Voxels with significant differences were observed in the right motor regions (pre-central gyrus; BA 4 and 6) as well as in somatosensory areas (right post-central gyrus; BA 2 and 3). In addition, significant voxels were detected in the right superior, middle, and inferior frontal gyri (BA 9, 6, 8, 10 and 46), in the right inferior parietal lobule (BA 40), and in the right cingulate gyrus (BA 24 and 32). Finally, toward the end of the time window, greater activation for real TMS (minus sham TMS) was observed in the right insula (BA 13).

On the other hand, analyses based on log of F-ratio (**Table 2** and **Figure 5**) revealed that real TMS (minus sham TMS) induced greater activation (significant voxels) mainly in the premotor (BA 6) and frontal regions (BA 9 and 8) of the stimulated left hemisphere (left middle frontal gyrus, left superior frontal gyrus, and left pre-central gyrus), in a time range roughly between 61 and 65 ms after stimulation. Furthermore, left frontal regions and sensorimotor networks showed significantly higher activations in a time interval roughly between 88 and 90 ms, and around 200 ms after real TMS (minus sham TMS). Significant voxels were observed in the left superior and middle frontal gyri (BA 10 and 46), while left middle and superior frontal gyri, pre- and post-central gyri, and the left inferior parietal lobule (BA 6, 8, 1, 2, 3, and 40) were more active in the subsequent time points. **Tables 1**, **2** report also the number of consecutive time-frames that resulted toward a significant activation, at a trend level ($p < 0.1$), of every maximal peak of activity highlighted from main analyses.

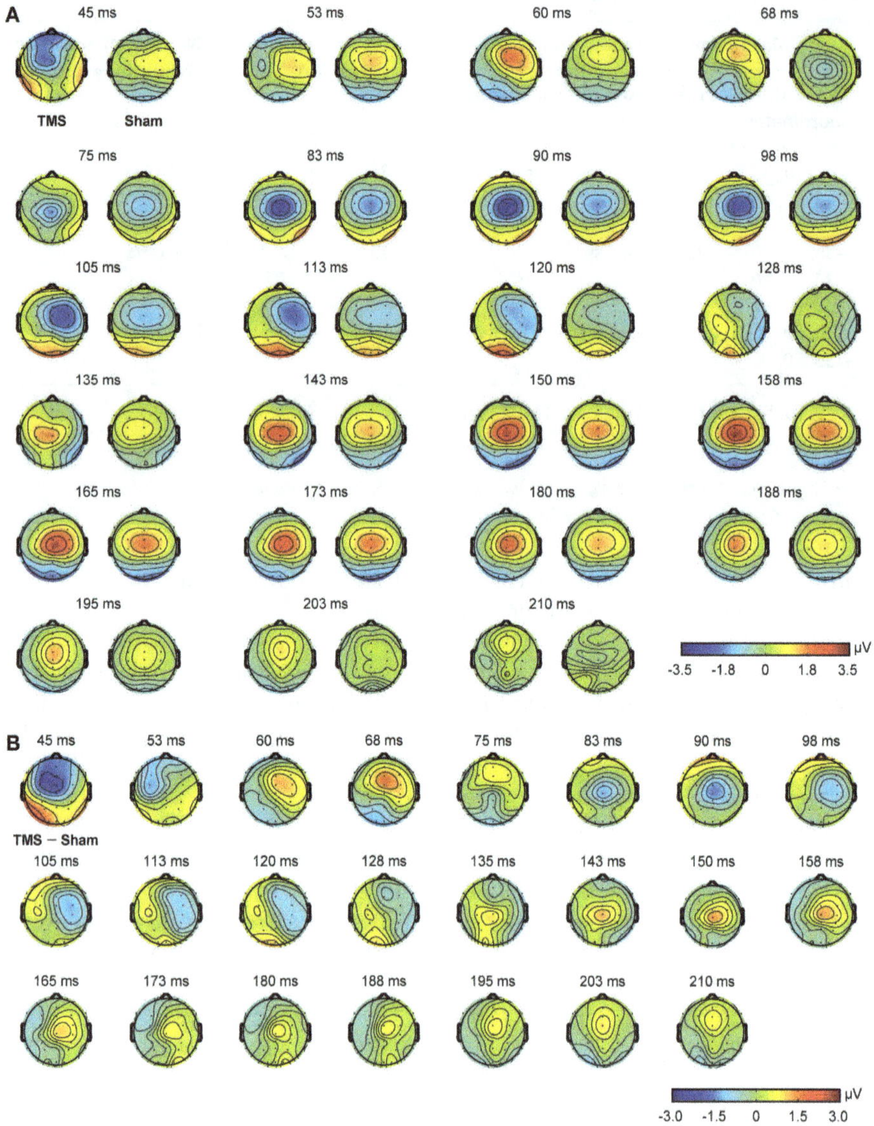

FIGURE 3 | Scalp topographies obtained from real TMS and sham conditions. Real TMS scalp topographies are shown on the left and sham topographies on the right **(A)**. Scalp topographies obtained from the direct comparison of real TMS and sham conditions are also shown **(B)**.

MEAN NEURAL ACTIVITY IN SPECIFIC TIME WINDOWS OF INTEREST

Mean activations in the three time windows of interest induced by real and sham TMS were compared with paired-sample non-parametric tests, using both *t*-statistic and log of F-ratio tests. **Tables 3, 4** summarize the main results, while **Figure 6** shows the main data over models of structural MRI.

T-statistic revealed significant differences only in the second time window of interest between 70 and 130 ms after real TMS (minus sham TMS) delivery. Analyses between 45 and 70 ms and between 130 and 213 ms after stimulus delivery did not reach the significance threshold. Significant voxels were mainly evident in the right hemisphere: the lingual gyrus, the middle and inferior occipital gyri, the fusiform gyrus, and the cuneus (BA 17, 18, 19, 23, 30). Moreover, in the same window, real TMS (minus sham TMS) induced significantly different activity in the left uncus, left parahippocampal gyrus (BA 28, 34, 35, 36), left pre-central gyrus, and in left middle and inferior frontal gyri (BA 6 and 9).

Statistical analyses based on log of F-ratio demonstrated significant differences between real TMS and sham conditions in two time windows (70–130 ms and 130–213 ms after stimulus delivery), while activity in the 45–70 ms time window did not reach the threshold for significance. After 70–130 ms, significant voxels were evident in the left hemisphere and also in the right hemisphere. Significant voxels in the real TMS condition (minus sham TMS) were observed bilaterally in the medial frontal gyrus, superior and middle frontal gyri, orbital gyrus and anterior cingulate cortex, and in the left cingulate, rectal, and inferior frontal gyri. These patterns of activity corresponded to BA 10, 6, 8, 9, 11, 32, and 46. When considering the time range between 130 and 213 ms, significant voxels were bilaterally evident in the superior

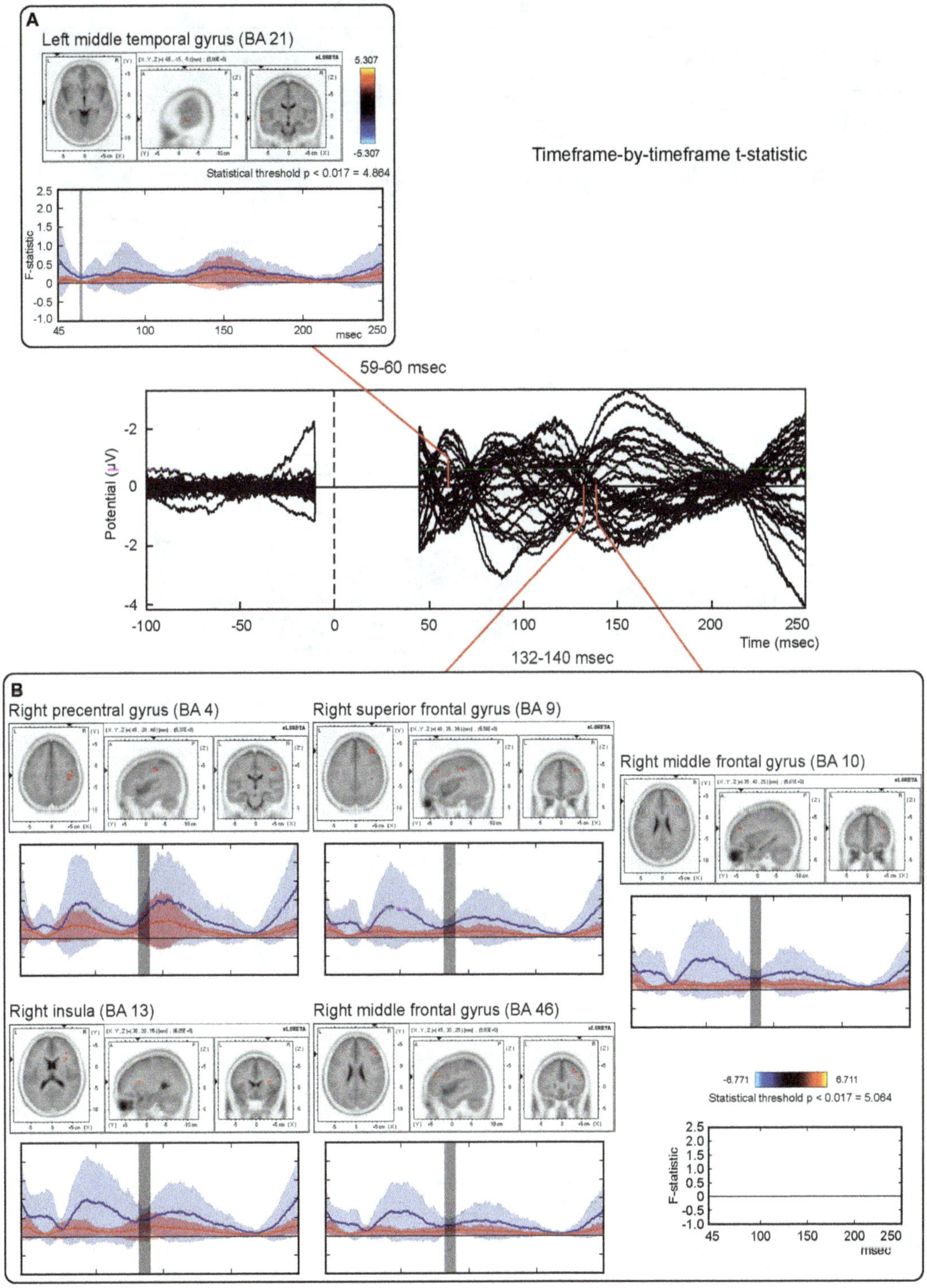

FIGURE 4 | Time-frame by time-frame sLORETA results (1). Principal sLORETA results obtained when considering a time-frame by time-frame analysis performed with *t*-statistic and comparing real TMS minus sham conditions. Images are plotted with respect to the time windows identified in a butterfly plot of the evoked potentials obtained from the real TMS condition. **(A)** Results obtained in the 59–60 ms time window. Activation with the maximal peak in the left middle temporal gyrus (BA 21) is shown. **(B)** Results obtained in the 132–140 ms time window. Activations with the maximal peaks in the right sensorimotor and frontal regions (BA 4, 9, 10, 13, and 46) are shown. The time course of the intensity of the signal in the source space is also shown. Specifically, real TMS signals for a specific peak (corresponding to a specific voxel) are indicated by a blue line (standard deviations are indicated by shadows of the same color). Sham signals for the same peak (and voxel) are indicated by a red line (standard deviations are indicated by shadows of the same color). The corresponding significant time-frames are indicated by gray shadows. It is very important to note that the intensity of the signal in the source space has, here, the form of an F-statistic, since sLORETA perform the standardized estimate of the cortical current density, expressed as a statistical value (F-distribution value; Pascual-Marqui, 2002).

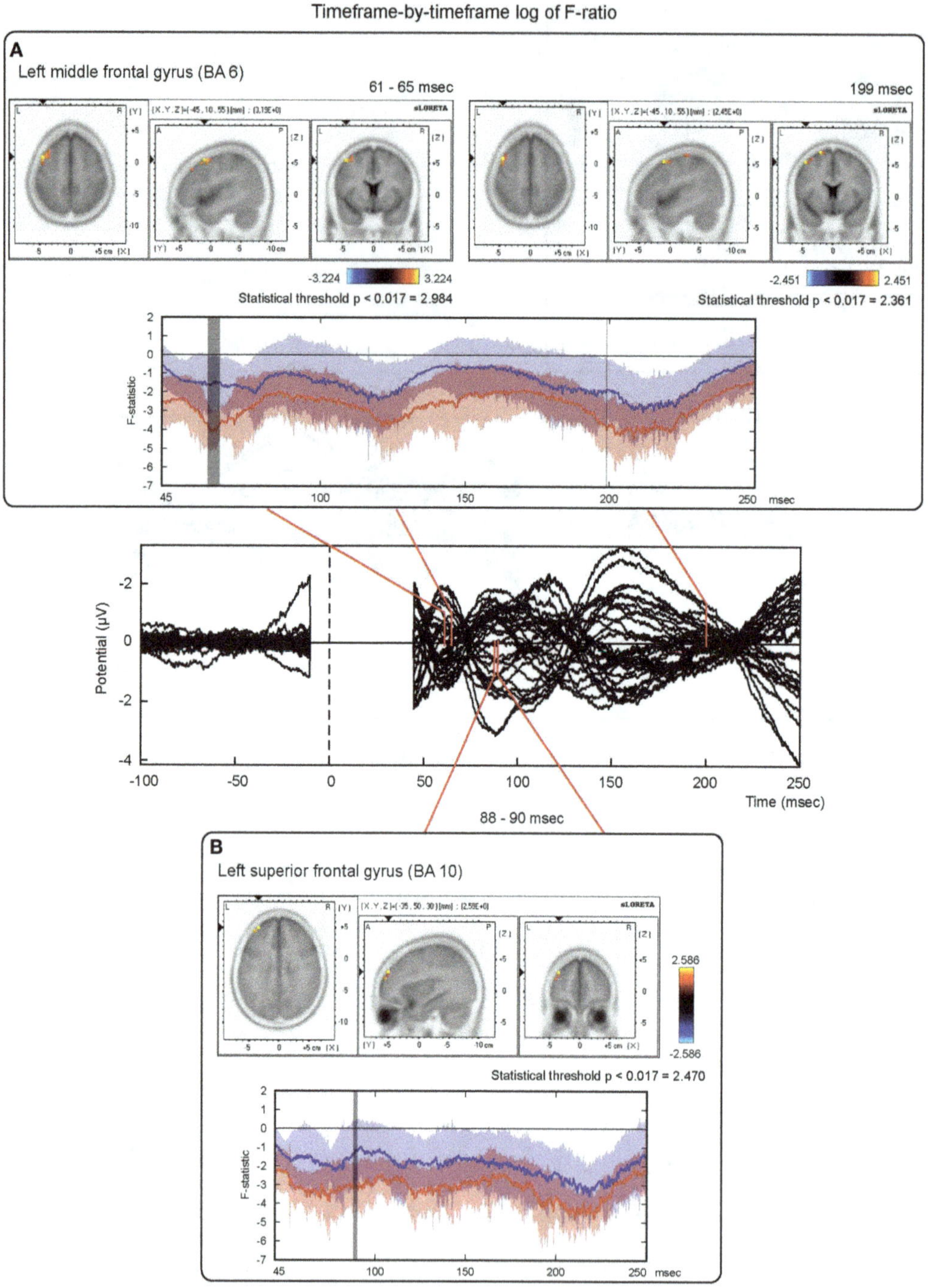

FIGURE 5 | Time-frame by time-frame sLORETA results (2). Principal sLORETA results obtained when considering a time-frame by time-frame analysis performed with log of F-ratio and comparing real TMS minus sham conditions. Images are plotted with respect to the time windows identified in a butterfly plot of the evoked potentials obtained from the real TMS condition. **(A)** Results obtained in the 61–65 ms time window and results obtained 199 ms after the delivery of TMS. Activations with the maximal peak in the left middle frontal gyrus (BA 6) are shown. **(B)** Results obtained in the 88–90 ms time window. Activation with the maximal peak of activation in the left superior frontal gyrus (BA 10) is shown. The time course of the intensity of the signal in the source space is also shown. Real TMS signals for a specific peak (corresponding to a specific voxel) are indicated by a blue line (standard deviations are indicated by shadows of the same color). Sham signals for the same peak (and voxel) are indicated by a red line (standard deviations are indicated by shadows of the same color). The corresponding significant time-frames are indicated by gray shadows. It is very important to note that the intensity of the signal in the source space has, here, the form of an F-statistic, since sLORETA perform the standardized estimate of the cortical current density, expressed as a statistical value (F-distribution value; Pascual-Marqui, 2002). It has negative values because they are the logarithmic transformation of source activation estimates.

Table 3 | Results from discrete time windows sLORETA analysis (mean neural activity, *t*-statistic).

Time of activation (ms)	Maximal peak of activation			Other significant voxels (BA)	Number of activated voxels
	X, Y, Z (MNI coordinates)	*BA*	Anatomical landmark		
45–70	N.S.	N.S.	N.S.	N.S.	N.S.
70–130	15, −95, 15	17	Right lingual gyrus	6 L, 9 L, 18 R, 19 R, 23 R, 28 L, 30 R, 34 L, 35 L, 36 L,	123
130–213	N.S.	N.S.	N.S.	N.S.	N.S.

Time of activation and location of maximal peaks that were significant are reported. The remaining significant voxels are also reported in BA. BA, Brodmann Area; L, left; R, right; N.S., Not Significant, results did not reach threshold for significance.

Table 4 | Results from discrete time windows sLORETA analysis (mean neural activity, log of F-ratio).

Time of activation (ms)	Maximal peak of activation			Other significant voxels (BA)	Number of activated voxels
	X, Y, Z (MNI coordinates)	*BA*	Anatomical landmark		
45–70	N.S.	N.S.	N.S.	N.S.	N.S.
70–130	−5, 65, 20	10	Left medial frontal gyrus	6 L/R, 8 L/R, 9 L/R, 10 R, 11 L/R, 32 L/R, 46 L	360
130–213	5, 30, 60	6	Right superior frontal gyrus	6 L, 8 L/R, 9 L	69

Time of activation and location of maximal peaks that were significant are reported. The remaining significant voxels are also reported in BA. BA, Brodmann Area; L, left; R, right; N.S., Not Significant, results did not reach threshold for significance.

frontal gyrus and medial frontal gyrus, as well as in the left middle frontal gyrus (BA 6, 8, 9).

ANATOMICAL LOCALIZATION OF THE STIMULATION SITE

Visual classification of brain gyri and sulci of a prototypical subject was performed on the basis of Duvernoy (1999) on an MRI scan. A vitamin E pill was used as fiducial and its position on the scalp allowed confirmation that the stimulation site successfully comprised the dorsal premotor cortex, as shown in the right panel of **Figure 1**. In this sense, we should also consider that the projection of particular EEG points on cortical surface could be estimated with an average standard deviation of 8 mm in a previous work by Okamoto et al. (2004).

DISCUSSION

SUMMARY OF RESULTS AND GENERAL INTERPRETATION

Our findings might depict the spatial and temporal long-range neural activity evoked by premotor cortex stimulation. In fact, PMd stimulation evoked significant activations in discrete and different time windows of interest, comprised in a larger window of analysis ranging from 45 ms to about 200 ms after stimulus delivery, which can be interpreted as evidence for the connectivity between the PMd and several other brain regions, mainly bilaterally within the frontal lobes, and with the posterior, occipital pole. Specifically, the main pattern of activity suggests stimulus propagation toward contralateral brain regions, mainly in the sensorimotor and frontal areas, within discrete time windows, together with the activation of more posterior, principally visual, brain areas. Moreover, a pattern of mainly ipsilateral activations was also found in sensorimotor and/or frontal structures. Thus, significant voxels were found both in the same hemisphere as well as contralaterally to the stimulation site. In the first case, both cortico-cortical connections and/or subcortical pathways possibly contributed to the pattern of activations (e.g., Zanon et al., 2010; Busan et al., 2012), whereas in the latter case the flow of TMS-induced activation was likely carried by transcallosal connections (Marconi et al., 2003).

Propagation of activity from the left premotor cortex has already been investigated using TMS/EEG (e.g., Casarotto et al., 2010; Korhonen et al., 2011). However, to the best of our knowledge, only discrete and early activations were considered (e.g., Casarotto et al., 2010), or the study focused on the methodological aspects of TMS/EEG (e.g., Korhonen et al., 2011). On the other hand, when TMS and/or TMS/EEG have been used to investigate the premotor/motor network, the propagation of activity from the primary motor cortex, rather than from PMd, was the main focus (e.g., Komssi et al., 2004; Esser et al., 2006).

The definition of connections among different areas is crucial not only to understand the functional organization of neural systems, but it can also be helpful to investigate disease mechanisms, as in the case of the spread of epileptic discharges to gather new information for planning surgical intervention (e.g., Engel et al., 2003).

Functional connections could be present between brain regions that are both directly linked by axonal fibers and/or through indirect pathways. Especially when a large interregional distance is involved, the latter may explain the degree of variance in functional connectivity that cannot be fully described by structural connectivity. Indeed, findings here reported could be more properly related with long-range neural activity. Moreover, this suggests that connectivity could be variable in time (e.g., Bestmann et al., 2008; Moisa et al., 2012) and different cortical

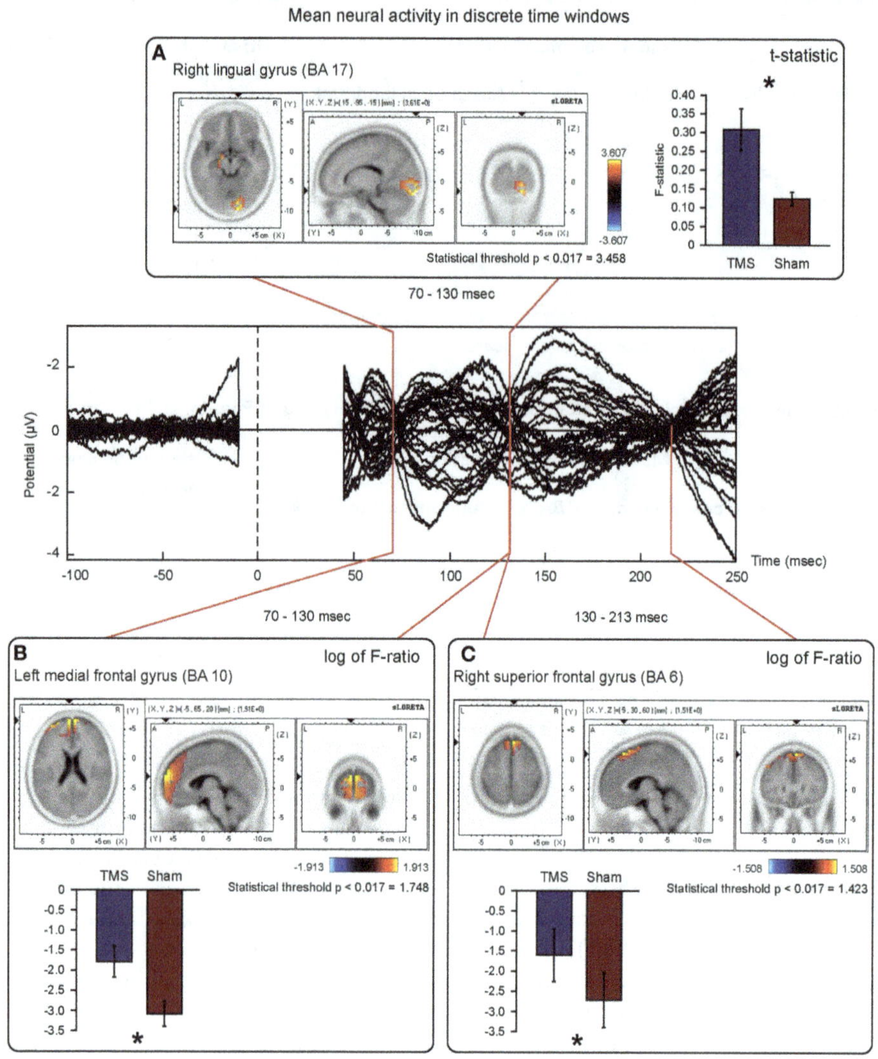

FIGURE 6 | Mean neural activity in discrete time windows of interest. Principal sLORETA results obtained when considering the mean of neural activity in discrete time windows and analysis performed with *t*-statistic **(A)** and log of F-ratio **(B,C)**. Statistics have been performed comparing the real TMS minus the sham conditions. Images are plotted with respect to the time windows identified in a butterfly plot of the evoked potentials obtained from the real TMS condition. **(A)** Mean results obtained in the 70–130 ms time window with *t*-statistic. Activation with the maximal peak in the right lingual gyrus (BA 17) is shown. **(B)** Mean results obtained in the 70–130 ms time window with log of F-ratio. Activation with the maximal peak in the left medial frontal gyrus (BA 10) is shown. **(C)** Mean results obtained in the 130–213 ms time window with log of F-ratio. Activation with the maximal peak in the right superior frontal gyrus (BA 6) is shown. The mean intensity of the signal in the source space in the time window of interest is also shown. Averaged real TMS signal for a specific peak (corresponding to a specific voxel) is indicated by a blue bar (standard deviations are also indicated). Averaged sham signal for the same peak (and voxel) is indicated by a red bar (standard deviations are also indicated). It is very important to note that the intensity of the signal in the source space has, here, the form of an F-statistic, since sLORETA perform the standardized estimate of the cortical current density, expressed as a statistical value (F-distribution value; Pascual-Marqui, 2002). It has negative values in panels **(B)** and **(C)** because they represent the logarithmic transformation of mean source activation estimates. Asterisks indicate a significant difference between conditions.

regions could work together forming functional connections according to the specific tasks they have to process. In this view, the PMd may form a functional network with frontal, parietal, and/or occipital cortical regions, varying with specific type of processes, like for example the planning of internally-paced rather than visually-guided sequence of movements (e.g., Bestmann et al., 2008; Moisa et al., 2012).

In the present study, several components characterized the electrical potentials evoked by PMd stimulation, namely the P60, the N95 and the P160, as described in the Results section. They are similar to those previously described in other TMS/EEG experiments, where TMS was applied to different regions of cortex (Paus et al., 2001; Komssi et al., 2002, 2004; Bonato et al., 2006; Lioumis et al., 2009; Zanon et al., 2010; Ferreri et al., 2011; Busan et al., 2012). Consistent with previous studies, EEG deviations from pre-stimulus baseline could be induced by activation of local and remote cortical neurons and/or synchronization of ongoing activity (e.g., Paus et al., 2001; Groppa et al., 2013). Further components should not be excluded, and in particular in the time windows not considered in the present analysis, for example those between 0 and 45 ms, which were removed because the recorded potentials were still corrupted by the electric artifact induced by the strong magnetic pulse.

PROPAGATION OF ACTIVITY TOWARD CONTRALATERAL REGIONS

The novelty of the present investigation relies on the long-range of the spatial and temporal profile of the activity propagation that was evoked when stimulating the dorsal premotor cortex in the left hemisphere. Furthermore, it provides new evidence to the presence of homo- and heterotopic projections that underpin the exchange of information inside the hemispheres and between them.

Stimulation of the left PMd showed, at about 130 ms from stimulus delivery, long-range contralateral activations mainly in the frontal and sensorimotor cortices (see **Figure 4B**). The present findings partially confirm what was already observed when investigating PMd connectivity with different techniques. For example, when TMS was applied on PMd during functional MRI (fMRI), a significant BOLD signal increase was observed in regions such as the contralateral PMd, bilateral premotor ventral regions, somatosensory cortex or the supplementary motor area, as well as in subcortical regions, such as the cerebellum and/or the caudate nucleus (e.g., Bestmann et al., 2005).

Contralateral propagation of activity during TMS/EEG co-registration was observed by Komssi et al. (2002) by stimulation of the left sensorimotor cortex, detecting activity in contralateral homologue brain regions, especially when considering the first 30 ms after the delivery of TMS and ipsilateral activations mainly in the sensorimotor structures and parietal lobe. In this regard, Ilmoniemi et al. (1997) showed activation of the contralateral homologous cortex about 20 ms after the delivery of the magnetic stimulus over central regions. Interestingly, observations similar to those reported in the present study (e.g., the transmission of the signal toward contralateral sensorimotor and frontal regions in discrete time windows of interest), were also obtained by Massimini et al. (2005) using a similar eyes-closed approach. For instance, they found contralateral activation of frontal networks when stimulating a dorsal premotor region in the right hemisphere, also in comparable time windows of interest. They could speculatively represent late and reverberant communications between frontal and sensorimotor regions of the two hemispheres, which are commonly active in the performing of specific tasks, like for example motor/cognitive tasks (e.g., Bestmann et al., 2008), and here engaged in the considered time window of interest by the initial and particular mental state of the brain (i.e., resting with closed eyes). Casarotto et al. (2010), in a study designed to evaluate the sensitivity and the repeatability of induced TEPs, performed a TMS/EEG investigation stimulating a very medial left dorsal premotor/supplementary motor region. The analysis of the neural generators (until 80 ms after stimulus delivery) showed that activations mainly propagated around the site of stimulation and toward more frontal regions with respect to contralateral and/or posterior regions. Finally, Iwahashi et al. (2008) observed the propagation of activity in a very early time window (about 20 ms after the stimulation of motor and parietal regions in both hemispheres) toward various anterior and posterior regions of the contralateral hemisphere, especially when stimulating motor regions.

Although the activations found in the sensorimotor cortex could be related to a somatosensory/peripheral effect evoked by TMS (see Paus et al., 2001, for a discussion; Ruff et al., 2006), it was suggested that TEPs were not significantly contaminated by somatosensory/peripheral effects after left primary motor cortex stimulation (e.g., Paus et al., 2001). In any case, the possibility of a somatosensory/peripheral stimulation related with TMS should be always considered (e.g., Ruff et al., 2006).

PROPAGATION OF ACTIVITY TOWARD FRONTAL REGIONS

Our findings suggest a pattern of activations that could appear, at a first view, mainly evident in the left hemisphere (**Figure 5**) in sensorimotor and/or frontal structures. The suggested connectivity among PMd and regions in the frontal and/or pre-frontal cortex is in agreement with the hypothesis of a rostro-caudal axis in the organization of the premotor cortex. According to this theory, rostral subdivisions are mainly involved in abstract and higher-order processes, while the caudal ones are mainly involved in low-order and motor-related processes (e.g., Gangitano et al., 2008; Goulas et al., 2012; Nee and Brown, 2012). More specifically, the rostral portion of the dorsal premotor cortex could be also seen as pre-PMd, while its caudal portion could be indicated as the proper PMd. This might reflect a parallelism between these areas and the pre-supplementary motor area (pre-SMA)/SMA complex. Thus, the pre-PMd seems to be preferentially involved in the cognitive aspects of brain functioning and more interconnected with other frontal regions, while the proper PMd seems to be more tightly connected with the motor aspects of behavior, such as the spatial and temporal characteristics of muscle activation (e.g., Picard and Strick, 2001; Matsumoto et al., 2003). As a consequence, activations related to higher-order processing, as could be the case of conditional visuo–motor associations, response selection, or motor imagery, should be mainly located in the pre-PMd (Grafton et al., 1998; Toni et al., 1999; Gerardin et al., 2000; Sakai et al., 2000), even if there is also substantial evidence suggesting an overlap between premotor regions that are important for both cognitive and motor tasks (Rottschy et al., 2012). Along these lines, the significant voxels we observed in regions in the frontal pole could be activated by the stimulation of rostral portions of PMd that are preferentially interconnected with more frontal brain regions (e.g., Barbas and Pandya, 1987; Lu et al., 1994). These regions could be involved in allocation of cognitive resources, selection of appropriate motor responses, and/or concurrent inhibition of unneeded ones (Chambers et al., 2007; Duque et al., 2012), speculatively supporting long-range timing of interactions, as in the present work.

The present pattern of results (e.g., the flowing of communication among different premotor and frontal regions) could also partially represent an interchange of information that could intervene between different eye fields that may be present in these regions of cortex (e.g., Luppino and Rizzolatti, 2000; see also **Figures 5A, 6C**). Finally, the dorsal premotor cortex could modulate the activity of the ventral premotor one: in fact, both areas could be interconnected (e.g., Goulas et al., 2012).

PROPAGATION OF ACTIVITY TOWARD POSTERIOR BRAIN REGIONS

We observed propagation of activity from PMd to posterior, mainly visual, brain regions (**Figure 6A**), in agreement with the already mentioned observations of Massimini et al. (2005) and Iwahashi et al. (2008). In this sense, also findings reported by Chouinard et al. (2003) suggest the possibility that motor regions might influence the activity of posterior brain regions mainly related to vision. The antero-posterior communications within the brain have been viewed as reciprocal, allowing not only the serial but also the recursive coding of information (e.g., Paus et al., 1997; Battaglia-Mayer et al., 1998; Massimini et al., 2005). Accordingly, concurrent serial and parallel processing in the human brain is present during integration of inputs that are necessary to perform, for example, visually-guided behaviors (e.g., Busan et al., 2009b; Hinkley et al., 2011). With regards to the PMd, this cortical region is presumed to be part of a network comprising the premotor cortex and superior parietal lobule whose activities underpin the parallel and recursive exchange of information (e.g., Battaglia-Mayer et al., 2003; Naranjo et al., 2007; Moisa et al., 2012; Rottschy et al., 2012). This model could be further supported by the present finding that posterior brain regions are activated in a time window between 70 and 130 ms after the delivery of TMS on PMd. Furthermore, the neurobiological substrate of this exchange of information can be the dorsal visual stream (Colby et al., 1988; Tanne et al., 1995; Rizzolatti and Matelli, 2003; Milner and Goodale, 2006) or the occipito-frontal fascicle (Jellison et al., 2004; Makris et al., 2007; Forkel et al., 2012) in this particular time window of interest.

By using the same approach, Casali et al. (2010) showed that a maximum spread of activation in the ipsilateral frontal cortex occurred in a time interval roughly between 70 and 100 ms after the stimulation of left superior occipital regions. Moreover, intracranial recordings in monkeys (Schroeder et al., 1998; Lamme and Roelfsema, 2000) and humans (Gaillard et al., 2009) have also demonstrated that visual stimulation could result in a posterior to anterior propagation of neural activity that reached the ipsilateral frontal lobe at latencies mainly between 120 and 150 ms. It is likely that these networks and circuits are indeed more complex (e.g., Zanon et al., 2010; Busan et al., 2012), as fascicles are simply physical links.

Taken together, these data support the view that different regions in the brain have different patterns of connectivity with the bilateral ventral and dorsal extrastriate cortex, which might be the basis of the differential organization of action and/or cognition (Rottschy et al., 2012). In the present work, the prevailing stimulation of the rostral PMd would likely involve regions that are compatible with eye-related neural activity, as for example frontal eye fields (FEF; Paus et al., 1997; Ruff et al., 2009), supplementary eye fields (Luppino and Rizzolatti, 2000; Amiez and Petrides, 2009), premotor/cingulate eye fields with the elicitation of other eye-related activities induced by premotor stimulation (Amiez and Petrides, 2009). Interestingly, Hinkley et al. (2011) showed that early high-gamma activity over the FEF during the saccade preparation moved toward the visual cortex during saccade execution. Overall, these observations suggest the presence of a connection between these regions (Paus et al., 1997; Ruff et al., 2006, 2009).

In the present study, magnetic stimuli were delivered to subjects who had their eyes closed. Therefore, the spread of activity should be considered in the light of the state-dependent theory (e.g., Silvanto and Muggleton, 2008). The findings presented herein were obtained starting from a condition that could be considered as similar to a "default mode" neural condition (e.g., Raichle et al., 2001; Raichle and Snyder, 2007; Greicius et al., 2009). In recent years, a growing body of evidence has supported the hypothesis of the existence of long-range brain networks with interdependent activities, which likely underpins mental processes (Bressler and Menon, 2010). Because these networks are identified both at rest and/or during the execution of active tasks, each might represent a distinct and intrinsically organized functional network (Calhoun et al., 2008; Smith et al., 2009). In this light, we suggest that TMS should have activated remote brain areas that could be part of the same functional network. This hypothesis could explain the similar results (e.g., activation of posterior brain regions) we obtained after stimulation of other cortical regions that could be part of the same network (Busan et al., 2012).

LIMITATIONS OF THE STUDY

TMS/EEG is a challenging technique, mainly because the magnetic stimulus induces a strong electric artifact that corrupts the EEG traces for some ms after stimulus delivery (Virtanen et al., 1999; Rogasch and Fitzgerald, 2013). For this reason, in most of the previous TMS/EEG studies, the analysis of recorded electric potentials started several ms after the delivery of the TMS pulse (e.g., Komssi et al., 2002; Litvak et al., 2007; Zanon et al., 2010; Busan et al., 2012). Nevertheless, the TMS/EEG technique allows investigation of the neural changes that happen in brain regions that are related to the stimulated area by means of direct and/or indirect links (Ilmoniemi et al., 1997; Massimini et al., 2005; Daskalakis et al., 2012).

In addition, one should consider that TMS evokes not only responses directly related to the magnetic stimulation, but also potentials due to acoustic and somatic stimulations. In this study, two components were principally observed on central electrodes, named N95 and P160, and could be mainly related to acoustic stimulation related to TMS delivery (Nikouline et al., 1999). In fact, similar components were observed both after real and sham TMS (slightly reduced in amplitude in the sham condition). In any case, this observation suggests that sham TMS could be a reliable control for acoustic stimulation related to TMS delivery. On the other hand, a reliable control for the somatic sensation related to TMS is difficult to obtain. TMS evoked a tactile sensation on the scalp and excitation of sensory receptors might activate the somatosensory cortex, for example through the trigeminal pathway, thus confounding the results such as EEG source imaging. Nonetheless, the present significant activations for real TMS were not clearly compatible with the results reported in studies that investigated the neuronal sources of sensorimotor evoked potentials related to trigeminal activations (e.g., Ohla et al., 2010). Thus, even if we attempted to eliminate the majority of artifacts, also by using ICA, a gold-standard method (Jung et al., 2000), the possibility remains that some artifacts, even if reduced in strength, were still present in the data collected. Moreover, even if we eliminated the major part of the TMS-induced artifacts by cutting the first 45 ms of post-stimulus EEG traces, and other artifacts by visual inspection and ICA, slower TMS artifacts might still be present in the acquired data. Linear detrend (e.g., Van Der Werf and Paus, 2006; Zanon et al., 2010) was used to partially correct for this problem, but all these elements should be taken into account. Thus, the possibility remains that some of the present patterns of activations could be related to and/or influenced by a series of unspecific effects of the magnetic stimulation that could be difficult to individuate and control in a reliable manner. Also for these reasons, the present paradigm might not have revealed some activations that could be part of the network.

The present findings should be considered as based on long-range neural activity, both from a spatial and temporal point of view. As a consequence, present findings could rely on polysynaptic and task-dependent networks, characterized by state-dependent, flexible bindings. Thus, different regions, connections and networks could be highlighted if different paradigms were applied (e.g., Bestmann et al., 2008). Indeed, during motor activity or cognitive tasks, PMd could be differently connected with other brain areas, resulting in networks that are different from what has been here observed. Thus, the present work might have revealed one of the possible, task-dependent and long-range networks related with PMd activation.

Finally, the possible spatial limitations of the EEG and the fact that the reconstruction of EEG sources is an inferential process, based on assumptions and a 3D model of the conductive volumes for solving the ill-posed inverse problem should be considered (Bai et al., 2007).

CONCLUSIONS

In conclusion, the present study corroborates and extends previous findings on the connectivity of PMd. In particular, our results shed light on the late temporal dynamics and connectivity among left PMd and mainly contralateral and posterior regions of the brain in right handed healthy humans.

ACKNOWLEDGMENTS

This work received partial financial support from the Italian Ministry for Education, University, and Research (MIUR). The authors are grateful to Dr. Francesco Bez, Dr. Alberto Della Mora, Dr. Gabriele Garbin and Dr. Veronica Guerra for help and support. We are also grateful to the Reviewers and their suggestions, allowing an increase in the readability of the manuscript.

REFERENCES

Amiez, C., and Petrides, M. (2009). Anatomical organization of the eye fields in the human and non-human primate frontal cortex. Prog. Neurobiol. 89, 220–230. doi: 10.1016/j.pneurobio.2009.07.010

Bai, X., Towle, V. L., He, E. J., and He, B. (2007). Evaluation of cortical current density imaging methods using intracranial electrocorticograms and functional MRI. Neuroimage 35, 598–608. doi: 10.1016/j.neuroimage.2006.12.026

Barbas, H., and Pandya, D. N. (1987). Architecture and frontal cortical connections of the premotor cortex (area 6) in the rhesus monkey. J. Comp. Neurol. 256, 211–228. doi: 10.1002/cne.902560203

Battaglia-Mayer, A., Caminiti, R., Lacquaniti, F., and Zago, M. (2003). Multiple lev- els of representation of reaching in the parieto-frontal network. Cereb. Cortex 13, 1009–1022. doi: 10.1093/cercor/13.10.1009

Battaglia-Mayer, A., Ferraina, S., Marconi, B., Bullis, J. B., Lacquaniti, F., Burnod, Y., et al. (1998). Early motor influences on visuomotor transformations for reaching: a positive image of optic ataxia. Exp. Brain Res. 123, 172–189. doi: 10.1007/s002210050559

Bestmann, S., Baudewig, J., Siebner, H. R., Rothwell, J. C., and Frahm, J. (2005). BOLD MRI responses to repetitive TMS over human dorsal premotor cortex. Neuroimage 28, 22–29. doi: 10.1016/j.neuroimage.2005.05.027

Bestmann, S., Swayne, O., Blankenburg, F., Ruff, C. C., Haggard, P., Weiskopf, N., et al. (2008). Dorsal premotor cortex exerts state-dependent causal influences on activity in contralateral primary motor and dorsal premotor cortex. Cereb. Cortex 18, 1281–1291. doi: 10.1093/cercor/bhm159

Bonato, C., Miniussi, C., and Rossini, P. M. (2006). Transcranial magnetic stim- ulation and cortical evoked potentials: a TMS/EEG co-registration study. Clin. Neurophysiol. 117, 1699–1707. doi: 10.1016/j.clinph.2006.05.006

Bressler, S. L., and Menon, V. (2010). Large-scale brain networks in cogni- tion: emerging methods and principles. Trends Cogn. Sci. 14, 277–290. doi: 10.1016/j.tics.2010.04.004

Brett, M., Johnsrude, I. S., and Owen, A. M. (2002). The problem of functional localization in the human brain. Nat. Rev. Neurosci. 3, 243–249. doi: 10.1038/nrn756

Busan, P., Barbera, C., Semenic, M., Monti, F., Pizzolato, G., Pelamatti, G., et al. (2009a). Effect of transcranial magnetic stimulation (TMS) on parietal and pre- motor cortex during planning of reaching movements. PLoS ONE 4:e4621. doi: 10.1371/journal.pone.0004621

Busan, P., Monti, F., Semenic, M., Pizzolato, G., and Battaglini, P. P. (2009b). Parieto-occipital cortex and planning of reaching movements: a transcra- nial magnetic stimulation study. Behav. Brain Res. 201, 112–119. doi: 10.1016/j.bbr.2009.01.040

Busan, P., Zanon, M., Vinciati, F., Monti, F., Pizzolato, G., and Battaglini, P. P. (2012). Transcranial magnetic stimulation and preparation of visually-guided reaching movements. Front. Neuroeng. 5:18. doi: 10.3389/fneng.2012.00018

Calhoun, V. D., Kiehl, K. A., and Pearlson, G. D. (2008). Modulation of temporally coherent brain networks estimated using ICA at rest and during cognitive tasks.

Hum. Brain Mapp. 29, 828–838. doi: 10.1002/hbm.20581

Caminiti, R., Genovesio, A., Marconi, B., Mayer, A. B., Onorati, P., Ferraina, S., et al. (1999). Early coding of reaching: frontal and parietal association connections of parieto-occipital cortex. Eur. J. Neurosci. 11, 3339–3345. doi: 10.1046/j.1460- 9568.1999.00801.x

Casali, A. G., Casarotto, S., Rosanova, M., Mariotti, M., and Massimini, M. (2010).

General indices to characterize the electrical response of the cerebral cortex to TMS. Neuroimage 49, 1459–1468. doi: 10.1016/j.neuroimage.2009.09.026

Casarotto, S., Romero Lauro, L. J., Bellina, V., Casali, A. G., Rosanova, M., Pigorini, A., et al. (2010). EEG responses to TMS are sensitive to changes in the per- turbation parameters and repeatable over time. PLoS ONE 5:e10281. doi: 10.1371/journal.pone.0010281

Chambers, C. D., Bellgrove, M. A., Gould, I. C., English, T., Garavan, H., McNaught, E., et al. (2007). Dissociable mechanisms of cognitive control in prefrontal and premotor cortex. J. Neurophysiol. 98, 3638–3647. doi: 10.1152/jn.00685.2007

Chouinard, P. A., Van Der Werf, Y. D., Leonard, G., and Paus, T. (2003). Modulating neural networks with transcranial magnetic stimulation applied over the dor- sal premotor and primary motor cortices. J. Neurophysiol. 90, 1071–1083. doi: 10.1152/jn.01105.2002

Colby, C. L., Gattass, R., Olson, C. R., and Gross, C. G. (1988). Topographical orga- nization of cortical afferents to extrastriate visual area PO in the macaque: a dual tracer study. J. Comp. Neurol. 269, 392–413. doi: 10.1002/cne.902690307

Daskalakis, Z. J., Farzan, F., Radhu, N., and Fitzgerald, P. B. (2012). Combined tran- scranial magnetic stimulation and electroencephalography: its past, present and future. Brain Res. 1463, 93–107. doi: 10.1016/j.brainres.2012.04.045

Davare, M., Andres, M., Cosnard, G., Thonnard, J. L., and Olivier, E. (2006).

Dissociating the role of ventral and dorsal premotor cortex in precision grasp- ing. J. Neurosci. 26, 2260–2268. doi: 10.1523/JNEUROSCI.3386-05.2006

Delorme, A., and Makeig, S. (2004). EEGLAB: an open source toolbox for anal- ysis of single-trial EEG dynamics including independent component analysis.

J. Neurosci. Methods 134, 9–21. doi: 10.1016/j.jneumeth.2003.10.009

Duque, J., Labruna, L., Verset, S., Olivier, E., and Ivry, R. B. (2012). Dissociating the role of prefrontal and premotor cortices in controlling inhibitory mechanisms during motor preparation. J. Neurosci. 32, 806–816. doi: 10.1523/JNEUROSCI.4299-12.2012

Duvernoy, H. M. (1999). The Human Brain. Surface, Blood Supply, and Three-Dimensional Sectional Anatomy. 2nd Edn. Wien: Springer-Verlag. doi: 10.1007/978-3-7091-6792-2

Engel, J. Jr.,Wiebe, S., French, J., Sperling, M., Williamson, P., Spencer, D., et al. (2003). Practice parameter: temporal lobe and localized neocortical resections for epilepsy: report of the Quality Standards Subcommittee of the American Academy of Neurology, in association with the American Epilepsy Society and the American Association of Neurological Surgeons. Neurology 60, 538–547. doi: 10.1212/01.WNL.0000055086.35806.2D

Esser, S. K., Huber, R., Massimini, M., Peterson, M. J., Ferrarelli, F., and Tononi, G. (2006). A direct demonstration of cortical LTP in humans: a combined TMS/EEG study. Brain Res. Bull. 69, 86–94. doi: 10.1016/j.brainresbull.2005.11.003

Ferreri, F., Pasqualetti, P., Maatta, S., Ponzo, D., Ferrarelli, F., Tononi,

G., et al. (2011). Human brain connectivity during single and paired pulse transcranial magnetic stimulation. Neuroimage 54, 90–102. doi: 10.1016/j.neuroimage.2010.07.056

Forkel, S. J., Thiebaut de Schotten, M., Kawadler, J. M., Dell'Acqua, F., Danek, A., and Catani, M. (2012). The anatomy of fronto-occipital connections from early blunt dissections to contemporary tractography. Cortex. doi: 10.1016/j.cortex.2012.09.005. [Epub ahead of print].

Frantseva, M., Cui, J., Farzan, F., Chinta, L. V., Perez Velazquez, J. L., and Daskalakis, Z. J. (2012). Disrupted cortical conductivity in schizophrenia: TMS–EEG study.

Cereb. Cortex. doi: 10.1093/cercor/bhs304. [Epub ahead of print].

Fuchs, M., Kastner, J., Wagner, M., Hawes, S., and Ebersole, J. S. (2002). A standard- ized boundary element method volume conductor model. Clin. Neurophysiol. 113, 702–712. doi: 10.1016/S1388-2457(02)00030-5

Gaillard, R., Dehaene, S., Adam, C., Clémenceau, S., Hasboun, D., Baulac, M., et al. (2009). Converging intracranial markers of conscious access. PLoS Biol. 7:e61. doi: 10.1371/journal.pbio.1000061

Galletti, C., Kutz, D. F., Gamberini, M., Breveglieri, R., and Fattori, P. (2003). Role of the medial parieto-occipital cortex in the control of reaching and grasping movements. Exp. Brain Res. 153, 158–170. doi: 10.1007/s00221-003-1589-z

Gangitano, M., Mottaghy, F. M., and Pascual-Leone, A. (2008). Release of premotor activity after repetitive transcranial magnetic stimulation of prefrontal cortex. Soc. Neurosci. 3, 289–302. doi: 10.1080/17470910701516838

Gerardin, E., Sirigu, A., Lehéricy, S., Poline, J. B., Gaymard, B., Marsault, C., et al. (2000). Partially overlapping neural networks for real and imagined hand movements. Cereb. Cortex 10, 1093–1104. doi: 10.1093/cercor/10.11.1093

Goodale, M. A. (1988). Hemispheric differences in motor control. Behav. Brain Res. 30, 203–214. doi: 10.1016/0166-4328(88)90149-0

Goulas, A., Uylings, H. B., and Stiers, P. (2012). Unravelling the intrinsic functional organization of the human lateral frontal cortex: a parcellation scheme based on resting state fMRI. J. Neurosci. 32, 10238–10252. doi: 10.1523/JNEUROSCI.5852-11.2012

Grafton, S. T., Fadiga, L., Arbib, M. A., and Rizzolatti, G. (1997). Premotor cor- tex activation during observation and naming of familiar tools. Neuroimage 6, 231–236. doi: 10.1006/nimg.1997.0293

Grafton, S. T., Fagg, A. H., and Arbib, M. A. (1998). Dorsal premotor cor- tex and conditional movement selection: a PET functional mapping study. J. Neurophysiol. 79, 1092–1097.

Greicius, M. D., Supekar, K., Menon, V., and Dougherty, R. F. (2009). Resting-state functional connectivity reflects structural connectivity in the default mode network. Cereb. Cortex 19, 72–78. doi: 10.1093/ cercor/bhn059

Groppa, S., Muthuraman, M., Otto, B., Deuschl, G., Siebner, H. R., and Raethjen, J. (2013). Subcortical substrates of TMS-induced modulation of the cortico- cortical connectivity. Brain Stimul. 6, 138–146. doi: 10.1016/j.brs.2012.03.014

Hagmann, P., Cammoun, L., Gigandet, X., Meuli, R., Honey, C. J., and Wedeen, V. J. (2008). Mapping the structural core of human cerebral cortex. PLoS Biol. 6:e159. doi: 10.1371/journal.pbio.0060159

Hamidi, M., Johnson, J. S., Feredoes, E., and Postle, B. R. (2011). Does high-frequency repetitive transcranial magnetic stimulation produce residual and/or cumulative effects within an experimental session? Brain Topogr. 23, 355–367. doi: 10.1007/s10548-010-0153-y

He, B., Yang, L., Wilke, C., and Yuan, H. (2011). Electrophysiological imaging of brain activity and connectivity-challenges and opportunities. IEEE Trans. Biomed. Eng. 58, 1918–1931. doi: 10.1109/TBME.2011.2139210

Herwig, U., Satrapi, P., and Schönfeldt-Lecuona, C. (2003). Using the international 10-20 EEG system for positioning of transcranial magnetic stimulation. Brain Topogr. 16, 95–99. doi: 10.1023/B:BRAT.0000006333.93597.9d

Hinkley, L. B., Nagarajan, S. S., Dalal, S. S., Guggisberg, A. G., and Disbrow, E. A. (2011). Cortical temporal dynamics of visually guided behavior. Cereb. Cortex 21, 519–529. doi: 10.1093/cercor/bhq102

Hoshi, E., and Tanji, J. (2006). Differential involvement of neurons in the dorsal and ventral premotor cortex during processing of visual signals for action planning. J. Neurophysiol. 95, 3596–3616. doi: 10.1152/jn.01126.2005

Huang, Y. Z., Rothwell, J. C., Lu, C. S., Wang, J., Weng, Y. H., Lai, S. C., et al. (2009). The effect of continuous theta burst stimulation over premotor cortex on cir- cuits in primary motor cortex and spinal cord. Clin. Neurophysiol. 120, 796–801. doi: 10.1016/j.clinph.2009.01.003

Iacoboni, M. (2006). Visuo-motor integration and control in the human posterior parietal cortex: evidence from TMS and fMRI. Neuropsychologia 44, 2691–2699. doi: 10.1016/j.neuropsychologia.2006.04.029

Ilmoniemi, R. J., and Kicic, D. (2010). Methodology for combined TMS and EEG.

Brain Topogr. 22, 233–248. doi: 10.1007/s10548-009-0123-4

Ilmoniemi, R. J., Virtanen, J., Ruohonen, J., Karhu, J., Aronen, H. J., Näätänen, R., et al. (1997). Neuronal responses to magnetic stimulation reveal cortical reactivity and connectivity. Neuroreport 8, 3537–3540. doi: 10.1097/00001756- 199711100-00024

Ilmoniemi, R., and Karhu, J. (2008). "TMS and electroencephalography: methods and current advances," in The Oxford handbook of transcranial stimulation, eds E. M. Wassermann, C. M. Epstein, U. Ziemann, T. Paus, and S. H. Lisanby (New York, NY: Oxford University Press Inc.), 593–608.

Iwahashi, M., Arimatsu, T., Ueno, S., and Iramina, K. (2008). "Differences in evoked EEG by transcranial magnetic stimulation at various stimulus points on the head," in 30th Annual International IEEE EMBS Conference, (Vancouver), 2570–2573.

Janssen, L., Meulenbroek, R. G. J., and Steenbergen, B. (2011). Behavioral evi- dence for left-hemisphere specialization of motor planning. Exp. Brain Res. 209, 65–72. doi: 10.1007/s00221-010-2519-5

Jellison, B. J., Field, A. S., Medow, J., Lazar, M., Salamat, M. S., and Alexander, A. L. (2004). Diffusion tensor imaging of cerebral white matter: a pictorial review of physics, fiber tract anatomy, and tumor imaging patterns. Am. J. Neuroradiol. 25, 356–369.

Julkunen, P., Pääkkönen, A., Hukkanen, T., Könönen, M., Tiihonen, P., Vanhatalo, S., et al. (2008). Efficient reduction of stimulus artefact in TMS–EEG by epithe- lial short-circuiting by minipunctures. Clin. Neurophysiol. 119, 475–481. doi: 10.1016/j.clinph.2007.09.139

Jung, T. P., Makeig, S., Humphries, C., Lee, T. W., McKeown, M. J., Iragui, V., et al. (2000). Removing electroencephalographic artifacts by blind source separation. Psychophysiology 37, 163–178. doi: 10.1111/1469-8986.3720163

Jurcak, V., Tsuzuki, D., and Dan, I. (2007). 10/20, 10/10, and 10/5 systems revisited: their validity as relative head-surface-based positioning systems. Neuroimage 34: 1600–1611. doi: 10.1016/j.neuroimage.2006.09.024

Komssi, S., Aronen, H. J., Huttunen, J., Kesäniemi, M., Soinne, L., Nikouline, V. V., et al. (2002). Ipsi- and contralateral EEG reactions to transcranial magnetic stimulation. Clin. Neurophysiol. 113, 175–184. doi: 10.1016/S1388-2457(01)00721-0

Komssi, S., and Kahkonen, S. (2006). The novelty value of the combined use of electroencephalography and transcranial magnetic stimulation for neu- roscience research. Brain Res. Rev. 52, 183–192. doi: 10.1016/j.brainresrev. 2006.01.008

Komssi, S., Kähkönen, S., and Ilmoniemi, R. J. (2004). The effect of stimulus inten- sity on brain responses evoked by transcranial magnetic stimulation. Hum. Brain Mapp. 21, 154–164. doi: 10.1002/ hbm.10159

Korhonen, R. J., Hernandez-Pavon, J. C., Metsomaa, J., Mäki, H., Ilmoniemi, R. J., and Sarvas, J. (2011). Removal of large muscle artifacts from transcranial magnetic stimulation-evoked EEG by independent component analysis. Med. Biol. Eng. Comput. 49, 397–407. doi: 10.1007/s11517-011-0748-9

Kurata, K. (1991). Corticocortical inputs to the dorsal and ventral aspects of the premotor cortex of macaque monkeys. Neurosci. Res. 12, 263–280. doi: 10.1016/0168-0102(91)90116-G

Lamme, V. A., and Roelfsema, P. R. (2000). The distinct modes of vision offered by feedforward and recurrent processing. Trends Neurosci. 23, 571–579. doi: 10.1016/S0166-2236(00)01657-X

Lancaster, J. L., Woldorff, M. G., Parsons, L. M., Liotti, M., Freitas, C. S., Rainey, L., et al. (2000). Automated Talairach Atlas labels for func- tional brain mapping. Hum. Brain Mapp. 10, 120–131. doi: 10.1002/1097-0193(200007)10:3<120::AID-HBM30>3.0.CO;2-8

Lioumis, P., Kicic, D., Savolainen, P., Makela, J. P., and Kähkönen, S. (2009). Reproducibility of TMS-evoked EEG responses. Hum. Brain Mapp. 30, 1387–1396. doi: 10.1002/hbm.20608

Litvak, V., Komssi, S., Scherg, M., Hoechstetter, K., Classen, J., Zaaroor, M., et al. (2007). Artifact correction and source analysis of early electroencephalographic responses evoked by transcranial magnetic stimulation over primary motor cortex. Neuroimage 37, 56–70. doi: 10.1016/j. neuroimage.2007.05.015

Lu, M. T., Preston, J. B., and Strick, P. L. (1994). Interconnections between the pre- frontal cortex and the premotor areas in the frontal lobe. J. Comp. Neurol. 341, 375–392. doi: 10.1002/cne.903410308

Luppino, G., and Rizzolatti, G. (2000). The organization of the frontal motor cortex. News Physiol. Sci. 15, 219–224.

Makris, N., Papadimitriou, G. M., Sorg, S., Kennedy, D. N., Caviness, V. S., and Pandya, D. N. (2007). The occipitofrontal fascicle in humans: a quantitative, in vivo, DT-MRI study. Neuroimage 37, 1100–1111. doi: 10.1016/j.neuroimage.2007.05.042

Manganotti, P., and Del Felice, A. (2013). New perspectives in transcranial mag-netic stimulation: epilepsy, consciousness and the perturbational approach. Behav. Neurol. 27, 155–167. doi: 10.3233/ BEN-2012-120263

Marconi, B., Genovesio, A., Giannetti, S., Molinari, M., and Caminiti, R. (2003). Callosal connections of dorso-lateral premotor cortex. Eur. J. Neurosci. 18, 775–788. doi: 10.1046/j.1460-9568.2003.02807.x

Massimini, M., Ferrarelli, F., Huber, R., Esser, S. K., Singh, H., and Tononi, G. (2005). Breakdown of cortical effective connectivity during sleep. Science 309, 2228–2232. doi: 10.1126/science.1117256

Matelli, M., and Luppino, G. (2001). Parietofrontal circuits for action and space perception in the macaque monkey. Neuroimage 14, S27–S32. doi: 10.1006/ nimg.2001.0835

Matsumoto, R., Ikeda, A., Ohara, S., Matsuhashi, M., Baba, K., Yamane, F., et al. (2003). Motor-related functional subdivisions of human lateral premotor cor- tex: epicortical recording in conditional visuomotor task. Clin. Neurophysiol. 114, 1102–1115. doi: 10.1016/S1388-2457(03)00065-8

Matsumoto, R., Nair, D. R., LaPresto, E., Bingaman, W., Shibasaki, H., and Luders, H. O. (2007). Functional connectivity in human cortical motor system: a cortico-cortical evoked potential study. Brain 130, 181–197. doi: 10.1093/ brain/awl257

Mazziotta, J., Toga, A., Evans, A., Fox, P., Lancaster, J., Zilles, K., et al. (2001). A probabilistic atlas and reference system for the human brain: International Consortium for Brain Mapping (ICBM). Philos. Trans. R. Soc. Lond. B Biol. Sci. 356, 1293–1322. doi: 10.1098/ rstb.2001.0915

Michel, C. M., Murray, M. M., Lantz, G., Gonzalez, S., Spinelli, L., and Grave de Peralta, R. (2004). EEG source imaging. Clin. Neurophysiol. 115, 2195–2222. doi: 10.1016/j.clinph.2004.06.001

Milner, D., and Goodale, M. (2006). The Visual Brain in Action. Oxford, USA: Oxford University Press. doi: 10.1093/

acprof:oso/9780198524724.001.0001 Miniussi, C., and Thut, G. (2010). Combining TMS and EEG offers new prospects in cognitive neuroscience. Brain Topogr. 22, 249–256. doi: 10.1007/s10548-009-0083-8

Moisa, M., Siebner, H. R., Pohmann, R., and Thielscher, A. (2012). Uncovering a context-specific connectional fingerprint of human dorsal premotor cortex. J. Neurosci. 32, 7244–7252. doi: 10.1523/ JNEUROSCI.2757-11.2012

Mütanen, T., Mäki, H., and Ilmoniemi, R. J. (2013). The effect of stimulus parameters on TMS-EEG muscle artifacts. Brain Stimul. 6, 371–376. doi: 10.1016/j.brs.2012.07.005

Naranjo, J. R., Brovelli, A., Longo, R., Budai, R., Kristeva, R., and Battaglini,

P. P. (2007). EEG dynamics of the frontoparietal network during reaching preparation in humans. Neuroimage 34, 1673–1682. doi: 10.1016/j.neuroimage.2006.07.049

Nee, D. E., and Brown, J. W. (2012). Rostral-caudal gradients of abstraction

revealed by multi-variate pattern analysis of working memory. Neuroimage 63, 1285–1294. doi: 10.1016/j.neuroimage.2012.08.034

Nichols, T. E., and Holmes, P. A. (2002). Nonparametric permutation tests for func- tional neuroimaging; a primer with examples. Hum. Brain Mapp. 15, 1–25. doi: 10.1002/ hbm.1058

Nikouline, V., Ruohonen, J., and Ilmoniemi, R. J. (1999). The role of the coil click in TMS assessed with simultaneous EEG. Clin. Neurophysiol. 110, 1325–1328. doi: 10.1016/S1388-2457(99)00070-X

Ohla, K., Toepel, U., le Coutre, J., and Hudry, J. (2010). Electrical neu- roimaging reveals intensity-dependent activation of human cortical gustatory and somatosensory areas by electric taste. Biol. Psychol. 85, 446–455. doi: 10.1016/j. biopsycho.2010.09.007

Okamoto, M., Dan, H., Sakamoto, K., Takeo, K., Shimizu, K., Kohno, S., et al.

(2004). Three-dimensional probabilistic anatomical cranio-cerebral correlation via the international 10-20 system oriented for transcranial functional brain mapping. Neuroimage 21, 99–111. doi: 10.1016/j. neuroimage.2003.08.026

Oldfield, R. C. (1971). The assessment and analysis of handedness: the Edinburgh inventory. Neuropsychologia 9, 97–113. doi: 10.1016/0028-3932(71)90067-4 Oostenveld, R., and Praamstra, P. (2001). The five percent electrode system for high-resolution EEG and ERP measurements. Clin. Neurophysiol. 112, 713–719. doi: 10.1016/S1388-2457(00)00527-7

Pascual-Marqui, R. D. (2002). Standardized low resolution brain electromagnetic tomography: a new method for localizing electrical activity in the brain. Int. J. Psychophysiol. 18, 49–65. doi: 10.1016/0167-8760(84)90014-X

Paus, T., Jech, R., Thompson, C. J., Comeau, R., Peters, T., and Evans, A. C. (1997). Transcranial magnetic stimulation during positron emission tomography: a new method for studying connectivity of the human cerebral cortex. J. Neurosci. 17, 3178–3184.

Paus, T., Sipila, P. K., and Strafella, A. P. (2001). Synchronization of neuronal activity in the human primary motor cortex by transcranial magnetic stimulation: an EEG study. J. Neurophysiol. 86, 1983–1990.

Picard, N., and Strick, P. L. (2001). Imaging the premotor areas. Curr. Opin. Neurobiol. 11, 663–672. doi: 10.1016/S0959-4388(01)00266-5

Raichle, M. E., MacLeod, A. M., Snyder, A. Z., Powers, W. J., Gusnard, D. A., and Shulman, G. L. (2001). A default mode of brain function. Proc. Natl. Acad. Sci. U.S.A. 98, 676–682. doi: 10.1073/ pnas.98.2.676

Raichle, M. E., and Snyder, A. Z. (2007). A default mode of brain function: a brief history of an evolving idea. Neuroimage 37, 1083–1090. doi: 10.1016/j. neuroimage.2007.02.041

Rizzolatti, G., and Luppino, G. (2001). The cortical motor system. Neuron 31, 889–901. doi: 10.1016/S0896-6273(01)00423-8

Rizzolatti, G., Luppino, G., and Matelli, M. (1998). The organization of the cortical motor system: new concepts. Electroenceph. Clin. Neurophysiol. 106, 283–296. doi: 10.1016/S0013-4694(98)00022-4

Rizzolatti, G., and Matelli, M. (2003). Two different streams from the dorsal visual system: anatomy and functions. Exp. Brain Res. 153, 146–157. doi: 10.1007/s00221-003-1588-0

Rogasch, N. C., and Fitzgerald, P. B. (2013). Assessing cortical network properties using TMS-EEG. Hum. Brain Mapp. 34, 1652–1669. doi: 10.1002/hbm.22016 Rossini, P. M., Barker, A. T., Berardelli, A., Caramia, M. D., Caruso, G., Cracco, R. G., et al. (1994). Non-invasive electrical and magnetic stimulation of the brain, spinal cord and roots: basic principles and procedures for routine clinical appli- cation. Report of an IFCN committee. Electroencephalogr. Clin. Neurophysiol. 91, 79–92. doi: 10.1016/0013-4694(94)90029-9

Rossi, S., Hallet, M., Rossini, P. M., Pascual-Leone, A., and The Safety of TMS.

Consensus Group (2009). Safety, ethical considerations, and application guide- lines for the use of transcranial magnetic stimulation in clinical practice and research. Clin. Neurophysiol. 120, 2008–2039. doi: 10.1016/j.clinph.2009.08.016 Rottschy, C., Caspers, S., Roski, C., Reetz, K., Dogan, I., Schulz, J. B., et al. (2012). Differentiated parietal connectivity of frontal regions for "what" and "where" memory . Brain Struct. Funct. 218, 1551–1567. doi: 10.1007/s00429-012-0476-4 Ruff, C. C., Blankenburg, F., Bjoertomt, O., Bestmann, S., Freeman, E., Haynes, J. D., et al. (2006). Concurrent TMS-fMRI and psychophysics reveal frontal influences on human retinotopic visual cortex. Curr. Biol. 16, 1479–1488. doi: 10.1016/j.cub.2006.06.057

Ruff, C. C., Blankenburg, F., Bjoertomt, O., Bestmann, S., Weiskopf, N., and Driver, J. (2009). Hemispheric differences in frontal and pari- etal influences on human occipital cortex: Direct confirmation with concurrent TMS-fMRI. J. Cogn. Neurosci. 21, 1146–1161. doi: 10.1162/ jocn.2009.21097

Rushworth, M. F. S., Johansen-Berg, H., Göbel, S. M., and Devlin, J. T. (2003). The left parietal and premotor cortices: motor attention and selection. Neuroimage 20, S89–S100. doi: 10.1016/j.neuroimage.2003.09.011

Sakai, K., Hikosaka, O., Takino, R., Miyachi, S., Nielsen, M., and Tamada, T. (2000). What and when: parallel and convergent processing in motor control. J. Neurosci. 20, 2691–2700.

Schroeder, C. E., Mehta, A. D., and Givre, S. J. (1998). A spatiotemporal profile of visual system activation revealed by current source density analysis in the awake macaque. Cereb. Cortex 8, 575–592. doi: 10.1093/cercor/8.7.575

Sekiguchi, H., Takeuchia, S., Kadotac, H., Kohnob, Y., and Nakajima, Y. (2011). TMS-induced artifacts on EEG can be reduced by rearrangement of the elec- trode's lead wire before recording. Clin. Neurophysiol. 122, 984–990. doi: 10.1016/j.clinph.2010.09.004

Shipp, S., Blanton, M., and Zeki, S. (1998). A visuo-somatomotor pathway

through superior parietal cortex in the macaque monkey: cortical connections of areas V6 and V6A. Eur. J. Neurosci. 10, 3171–3193. doi: 10.1046/j.1460- 9568.1998.00327.x

Silvanto, J., and Muggleton, N. G. (2008). New light through old windows: mov- ing beyond the "virtual lesion" approach to transcranial magnetic stimulation. Neuroimage 39, 549–552. doi: 10.1016/j.neuroimage.2007.09.008

Smith, S. M., Fox, P. T., Miller, K. L., Glahn, D. C., Fox, P. M., Mackay, C. E., et al. (2009). Correspondence of the brain's functional architecture dur- ing activation and rest. Proc. Natl. Acad. Sci. U.S.A. 106, 13040–13045. doi: 10.1073/pnas.0905267106

Steinsträter, O., Sommer, J., Deppe, M., and Knecht, S. (2002). The Münster T2T-Converter. Available online at: http://wwwneuro03.uni-muenster.de/ger/t2tconv/

Tanne, J., Boussaoud, D., Boyer-Zeller, N., and Rouiller, E. M. (1995). Direct visual pathways for reaching movements in the macaque monkey. Neuroreport 7, 267–272.

Toni, I., Schluter, N. D., Josephs, O., Friston, K., and Passingham, R. E. (1999).

Signal-, set- and movement-related activity in the human brain: an event related fMRI study. Cereb. Cortex 9, 35–49. doi: 10.1093/cercor/9.1.35

Van Der Werf, Y. D., and Paus, T. (2006). The neural response to transcranial magnetic stimulation of the human motor cortex. I. Intracortical and cortico- cortical contributions. Exp. Brain Res. 175, 231–245. doi: 10.1007/s00221-006-0551-2

Veniero, D., Bortoletto, M., and Miniussi, C. (2009). TMS-EEG co-registration: on TMS-induced artifact. Clin. Neurophysiol. 120, 1392–1399. doi: 10.1016/j.clinph.2009.04.023

Vingerhoets, G., Alderweireldt, A. S., Vandemaele, P., Cai, Q., Van der Haegen, L., Brysbaert, M., et al. (2013). Praxis and language are linked: Evidence from co-lateralization in individuals with atypi- cal language dominance. Cortex 49, 172–183. doi: 10.1016/j.cortex. 2011.11.003

Virtanen, J., Ruohonen, J., Naatanen, R., and Ilmoniemi, R. J. (1999).

Instrumentation for the measurement of electric brain responses to transcra- nial magnetic stimulation. Med. Biol. Eng. Comput. 37, 322–326. doi: 10.1007/ BF02513307

Wassermann, E. M. (1998). Risk and safety of repetitive transcranial magnetic stimulation: report and suggested guidelines from the International Workshop on the Safety of Repetitive Transcranial Magnetic Stimulation, June 5–7, 1996. Electroencephalogr. Clin. Neurophysiol. 108, 1–16. doi: 10.1016/S0168-5597 (97)00096-8

Zanon, M., Busan, P., Monti, F., Pizzolato, G., and Battaglini, P. P. (2010). Cortical connections between dorsal and ventral visual streams in humans: evidence by TMS/EEG co-registration. Brain Topogr. 22, 307–317. doi: 10.1007/s10548-009- 0103-8

2

Dorsolateral prefrontal transcranial magnetic stimulation in patients with major depression locally affects alpha power of REM sleep

Maria Concetta Pellicciari[1], Susanna Cordone[2], Cristina Marzano[2], Stefano Bignotti[1], Anna Gazzoli[1], Carlo Miniussi[1,3] and Luigi De Gennaro[2]*

[1] Cognitive Neuroscience Section, IRCCS Centro San Giovanni di Dio Fatebenefratelli, Brescia, Italy
[2] Department of Psychology, University of Rome Sapienza, Rome, Italy
[3] Department of Clinical and Experimental Sciences, National Institute of Neuroscience, University of Brescia, Brescia, Italy

***Correspondence:**
Luigi De Gennaro, Dipartimento di Psicologia - Sezione di Neuroscienze, Università di Roma "Sapienza," Via dei Marsi, 78, 00185 Roma, Italy
e-mail: luigi.degennaro@uniroma1.it

Sleep alterations are among the most important disabling manifestation symptoms of Major Depression Disorder (MDD). A critical role of sleep importance is also underlined by the fact that its adjustment has been proposed as an objective marker of clinical remission in MDD. Repetitive transcranial magnetic stimulation (rTMS) represents a relatively novel therapeutic tool for the treatment of drug-resistant depression. Nevertheless, besides clinical evaluation of the mood improvement after rTMS, we have no clear understanding of what are the neurophysiological correlates of such treatment. One possible marker underlying the clinical outcome of rTMS in MDD could be cortical changes on wakefulness and sleep activity. The aim of this open-label study was to evaluate the efficacy of a sequential bilateral rTMS treatment over the dorsolateral prefrontal cortex (DLPFC) to improve the mood in MDD patients, and to determine if rTMS can induce changes on the sleep structure, and if those changes can be used as a surrogate marker of the clinical state of the patient. Ten drug-resistant depressed patients participated to ten daily sessions of sequential bilateral rTMS with a low-frequency TMS (1 Hz) over right-DLPFC and a subsequent high-frequency (10 Hz) TMS over left-DLPFC. The clinical and neurophysiological effects induced by rTMS were evaluated, respectively by means of the Hamilton Depression Rating Scale (HDRS), and by comparing the sleep pattern modulations and the spatial changes of EEG frequency bands during both NREM and REM sleep, before and after the real rTMS treatment. The sequential bilateral rTMS treatment over the DLPFC induced topographical-specific decrease of the alpha activity during REM sleep over left-DLPFC, which is significantly associated to the clinical outcome. In line with the notion of a left frontal hypoactivation in MDD patients, the observed local decrease of alpha activity after rTMS treatment during the REM sleep suggests that alpha frequency reduction could be considered as a marker of up-regulation of cortical activity induced by rTMS, as well as a surrogate neurophysiological correlate of the clinical outcome.

Keywords: major depression, repetitive transcranial stimulation, REM sleep, dorsolateral prefrontal cortex, alpha activity

INTRODUCTION

Major depression disorder (MDD) is considered not only a remarkable affliction for patients but also an economic burden for modern society (Luppa et al., 2007). The World Health Organization estimates that about 350 million people globally are affected by depression and that by 2030 it will rank as the largest contributor to disease. MDD represents a syndrome that encompasses many different symptoms which brutally affect several domains of the patient's life, with specific disturbances in mood, cognition and physical status. Among the physical symptoms, sleep alterations represent one of the most disabling manifestations of MDD and an early marker of the depression recurrence onset (Perlis et al., 1997; Baglioni et al., 2011). Insomnia, delayed sleep onset, non-restorative sleep with frequent awakenings during the night, and shorten duration of sleep are the most reported subjective complaints of MDD patients. Besides clinical observation, an altered macro- and micro-architecture of sleep characterizes the electroencephalographic (EEG) recordings of those patients (Lustberg and Reynolds, 2000; Armitage, 2007; Steiger and Kimura, 2010). An increase of rapid-eye-movement (REM) density, an increase of fast-frequency EEG activity, a prolongation of the first REM sleep period (Lauer et al., 1991; Riemann et al., 1994) with a reduction of sleep efficiency, an increase in REM sleep latency (Reynolds and Kupfer, 1987) and EEG slow-wave activity during non-REM sleep (NREM) (Mayers and Baldwin, 2005) represent the main neurophysiological correlates underlying subjective sleep complaints in the MDD.

Among EEG sleep disturbances, the REM sleep alterations are considered not only the main feature that characterize the sleep of depressed patients (Kupfer, 1976) as their adjustment are even used as biomarkers of disease remission. In that regard, several studies reported how antidepressant treatments have a clear-cut and immediate effects on REM sleep (Reynolds and Kupfer, 1987; Sandor and Shapiro, 1994; Sharpley and Cowen, 1995; Riemann et al., 2001), in terms of latency increase (Kupfer et al., 1981) and density decrease (Buysse et al., 1999), whereas the action on non-REM sleep are quite inconsistent (Sharpley and Cowen, 1995). Those data support the hypothesis of a specific link between REM sleep and depression.

Aiming at facing the drug-resistance in MDD, several non-pharmacological interventions have been proposed, including brain stimulation techniques [i.e., electroconvulsive therapy (ECT), deep brain stimulation (DBS)].

In the last decade, due to its ability to stimulate focally and non-invasively cortical brain areas (George et al., 2013), repetitive transcranial magnetic stimulation (rTMS) has been introduced for the treatment of medication refractory depression. TMS can induce a transient and painless electro-magnetic field through the skull, allowing the depolarization of the cortical neurons under the stimulated scalp location, and into connected areas (Li et al., 2010). Specifically, rTMS allows to modulate the cortical excitability, in a specific frequency-manner, with changes that persist beyond the duration of rTMS application. If applied at high frequency (≥5 Hz), TMS has been shown to induce a cortical excitability increase, while at low frequency (≤1 Hz) it induces a cortical excitability decrease.

Functional neuroimaging studies suggested that the prefrontal cortex, with its specific involvement in mood regulation, should be the cortical target of rTMS treatment in depression (Padberg and George, 2009). A typical abnormality observed in the cortical activity of major depressed patients is represented by prefrontal cortex asymmetry, with hypoactivity in the left dorsolateral prefrontal cortex (L-DLPFC) and relative hyperactivity of the right DLPFC (R-DLPCF) (Drevets, 2000; Walter et al., 2007; Grimm et al., 2008). That characteristical activation pattern has been shown both by examining resting cerebral glucose metabolism and blood flow with PET (Drevets et al., 1997; Videbech et al., 2002) and with EEG (Bruder et al., 1997; Debener et al., 2000; Allen et al., 2004). In agreement with those findings, several studies support the hypothesis that rTMS can increase with high frequencies and dampening with low frequencies the DLPFC excitability, rebalancing the altered functioning of the L-DLPFC and R-DLPFC, respectively involved as neurophysiological mediators of positive and negative mood (Silberman and Weingartner, 1986; Davidson, 1992). The clinical efficacy of rTMS for the treatment of the MDD (George et al., 2013), has been validated utilizing both unilateral (Lisanby et al., 2009; Pallanti et al., 2010) and bilateral approach, i.e., low frequency right-sided and high frequency left-sided over DLPFC (Fitzgerald et al., 2006). The latter is considered more effective for the treatment of major depression due the potential additive effect of both frequency stimulations, provided sequentially (Blumberger et al., 2012).

Although the clinical outcome of rTMS in depressed patients is relatively established, few studies have investigated the EEG effects of a rTMS treatment in depressed patients, in terms of cortical frequency changes, on wakefulness (Funk and George, 2008; Valiulis et al., 2012) and sleep activity (Saeki et al., 2012). In a recent study, Saeki et al. (2012), focusing their attention on slow wave activity (SWA) and sleep spindle activity, highlighted a local increase of SWA during NREM sleep and no change in REM sleep parameters after five sessions of high frequency rTMS to the left DLPFC.

Considering the role of other frequency bands, specifically the alpha activity as a cortical hypoactivity marker of depression syndrome, we hypothesized that the study of sleep changes induced by rTMS on all frequency bands, could allow to identify the biomarkers of the clinical remission and to better disclose the sleep neurophysiological correlates which could contribute to the improvement in clinical outcome observed in depressed drug resistant patients.

In the present open-label study, we aimed at verifying three outcomes. First, we wanted to evaluated the efficacy of a 10-days sequential bilateral rTMS treatment over the DLPFC to modulate mood in the MDD drug resistant patients, as assessed by the Hamilton Depression Rating Scale (HDRS). The second aspect was to evaluate if it was possible to induce changes on macro and micro-structure of sleep by means of rTMS, assessed by scoring EEG sleep recordings. Finally, we aimed at exploring the possible correlation between the clinical outcome and the neurophysiological changes.

According to these aims, sequential bilateral rTMS to DLPFC in treatment-resistant depressed patients, with a low-frequency TMS (1 Hz) over R-DLPFC and a subsequent high-frequency (10 Hz) TMS over L-DLPFC was applied. Spatial changes of EEG frequency bands were investigated by comparing maps not only of all EEG power bands but also of Hz-by-Hz EEG power values before and after rTMS treatment, during both NREM and REM sleep. The choice to investigate the cortical topography of REM and NREM sleep separately was dictated by the interest to differentiate the neuromodulator effects induced by rTMS on these sleep stages, considering their specific involvement and reciprocal relationship in the pathophysiological changes of depression (Armitage, 2007). Finally, the magnitude of the relative EEG sleep changes after rTMS was correlated with the changes of HDRS with the aim to identify if EEG sleep changes can be considered a biomarker of clinical outcome.

MATERIALS AND METHODS

PATIENTS

Ten patients (5 males and 5 females, of mean age 52.8 ± 6.3 years, range 42–63 years) were included in this study. All of them had a diagnosis of MDD, formulated by an expert psychiatrist on the basis of a structured clinical interview for DSM-IV Axis I (SCID-I) according to the diagnostic and statistical manual of the American Psychiatric Association (APA. Diagnostic and statistical manual of mental disorders. 4th—TR ed. Washington, DC: APA Press; 2000). The MDD patients had no psychiatric comorbidity according to DSM-IV criteria, history of neurological disorders, epilepsy or substance abuse and contraindication for TMS (Rossi et al., 2009). For none of them the previous clinical outcome showed any improvement following the pharmacological antidepressant treatment. The pharmacological treatments are detailed in **Table 1**.

Patients with primary sleep disorders (International Classification of Sleep Disorders, 2nd Edition- ICSD-2, 2005) as evaluated by polysomnographic recordings during an adaptation night in our laboratory, were excluded from the study.

Additional inclusion criteria were: a score ≥17 at the 21 items HDRS, or clinical improvement ≤50% obtained on the HDRS obtained and absence of improvement at the Clinical Global Impression (CGI) during the drug treatment with at least two classes of antidepressant drugs in standard doses for a period of at least 2 months. Prior to the inclusion, all patients had had a period of constant medication for 2 months and continued the same medication at the enrolment and for the full duration of the study. Therefore, pharmacological dosages were kept constant during the treatment. None of the patients received additional non pharmacological treatments, such as psychotherapy, during the study.

This study was approved by the CEIOC Ethics Committee of IRCCS Centro San Giovanni di Dio Fatebenefratelli, Brescia, Italy. Prior the beginning of the study and after a complete description of it, written informed consent was obtained from each patient.

PROCEDURE

None of the patients was familiar with the rTMS procedure. An open-label experimental design was used in the present study. Therefore, before the real treatment, each patient was subjected to a 3 days administration of a sham rTMS treatment applied over the parietal cortex, to allow their adaptation to the experimental setting (specifically, to the noise of rTMS). The real rTMS treatment consisted of 10 daily sessions of stimulation (Monday through Friday), for two weeks. Each subject underwent the stimulations at the same time each day, in the late afternoon. Before the real rTMS treatment and the following day the end of the whole treatment, the clinical symptoms were evaluated by means of the HDRS. An expert psychiatrist blind to the treatment performed the clinical rating. As reported above, the pharmacological treatment was kept constant during the rTMS treatment.

Each patient participated in the study for five nights. The sleep recordings, carried out in a sound-proof room, were scheduled in the adaptation night followed by a baseline night (BSL) in correspondence respectively of the second and third session of sham pre-treatment, and three nights during the real rTMS treatment, respectively after the first (R1), the ninth (re-adaptation night—R2) and tenth (final treatment—R3) rTMS session. Before the sleep recordings, all patients were stimulated 60 min before light off. Time in bed after lights off was ~7 h.

Table 1 | Concomitant pharmacological medications are detailed for all patients.

Pharmacological treatment	Patients (n = 10)
BZD + SNRI	1
BZD + SNRI + Aneuro	3
BZD + SNRI + Tneuro	1
BZD + SNRI + TCA	1
BZD + SNRI + TCA + Aneuro + MS	1
BZD + TCA + MS	1
BZD + SSRI + SARI + Aneuro	1
SSRI + Tneuro	1

BZD, benzodiazepines; Antidepressants: SSRI, selective serotonin reuptake inhibitors; SNRI, serotonin-noradrenalin reuptake inhibitors; SARI, serotonin2-antagonists/serotonin reuptake inhibitors; TCA, tricyclic antidepressants; Antipsychotics: Tneuro, typical neuroleptic; Aneuro, atypical neuroleptic; MS, mood stabilizer.

TRANSCRANIAL MAGNETIC STIMULATION

rTMS was delivered by a Magstim Super Rapid Magnetic Stimulator (50 Hz—biphasic, four boosters) with a standard double 70-mm coil (Magstim Company Limited, Whitland, UK). We alternated two coils, in order to allow cooling during the repetitive stimulation without interruption. Before starting the rTMS treatment, the motor threshold (MT) was determined for each subject, respectively over the left and right motor area, following international standards (Rossini et al., 1994).

Aiming to align all patients into a balanced baseline state, a sham rTMS treatment was employed in the 3 days before real rTMS. For sham treatment, a 25-mm thick plywood shield, build to appear as an integral part of the apparatus, was interposed between the coil itself and the scalp, separating the two. Moreover, the ventral surface of the coil, from which the magnetic field was delivered, was upside down and the stimulus intensity was at 110% of MT. In the sham session, 1200 pulses at 1 Hz frequency for 20 s, with an inter-train interval of 10 s, were delivered over the parietal cortex. The real rTMS treatment was delivered at 110% of MT on the frontal scalp area overlying the R-DLPFC and L-DLPFC. For the identification of the stimulated brain areas, the left and right DLPFCs were localized on the basis of a reconstruction of cerebral cortex in the Talairach coordinate system using the SofTaxic neuronavigation system (EMS, Bologna, Italy www.softaxic.com). Using this system, we marked the stimulation sites over the left and the right DLPFC, coinciding with Brodmann areas 46. These localizations were in accordance to previous reports (e.g., Saeki et al., 2012).

The coil was placed tangentially to the scalp with the handle pointing backwards and laterally at about a 45° angle away from the midsagittal axis of the patient' heads and oriented to elicit a postero lateral anteromedial current flow in the brain tissue. The rTMS was first applied at low frequency over the R-DLPFC and then at high frequency over the L-DLPFC.

Low frequency rTMS consisted of 60 trains of stimuli at 1 Hz frequency for 20 s with an inter-train interval of 10 s. High frequency rTMS consisted of 60 trains of stimuli at 10 Hz frequency for 2 s, with an inter-train interval of 28 s. An interval of ~30 min separated the two sessions. Each session lasted ~30 min and the total number of pulses was the same between the two stimulation paradigms (in total 1200 pulses both for the 1 Hz-TMS and that for the 10 Hz-TMS). These parameters are in line with safety recommendations for rTMS (Wassermann, 1998; Wassermann and Lisanby, 2001).

POLYSOMNOGRAPHIC RECORDINGS

A BrainAmp Recorder System (BrainAmp 32 channel, BrainProducts GmbH, Munich, Germany) was used for polygraphic recordings. EEG signals were high pass filtered with a time constant of 0.3 s and low pass filtered at 70 Hz, and digitized at a sampling rate of 250 Hz. The nineteen unipolar EEG derivations of the international 10–20 system (Fp1, Fp2, F7, F8, F3, F4, Fz, C4, C3, Cz, P3, P4, Pz, T4, T6, T3, T5, O1, O2) were recorded from scalp electrodes. Additional electrodes were used as the ground and reference. The ground electrode was placed in the midfrontal (Fpz) position. The reference electrode was placed from a left mastoid, while recordings obtained from right mastoid electrode was used off-line to re-reference the scalp recordings. Ten additional unipolar EEG derivations were recorded. One electrode was positioned exactly over the individual right DLPFC (R-DLPFC), and other four electrodes were placed around this point in each orthogonal direction at a distance of 1 cm. The R-hotspot (R-DLFPC) resulted very close to the F3 electrode of the 10–20 system. As a denotation, the four orthogonal positions will be indicated as "anterior to right dorsolateral prefrontal cortex" (aR-DLPFC), "medial to right DLPFC" (mR-DLPFC), "posterior to right DLPFC" (pR-DLPFC), and "lateral to right DLPFC" (lR-DLPFC). The same montage and denotation was also used for the left dorsolateral prefrontal cortex (L-DLPFC, aL-DLPFC, mL-DLPFC, pL-DLPFC, and lL-DLPFC). Horizontal and vertical eye movements were detected by recording the electro-oculogram (EOG) in order to monitor subject behavior on-line and reject, off-line, trials with ocular artifacts. The submental electromyogram was recorded with a time constant of 0.03 s. Bipolar horizontal eye movements were recorded with a time constant of 1 s. The bipolar horizontal electrooculogram was recorded from electrodes placed about 1 cm from the medial and lateral canthi of the dominant eye. Impedance for all electrodes was kept below 5 kΩ.

DATA ANALYSIS

Clinical data analysis

The effect of the rTMS treatment on the clinical outcome (HDRS) was assessed by means of an analysis of variance (ANOVA), in which the clinical data at BSL and at R3 nights were compared.

Sleep measures

Sleep stages of BSL and R3 nights were visually scored in 20 s epochs, according to the standard criteria (Rechtschaffen and Kales, 1968). The following were considered as dependent variables: (a) stage 1 latency; (b) stage 2 latency; (c) REM latency; (d) percentage of stage 1; (e) percentage of stage 2; (f) percentage of REM sleep; (g) wakefulness after sleep onset (WASO), expressed as the intra-sleep time (min) spent awake; (h) number of awakenings (the number of >10 s episodes of WASO); (i) number of arousals (the number of <10 s episodes of WASO); (j) total sleep time (TST), defined as the sum of time spent in stage 1, stage 2, SWS, and REM; (k) total bedtime (TBT); (l) sleep efficiency index (SEI = TST/TBT × 100). The polysomnographic EEG measures were submitted to one-way repeated measure ANOVAs, comparing BSL, and R3 nights.

Quantitative analysis of sleep EEG

The polygraphic signals (29 EEG channels, EOG, and electromyography) were low pass filtered at 30 Hz, analog to digital converted on-line with a sampling rate of 128 Hz, and stored on the disk of a personal computer. Ocular and muscle artifacts were excluded off-line by visual inspection. We investigated the 0.50–25.00 Hz frequency range, computing the power spectra by a Fast Fourier Transform routine for 4 s periodgrams. Before conducting the statistical analyses, the data were reduced to the traditional EEG bands of sleep, by collapsing adjacent 0.25-Hz bins: delta (0.50–4.75 Hz), theta (5.00–7.75 Hz), alpha (8.00–11.75 Hz), sigma (12.00–15.75 Hz), and beta (15.00–24.75 Hz). The power spectra were calculated separately for the NREM sleep (stage 2 + 3 + 4) and the REM sleep. These EEG power values were considered as dependent measures. The values were log-transformed, color coded, plotted at the corresponding position on the planar projection of the scalp surface, and interpolated (biharmonic spline) between electrodes.

The EEG power maps were computed separately for the BSL and the R3 nights, and separately for NREM and REM sleep. Then, power values of the BSL vs. R3 nights were compared for each band and scalp location by means of paired *t*-tests. Finally, the statistical maps of the *t*-value comparisons were color coded and plotted separately for NREM and REM sleep.

The Bonferroni correction for multiple comparisons was applied. Considering the mean correlation between the variables of the NREM sleep ($r = 0.49$), the alpha level was then adjusted to ≤ 0.0039 ($t \geq 3.84$). Similarly, considering the mean correlation between the variables of the REM sleep ($r = 0.57$), the alpha level was then adjusted to ≤ 0.0059 ($t \geq 3.58$).

RESULTS

CLINICAL DATA

The analysis on the HDRS scores revealed a significant improvement of the clinical status as a consequence of the rTMS treatment [BSL = 22.2, ± 2.15; R3 = 15.7, ± 5.46; $F_{(1, 9)} = 14.16$; $p = 0.0045$]. As shown in **Figure 1**, nine out of ten patients improved at HDRS after the rTMS treatment, and their mean percentage decrease was 35.0% (±13%).

POLYSOMNOGRAPHY

Table 2 reports the results of the analyses of variance on polysomnographic (PSG) variables. The macrostructural variables of sleep pointed to a lack of significant differences between baseline and post-treatment nights (R3), with the exception of a slight reduction of the time spent in WASO (BSL = 76.9 min, ± 54.4; R3 = 52.6 min, ±31.4). Notably, there was no change in the measures of latency and of time spent in the REM sleep.

QUANTITATIVE ANALYSIS OF EEG

NREM sleep

Figure 2 shows the EEG activity in the NREM sleep, averaged over all the 29 scalp locations during baseline and post-treatment sleep. Power maps of both nights indicated stable patterns within different frequency ranges, and the data of maxima and minima exhibited the typical features of power spectra during the NREM sleep. The delta and alpha bands showed a frontal midline predominance and minimum values over the temporal regions. In the theta band, the highest values were at the fronto-central midline areas, while the sigma band showed a centro-parietal maxima. These topographical maps were substantially stable in the different conditions. The lower part of the figure reports the results of the statistical comparisons, and no significant difference was highlighted for any frequency band and scalp location as a consequence of rTMS sessions.

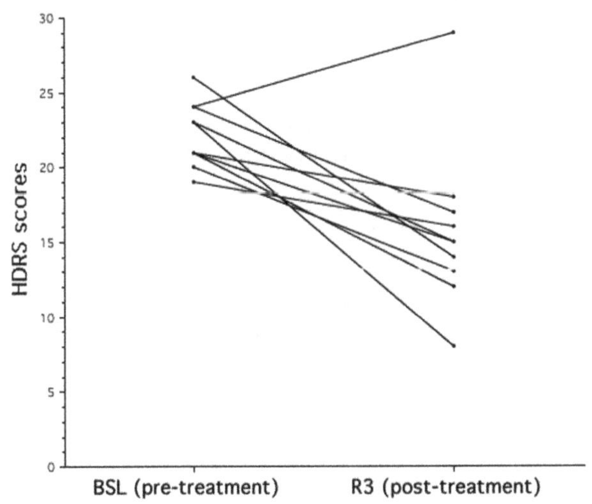

FIGURE 1 | The effects of rTMS on mood in patients with major depression. Individual Hamilton Depression Rating Scale (HDRS) score evaluated at baseline (BSL) and after rTMS treatment (R3). After rTMS there is a significant decrease of HDRS score that corresponds to a clinical status improvement.

REM sleep

Similarly, **Figure 3** shows EEG activity in REM sleep during the BSL and R3 nights. The same stable patterns within different frequency bands were roughly maintained in REM sleep, with the notable exception of the 8–15 Hz range. Topographical maps confirmed a prevalence of the delta band at frontal midline similar to NREM sleep, with minimum values over the temporal regions. In the theta band, the highest values were at the fronto-central midline areas, while the alpha and sigma bands showed a centro-parietal maxima. Both the sigma and beta activity showed minimal values in correspondence of the temporal sites.

The lower part of the figure reports the results of the statistical comparisons, which pointed to a significant decrease of the alpha power ($t = -3.79$; $p = 0.0043$) over the lL-DLPFC site in the R3 compared to the BSL night.

A further analysis of EEG changes with a 1-Hz frequency resolution, aimed to refine the significant difference found for the alpha band, clearly showed that the decrease of EEG activity during REM sleep, mainly regarded the 9 (9.00–9.75 Hz) and 10 (10.00–10.75 Hz) Hz bins. The statistical maps comparing the BSL and the R3 nights showed that even for those frequency bins the observed differences were significant (**Figure 4**). Specifically, we observed a significant decrease in the alpha band on lL-DLPFC, respectively at 9 Hz ($t = -4.14$; $p = 0.0025$) and at 10 Hz ($t = -4.12$; $p = 0.0026$).

RELATION BETWEEN EEG CHANGES AND CLINICAL IMPROVEMENT

According to the findings of the topographical analyses, the main questions remains: "Is the EEG difference associated to the extent clinical improvement?" For this reason, we assessed the correlation between the magnitude of decreased alpha activity in

Table 2 | Means and standard deviations (*SD*) of the polysomnographic variables, before (BSL) and after rTMS treatment (R3), based on visual scoring for all patients.

Variables	BSL		R3		$F_{(1, 9)}$	*P*
	Mean	*SD*	Mean	*SD*		
Stage 1 latency (min)	32.17	27.27	27.36	29.12	0.63	0.45
Stage 2 latency (min)	35.63	30.23	29.80	31.20	0.61	0.45
REM latency (min)	129.90	21.12	122.50	46.68	0.38	0.55
Stage 1 (%)	17.41	16.74	16.99	14.01	0.02	0.88
Stage 2 (%)	66.76	20.55	64.17	18.69	0.94	0.36
REM (%)	15.83	9.41	18.84	6.37	1.76	0.21
WASO (min)	76.88	54.44	52.62	31.35	4.09	0.07
Awakenings (#)	24.20	13.98	21.30	8.65	0.91	0.36
Arousals (#)	82.80	51.42	85.70	53.16	0.22	0.65
TST (min)	414.40	65.62	420.83	69.55	0.13	0.73
TBT (min)	573.23	148.67	501.97	36.98	2.47	0.15
SEI % (TST/TBT)	75.68	18.55	83.74	12.24	2.08	0.18

The results of one-way repeated measure analyses of variance are also reported. No significant difference is present between BSL and R3, with the exception of a slight reduction of wakefulness after sleep onset. REM, rapid eye movement; WASO, wake after sleep onset; TST, total sleep time; TBT, total bed time; SEI, sleep efficiency index.

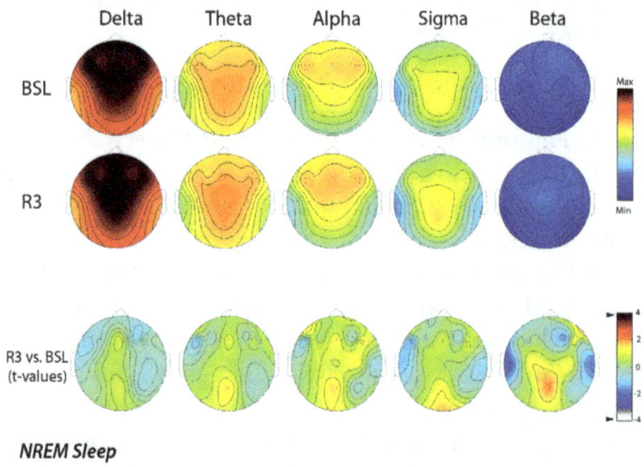

FIGURE 2 | Topographic distribution of EEG power during NREM sleep of the baseline night (BSL) and of the night after the rTMS treatment (R3). Average values are normalized by total power, color-coded, plotted at the corresponding position on the planar projection of the scalp surface and interpolated (biharmonic spline) between electrodes. The maps are based on the 19 unipolar EEG derivations of the international 10–20 system with averaged mastoid reference, and on 10 additional derivations, positioned in both hemispheres respectively over left and right dorsolateral prefrontal cortex and in each orthogonal direction at a distance of 1 cm from the hotspot (electrode positions indicated by dots). In the upper part, the first two rows show the absolute EEG power during NREM sleep of the baseline night (BSL) of the night after the rTMS treatment (R3). Maps are plotted for the following EEG bands: delta (0.50–4.75 Hz), theta (5.00–7.75 Hz), alpha (8.00–11.75 Hz), sigma (12.00–15.75 Hz), and beta (15.00–24.75 Hz). To optimize the contrast, each map was scaled separately between minimal (min) and maximal (max) power values. In the lower part, the statistical maps (*t*-values maps) of the comparison between R3 vs. BSL are illustrated for each frequency band (positive *t*-values indicate a prevalence of the first over the second term). Please note that the color code reports the actual *t*-values (the two-tailed level of significance of $p = 0.0039$, after the Bonferroni correction, corresponds to a $t = 3.84$).

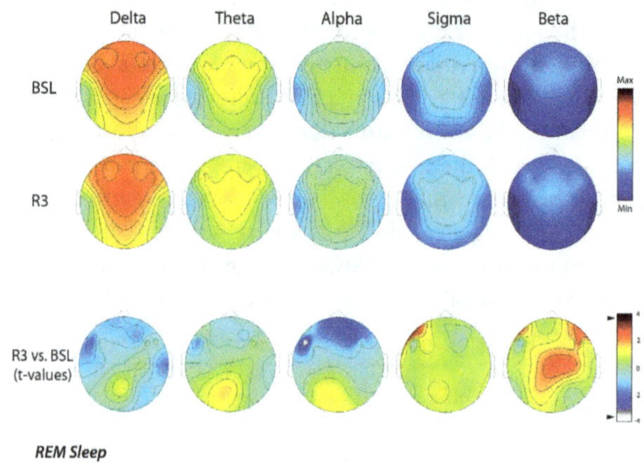

FIGURE 3 | Topographic distribution of EEG power during REM sleep of the baseline night (BSL) and of the night after the rTMS treatment (R3). Average values are normalized by total power, color-coded, plotted at the corresponding position on the planar projection of the scalp surface and interpolated (biharmonic spline) between electrodes. The maps are based on the 19 unipolar EEG derivations of the international 10–20 system with averaged mastoid reference, and on 10 additional derivations, positioned in both hemispheres respectively over left and t right dorsolateral prefrontal cortex and in each orthogonal direction at a distance of 1 cm from the hotspot (electrode positions indicated by dots). In the upper part, the first two rows show the absolute EEG power during REM sleep of the baseline night (BSL) and of the night after the rTMS treatment (R3). Each columns reports maps of the EEG power in the delta, theta, alpha, sigma, and beta frequency ranges. To optimize the contrast, each map was scaled separately between minimal (min) and maximal (max) power values. In the lower part, the statistical maps (*t*-values maps) of the comparison between R3 vs. BSL are illustrated for each frequency band (positive *t*-values indicate a prevalence of the first over the second term). Please note that the color code reports the actual *t*-values (the two-tailed level of significance of $p = 0.0059$, after the Bonferroni correction, corresponds to a $t = 3.58$). Specifically, the alpha power decreased significantly ($t = -3.79$; $p = 0.0043$) during REM sleep at R3 respect to BSL night on lL-DLPFC.

REM sleep at the lL-DLPFC site and the corresponding clinical improvement (in 9 out 10 patients), as expressed by the post-treatment minus pre-treatment HDRS scores. As shown in **Figure 5**, a significant correlation ($r = 0.74$), although on a small sample size, was highlighted with larger decreases of alpha activity in REM sleep associated to larger clinical improvements.

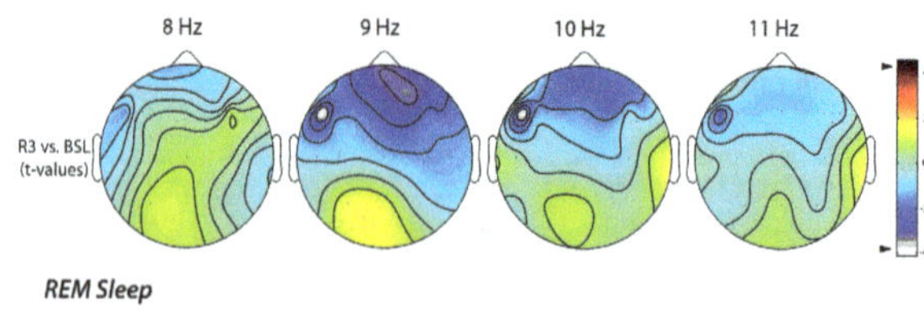

FIGURE 4 | Topographic statistical distribution of the change in alpha power (8.00–11.75 Hz), assessed by comparing (*t*-tests) R3 and baseline nights, for the REM sleep. Values are expressed in terms of *t*-values: negative t-values indicate a decrease at R3 over the baseline night. Filled white circles indicate electrodes showing a significant difference. The analysis of EEG changes with a 1-Hz frequency resolution highlighted an alpha power decrease on lL-DLPFC both to 9 Hz ($t = -4.14$; $p = 0.0025$) and to 10 Hz ($t = -4.12$; $p = 0.0026$).

DISCUSSION

The present study was aimed at evaluating the clinical efficacy of a sequential bilateral rTMS treatment in patients with treatment-resistant MDD and to assess the rTMS-induced macro- and microstructural sleep changes. Keeping in mind the limitations of our open-label design, we observed that rTMS treatment with high frequency over L-DLPFC and low frequency over R-DLPFC was able to induce antidepressant effects. The application of rTMS induced a significant decrease of HDRS score, a clinical marker of mood improvement. Despite no changes detected in the sleep macrostructure after the treatment, a frequency-dependent rTMS effect was observed on the microstructural REM sleep pattern. Specifically, the rTMS induced an alpha power decrease in the REM sleep over the L-DLPFC, that resulted strongly correlated to the clinical outcome.

The observed clinical improvement was in accordance with previous studies that demonstrated the antidepressant efficacy of rTMS (George et al., 2000; Burt et al., 2002; Grunhaus et al., 2003; Fitzgerald et al., 2009). The inclusion of patients with a diagnosis of medication-resistant depression, in our study, could

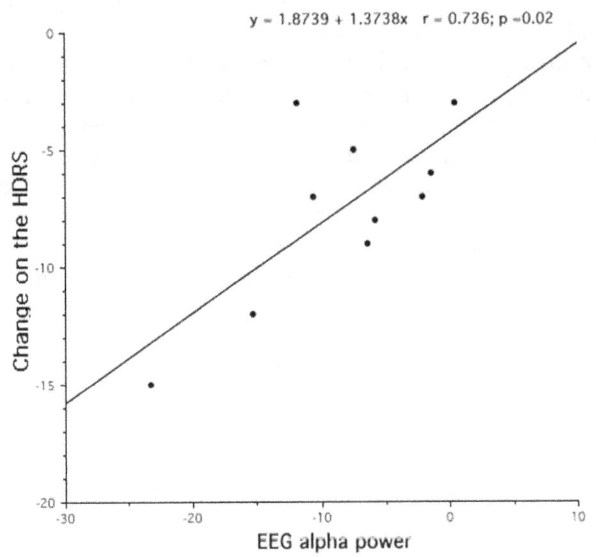

FIGURE 5 | Changes after rTMS treatment in REM alpha power and clinical improvement, assessed by Hamilton Depression Rating Scale (HDRS). After 10 days of treatment, the decrease of REM alpha power results strongly correlated to the treatment outcome.

have limited the magnitude of the therapeutic response, as those patients show a lower response rate to antidepressant intervention compared to non-treatment-resistant patients (Fitzgerald, 2003; Fregni et al., 2006; Brakemeier et al., 2007; Padberg and George, 2009). Even if the mean HDRS response rate decrease was statistically significant while not clinically relevant, declining from very severe and severe depression before the treatment to moderate and mild depression after the treatment, our results should be interpreted positively as the mean percentage of improvements in HDRS score is 35% after rTMS in nine out of ten non-responders patients. To that regard, we hypothesized that the lack of clinical improvement of the non-responder patient to rTMS treatment could be due to his older age, considering the inverse relationship between age and antidepressant response (Manes et al., 2001; Fregni et al., 2006); however the direct assessment of the relation between older age and cortical atrophy has not been viable in the current protocol. The impact of atrophy, in fact, increasing the distance of the coil from the prefrontal cortex (Kozel et al., 2000) would decrease the strength of the induced electrical current and limit the effectiveness of treatment. Probably, a rTMS dose adjusted to overcome cortical atrophy or a more long TMS course (Lisanby et al., 2009) could have been more effective for that patient.

Our clinical results support the notion that the sequential bilateral rTMS combining high frequency left-side and low frequency right-side is an effective antidepressant treatment (Fitzgerald et al., 2006), even though by a point of view of sleep pattern we did not found any macrostructural correlate to that outcome. Considering the role of the REM sleep as a diagnostic and prognostic biological marker of depression, the absence of changes observed on the sleep macrostructure should be considered unexpected. Some changes on the REM variables after the rTMS treatment was expected in the direction of inhibition of REM sleep, manifested by an increase of its latency and a decrease of its amount. However, those changes are frequently observed in the between-subjects protocols that compare the data of depressed patients with those of healthy control subjects (Giles et al., 1993). We hypothesized that with the within-subjects protocol used in this study, it was unlikely to observe evident changes in sleep parameters, like the REM sleep latency or density, that could be well stabilized by depressive disorder, representing a "trait" characteristic (Rush et al., 1986; Giles et al., 1989; Tsuno et al., 2005; Rao and Poland, 2008; Pillai et al., 2011). Moreover, our results confirm the previous findings pointing out how some EEG sleep structural measures remain stable even after pharmacological (Steiger et al., 1989; Kupfer et al., 1994; Murck et al., 2003), non-pharmacological antidepressant treatment (Thase et al., 1998) or combined therapy (Giles et al., 1993).

Although we did not find any changes in the REM macrostructural variables, the main result of the present study regards a specific modulation of the cortical activity during the REM sleep. The observed decrease of cortical activity in the alpha band during the REM sleep after rTMS treatment could represent a specific microstructural marker of depression's remission.

From lesion and neuroimaging studies (Baxter et al., 1989; Martinot et al., 1990; Henriques and Davidson, 1991; Bench et al., 1992; Biver et al., 1994), it is well established as major depression is considered as a hypoactivity syndrome associated with reduced left prefrontal metabolism and cortical dysfunction, in terms of cortical activation decrease (Drevets, 2000; for a review see, Koenigs and Grafman, 2009). Several studies have reported that a marker of this dysregulation could be identified in the alpha power increase, given the inverse relationship between EEG alpha and neural activity, and the consequent role of alpha activity as an inhibitory oscillatory rhythm (Henriques and Davidson, 1990, 1991; Pollock and Schneider, 1990; Ricardo-Garcell et al., 2009; Kemp et al., 2010). Even though the lack of a control healthy group does not allow us to verify if our patients were characterized by a left hypoactivity syndrome (Lubar et al., 2003; Jaworska et al., 2012), our results can be explained by that model. Regarding the alpha power decrease observed during the REM sleep and localized over the left cortex stimulated with high frequency rTMS, we hypothesized that such rTMS frequency, increasing the cortical excitability, might act toward normalizing the DLPFC dysregulation, expressed by the cortical activity modulation observed during the REM sleep. That result is strongly in line with the increase of the cortical excitability after the high frequency rTMS (Fitzgerald et al., 2002; Hallett and Rothwell, 2011). Our results confirm the previous findings that the decrease of the frontal hypoactivity, probably in terms of cortical activity's normalization, could represent the underlying mechanism by which not only antidepressant drugs (Baxter et al., 1989; Mayberg et al., 2000) but also high frequency TMS fosters improvements in depressive disorder, as highlighted by the higher cerebral blood flow values and the cortical excitability increase (George et al., 1999, 2000; Teneback et al., 1999; Speer et al., 2000; Nahas et al., 2001; Rossini et al., 2010). We hypothesize that the high frequency rTMS, stimulating the underlying cortical region and changing the activity of the corresponding neural tissue, could determine an up-regulation of the local activity (Chen, 2000; Fitzgerald et al., 2002). Specifically, the antidepressant effect of the high frequency TMS could be the result of a re-activation of hypofunctional L-DLPFC, in terms of increase of cortical activity, and the neurophysiological biomarker of this effect could be objectified in the decrease of local alpha activity during REM sleep. Our result is strongly in line with the recent hypothesis that rTMS alters and resets cortical oscillators, regulating the intrinsic cerebral rhythms and restoring normal brain function (Leuchter et al., 2013). In particular, the high frequency rTMS could act as an exogenous input, affecting the cortical components, normalizing the intrinsic brain activity and ameliorating the depressive symptoms.

Moreover, the high frequency rTMS could modulate not only the local neuronal firing rate, depolarizing the excitability of neurons, but could also produce a therapeutic effect through the modulation of the monoaminergic receptors involved in the REM sleep. In that regard, an attractive hypothesis to explain both the antidepressant effects induced by rTMS and the REM sleep modulations could be identified in the involvement of serotoninergic mechanisms (Cohrs et al., 1998; Ben-Shachar et al., 1999; Gur et al., 2000; Post and Keck, 2001; Adrien, 2002; Padberg and George, 2009; Baeken et al., 2011). These mechanisms are the same that are involved in other pharmacological (Maudhuit et al., 1997) and non-pharmacological (i.e., total or REM sleep deprivation) (Prevot et al., 1996) antidepressant interventions.

Regarding the bidirectional relationship between sleep disturbance and depression (Riemann et al., 2001; Tsuno et al., 2005) and even though the connection between sleep modifications and clinical improvement have not yet been established, two possible scenarios could be hypothesized to explain our results. In the first one, the rTMS treatment could have acted modulating the clinical symptoms and their improvement could causally affect the EEG sleep topography. In the second one, the rTMS-induced effects on sleep cortical activity could represent the physiological framework, underlying the clinical outcome. Although our results do not allow us to clearly discriminate whether the alpha activity change observed during REM sleep after rTMS treatment was the trigger for the clinical improvement or only an its passive consequence, we speculate that the topographical sleep change was causally determined by the clinical improvement induced by rTMS treatment, representing a neurophysiological correlate of clinical outcome.

The main neurophysiological results of the present study, namely an alpha decrease during the REM sleep in the same frequency range of high frequency rTMS applied in this protocol (i.e., 10 Hz) allow us to speculate that high frequency rTMS could act by saturating the local alpha power and producing an excitability increase functional to remission of the depressive disorder. A similar change in the alpha band was observed in REM sleep after a protocol of sleep deprivation (Roth et al., 1999; Marzano et al., 2010), supporting such frequency as a quantitative and distinctive marker of REM sleep. In that regard, we speculate that the alpha frequency decrease could represent a biological marker of the sleep pressure for the REM sleep, as the delta power represents a well-recognized index of sleep homeostasis for the NREM sleep (Tononi and Cirelli, 2006).

Another important issue is the topography-specificity of the alpha change between the stimulated DLPFCs. Even though no sleep frequency changes were observed over the right stimulated cortex, we speculate that the topographical effect over the L-DLPFC didn't exclude a sequential effect of low frequency rTMS applied over the R-DLPFC cortex, most probably through trans-synaptic connections (Paus et al., 1997; Nahas et al., 2001). Probably, the application of low frequency before the high frequency rTMS may have contributed to prime the effects observed over the left cortex, determining a synergetic effect on the clinical outcome (Fitzgerald et al., 2006) even though no detectable at cortical level.

Finally, even though our study was focused on all EEG frequency bands, our results are partially in agreement with the only study in which the sleep electrophysiological effects induced by rTMS treatment on patients with a major depressive episode were investigated (Saeki et al., 2012). Regarding NREM sleep, in this latter study a delta power increase at left DLFPC was observed after the initial five rTMS sessions, but not after the total 10 rTMS sessions. In agreement to these authors, also our negative finding on SWA during NREM sleep after 10 rTMS sessions could be due to the involvement of homeostatic regulation mechanism. On the other hand, the discrepancy of results during REM sleep, when we observed a local decrease of alpha activity, could be due to their focus on two specific EEG frequency bands (slow wave and spindle activity), not considering all sleep bands.

Several limitations need to be addressed. The first limitation was the experimental design. The open-label experimental design and the lack of a sham comparison group (with subsequent sleep recordings) doesn't allow us to thoroughly exclude a placebo effect in the clinical response of our patients (Miniussi et al., 2005), though the observed linear relationship between EEG and HDRS changes suggests a specificity of the relationship.

Moreover, our sample size was relatively small and the patients were all under pharmacological therapy during rTMS treatment, making it impossible to evaluate the clinical and neurophysiological effect of rTMS as stand-alone treatment. In that regard, the non-suspension of the drug treatment could be responsible for the lack of significant macrostructural differences, highlighted both in the REM (in terms of latency and density) and the NREM sleep. Specifically, it is well known how the REM sleep duration is reduced by the antidepressant drug action until to its suppression (Holshoe, 2009), and how the NREM sleep, and in particular the sigma band and SWA are affected by benzodiazepines (e.g., Bastien et al., 2003). Only additional studies with a wider patient sample and patients pharmacological washing out, as well as a sham condition may allow a better understanding of the macro- and microstructural effects induced by rTMS treatment on depressive disorder.

CONCLUSION

Concluding, in line with the theory of the left frontal hypoactivation during the rest in depression, the observed local decrease of alpha activity after rTMS treatment during the REM sleep confirms the possibility of identifying that EEG frequency as a marker of the cortical activity up-regulation induced by high frequency rTMS as well as a neurophysiological correlate of clinical outcome, providing also an important information regarding the underlying neuronal circuit responsible of antidepressant response. The observed correlation between cortical activity modulation and clinical response indicate clearly that these results are not respectively related to a TMS-induced brain activation independent of the treatment response or to the antidepressant response to rTMS but are determined by their causal and direct relationship. This is the first study, to our knowledge, that combining clinical rTMS-induced effects and neurophysiological evaluation of the EEG sleep changes after a long-term treatment, allows to delineate not only the behavioral outcome, but also the involved sleep cortical circuits, showing that the antidepressant effects of rTMS might be mediated by a significant sleep influence. We conclude that rTMS, and specifically the high frequency stimulation, can represent a relevant strategy in the modulation of hypoactivity syndrome, like in MDD and that the study of the microstructural sleep pattern represents a potential tool for understanding the neurophysiological mechanisms of the mood disorders and their possible regulation. Finally, we propose the left frontal alpha frequency of the REM sleep as a state-dependent marker for depression and its remission.

ACKNOWLEDGMENTS

The authors are grateful to Mrs Claudia Fracassi and Dr Cornelia Pirulli for their help in data collection and the Italian Ministry of Health, Grant RF 05/56 to Cristina Marzano and Ricerca Corrente, for the financial support.

REFERENCES

Adrien, J. (2002). Neurobiological bases for the relation between sleep and depression. *Sleep Med. Rev.* 6, 341–351.

Allen, J. J., Urry, H. L., Hitt, S. K., and Coan, J. A. (2004). The stability of resting frontal electroencephalographic asymmetry in depression. *Psychophysiology* 41, 269–280. doi: 10.1111/j.1469-8986.2003.00149.x

Armitage, R. (2007). Sleep and circadian rhythms in mood disorders. *Acta Psychiatr. Scand. Suppl.* 433, 104–115. doi: 10.1111/j.1600-0447.2007.00968.x

Baeken, C., De Raedt, R., Bossuyt, A., Van Hove, C., Mertens, J., Dobbeleir, A., et al. (2011). The impact of HF-rTMS treatment on serotonin(2A) receptors in unipolar melancholic depression. *Brain Stimul.* 4, 104–111. doi: 10.1016/j.brs.2010.09.002

Baglioni, C., Battagliese, G., Feige, B., Spiegelhalder, K., Nissen, C., Voderholzer, U., et al. (2011). Insomnia as a predictor of depression: a meta-analytic evaluation of longitudinal epidemiological studies. *J. Affect. Disord.* 135, 10–19. doi: 10.1016/j.jad.2011.01.011

Bastien, C. H., LeBlanc, M., Carrier, J., and Morin, C. M. (2003). Sleep EEG power spectra, insomnia, and chronic use of benzodiazepines. *Sleep* 26, 313–317

Baxter, L. R. Jr, Schwartz, J. M., Phelps, M. E., Mazziotta, J. C., Guze, B. H., Selin, C. E., et al. (1989). Reduction of prefrontal cortex glucose metabolism common to three types of depression. *Arch. Gen. Psychiatry* 46, 243–250. doi: 10.1001/archpsyc.1989.01810030049007

Bench, C. J., Friston, K. J., Brown, R. G., Scott, L. C., Frackowiak, R. S., and Dolan, R. J. (1992). The anatomy of melancholia–focal abnormalities of cerebral blood flow in major depression. *Psychol. Med.* 22, 607–615. doi: 10.1017/S003329170003806X

Ben-Shachar, D., Gazawi, H., Riboyad-Levin, J., and Klein, E. (1999). Chronic repetitive transcranial magnetic stimulation alters beta-adrenergic and 5-HT2 receptor characteristics in rat brain. *Brain Res.* 816, 78–83. doi: 10.1016/S0006-8993(98)01119-6

Biver, F., Goldman, S., Delvenne, V., Luxen, A., De Maertelaer, V., Hubain, P., et al. (1994). Frontal and parietal metabolic disturbances in unipolar depression. *Biol. Psychiatry* 36, 381–388. doi: 10.1016/0006-3223(94)91213-0

Blumberger, D. M., Tran, L. C., Fitzgerald, P. B., Hoy, K. E., and Daskalakis, Z. J. (2012). A randomized double-blind sham-controlled study of transcranial direct current stimulation for treatment-resistant major depression. *Front. Psychiatry* 3:74. doi: 10.3389/fpsyt.2012.00074

Brakemeier, E. L., Luborzewski, A., Danker-Hopfe, H., Kathmann, N., and Bajbouj, M. (2007). Positive predictors for antidepressive response to prefrontal repetitive transcranial magnetic stimulation (rTMS). *J. Psychiatr. Res.* 41, 395–403. doi: 10.1016/j.jpsychires.2006.01.013

Bruder, G. E., Fong, R., Tenke, C. E., Leite, P., Towey, J. P., Stewart, J. E., et al. (1997). Regional brain asymmetries in major depression with or without an anxiety disorder: a quantitative electroencephalographic study. *Biol. Psychiatry* 41, 939–948. doi: 10.1016/S0006-3223(96)00260-0

Burt, T., Lisanby, S. H., and Sackeim, H. A. (2002). Neuropsychiatric applications of transcranial magnetic stimulation: a meta analysis. *Int. J. Neuropsychopharmacol.* 5, 73–103. doi: 10.1017/S1461145702002791

Buysse, D. J., Kupfer, D. J., Cherry, C., Stapf, D., and Frank, E. (1999). Effects of prior fluoxetine treatment on EEG sleep in women with recurrent depression. *Neuropsychopharmacology* 21, 258–267. doi: 10.1016/S0893-133X(99)00025-1

Chen, R. (2000). Studies of human motor physiology with transcranial magnetic stimulation. *Muscle Nerve Suppl.* 9, S26–S32.

Cohrs, S., Tergau, F., Riech, S., Kastner, S., Paulus, W., Ziemann, U., et al. (1998). High-frequency repetitive transcranial magnetic stimulation delays rapid eye movement sleep. *Neuroreport* 9, 3439–3443. doi: 10.1097/00001756-199810260-00019

Davidson, R. J. (1992). Anterior cerebral asymmetry and the nature of emotion. *Brain Cogn.* 20, 125–151. doi: 10.1016/0278-2626(92)90065-T

Debener, S., Beauducel, A., Nessler, D., Brocke, B., Heilemann, H., and Kayser, J. (2000). Is resting anterior EEG alpha asymmetry a trait marker for depression. Findings for healthy adults and clinically depressed patients. *Neuropsychobiology* 41, 31–37. doi: 10.1159/000026630

Drevets, W. C. (2000). Functional anatomical abnormalities in limbic and prefrontal cortical structures in major depression. *Prog. Brain Res.* 126, 413–431. doi: 10.1016/S0079-6123(00)26027-5

Drevets, W. C., Price, J. L., Simpson, J. R. Jr., Todd, R. D., Reich, T., and Vannier, M. (1997). Subgenual prefrontal cortex abnormalities in mood disorders. *Nature* 386, 824–827. doi: 10.1038/386824a0

Fitzgerald, P. (2003). Is it time to introduce repetitive transcranial magnetic stimulation into standard clinical practice for the treatment of depressive disorders. *Aust. N.Z. J. Psychiatry* 37, 5–11. discussion: 12–14. doi: 10.1046/j.1440-1614.2003.01115.x

Fitzgerald, P. B., Benitez, J., de Castella, A., Daskalakis, Z. J., Brown, T. L., and Kulkarni, J. (2006). A randomized, controlled trial of sequential bilateral repetitive transcranial magnetic stimulation for treatment-resistant depression. *Am. J. Psychiatry* 163, 88–94. doi: 10.1176/appi.ajp.163.1.88

Fitzgerald, P. B., Brown, T. L., and Daskalakis, Z. J. (2002). The application of transcranial magnetic stimulation in psychiatry and neurosciences research. *Acta Psychiatr. Scand.* 105, 324–340. doi: 10.1034/j.1600-0447.2002.1r179.x

Fitzgerald, P. B., McQueen, S., Herring, S., Hoy, K., Segrave, R., Kulkarni, J., et al. (2009). A study of the effectiveness of high-frequency left prefrontal cortex transcranial magnetic stimulation in major depression in patients who have not responded to right-sided stimulation. *Psychiatry Res.* 169, 12–15. doi: 10.1016/j.psychres.2008.06.017

Fregni, F., Boggio, P. S., Nitsche, M. A., Rigonatti, S. P., and Pascual-Leone, A. (2006). Cognitive effects of repeated sessions of transcranial direct current stimulation in patients with depression. *Depress. Anxiety* 23, 482–484. doi: 10.1002/da.20201

Funk, A. P., and George, M. S. (2008). Prefrontal EEG asymmetry as a potential biomarker of antidepressant treatment response with transcranial magnetic stimulation (TMS): a case series. *Clin.*

EEG Neurosci. 39, 125–130. doi: 10.1177/155005940803900306

George, M. S., Nahas, Z., Kozel, F. A., Goldman, J., Molloy, M., and Oliver, N. (1999). Improvement of depression following transcranial magnetic stimulation. *Curr. Psychiatry Rep.* 1, 114–124. doi: 10.1007/s11920-999-0020-2

George, M. S., Nahas, Z., Molloy, M., Speer, A. M., Oliver, N. C., Li, X. B., et al. (2000). A controlled trial of daily left prefrontal cortex TMS for treating depression. *Biol. Psychiatry* 48, 962–970. doi: 10.1016/S0006-3223(00)01048-9

George, M. S., Taylor, J. J., and Short, E. B. (2013). The expanding evidence base for rTMS treatment of depression. *Curr. Opin. Psychiatry* 26, 13–18. doi: 10.1097/YCO.0b013e32835ab46d

Giles, D. E., Etzel, B. A., Reynolds, C. F. 3rd., and Kupfer, D. J. (1989). Stability of polysomnographic parameters in unipolar depression: a cross-sectional report. *Biol. Psychiatry* 25, 807–810. doi: 10.1016/0006-3223(89)90256-4

Giles, D. E., Jarrett, R. B., Rush, A. J., Biggs, M. M., and Roffwarg, H. P. (1993). Prospective assessment of electroencephalographic sleep in remitted major depression. *Psychiatry Res.* 46, 269–284. doi: 10.1016/0165-1781(93)90095-X

Grimm, S., Beck, J., Schuepbach, D., Hell, D., Boesiger, P., Bermpohl, F., et al. (2008). Imbalance between left and right dorsolateral prefrontal cortex in major depression is linked to negative emotional judgment: an fMRI study in severe major depressive disorder. *Biol. Psychiatry* 63, 369–376. doi: 10.1016/j.biopsych.2007.05.033

Grunhaus, L., Schreiber, S., Dolberg, O. T., Polak, D., and Dannon, P. N. (2003). A randomized controlled comparison of electroconvulsive therapy and repetitive transcranial magnetic stimulation in severe and resistant nonpsychotic major depression. *Biol. Psychiatry* 53, 324–331. doi: 10.1016/S0006-3223(02)01499-3

Gur, E., Lerer, B., Dremencov, E., and Newman, M. E. (2000). Chronic repetitive transcranial magnetic stimulation induces subsensitivity of presynaptic serotonergic autoreceptor activity in rat brain. *Neuroreport* 11, 2925–2929. doi: 10.1097/00001756-200009110-00019

Hallett, M., and Rothwell, J. (2011). Milestones in clinical neurophysiology. *Mov. Disord.* 26, 958–967. doi: 10.1002/mds.23572

Henriques, J. B., and Davidson, R. J. (1990). Regional brain electrical asymmetries discriminate between previously depressed and healthy control subjects. *J. Abnorm. Psychol.* 99, 22–31. doi: 10.1037/0021-843X.99.1.22

Henriques, J. B., and Davidson, R. J. (1991). Left frontal hypoactivation in depression. *J. Abnorm. Psychol.* 100, 535–545. doi: 10.1037/0021-843X.100.4.535

Holshoe, J. M. (2009). Antidepressants and sleep: a review. *Perspect. Psychiatr. Care* 45, 191–197. doi: 10.1111/j.1744-6163.2009.00221.x

Jaworska, N., Blier, P., Fusee, W., and Knott, V. (2012). Alpha Power, alpha asymmetry and anterior cingulate cortex activity in depressed males and females. *J. Psychiatr. Res.* 46, 1483–1491. doi: 10.1016/j.jpsychires.2012.08.003

Kemp, A. H., Griffiths, K., Felmingham, K. L., Shankman, S. A., Drinkenburg, W., Arns, M., et al. (2010). Disorder specificity despite comorbidity: resting EEG alpha asymmetry in major depressive disorder and post-traumatic stress disorder. *Biol. Psychol.* 85, 350–354. doi: 10.1016/j.biopsycho.2010.08.001

Koenigs, M., and Grafman, J. (2009). The functional neuroanatomy of depression: distinct roles for ventromedial and dorsolateral prefrontal cortex. *Behav. Brain Res.* 201, 239–243. doi: 10.1016/j.bbr.2009.03.004

Kozel, F. A., Nahas, Z., deBrux, C., Molloy, M., Lorberbaum, J. P., Bohning, D., et al. (2000). How coil-cortex distance relates to age, motor threshold, and antidepressant response to repetitive transcranial magnetic stimulation. *J. Neuropsychiatry Clin. Neurosci.* 12, 376–384. doi: 10.1176/appi.neuropsych.12.3.376

Kupfer, D. J. (1976). REM latency: a psychobiologic marker for primary depressive disease. *Biol. Psychiatry* 11, 159–174.

Kupfer, D. J., Ehlers, C. L., Frank, E., Grochocinski, V. J., McEachran, A. B., and Buhari, A. (1994). Persistent effects of antidepressants: EEG sleep studies in depressed patients during maintenance treatment. *Biol. Psychiatry* 35, 781–793. doi: 10.1016/0006-3223(94)91140-1

Kupfer, D. J., Spiker, D. G., Coble, P. A., Neil, J. F., Ulrich, R., and Shaw, D. H. (1981). Sleep and treatment prediction in endogenous depression. *Am. J. Psychiatry* 138, 429–434.

Lauer, C. J., Riemann, D., Wiegand, M., and Berger, M. (1991). From early to late adulthood. Changes in EEG sleep of depressed patients and healthy volunteers. *Biol. Psychiatry* 29, 979–993. doi: 10.1016/0006-3223(91)90355-P

Leuchter, A. F., Cook, I. A., Jin, Y., and Phillips, B. (2013). The relationship between brain oscillatory activity and therapeutic effectiveness of transcranial magnetic stimulation in the treatment of major depressive disorder. *Front. Hum. Neurosci.* 7:37. doi: 10.3389/fnhum.2013.00037

Li, C., Wang, S., Hirvonen, J., Hsieh, J., Bai, Y., Hong, C., et al. (2010). Antidepressant mechanism of add-on repetitive transcranial magnetic stimulation in medication-resistant depression using cerebral glucose metabolism. *J. Affect. Disord.* 127, 219–229. doi: 10.1016/j.jad.2010.05.028

Lisanby, S. H., Husain, M. M., Rosenquist, P. B., Maixner, D., Gutierrez, R., Krystal, A., et al. (2009). Daily left prefrontal repetitive transcranial magnetic stimulation in the acute treatment of major depression: clinical predictors of outcome in a multisite, randomized controlled clinical trial. *Neuropsychopharmacology* 34, 522–534. doi: 10.1038/npp.2008.118

Lubar, J. F., Congedo, M., and Askew, J. H. (2003). Low-resolution electromagnetic tomography (LORETA) of cerebral activity in chronic depressive disorder. *Int. J. Psychophysiol.* 49, 175–185. doi: 10.1016/S0167-8760(03)00115-6

Luppa, M., Heinrich, S., Angermeyer, M. C., Konig, H. H., and Riedel-Heller, S. G. (2007). Cost-of-illness studies of depression: a systematic review. *J. Affect. Disord.* 98, 29–43. doi: 10.1016/j.jad.2006.07.017

Lustberg, L., and Reynolds, C. F. (2000). Depression and insomnia: questions of cause and effect. *Sleep Med. Rev.* 4, 253–262. doi: 10.1053/smrv.1999.0075

Manes, F., Jorge, R., Morcuende, M., Yamada, T., Paradiso, S., and Robinson, R. G. (2001). A controlled study of repetitive transcranial magnetic stimulation as a treatment of depression in the elderly. *Int. Psychogeriatr.* 13, 225–231. doi: 10.1017/S1041610201007608

Martinot, J. L., Hardy, P., Feline, A., Huret, J. D., Mazoyer, B., Attar-Levy, D., et al. (1990). Left prefrontal glucose hypometabolism in the depressed state: a confirmation. *Am. J. Psychiatry* 147, 1313–1317.

Marzano, C., Ferrara, M., Curcio, G., and De Gennaro, L. (2010). The effects of sleep deprivation in humans: topographical electroencephalogram changes in non-rapid eye movement (NREM) sleep versus REM sleep. *J. Sleep Res.* 19, 260–268. doi: 10.1111/j.1365-2869.2009.00776.x

Maudhuit, C., Prevot, E., Dangoumau, L., Martin, P., Hamon, M., and Adrien, J. (1997). Antidepressant treatment in helpless rats: effect on the electrophysiological activity of raphe dorsalis serotonergic neurons. *Psychopharmacology (Berl.)* 130, 269–275. doi: 10.1007/s002130050239

Mayberg, H. S., Brannan, S. K., Tekell, J. L., Silva, J. A., Mahurin, R. K., McGinnis, S., et al. (2000). Regional metabolic effects of fluoxetine in major depression: serial changes and relationship to clinical response. *Biol. Psychiatry* 48, 830–843. doi: 10.1016/S0006-3223(00)01036-2

Mayers, A. G., and Baldwin, D. S. (2005). Antidepressants and their effect on sleep. *Hum. Psychopharmacol.* 20, 533–559. doi: 10.1002/hup.726

Miniussi, C., Bonato, C., Bignotti, S., Gazzoli, A., Gennarelli, M., Pasqualetti, P., et al. (2005). Repetitive transcranial magnetic stimulation (rTMS) at high and low frequency: an efficacious therapy for major drug-resistant depression? *Clin. Neurophysiol.* 116, 1062–1071. doi: 10.1016/j.clinph.2005.01.002

Murck, H., Nickel, T., Kunzel, H., Antonijevic, I. A., Schill, J., Zobel, A., et al. (2003). State markers of depression in sleep EEG: dependency on drug and gender in patients treated with tianeptine or paroxetine. *Neuropsychopharmacology* 28, 348–358. doi: 10.1038/sj.npp.1300029

Nahas, Z., Teneback, C. C., Kozel, A., Speer, A. M., DeBrux, C., Molloy, M., et al. (2001). Brain effects of TMS delivered over prefrontal cortex in depressed adults: role of stimulation frequency and coil-cortex distance. *J. Neuropsychiatry Clin. Neurosci.* 13, 459–470. doi: 10.1176/appi.neuropsych.13.4.459

Padberg, F., and George, M. S. (2009). Repetitive transcranial magnetic stimulation of the prefrontal cortex in depression. *Exp. Neurol.* 219, 2–13. doi: 10.1016/j.expneurol.2009.04.020

Pallanti, S., Bernardi, S., Di Rollo, A., Antonini, S., and Quercioli, L. (2010). Unilateral low frequency versus sequential bilateral repetitive transcranial magnetic stimulation: is simpler better for treatment of resistant depression? *Neuroscience* 167, 323–328.

Paus, T., Jech, R., Thompson, C. J., Comeau, R., Peters, T., and Evans, A. C. (1997). Transcranial magnetic stimulation during positron emission tomography: a new method for studying connectivity of the human cerebral cortex. *J. Neurosci.* 17, 3178–3184.

Perlis, M. L., Giles, D. E., Buysse, D. J., Thase, M. E., Tu, X., and Kupfer, D. J. (1997). Which depressive symptoms are related to which sleep electroencephalographic variables? *Biol. Psychiatry* 42, 904–913.

Pillai, V., Kalmbach, D. A., and Ciesla, J. A. (2011). A meta analysis of electroencephalographic sleep in depression: evidence for genetic biomarkers. *Biol. Psychiatry* 70, 912–919. doi: 10.1016/j.biopsych.2011.07.016

Pollock, V. E., and Schneider, L. S. (1990). Quantitative, waking EEG research on depression. *Biol. Psychiatry* 27, 757–780. doi: 10.1016/0006-3223(90)90591-O

Post, A., and Keck, M. E. (2001). Transcranial magnetic stimulation as a therapeutic tool in psychiatry: what do we know about the neurobiological mechanisms? *J. Psychiatr. Res.* 35, 193–215. doi: 10.1016/S0022-3956(01)00023-1

Prevot, E., Maudhuit, C., Le Poul, E., Hamon, M., and Adrien, J. (1996). Sleep deprivation reduces the citalopram-induced inhibition of serotoninergic neuronal firing in the nucleus raphe dorsalis of the rat. *J. Sleep Res.* 5, 238–245. doi: 10.1111/j.1365-2869.1996.00238.x

Rao, U., and Poland, R. E. (2008). Electroencephalographic sleep and hypothalamic-pituitary-adrenal changes from episode to recovery in depressed adolescents. *J. Child Adolesc. Psychopharmacol.* 18, 607–613. doi: 10.1089/cap.2008.034

Rechtschaffen, A., and Kales, A. (1968). *A Manual of Standardized Terminology, Techniques and Scoring System for Sleep Stages of Human Subjects.* Los Angeles, CA: UCLA Brain Information Service.

Reynolds, C. F. 3rd., and Kupfer, D. J. (1987). Sleep research in affective illness: state of the art circa 1987. *Sleep* 10, 199–215.

Ricardo-Garcell, J., Gonzalez-Olvera, J. J., Miranda, E., Harmony, T., Reyes, E., Almeida, L., et al. (2009). EEG sources in a group of patients with major depressive disorders. *Int. J. Psychophysiol.* 71, 70–74. doi: 10.1016/j.ijpsycho.2008.07.021

Riemann, D., Berger, M., and Voderholzer, U. (2001). Sleep and depression–results from psychobiological studies: an overview. *Biol. Psychol.* 57, 67–103. doi: 10.1016/S0301-0511(01)00090-4

Riemann, D., Schnitzler, M., Hohagen, F., and Berger, M. (1994). Depression and sleep–the status of current research. *Fortschr. Neurol. Psychiatr.* 62, 458–478. doi: 10.1055/s-2007-1002303

Rossi, S., Hallett, M., Rossini, P. M., Pascual-Leone, A., and Safety of TMS Consensus Group, (2009). Safety, ethical considerations, and application guidelines for the use of transcranial magnetic stimulation in clinical practice and research. *Clin. Neurophysiol.* 120, 2008–2039. doi: 10.1016/j.clinph.2009.08.016

Rossini, D., Lucca, A., Magri, L., Malaguti, A., Smeraldi, E., Colombo, C., et al. (2010). A symptom-specific analysis of the effect of high-frequency left or low-frequency right transcranial magnetic stimulation over the dorsolateral prefrontal cortex in major depression. *Neuropsychobiology* 62, 91–97. doi: 10.1159/000315439

Rossini, P. M., Barker, A. T., Berardelli, A., Caramia, M. D., Caruso, G., Cracco, R. Q., et al. (1994). Non-invasive electrical and magnetic stimulation of the brain, spinal cord and roots: basic principles and procedures for routine clinical application. Report of an IFCN committee. *Electroencephalogr. Clin. Neurophysiol.* 91, 79–92. doi: 10.1016/0013-4694(94)90029-9

Roth, C., Achermann, P., and Borbely, A. A. (1999). Alpha activity in the human REM sleep EEG: topography and effect of REM sleep deprivation. *Clin. Neurophysiol.* 110, 632–635. doi: 10.1016/S1388-2457(98)00060-1

Rush, A. J., Erman, M. K., Giles, D. E., Schlesser, M. A., Carpenter, G., Vasavada, N., et al. (1986). Polysomnographic findings in recently drug-free and clinically remitted depressed patients. *Arch. Gen. Psychiatry* 43, 878–884. doi: 10.1001/archpsyc.1986.01800090068009

Saeki, T., Nakamura, M., Hirai, N., Noda, Y., Hayasaka, S., Iwanari, H., et al. (2012). Localized potentiation of sleep slow-wave activity induced by prefrontal repetitive transcranial magnetic stimulation in patients with a major depressive episode. *Brain Stimul.* 6, 390–396. doi: 10.1016/j.brs.2012.08.004

Sandor, P., and Shapiro, C. M. (1994). Sleep patterns in depression and anxiety: theory and pharmacological effects. *J. Psychosom. Res.* 38(Suppl. 1), 125–139. doi: 10.1016/0022-3999(94)90143-0

Sharpley, A. L., and Cowen, P. J. (1995). Effect of pharmacologic treatments on the sleep of depressed patients. *Biol. Psychiatry* 37, 85–98. doi: 10.1016/0006-3223(94)00135-P

Silberman, E. K., and Weingartner, H. (1986). Hemispheric lateralization of functions related to emotion. *Brain Cogn.* 5, 322–353. doi: 10.1016/0278-2626(86)90035-7

Speer, A. M., Kimbrell, T. A., Wassermann, E. M., D Repella, J, Willis, M W, Herscovitch, P, et al. (2000). Opposite effects of high and low frequency rTMS on regional brain activity in depressed patients. *Biol. Psychiatry* 48, 1133–1141. doi: 10.1016/S0006-3223(00)01065-9

Steiger, A., and Kimura, M. (2010). Wake and sleep EEG provide biomarkers in depression. *J. Psychiatr. Res.* 44, 242–252. doi: 10.1016/j.jpsychires.2009.08.013

Steiger, A., von Bardeleben, U., Herth, T., and Holsboer, F. (1989). Sleep EEG and nocturnal secretion of cortisol and growth hormone in male patients with endogenous depression before treatment and after recovery. *J. Affect. Disord.* 16, 189–195. doi: 10.1016/0165-0327(89)90073-6

Teneback, C. C., Nahas, Z., Speer, A. M., Molloy, M., Stallings, L. E., Spicer, K. M., et al. (1999). Changes in prefrontal cortex and paralimbic activity in depression following two weeks of daily left prefrontal TMS. *J. Neuropsychiatry Clin. Neurosci.* 11, 426–435.

Thase, M. E., Howland, R. H., and Friedman, E. S. (1998). Treating antidepressant nonresponders with augmentation strategies: an overview. *J. Clin. Psychiatry* 59 (Suppl. 5), 5–12. discussion: 13–15.

Tononi, G., and Cirelli, C. (2006). Sleep function and synaptic homeostasis. *Sleep Med. Rev.* 10, 49–62. doi: 10.1016/j.smrv.2005.05.002

Tsuno, N., Besset, A., and Ritchie, K. (2005). Sleep and depression. *J. Clin. Psychiatry* 66, 1254–1269. doi: 10.4088/JCP.v66n1008

Valiulis, V., Gerulskis, G., Dapsys, K., Vistartaite, G., Siurkute, A., and Maciulis, V. (2012). Electrophysiological differences between high and low frequency rTMS protocols in depression treatment. *Acta Neurobiol. Exp. (Wars)* 72, 283–295.

Videbech, P., Ravnkilde, B., Pedersen, T. H., Hartvig, H., Egander, A., Clemmensen, K., et al. (2002). The Danish PET/depression project: clinical symptoms and cerebral blood flow. A regions-of-interest analysis. *Acta Psychiatr. Scand.* 106, 35–44. doi: 10.1034/j.1600-0447.2002.02245.x

Walter, H., Wolf, R. C., Spitzer, M., and Vasic, N. (2007). Increased left prefrontal activation in patients with unipolar depression: an event-related, parametric, performance-controlled fMRI study. *J. Affect. Disord.* 101, 175–185. doi: 10.1016/j.jad.2006.11.017

Wassermann, E. M. (1998). Risk and safety of repetitive transcranial magnetic stimulation: report and suggested guidelines from the international workshop on the safety of repetitive transcranial magnetic stimulation, June 5-7, 1996. *Electroencephalogr. Clin. Neurophysiol.* 108, 1–16. doi: 10.1016/S0168-5597(97)00096-8

Wassermann, E. M., and Lisanby, S. H. (2001). Therapeutic application of repetitive transcranial magnetic stimulation: a review. *Clin. Neurophysiol.* 112, 1367–1377. doi: 10.1016/S1388-2457(01)00585-5

3

Long-latency TMS-evoked potentials during motor execution and inhibition

Kentaro Yamanaka[1] *, Hiroshi Kadota [2,3] and Daichi Nozaki [2]

[1] Graduate School of Human Life Sciences, Showa Women's University, Tokyo, Japan
[2] Graduate School of Education, The University of Tokyo, Tokyo, Japan
[3] Research Institute, Kochi University of Technology, Kochi, Japan

Correspondence:
Kentaro Yamanaka, Graduate School of Human Life Sciences, Showa Women's University, 1-7 Taishido, Setagaya-ku, Tokyo 154-8533, Japan
e-mail: kentaro@swu.ac.jp

Transcranial magnetic stimulation (TMS) has often been used in conjunction with electroencephalography (EEG), which is effective for the direct demonstration of cortical reactivity and corticocortical connectivity during cognitive tasks through the spatio-temporal pattern of long-latency TMS-evoked potentials (TEPs). However, it remains unclear what pattern is associated with the inhibition of a planned motor response. Therefore, we performed TMS-EEG recording during a go/stop task, in which participants were instructed to click a computer mouse with a right index finger when an indicator that was moving with a constant velocity reached a target (go trial) or to avoid the click when the indicator randomly stopped just before it reached the target (stop trial). Single-pulse TMS to the left (contralateral) or right (ipsilateral) motor cortex was applied 500 ms before or just at the target time. TEPs related to motor execution and inhibition were obtained by subtractions between averaged EEG waveforms with and without TMS. As a result, in TEPs induced by both contralateral and ipsilateral TMS, small oscillations were followed by a prominent negative deflection around the TMS site peaking at approximately 100 ms post-TMS (N100), and a less pronounced later positive component (LPC) over the broad areas that was centered at the midline-central site in both go and stop trials. However, compared to the pattern in go and stop trials with TMS at 500 ms before the target time, N100 and LPC were differently modulated in the go and stop trials with TMS just at the target time. The amplitudes of both N100 and LPC decreased in go trials, while the amplitude of LPC decreased and the latency of LPC was delayed in both go and stop trials. These results suggested that TMS-induced neuronal reactions in the motor cortex and subsequent their propagation to surrounding cortical areas might change functionally according to task demand when executing and inhibiting a motor response.

Keywords: transcranial magnetic stimulation, electroencephalography, motor-evoked potentials, motor cortex, execution, inhibition

INTRODUCTION

Transcranial magnetic stimulation (TMS; Barker et al., 1985) is a powerful tool that allows for the non-invasive investigation of the functional state of the cerebral cortex and corticomotoneuronal (CM) pathways (Hallett, 2000, 2007; Walsh and Cowey, 2000; Reis et al., 2008). Motor evoked potentials (MEP) that are induced in hand muscles after TMS over the motor cortex can be modulated during various motor tasks. For example, premovement MEP enhancements within 100 ms before response onset have been reported in many previous studies (Starr et al., 1988; Pascual-Leone et al., 1992; Chen et al., 1998; Leocani et al., 2000; Yamanaka et al., 2002). In contrast, the transient suppression of MEPs has been demonstrated during no-go trials of go/no-go tasks (Hoshiyama et al., 1996, 1997; Leocani et al., 2000; Yamanaka et al., 2002) and during the stop trials of stop-signal tasks (Badry et al., 2009; van den Wildenberg et al., 2010). The results of those studies have suggested that such MEP changes might primarily reflect modulations of CM excitability according to task demand.

Transcranial magnetic stimulation has often been used in combination with electroencephalographic (EEG) recordings (Ilmoniemi et al., 1997). This combined TMS-EEG technique makes it possible to investigate cortical reactivity and corticocortical connectivity from the spatiotemporal patterns of TMS-evoked potentials (TEP), which consist of peaks of negative/positive oscillations lasting about 300 ms (Komssi and Kähkönen, 2006; Ilmoniemi and Kičić, 2010). Although the functional meaning and cortical origin of the TEP peaks are not completely understood, a prominent long-latency negative peak has been commonly observed when TMS is delivered over the motor cortex in many previous studies (Paus et al., 2001; Nikulin et al., 2003; Komssi et al., 2004; Bonato et al., 2006; Kičić et al., 2008; Bonnard et al., 2009; Lioumis et al., 2009; Ferreri et al., 2011, 2012; Rogasch et al., 2013). This reproducible large negative peak at about 100 ms after the TMS pulse is named N1 or N100.

Previous studies have demonstrated that TEPs are modulated in various conditions, including arousal states (Massimini et al., 2005, 2007) and during the performance of motor tasks (Nikulin et al., 2003; Kičić et al., 2008; Bonnard et al., 2009). Nikulin et al. (2003) have reported that the N100 peak that is induced by TMS over the motor cortex that is contralateral to the response hand is attenuated during a visually triggered motor response task. Kičić et al. (2008) have demonstrated that such N100 attenuation is observed during visually triggered motor response tasks with not only contralateral, but also ipsilateral, hand responses, although it is smaller in the ipsilateral hand response. These studies have commonly indicated that, during motor preparation and/or execution periods, MEP amplitudes increase, but the N100 amplitudes in TEPs to the motor cortex decrease. That is, the N100 of the TEPs to the motor cortex might be associated with cortical inhibitory processes (Nikulin et al., 2003; Bender et al., 2005; Kähkönen and Wilenius, 2007; Kičić et al., 2008). However, it is still unknown how the N100 in TEPs is modulated when inhibiting a planned motor response.

Human neuroimaging studies have reported that a scattering of cortical regions, comprised mesial, medial, and inferior frontal and parietal cortices, as well as motor cortex, were activated during tasks with motor inhibition (Garavan et al., 1999; Liddle et al., 2001; Rubia et al., 2001; Watanabe et al., 2002; Wager et al., 2005). However, the detailed time course of the motor inhibitory activities cannot be revealed by neuroimaging studies mainly due to the limitations of temporal resolution. Moreover, direct relationships between the motor cortex and motor inhibitory regions cannot be revealed by them. On the other hand, TMS-EEG study can be used for assessing cortical reactivity and corticocortical connectivity at the time when TMS is delivered.

Therefore, we conducted TMS-EEG recordings during a timing-coincident go/stop task (Coxon et al., 2006, 2007) and examined the differences in TEPs at the time of motor execution and inhibition. We especially focused on the N100 and the subsequent late positive component (LPC) in this study.

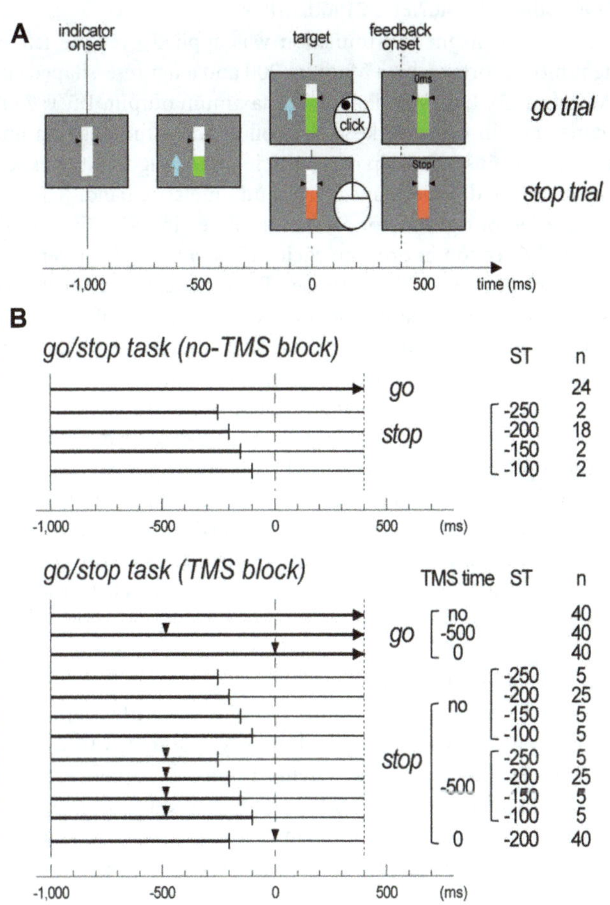

FIGURE 1 | Task designs of experiments. (A) Illustrations of the display for the go/stop task. The trial type is noted on the right side, and the time scale is displayed at the bottom. **(B)** Illustrations of trial structure for the go/stop task with and without transcranial magnetic stimulation (TMS). The time scale is displayed at the bottom. The vertical lines at −1,000 ms represent the indicator onset, the vertical dashed lines at 0 ms represent the target, and the vertical dotted lines represent the feedback onset. The small triangles represent the time points at which TMS was delivered (TMS time). The trial type is noted on the right side, with the TMS time, stop time (ST), and total number of trials. In the stop trials, the time points at which an indicator stopped are shown with vertical thin bars.

MATERIALS AND METHODS

PARTICIPANTS

Six right-handed healthy volunteers (six men, 27.9 ± 5.7 years) participated in contralateral-TMS session (over the left hemisphere). Another six right-handed healthy volunteers (one woman and five men, 26.9 ± 4.7 years) participated in the ipsilateral-TMS session (over the right hemisphere). All participants provided their informed consent, and the experimental procedures were approved by the local ethics committee of the Graduate School of Education at the University of Tokyo.

TASK SETTING

All participants conducted a timing-coincident go/stop task (**Figure 1A**). In the task, each trial began with presentation of a white bar against a gray background with two small black triangles indicating a target at the center of the display. After 600 ms, a green indicator moved upward from the bottom of the bar at a constant rate, reaching the target (black triangles) in 1,000 ms and the top of the bar in 1,400 ms. The time point at which the indicator began moving upward was referred to as the indicator onset. Participants were instructed to click the mouse in order to stop the moving green indicator at the target (referred to as go trials). In half of the trials, the moving green indicator unexpectedly stopped and turned red just before it reached the target. The participant was instructed to withhold their click when the moving green indicator stopped and turned red (referred to as stop trials). The time point at which the indicator stopped (stop time: ST) was set at −250, −200, −150, and −100 ms relative to the target. In each go and stop trial, after 1,400 ms of the indicator onset, visual feedback about a participant's performance [response time (RT) relative to target (ms) or "miss" for go trials; "stop!!" or "false alarm" with RT (ms) for stop trials] was presented for 500 ms on the central bar. This constant time setting was used to prevent participants' eye blinks before the visual feedback onset. The participant was informed that the indicator in some trials would be easy to stop, and that it would be more difficult or impossible to stop in other trials because it would be too close to the target.

TRANSCRANIAL MAGNETIC STIMULATION

Transcranial magnetic stimulation was applied over the left or right motor cortex with a Magstim 200 and a figure-8-shaped coil (Magstim Co. Ltd., Whitland, UK; maximum output, 1.5 T; 7 cm diameters). In order to keep the coil at the same position and direction against the scalp of a participant throughout the experiment, we used a mechanical arm and an elastic band. The coil over the left or right motor cortex was placed in the optimal position and direction in order to elicit MEPs in the right or left first dorsal interosseous (FDI) muscle. TMS intensity was expressed as a percentage of the motor threshold [MT; ±% of the maximal stimulator output: mean ± standard deviation (SD) for all participants], which was defined as the minimum intensity necessary to induce MEPs over 50 μV in the resting FDI muscle in at least three of five trials. TMS intensity in the experiment was set to the suprathreshold (120% of MT) in order to obtain MEPs of matched amplitudes (approximately 1.0 mV) in the resting FDI muscle. Coil position and MT were repeatedly checked and maintained throughout the experiment. All participants wore earplugs during the entire experiment to reduce the auditory click produced by the TMS coil.

EEG AND EMG RECORDINGS

During the performance of the go/stop task, EEG, and electromyograms (EMG) were continuously acquired with a TMS-compatible EEG recording system (BrainAmp, Brain Products GmbH, Munich, Germany). EEG was recorded from 61 Ag/AgCl surface electrodes that were mounted on an elastic cap and that corresponded to the modified International 10–20 System of electrode placement, and four additional electrodes were attached to the forehead, left, and right ears, and the site beneath the left eye. In order to reduce the TMS-induced artifacts, we used the electrode lead wire rearrangement technique (Sekiguchi et al., 2011). The data were recorded against a reference electrode that was placed on the forehead and later re-referenced offline to the averaged value of the earlobes. The data from the site beneath the left eye was used for monitoring eye blink and eye movement. EMG was recorded from the right or left FDI muscle with Ag/AgCl surface electrodes. Electrode impedance was maintained below 10 kΩ. EEG and EMG signals were amplified and filtered (bandpass settings: 0.5–100 Hz for EEG signals and 50–300 Hz for EMG signals) and continuously stored with a trigger signal from the computer that indicated task onset and TMS trigger at a sampling rate of 1,000 Hz for the offline analysis. In the offline analysis, we resampled all data at a rate of 500 Hz.

EXPERIMENTAL PROCEDURES

Participants were comfortably seated on a chair in an electrically shielded room facing a 12.1-in. computer display (screen resolution, 1,280 × 800 pixels; refresh rate, 60 Hz), and she/he placed her/his right index finger on the main (left) button of a computer mouse. Then, she/he was lectured about the go/stop task, and she/he practiced it. After completing the experimental settings for the EEG and EMG recordings and TMS, participants first conducted 1 block of the go/stop task without TMS. This no-TMS block was conducted in order to assess task performance and record electrophysiological signals during the go/stop task without TMS. There were 48 trials in total, 24 go and 24 stop. The intertrial intervals were 4.5 s. For the stop trials, the indicator stopped randomly at an ST of −250, −200, −150, and −100 ms with 2, 2, 18, and 2 trials for each ST. Next, the participants conducted five blocks of the go/stop task with TMS. There were 240 trials in total, 120 go, and 120 stop. The intertrial intervals were 7.5 s, and the interblock intervals were about 3 min. In both the go and stop trials, TMS was randomly delivered at a TMS time of −500 and 0 ms relative to the target, with a total of 80 trials, 40 go and 40 stop, for each TMS time. That is, TMS was not delivered in 40 go and 40 stop trials in these five TMS blocks. We adopted a TMS time of −500 ms as a motor preparatory period for participants' brain processes not to separate into go and stop, while a TMS time of 0 ms was adopted as the period for motor execution or inhibition. For the stop trials, the indicator stopped consistently at an ST of −200 ms in the stop trials with TMS at a TMS time of 0 ms or randomly at an ST of −250, −200, −150, and −100 ms, with 5, 5, 25, and 5 trials for each ST, in the stop trials with TMS at a TMS time of −500 ms or without TMS. Although the ratio of each ST that appeared in the stop trials in five TMS blocks was different at each TMS time, it was totally equal to those in a no-TMS block (8.3, 8.3, 75, and 8.3% for each ST). This biased setting in ST and TMS time was used to increase the number of stop trials with TMS at a TMS time of 0 m and at an ST of −200 ms for the EEG averaging procedure. None of the participants noticed this biased ST setting during the experiments. The numbers of trials in each ST and TMS time condition are shown in **Figure 1B**.

PERFORMANCE DATA

Because the task performance in the trials with TMS was changed by the effects of TMS (an appearance of MEP and a silent period), we used only trials of the go/stop task without TMS for task performance assessments. In order to exclude premature responses and misses in the go trials, outlying RTs were discarded with the following criteria: <−100 and >150 ms in the go trials (0.7% for six subjects in the contralateral-TMS experiment and 0.5% for six subjects in the ipsilateral-TMS experiment). The means and SDs of the RTs were then calculated for each participant and trial condition. For the stop trials, the percentage of correct responses (% correct) was calculated for each participant and ST. Next, the ST for which the probability of successful stopping was 50% (50% ST) was determined with the least-square fitting curve to the sigmoid function. The 50% ST was subtracted from the mean go RT in order to determine the stop-signal reaction time (SSRT), which is the estimated time required for unobservable stop processes based on a *race model* (Logan and Cowan, 1984; Logan et al., 1984; Verbruggen and Logan, 2008).

MEP DATA

For each trial with TMS, the peak-to-peak MEP amplitudes were measured from the EMG data. Stop trials with false alarm responses were excluded from the MEP analysis. The mean MEP amplitudes were calculated for each participant, trial condition (go or stop), and TMS time (−500 or 0 ms). Finally, the group mean MEP amplitudes were calculated for each trial condition and TMS time.

EEG DATA PROCESSING

The data from the 61-channel scalp EEG (and 1-channel eye-related potential) in all conditions were first segmented in epochs from 1,500 ms before and 1,000 ms after the target time, and all of the segmented data was bunched together for each subject. Next, an independent component (IC) analysis with extended infomax algorithm (Bell and Sejnowski, 1995; Lee et al., 1999) was applied to the EEG data in order to identify and remove the components reflecting TMS-related artifacts and eye-blink- and/or eye-movement-related activities (Jung et al., 2000a,b; Johnson et al., 2012). From the 62 extracted independent components (ICs), the TMS-related ICs were chosen mainly by their time courses; the variance value of the IC during a time period of 20 ms just after the TMS was 20 times larger than those during the rest of the time periods and during no-TMS trials. The results suggested that such ICs impulsively induced huge potentials only when the TMS pulse was delivered. Eye-blink- and eye-movement-related activities were also determined by the time courses, which indicated their inactivation during a task, and scalp topographies of the projection maps, which provided their origin on the edge of anterior sites. Based on these criteria, we could effectively remove TMS-related [11.4 ± 2.7 (mean $\pm$ SD for all participants)], eye-blink-related (1 ± 0), and eye-movement-related (0.8 ± 0.4) components and obtain EEG waveforms with little distortion, at least during the time period with two large long-latency TEP components (see **Figure A1** in Appendix).

The artifact-removed EEG data was low-pass filtered below 40 Hz. Next, after the baseline correction (during the 500 ms before indicator onset), they were separately averaged for 2 trial (go/stop) $\times$ 3 TMS time (no-TMS/TMS at -500 ms/TMS at 0 ms) $\times$ 2 TMS side (contralateral/ipsilateral) conditions for each participant. For no-TMS stop trials, EEG data were averaged only in stop trials with an ST of -200 ms because the number of trials with STs of -250, -150, and -100 ms was so small for the averaging procedure. However, for stop trials with a TMS at -500 ms, the EEG data were collectively averaged in all stop trials with STs of -250, -200, -150, and -100 ms because the averaged EEGs around the TMS time (-500 ms) were little affected by the differences in the STs. Finally, in order to extract the TEP during the performance of the go/stop task, the averaged EEG waveforms in no-TMS go or stop trials were subtracted from those in go or stop trials with TMS at -500 or 0 ms (Nikulin et al., 2003; Kičić et al., 2008). For the figure representations, we obtained 61-channel grand-mean-averaged EEGs in no-TMS trials for 2 trial $\times$ 2 TMS side conditions and 61-channel grand-mean TEPs for 2 trial $\times$ 2 TMS time $\times$ 2 TMS side conditions.

The amplitudes and latencies of the two long-latency components (N100 and LPC) were determined as follows. First, we determined the regions of interest (ROIs) for N100 and LPC from the TEP waveforms and scalp topographies (see **Figures 5** and **6**). Since the distributions of the N100 were lateralized to the stimulated hemisphere, the ROIs of the N100 were defined as nine electrodes around FC1 (F3, F1, Fz, FC3, FC1, FCz, C3, C1, and Cz) in the contralateral TMS condition and nine electrodes around FC2 (Fz, F2, F4, FCz, FC2, FC4, Cz, C2, and C4) in the ipsilateral TMS condition. On the other hand, the ROI of the LPC was defined as nine electrodes around Cz (FC1, FCz, FC2, C1, Cz, C2, CP1, CPz, and CP2) in both TMS side conditions. In the averaged waveforms in the ROI of the N100, the amplitudes and latencies were measured at the largest negative peak during 80–120 ms after TMS. In the averaged waveforms in the ROI of the LPC, amplitudes, and latencies were also measured at the largest positive peak during 120–300 ms after TMS.

STATISTICAL ANALYSIS

The main purpose of this study was to examine the effects of 2 trial (go or stop) $\times$ 2 TMS time (-500 or 0 ms) $\times$ 2 TMS side (contralateral or ipsilateral) conditions on the TEPs and MEPs during the performance of a go/stop task. In addition, we needed to confirm the effects of TMS sides on task performance (mean go RT, 50% ST, and SSRT in no-TMS trials). Task performances were compared by two-sample t-tests between the contralateral and ipsilateral TMS conditions. Mean MEP amplitudes and the N100 and LPC amplitudes and latencies for the $2 \times 2 \times 2$ conditions were submitted to three-way mixed factorial ANOVAs with within-participant factors of trial and TMS time and the between-participants factor of TMS side. If necessary, *post hoc* multiple comparisons were conducted by using paired t-tests with Bonferroni correction. The level of significance that was used for all of the tests was $p < 0.05$.

RESULTS

TASK PERFORMANCE

In both the contralateral and ipsilateral TMS conditions, all participants could click close to but a little behind the target in the no-TMS go trials, and the longer the time until the target, the more successfully they could stop their clicking in the no-TMS stop trials (**Figure 2A**). For the mean go RTs (contralateral, 16.0 ± 5.1 ms; ipsilateral, 16.7 ± 11.0 ms), 50% STs (contralateral, -157.1 ± 16.0 ms; ipsilateral, -167.9 ± 11.7 ms), and SSRTs (contralateral, 173.0 ± 14.2 ms; ipsilateral, 184.6 ± 13.6 ms) in the no-TMS trials, no significant differences were observed between the contralateral and ipsilateral TMS conditions (**Figure 2B**). These results indicated that task performances in the go/stop task were not very different between the participants in the contralateral and ipsilateral TMS conditions.

MEP AMPLITUDE

Mean MEP amplitudes increased only in the go trials with the contralateral TMS at 0 ms, and there were not much differences in the mean MEP amplitudes in the other seven conditions (**Figure 3**). The mixed factorial ANOVA of the mean MEP amplitudes revealed significant within-participant effects of trial [$F(1, 10) = 17.7$, $p < 0.01$] and TMS time [$F(1, 10) = 11.4$, $p < 0.01$] and their significant interaction [$F(1, 10) = 17.4$, $p < 0.01$]. There were no significant between-participants effects of TMS side, while there were significant TMS side $\times$ TMS time [$F(1, 10) = 10.4$, $p < 0.01$], TMS side $\times$ trial [$F(1, 10) = 12.4$, $p < 0.01$], and TMS side $\times$ TMS time $\times$ trial [$F(1, 10) = 12.8$, $p < 0.01$] interactions. Therefore, *post hoc* multiple comparisons were conducted for all six pairs among 2 TMS time $\times$ 2 trial conditions separately for each TMS side. There were significant differences of mean MEP amplitudes in three pairs between go trial with TMS at 0 ms and the other

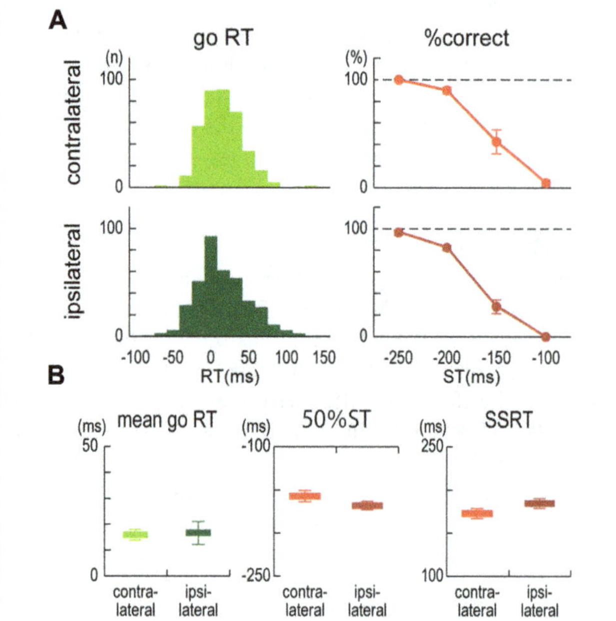

FIGURE 2 | Task performance. (A) Distributions of response time (RT) in go trials without TMS and the percentage of correct responses (% correct) in stop trials without TMS for each stop time (ST) that was obtained from six participants in contralateral (upper) and ipsilateral (lower) TMS conditions. RT denotes a clicking time relative to the target. **(B)** Group results of mean go RT (left), estimated 50% STs in stop trials (center), and stop-signal reaction times (SSRTs) in stop trials (right). The 50% ST is an estimated stop time in which the probability of successful stopping was 50%. SSRT is the estimated time required for an unobservable stop process. Error bars show standard error (SE).

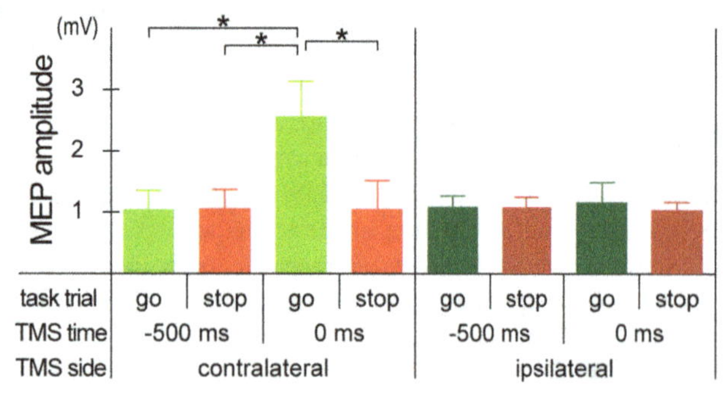

FIGURE 3 | Motor-evoked potential (MEP) amplitude. Group means (±SE) of MEP amplitudes during the go/stop task with contralateral (upper) and ipsilateral (lower) TMS at −500 and 0 ms. Error bars show standard error (SE). *$p < 0.05$; significant difference in *post hoc* multiple comparisons with Bonferroni corrected paired *t*-tests.

three conditions for the contralateral TMS condition, while there was no significant difference of mean MEP amplitudes in all six pairs for the ipsilateral TMS condition. These results indicated that MEP enlarged only in go trials with the contralateral TMS at 0 ms.

AVERAGED EEGS IN NO-TMS TRIALS

In the grand-mean-averaged EEG waveforms in no-TMS trials (**Figure 4**), gradual negative deflections over the fronto-central sites were observed as the target time approached in both go and stop trials. After the stop signal onset of −200 ms, the grand-mean-averaged EEG waveforms clearly differentiated between go and stop trials. Distinct negative–positive peaks over the frontocentral sites appeared around and after the target time in stop trials, while a mild positive peak over the centroparietal sites appeared after the target time in go trials. These waveforms in the no-TMS trials have been typically shown in the go and stop trials of the go/stop (or stop-signal) task (De Jong et al., 1990; Schmajuk et al., 2006).

TMS-EVOKED POTENTIALS

In the grand-mean TEPs of all 2 × 2 × 2 conditions (**Figure 5**), a prominent negative peak around the TMS sites was observed about 100 ms after the TMS onset (N100) after the short-latency, high-frequency oscillations. Then, a less pronounced positive deflection over the broad areas that was centered at the midline-central site appeared about 180–300 ms after TMS onset (LPC). Distinct large long-latency negative–positive deflections in TEPs have been typically shown in previous TMS-EEG studies (Paus et al., 2001; Nikulin et al., 2003; Komssi et al., 2004; Bonato et al., 2006; Kičić et al., 2008; Bonnard et al., 2009; Lioumis et al., 2009; Ferreri et al., 2011, 2012; Rogasch et al., 2013).

Regardless of the TMS sides, N100 amplitudes in go trials with TMS at 0 ms (contralateral, −14.0 ± 8.9 μV; ipsilateral, −11.5 ± 6.1 μV) were smaller than those in go trials with TMS at −500 ms (contralateral, −20.6 ± 12.4 μV; ipsilateral, −16.6 ± 9.7 μV), while there was not much difference in N100 amplitudes in stop trials with TMS at −500 ms (contralateral, −19.3 ± 10.8 μV; ipsilateral, −17.2 ± 9.1 μV) and 0 ms (contralateral, −19.6 ± 11.8 μV; ipsilateral, −16.4 ± 11.7 μV; **Figures 5** and **6**, upper). The mixed factorial ANOVA of N100 amplitudes revealed significant effects of trial [$F(1, 10) = 12.9$, $p < 0.01$] and TMS time [$F(1, 10) = 18.4$, $p < 0.01$] and a significant interaction of them [$F(1, 10) = 6.2$, $p < 0.05$]. However, it showed no significant effects of TMS side and second- and third-interactions, including TMS side. Therefore, *post hoc* multiple comparisons were conducted for all six pairs among 2 TMS time × 2 trial conditions without respect to the TMS side. There were significant differences in the N100 amplitudes in three pairs between go trial with TMS at 0 ms and the other three conditions. In contrast to the N100 amplitudes, there were not much differences in the N100 latencies among the 2 × 2 × 2 conditions (**Figure 6**, upper). The mixed factorial ANOVA of N100 latencies revealed neither significant main effects nor significant interactions. These results indicated that, regardless of the contralateral or ipsilateral TMS, N100 appeared at almost the same latencies, but it was attenuated only in go trials with TMS at 0 ms.

Regardless of the TMS sides, LPC amplitudes in go trials with TMS at 0 ms (contralateral, 8.4 ± 3.8 μV; ipsilateral, 14.0 ± 5.9 μV) were smaller than those in go trials with TMS at −500 ms (contralateral, 18.9 ± 7.1 μV; ipsilateral, 22.2 ± 8.5 μV), and LPC amplitudes in stop trials with TMS at 0 ms (contralateral, 11.9 ± 5.2 μV; ipsilateral, 12.9 ± 5.9 μV) were smaller than those in stop trials with TMS at −500 ms (contralateral, 19.5 ± 6.3 μV; ipsilateral, 22.9 ± 9.8 μV; **Figures 5** and **6**, lower). In addition, LPC latencies in the go and stop trials with TMS at 0 ms were larger than those in go and stop trials with TMS at −500 ms

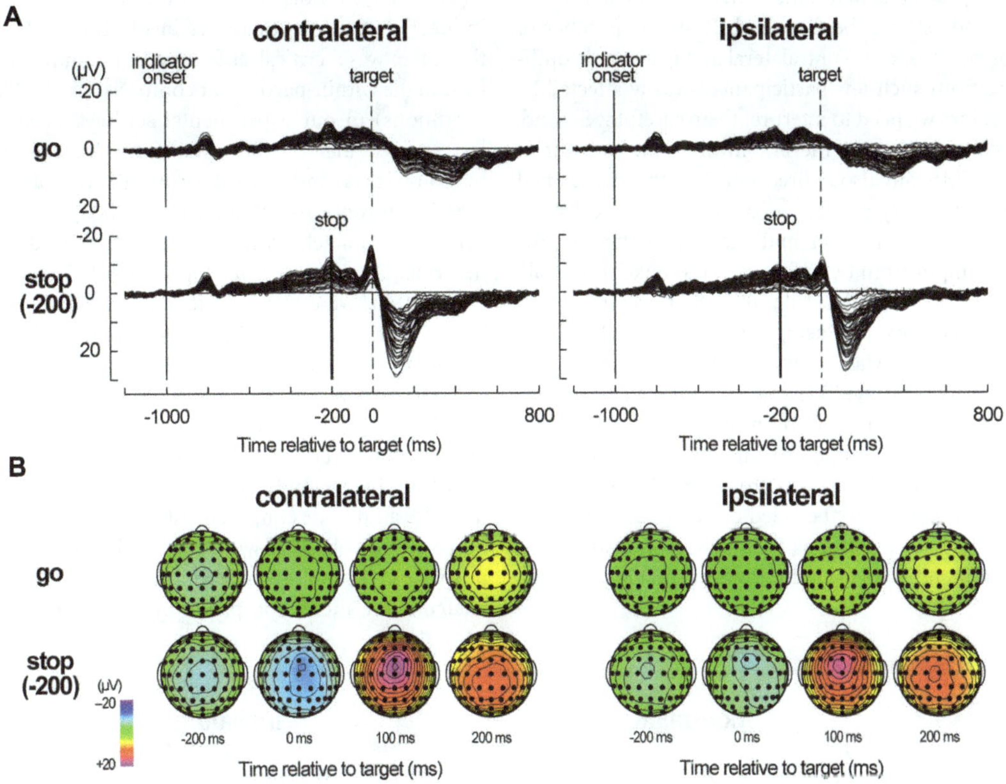

FIGURE 4 | Averaged electroencephalography (EEG) data in no-TMS trials. (A) Averaged EEG waveforms in no-TMS trials during a go/stop task for six participants in a contralateral-TMS session (left two panels) and for six participants in an ipsilateral-TMS session (right two panels). For stop trials, only the waveforms in stop trials with a stop time of −200 ms [stop(−200) trials] are displayed. The waveforms of all 61 sites are shown as thin black lines. The vertical thin lines represent indicator onset, the vertical dashed lines represent target time for the go task, and the vertical thick lines represent stop-signal onset. Time scales relative to target are displayed at the bottom. **(B)** Scalp topographies of averaged EEGs in the go and stop(−200) trials for six participants in a contralateral-TMS session (left 2 × 4 arrays) and for six participants in an ipsilateral-TMS session (right 2 × 4 arrays). The topographies are displayed only at −200, 0, 100, and 200 ms relative to target.

(**Figure 6**, lower). The mixed factorial ANOVA of LPC amplitudes revealed significant effects of TMS time [$F(1, 10) = 49.9, p < 0.01$] but no significant effects of trial and no significant interaction of trial × TMS time. Moreover, it also showed no significant effects of TMS side and second- and third-interactions including TMS side. Therefore, *post hoc* multiple comparisons were conducted for all six pairs among 2 TMS time × 2 trial conditions without respect to the TMS side. There were significant differences in the LPC amplitudes in four pairs between both go and stop trial with TMS at −500 ms and both go and stop trial with TMS at 0 ms. The mixed factorial ANOVA of LPC latencies revealed significant effects of TMS time [$F(1, 10) = 15.9$, $p < 0.01$] but no significant effects of trial and no significant interaction of trial × TMS time. Moreover, it also showed no significant effects of TMS side and second- and third-interactions including TMS side. Therefore, *post hoc* multiple comparisons were conducted for all six pairs among 2 TMS time × 2 trial conditions without respect to the TMS side. There were significant differences in the LPC latencies in two pairs between go and stop trial with TMS at −500 ms and stop trial with TMS at 0 ms. These results indicated that, regardless of contralateral or ipsilateral TMS, LPC was reduced and delayed in both go and stop trials with TMS at 0 ms.

DISCUSSION

In this study, we compared two distinct long-latency components of TEPs (N100 and LPC) at the preparatory, executive, and inhibitory periods during a go/stop task. Consequently, the N100 and LPC of the TEPs were obviously modulated depending on the TMS time and trial conditions. First, the task performance in no-TMS trials were typically shown in the go and stop trials of the go/stop (or stop-signal) task (Logan and Cowan, 1984; Logan et al., 1984; Coxon et al., 2006, 2007; Verbruggen and Logan, 2008). Next, the TEPs were obtained from the subtracted waveforms: the averaged EEG responses in go or stop trials without TMS were subtracted from those in go or stop trials with TMS, respectively. That is, the effects of overlapped event-related potentials during a go/stop task have been excluded from the TEP waveforms, indicating different spatiotemporal patterns of cortical responses to the TMS in a go or stop trial 500 ms before or just at the target time. Therefore, TEP modulations in the task conditions that were demonstrated in this study were considered to be representative of TMS-induced neuronal reactions in the motor cortex and subsequent their propagation to surrounding cortical areas during motor preparation, execution, and inhibition.

Before reaching such a conclusion, some methodological limitations of this study should be discussed. First, the number of participants was small (six for contralateral and ipsilateral condition each). Data from such few participants is easily affected by outliers and therefore we need to interpret them carefully. Second, the long-latency components of the TEP involved not only direct cortical effects of TMS, but also indirect effects that accompanied the TMS, such as auditory and bone-conduction sound by the coil click, somatosensory sensation on the scalp, and afferent proprioceptive/tactile input from twitching muscles (Nikouline et al., 1999; Tiitinen et al., 1999; Nikulin et al., 2003). Some recent studies have used a masking noise for reducing auditory coil-click perception (Tiitinen et al., 1999; Massimini et al., 2005, 2007; Bonnard et al., 2009; Ferreri et al., 2011, 2012; Rogasch et al., 2013). In contrast, we did not take any special precautions for these indirect effects except for the use of earplugs because such techniques will not eliminate all indirect TMS effects from the TEP waveforms completely. Therefore, it cannot be ruled out that the TEP modulations among the task conditions that were demonstrated in this study were influenced by the indirect effects that accompanied TMS.

However, considering the within-participant equivalence of the indirect TMS effects that were involved in TEPs, it was unlikely that there was a critical difference in the indirect TMS effects, at least in the within-participant comparisons (2 TMS time × 2 trial conditions) in our experimental settings. Next, previous studies reported that the EEG waveforms that were induced only by coil-click sounds (auditory N1-P2 complex) differed from the TEP waveforms (Nikulin et al., 2003). In this study, apart from approximately symmetric auditory evoked potentials (Mäkinen et al., 2005; Fuentemilla et al., 2006), TEP (especially N100) distributions were asymmetric and lateralized to the stimulated hemisphere (see **Figure 5**), suggesting that non-auditory effect might involve the TEPs. Finally, Paus et al. (2001) and Nikulin et al. (2003) have demonstrated that N100 amplitudes did not correlate with MEP amplitudes in target hand muscles, suggesting that the N100 might not be a predominant reflection of peripheral afferent sensation. In this study, N100 attenuation was accompanied with the MEP amplitude enhancement in the contralateral TMS condition but it was observed without the MEP amplitude enhancement in the ipsilateral TMS conditions. If the N100 attenuation was related to the afferent proprioceptive/tactile input from twitching

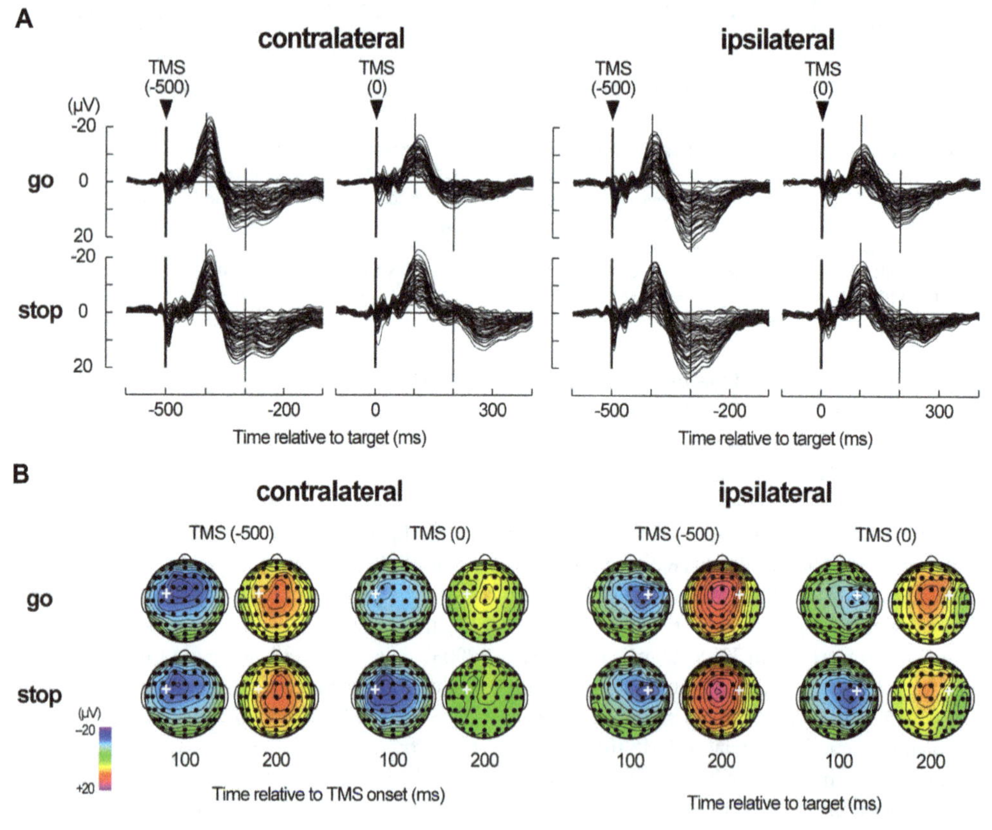

FIGURE 5 | TMS-evoked potentials. (A) TMS-evoked potentials (TEPs) during go/stop task with TMS at −500 and 0 ms for six participants in a contralateral-TMS session (left 2 × 2 panels) and with TMS at −500 and 0 ms for six participants in an ipsilateral-TMS session (right 2 × 2 panels). The vertical thick lines represent TMS onset, and the vertical thin lines represent 100 and 200 ms after the TMS onset. Time scales relative to target are displayed at the bottom. **(B)** The scalp topographies of TEPs in the go and stop trials for six participants in a contralateral-TMS session (two left 2 × 4 arrays) and for six participants in an ipsilateral-TMS session (two right 2 × 4 arrays). The bold white plus in each topography represents the TMS sites. The topographies are displayed only at 100 and 200 ms relative to TMS onset, corresponding approximately to N100 and later positive component (LPC), respectively.

muscles, it was developed differently in contralateral and ipsilateral TMS conditions. Therefore, it is unlikely that the N100 is a primary reflection of the reafferent proprioceptive/tactile input. When we take all things together, the N100 and LPC modulations among the task conditions seemed to be potential changes that originated from, at least in part, TMS-induced neuronal reactions in the motor cortex and subsequent their propagation to surrounding cortical areas.

The two long-latency TEP components (N100 and LPC) that we focused on corresponded to the last two dominant peaks in typical 300 ms-long waveforms that are induced by TMS to the motor cortex (Bonato et al., 2006; Komssi and Kähkönen, 2006; Lioumis et al., 2009; Ilmoniemi and Kičić, 2010; Ferreri et al., 2011, 2012). N100 has been demonstrated to be very sensitive to small changes in cortical excitability and therefore to be associated with cortical inhibitory process (Nikulin et al., 2003; Bender et al., 2005; Kähkönen and Wilenius, 2007; Kičić et al., 2008). Moreover, recent studies investigating the detailed characteristics of long-interval cortical inhibition induced in the MEPs and TEPs by paired-pulse TMS-EEG paradigms (Fitzgerald et al., 2009; Rogasch et al., 2013) have suggested that the N100 that is evoked by the conditioning TMS is consistent with the underlying mechanism that results in long-interval cortical inhibition of MEPs, which most likely involve $GABA_B$-mediated inhibition of cortical activity. However, Ferreri et al. (2011) have recently proposed that the long latency and wide distribution of LPC (P190) suggest the engagement of a reverberant corticosubcortical circuit.

The main finding of this study was the different N100 and LPC modulations between go and stop trials. Although there were not much differences between go and stop trials in the TEP waveforms that were induced by both contralateral and ipsilateral TMS at −500 ms, there were distinct differences between go and stop trials in those at 0 ms. These results indicated that the TEP waveforms were modulated by the underlying cortical and/or subcortical activities that were required for performing the go/stop task. N100 distribution was lateralized to the TMS site, and N100 amplitude was decreased only in go trials with both contralateral and ipsilateral TMS at 0 ms, which was in agreement with the results of previous studies (Nikulin et al., 2003; Kičić et al., 2008). This decrease of the N100 amplitudes on both sides during go trials might reflect decreased activity in the cortical inhibitory circuit for initiating and executing a planned motor response. Unlike in the case of the contralateral N100, the decrease in the ipsilateral N100 amplitude was not accompanied with an increase in MEP. This inconsistency in TEP and MEP modulations between contralateral and ipsilateral TMS might be due to a methodological difference: TEP is a method that is used for assessing cortical states directly from cortical responses against TMS while the MEP is a method that is used for assessing cortical states indirectly through muscle twitch, including spinal and peripheral effects. However, regardless of the TMS side, the N100 amplitudes in stop trials with TMS at 0 ms were similar in size to those in go and stop trials with TMS at 0 ms. These large N100s in preparatory (at −500 ms in go and stop trials) and inhibitory (at 0 ms in stop trials) periods might reflect enhanced activity in the cortical inhibitory circuit for waiting and inhibiting a planned motor response. As for LPC with TMS at 0 ms, amplitude was decreased and latency was delayed in both go and stop trials. Although LPC has been discussed less frequently than N100 in previous studies (Ferreri et al., 2011), these LPC modulations might also be associated with the state of reverberant corticosubcortical circuits during the performance of a go/stop task.

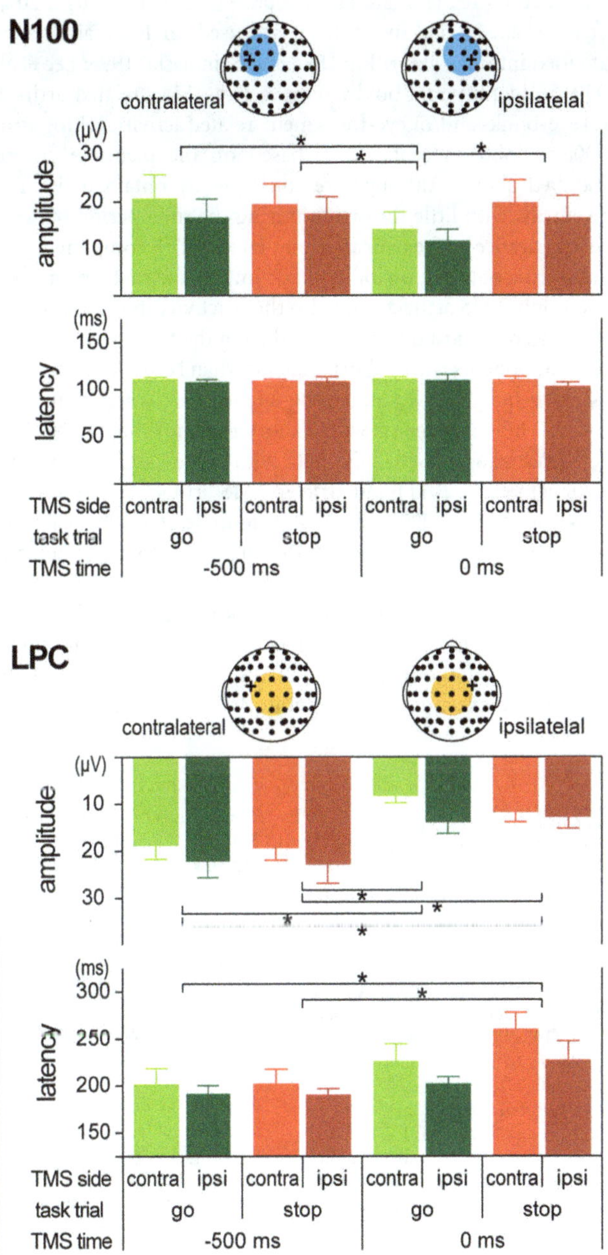

FIGURE 6 | Amplitudes and latencies of long-latency components in TMS-evoked potential (TEP). Group means (±SE) of N100 (upper) and LPC (lower) amplitudes and latencies during go/stop tasks with contralateral and ipsilateral TMS at −500 and 0 ms. Light blue and orange circles in the scalp electrode drawings represent regions of interest (ROIs). Error bars show standard error (SE). $*p < 0.05$, significant difference in *post hoc* multiple comparisons with Bonferroni corrected paired t-tests.

Recent studies on the short-latency component of TEPs have suggested that they can be used to evaluate reactivity in the stimulated cortex (Bonato et al., 2006; Veniero et al., 2010, 2013; Ferreri et al., 2011). In contrast, we used an IC analysis with extended infomax algorithm (Bell and Sejnowski, 1995; Lee et al., 1999) to identify and boldly remove large TMS-related artifacts and eye-blink- and/or eye-movement-related activities (Jung et al., 2000a,b; Johnson et al., 2012) based on the plausible criteria described above. Although we consequently obtained the TEP waveforms with little distortion during the time period between the appearance of the two large long-latency TEP components, we cannot rule out the possibility that components that were related to not only TMS artifacts, but also the reactivity in the stimulated cortex, were removed particularly during the time period for the TEP components with a shorter latency than N100. Therefore, we discussed only the two large long-latency TEP components and not the TEP components with a shorter latency than N100. Further investigations with EEG data with more careful recordings (Sekiguchi et al., 2011) and stricter TMS artifact-rejection criteria (Veniero et al., 2009) will allow us to understand short-latency cortical reactivity in the motor cortex during motor execution and inhibition.

In summary, we conducted combined TMS-EEG recordings during a go/stop task and compared the two dominant long-latency components of the TEPs (N100 and LPC) at the preparatory, executive, and inhibitory periods during go/stop tasks. Consequently, N100 and LPC were differently modulated in go and stop trials that were conducted with contralateral and ipsilateral TMS just at the target time. The N100 amplitude was decreased only in go trials while the LPC amplitude was decreased and the LPC latency was delayed in both go and stop trials. These results suggested that TMS-induced neuronal reactions in the motor cortex and subsequent their propagation to surrounding cortical areas might change functionally according to task demand in go and stop trials, that is, motor preparation, execution, and inhibition.

ACKNOWLEDGMENTS

This work was supported by Grant-in-Aid for Scientific Research (C; #22500529) from JSPS and Showa Women's University to Kentaro Yamanaka, Grants-in-Aid for Young Scientists (B; #22700590) from JSPS to Hiroshi Kadota, and Grant-in-Aid for Young Scientists (S; #20670008) from JSPS and the Funding Program for Next Generation World-Leading Researchers (#LS034) from JSPS to Daichi Nozaki.

REFERENCES

Badry, R., Mima, T., Aso, T., Nakatsuka, M., Abe, M., Fathi, D., et al. (2009). Suppression of human cortico-motoneuronal excitability during the stop-signal task. Clin. Neurophysiol. 120, 1717–1723. doi: 10.1016/j.clinph.2009.06.027

Barker, A. T., Jalinous, R., and Freeston, I. L. (1985). Non-invasive magnetic stimulation of human motor cortex. Lancet 325, 1106–1107. doi: 10.1016/S0140- 6736(85)92413-4

Bell, A. J., and Sejnowski, T. J. (1995). An information-maximization approach to blind separation and blind deconvolution. Neural Comput. 7, 1129–1159. doi: 10.1162/neco.1995.7.6.1129

Bender, S., Basseler, K., Sebastian, I., Resch, F., Kammer, T., Oelkers-Ax, R., et al. (2005). Transcranial magnetic stimulation evokes giant inhibitory potentials in children. Ann. Neurol. 58, 58–67. doi: 10.1002/ana.20521

Bonato, C., Miniussi, C., and Rossini, P. M. (2006). Transcranial magnetic stimulation and cortical evoked potentials: a TMS/EEG co-registration study. Clin. Neurophysiol. 117, 1699–1707. doi: 10.1016/j.clinph.2006.05.006

Bonnard, M., Spieser, L., Meziane, H. B., de Graaf, J. B., and Pailhous, J. (2009). Prior intention can locally tune inhibitory processes in the primary motor cortex: direct evidence from combined TMS-EEG. Eur. J. Neurosci. 30, 913–923. doi: 10.1111/j.1460-9568.2009.06864.x

Chen, R., Yaseen, Z., Cohen, L. G., and Hallett, M. (1998). Time course of corti- cospinal excitability in reaction time and self-paced movements. Ann. Neurol. 44, 317–325. doi: 10.1002/ana.410440306

Coxon, J. P., Stinear, C. M., and Byblow, W. D. (2006). Intracortical inhibition during volitional inhibition of prepared action. J. Neurophysiol. 95, 3371–3383. doi: 10.1152/jn.01334.2005

Coxon, J. P., Stinear, C. M., and Byblow, W. D. (2007). Selective inhibition of movement. J. Neurophysiol. 97, 2480–2489. doi: 10.1152/jn.01284.2006

De Jong, R., Coles, M. G., Logan, G. D., and Gratton, G. (1990). In search of the point of no return: the control of response processes. J. Exp. Psychol. Hum. Percept. Perform. 16, 164-182. doi: 10.1037/0096-1523.16.1.164

Ferreri, F., Pasqualetti, P., Määttä, S., Ponzo, D., Ferrarelli, F., Tononi, G., et al. (2011). Human brain connectivity during single and paired pulse transcranial magnetic stimulation. Neuroimage 54, 90–102. doi: 10.1016/j.neuroimage.2010.07.056

Ferreri, F., Ponzo, D., Hukkanen, T., Mervaala, E., Könönen, M., Pasqualetti, P., et al. (2012). Human brain cortical correlates of short-latency afferent inhibition: a combined EEG-TMS study. J. Neurophysiol. 108, 314–323. doi: 10.1152/jn.00796.2011

Fitzgerald, P. B., Maller, J. J., Hoy, K., Farzan, F., and Daskalakis, Z. J. (2009). GABA and cortical inhibition in motor and non-motor regions using com- bined TMS-EEG: a time analysis. Clin. Neurophysiol. 120, 1706–1710. doi: 10.1016/j.clinph.2009.06.019

Fuentemilla, L., Marco-Pallarés, J., and Grau, C. (2006). Modulation of spectral power and of phase resetting of EEG contributes differentlly to the gen- eration of auditory event-related potentials. Neuroimage 30, 909–916. doi: 10.1016/j.neuroimage.2005.10.036

Garavan, H., Ross, T. J., and Stein, E. A. (1999). Right hemispheric dominance of inhibitory control: an event related functional MRI study. Proc. Natl. Acad. Sci. U.S.A. 96, 8301–8306. doi: 10.1073/pnas.96.14.8301

Hallett, M. (2000). Transcranial magnetic stimulation and the human brain. Nature 406, 147–150. doi: 10.1038/35018000

Hallett, M. (2007). Transcranial magnetic stimulation: a primer. Neuron 55, 187– 199. doi: 10.1016/j.neuron.2007.06.026

Hoshiyama, M., Kakigi, R., Koyama, S., Takeshima, Y., Watanabe, S., and Shi- mojo, M. (1997). Temporal changes of pyramidal tract activities after decision of movement: a study using transcranial magnetic stimulation of the motor cortex in humans. Electroencephalogr. Clin. Neurophysiol. 105, 255–261. doi: 10.1016/S0924-980X(97)00019-2

Hoshiyama, M., Koyama, S., Kitamura, Y., Shimojo, M., Watanabe, S., and Kakigi, R. (1996). Effects of judgement process on \in go/no-go hand movement task. Neurosci. Res. 24, 427–430. doi: 10.1016/0168-0102(95)01013-0

Ilmoniemi, R. J., and Kicˇic´, D. (2010). Methodology for combined TMS and EEG.

Brain Topogr. 22, 233–248. doi: 10.1007/s10548-009-0123-4

Ilmoniemi, R. J., Virtanen, J., Ruohonen, J., Karhu, J., Aronen, H. J., Näätänen, R., et al. (1997). Neuronal responses to magnetic stimulation reveal cortical reactivity and connectivity. Neuroreport 8, 3537–3540. doi: 10.1097/00001756-199711100-00024

Johnson, J. S., Kundu, B., Casali, A. G., and Postle, B. R. (2012). Task-dependent changes in cortical excitability and effective connectivity: a combined TMS-EEG study. J. Neurophysiol. 107, 2383–2392. doi: 10.1152/jn.00707.2011

Jung, T.-P., Makeig, S., Humphries, C., Lee, T.-W., McKeown, M. J.,

Iragui, V., et al. (2000a). Removing electroencephalographic artifacts by blind source separation. Psychophysiology 37, 163–178. doi: 10.1111/1469-8986.3720163

Jung, T.-P., Makeig, S., Westerfield, M., Townsend, J., Courchesne, E., and Sejnowski, T. J. (2000b). Removal of eye activity artifacts from visual event-related poten- tials in normal and clinical subjects. Clin. Neurophysiol. 111, 1745–1758. doi: 10.1016/S1388-2457(00)00386-2

Kähkönen, S., and Wilenius, J. (2007). Effects of alcohol on TMS-evoked N100 responses. J. Neurosci. Methods 166, 104–108. doi: 10.1016/j.jneumeth. 2007.06.030

Kicˇic´, D., Lioumis, P., Ilmoniemi, R. J., and Nikulin, V. V. (2008). Bilateral changes in excitability of sensorimotor cortices during unilateral movement: combined elec- troencephalographic and transcranial magnetic stimulation study. Neuroscience 152, 1119–1129. doi: 10.1016/j. neuroscience.2008.01.043

Komssi, S., and Kähkönen, S. (2006). The novelty value of the combined use of electroencephalography and transcranial magnetic stimulation for neuroscience research. Brain Res. Rev. 52, 183–192. doi: 10.1016/j.brainresrev.2006.01.008

Komssi, S., Kähkönen, S., and Ilmoniemi, R. J. (2004). The effect of stimulus intensity on brain response evoked by transcranial magnetic stimulation. Hum. Brain Mapp. 21, 154–164. doi: 10.1002/ hbm.10159

Lee, T.-W., Grolami, M., and Sejnowski, T. J. (1999). Independent component analysis using an extended infomax algorithm for mixed subgaussian and super- gaussian sources. Neural Comput. 11, 417–441. doi: 10.1162/0899766993000 16719

Leocani, L., Cohen, L. G., Wassermann, E. M., Ikoma, K., and Hallett, M. (2000). Human corticospinal excitability evaluated with transcranial magnetic stimu- lation during different reaction time paradigms. Brain 123, 1161–1173. doi: 10.1093/brain/123.6.1161

Liddle, P. F., Kiehl, K. A., and Smith, A. M. (2001). Event related fMRI study of response inhibition. Hum. Brain Mapp. 12, 100–109. doi: 10.1002/1097-0193(200102)12:2<100::AID-HBM1007>3.0.CO;2-6

Lioumis, P., Kicˇic´, D., Savolainen, P., Mäkelä, J. P., and Kähkönen, S. (2009). Repro- ducibility of TMS-evoked EEG responses. Hum. Brain Mapp. 30, 1387–1396. doi: 10.1002/hbm.20608

Logan, G. D., Cowan, W. B., and Davis, K. A. (1984). On the ability to inhibit simple and choice reaction time responses: a model and a method. J. Exp. Psychol. Hum. Percept. Perform. 10, 276–291. doi: 10.1037/0096-1523.10.2.276

Logan, G. D., and Cowan, W. B. (1984). On the ability to inhibit thought and action: a theory of an act of control. Psychol. Rev. 91, 295–327. doi: 10.1037/0033- 295X.91.3.295

Mäkinen, V., Tiitinen, H., and May, P. (2005). Auditory event-related responses are generated independently of ongoing brain activity. Neuroimage 24, 961–968. doi: 10.1016/j. neuroimage.2004.10.020

Massimini, M., Ferrarelli, F., Esser, S. K., Riedner, B. A., Huber, R., Murphy, M., et al. (2007). Triggering sleep slow waves by transcranial magnetic stimulation. Proc. Natl. Acad. Sci. U.S.A. 104, 8496–8501. doi: 10.1073/ pnas.0702495104

Massimini, M., Ferrarelli, F., Huber, R., Esser, S. K., Singh, H., and Tononi, G. (2005). Breakdown of cortical effective connectivity during sleep. Science 309, 2228–2232. doi: 10.1126/science.1117256

Nikouline, V., Ruohonen, J., and Ilmoniemi, R. J. (1999). The role of the coil click in TMS assessed with simultaneous EEG. Clin. Neurophysiol. 110, 1325–1328. doi: 10.1016/S1388-2457(99)00070-X

Nikulin, V. V., Kicˇic´, D., Kähkönen, S., and Ilmoniemi, R. J. (2003). Modulation of electro-encephalographic responses to transcranial magnetic stimulation: evi- dence for changes in cortical excitability related to movement. Eur. J. Neurosci. 18, 1206–1212. doi: 10.1046/j.1460-9568.2003.02858.x

Pascual-Leone, A., Valls-Solé, J., Wassermann, E. M., Brasil-Neto, J. P., Cohen, L. G., and Hallett, M. (1992). Effects of focal transcranial magnetic stimulation on simple reaction time to acoustic, visual and somatosensory stimuli. Brain 115, 1045–1059. doi: 10.1093/ brain/115.4.1045

Paus, T., Sipila, P. K., and Strafella, A. P. (2001). Synchronization of neuronal activity in the human primary motor cortex by transcranial magnetic stimulation: an EEG study. J. Neurophysiol. 86, 1983–1990.

Reis, J., Swayne, O. B., Vandermeeren, Y., Camus, M., Dimyan, M. A., Harris- Love, M., et al. (2008). Contribution of transcranial magnetic stimulation to the understanding of cortical mechanisms involved in motor control. J. Physiol. 586, 325–351. doi: 10.1113/jphysiol.2007.144824

Rogasch, N. C., Daskalakis, Z. J., and Fitzgerald, P. B. (2013). Mechanisms underlying long-interval cortical inhibition in the human motor cortex: a TMS-EEG study. J. Neurophysiol. 109, 89–98. doi: 10.1152/jn.00762.2012

Rubia, K., Russell, T., Overmeyer, S., Brammer, M. J., Bullmore, E. T., Sharma, T., et al. (2001). Mapping motor inhibition: conjunctive brain activations across different versions of go/no-go and stop tasks. Neuroimage 13, 250–261. doi: 10.1006/nimg.2000.0685

Schmajuk, M., Liotti, M., Busse, L., and Woldorff, M. G. (2006). Electro-physiological activity underlying inhibitory control processes in normal adults. Neuropsychologia 44, 384–395. doi: 10.1016/j. neuropsychologia.2005.06.005

Sekiguchi, H., Takeuchi, S., Kadota, H., Kohno, Y., and Nakajima, Y. (2011). TMS-induced artifacts on EEG can be reduced by rearrangement of the elec- trode's lead wire before recording. Clin. Neurophysiol. 122, 984–990. doi: 10.1016/j. clinph.2010.09.004

Starr, A., Caramia, M., Zarola, F., and Rossini, P. M. (1988). Enhancement of motor cortical excitability in humans by non-invasive electrical stimulation appears prior to voluntary movement. Electroencephalogr. Clin. Neurophysiol. 70, 26–32. doi: 10.1016/0013-4694(88)90191-5

Tiitinen, H., Virtanen, J., Ilmoniemi, R. J., Kamppuri, J., Ollikainen, M., Ruohonen, J., et al. (1999). Separation of contamination caused by coil clicks from responses elicited by transcranial magnetic stimulation. Clin. Neurophysiol. 110, 982–985. doi: 10.1016/S1388-2457(99)00038-3

van den Wildenberg, W. P., Burle, B., Vidal, F., van der Molen, M. W., Ridderinkhof, K. R., and Hasbroucq, T. (2010). Mechanisms and dynamics of cortical motor inhibition in the stop-signal paradigm: a TMS Study. J. Cogn. Neurosci. 22, 225– 239. doi: 10.1162/jocn.2009.21248

Veniero, D., Bortoletto, M., and Miniussi, C. (2009). TMS-EEG co- registration: on TMS-induced artifact. Clin. Neurophysiol. 120, 1392–1399. doi: 10.1016/j. clinph.2009.04.023

Veniero, D., Bortoletto, M., and Miniussi, C. (2013). Cortical modulation of short-latency TMS-evoked potentials. Front. Hum. Neurosci. 6:352. doi: 010.3389/ fnhum.2012.00352

Veniero, D., Maioli, C., and Miniussi, C. (2010). Potentiation of short-latency cor- tical responses by high-frequency repetitive transcranial magnetic stimulation. J. Neurophysiol. 104, 1578–1588. doi: 10.1152/jn.00172.2010

Verbruggen, F., and Logan, G. D. (2008). Response inhibition in the stop-signal paradigm. Trends. Cogn. Sci. 12, 418–424. doi: 10.1016/j.tics.2008.07.005

Wager, T. D., Sylvester, C.-Y., Lacey, S. C., Nee, D. E., Franklin, M., and Jonides, J. (2005). Common and unique components of response inhibition revealed by fMRI. Neuroimage 27, 323–340. doi: 10.1016/j.neuroimage.2005.01.054

Walsh, V., and Cowey, A. (2000). Transcranial magnetic stimulation and cognitive neuroscience. Nat. Rev. Neurosci. 1, 73–79. doi: 10.1038/35036239

Watanabe, J., Sugiura, M., Sato, K., Maeda, Y., Matsue, Y., Fukuda, H., et al. (2002). The human prefrontal and parietal association cortices are involved in NO-GO performances: an event-related fMRI study. Neuroimage 17, 1207–1216. doi: 10.1006/nimg.2002.1198

Yamanaka, K., Kimura, T., Miyazaki, M., Kawashima, N., Nozaki, D., Nakazawa, K., et al. (2002). Human cortical activities during Go/NoGo tasks with opposite motor control paradigms. Exp. Brain. Res. 142, 301–307. doi: 10.1007/s00221-001-0943-2

APPENDIX

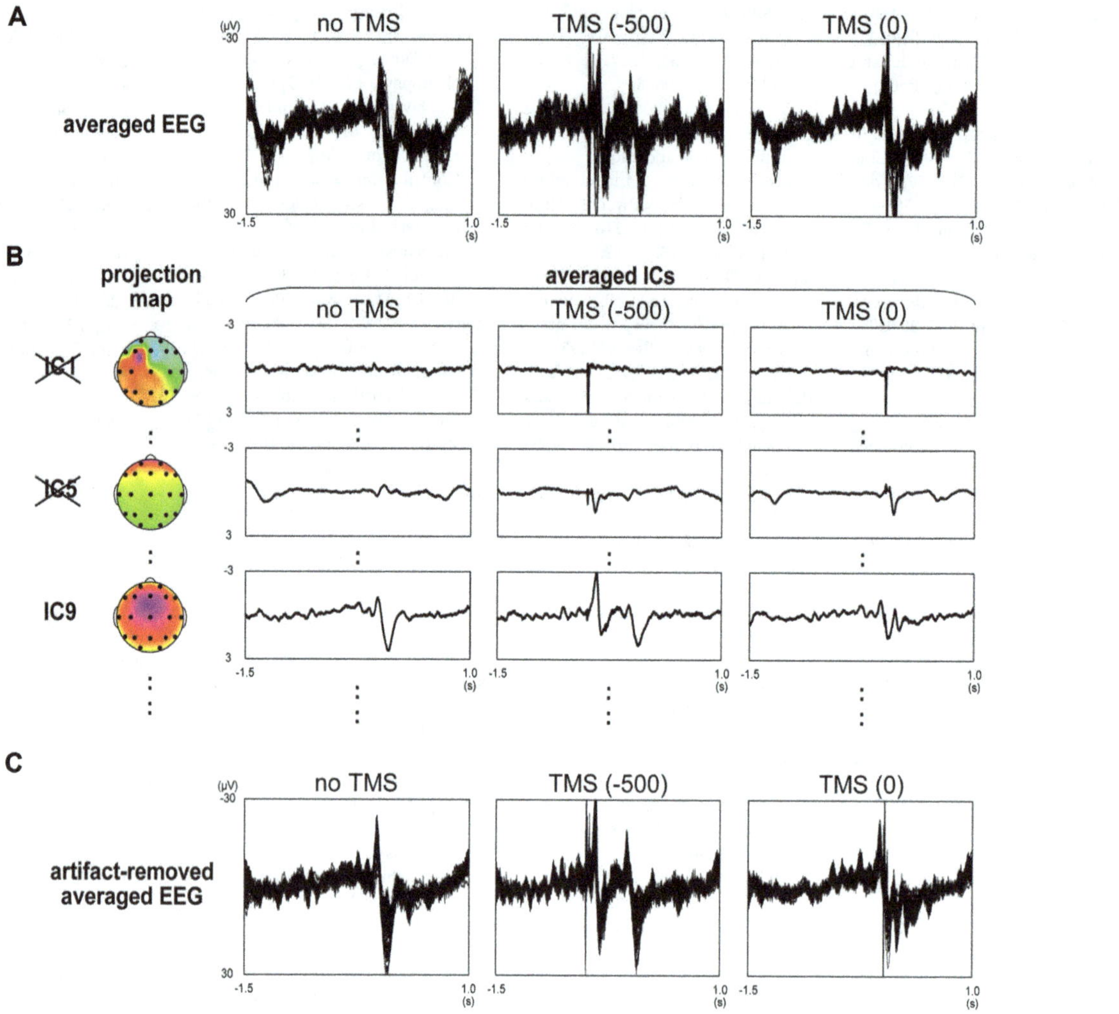

FIGURE A1 | Artifact rejection from TMS-EEG data by using independent component analysis in a typical participant. (A) Averaged EEG waveforms in no-TMS stop trials (left panel), stop trials with contralateral-TMS at −500 and 0 ms (middle and right panels) recorded from 61 surface electrodes. **(B)** Averaged independent component (IC) waveforms and their projection maps in no-TMS stop trials (left panel), stop trials with contralateral-TMS at −500 and 0 ms (middle and right panels) extracted from 61 EEG waveforms. In order of their variance size, the largest component (IC1), fifth largest component (IC5), and ninth largest component (IC9) were selectively shown. **(C)** Artifact-removed averaged EEG waveforms in no-TMS stop trials (left panel), stop trials with contralateral-TMS at −500 and 0 ms (middle and right panels).

4

Task-related modulation of effective connectivity during perceptual decision making: dissociation between dorsal and ventral prefrontal cortex

Rei Akaishi[1,2], Naoko Ueda[1] and Katsuyuki Sakai[1]*

[1] Department of Cognitive Neuroscience, Graduate School of Medicine, The University of Tokyo, Tokyo, Japan
[2] Department of Experimental Psychology, University of Oxford, Oxford, UK

***Correspondence:**
Katsuyuki Sakai, Department of Cognitive Neuroscience, Graduate School of Medicine, The University of Tokyo, 7-3-1 Hongo, Bunkyo-ku, Tokyo 113-0033, Japan
e-mail: ksakai@m.u-tokyo.ac.jp

The dorsal and ventral parts of the lateral prefrontal cortex have been thought to play distinct roles in decision making. Although its dorsal part such as the frontal eye field (FEF) is shown to play roles in accumulation of sensory information during perceptual decision making, the role of the ventral prefrontal cortex (PFv) is not well-documented. Previous studies have suggested that the PFv is involved in selective attention to the task-relevant information and is associated with accuracy of the behavioral performance. It is unknown, however, whether the accumulation and selection processes are anatomically dissociated between the FEF and PFv. Here we show that, by using concurrent TMS and EEG recording, the short-latency (20–40 ms) TMS-evoked potentials after stimulation of the FEF change as a function of the time to behavioral response, whereas those after stimulation of the PFv change depending on whether the response is correct or not. The potentials after stimulation of either region did not show significant interaction between time to response and performance accuracy, suggesting dissociation between the processes subserved by the FEF and PFv networks. The results are consistent with the idea that the network involving the FEF plays a role in information accumulation, whereas the network involving the PFv plays a role in selecting task relevant information. In addition, stimulation of the FEF and PFv induced activation in common regions in the dorsolateral and medial frontal cortices, suggesting convergence of information processed in the two regions. Taken together, the results suggest dissociation between the FEF and PFv networks for their computational roles in perceptual decision making. The study also highlights the advantage of TMS-EEG technique in investigating the computational processes subserved by the neural network in the human brain with a high temporal resolution.

Keywords: transcranial magnetic stimulation, electroencephalography, frontal eye field, ventral prefrontal cortex, perceptual decision making, accumulation, selection

INTRODUCTION

Perceptual decision making is understood as a process of accumulating task-relevant sensory information toward a decision threshold (Gold and Shadlen, 2007). It has been shown that neurons in the frontal eye field (FEF) as well as lateral intraparietal region of monkeys show build-up of activity after presentation of a noisy sensory stimulus until the behavioral response. These activity patterns are taken to reflect the information accumulation process. However, in imaging studies of humans, not only the FEF but also the ventral prefrontal cortex (PFv) around the posterior portion of the inferior frontal sulcus are shown to be active in discrimination of sensory stimuli (Binder et al., 2004; Pessoa and Padmala, 2005; Ploran et al., 2007; Thielscher and Pessoa, 2007; Kayser et al., 2010; Liu and Pleskac, 2011). It has been proposed that the PFv plays a role in allocation of attentional resources to maintain accuracy of decision making, possibly by sending selection signals to sensory areas to collect choice-relevant information (Corbetta and Shulman, 2002; Heekeren et al., 2008).

A crucial question here is whether the selection process in the PFv can be distinguished from information accumulation process in the FEF. It also remains open how the processes of information accumulation and selection interact in the decision network. To answer these questions, we used concurrent transcranial magnetic stimulation (TMS) and electroencephalography (EEG) recording (TMS-EEG) (Komssi and Kähkönen, 2006; Driver et al., 2009; Siebner et al., 2009; Miniussi and Thut, 2010; Reithler et al., 2011; Daskalakis et al., 2012; Rogasch and Fitzgerald, 2013), and examined neural network connectivity involving the FEF and PFv during perceptual decision making. A single pulse of TMS over a given cortical region induces spread of neural impulses from the stimulated region toward the anatomically connected regions (Ilmoniemi et al., 1997), and the pattern of neural impulse transmission changes depending on the state of local and inter-regional neural network downstream to the stimulated region (Massimini et al., 2005; Esser et al., 2009; Morishima et al., 2009; Akaishi et al., 2010). We reasoned that we can make inference about the cognitive or computational processes subserved by the network involving the stimulated region by analyzing experimental or behavioral factors that modulate the scalp distribution of TMS-evoked potentials in EEG (TMS-EPs). Because of the causal relationship between the stimulation and EEG responses, this technique of TMS-EEG reveals how the stimulated region interacts with other regions of the network. In the present study, we analyzed the TMS-EPs after stimulation of the FEF and PFv, and show double dissociation between the FEF and PFv for their roles in information accumulation and selection. We also show that the functional networks of the FEF and PFv overlap in the medial and dorsolateral prefrontal cortex.

MATERIALS AND METHODS

SUBJECTS

Twenty normal human subjects participated in the experiment with FEF stimulation (8 females; age: 20–42), and 13 in the experiment with PFv stimulation (6 females; age: 21–46). Written informed consents were obtained from all the subjects prior to the experiments. The study was approved by the ethics committee of the Graduate School of Medicine, the University of Tokyo.

BEHAVIORAL PARADIGM

Subjects performed a reaction time version of the two-direction motion discrimination task with manual response (**Figure 1A**).

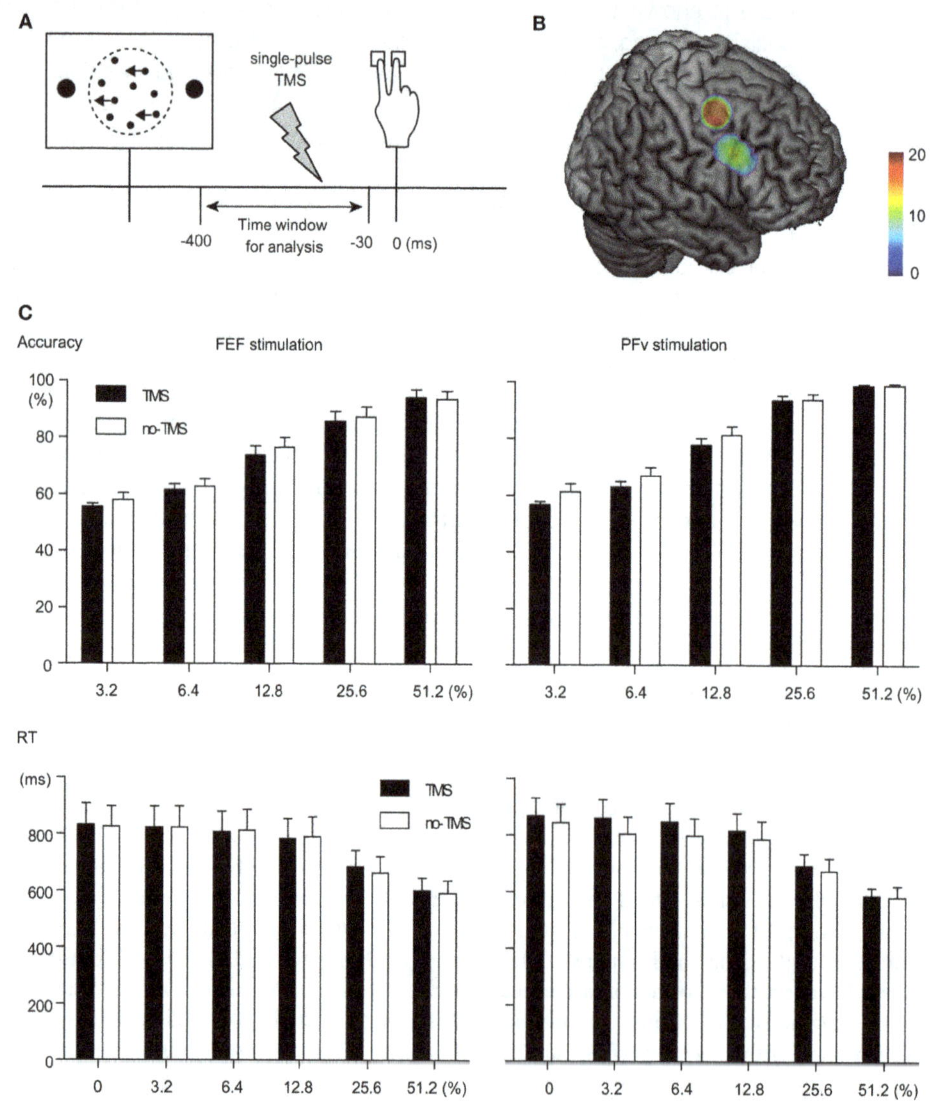

FIGURE 1 | TMS manipulation experiment. (A) Behavioral paradigm. A single-pulse TMS was given at variable timing between visual stimulus onset and behavioral response. Trials in which TMS was given within the time window between 30 and 400 ms before behavioral response were analyzed. **(B)** Stimulation sites rendered on a template MNI brain. Dorsal and ventral clusters indicate FEF and PFv stimulation sites, respectively. Color bar indicates the number of overlapped subjects. Note that the number of subjects was 20 and 13 for FEF and PFv stimulation, respectively. **(C)** TMS effects on behavior. Accuracy (top) and RT (bottom) for each motion coherence level (abscissa) are shown separately for FEF (left) and PFv stimulation (right).

The stimulus was a set of white dots (123.1 cd/m^2, size: 0.06° of visual angle, mean density of 49.6 dots/deg^2 *s) displayed within an invisible circular aperture (5° in diameter) at the center of a dark background (1.8 cd/m^2). The refresh rate of the monitor was 60 Hz. A subset of dots was offset from their original position every 50 ms to create apparent motion to the left or right at 5.0°/s and the remaining dots were moved to random locations. The percentage of the dots that were moving in the same direction was manipulated at 0, 3.2, 6.4, 12.8, 25.6, and 51.2%. Trials with 0% motion coherence were excluded from the analysis of TMS-EPs because the accuracy of performance cannot be examined. The direction of motion and motion coherence level were pseudo-randomized within an experimental session, such that the same number of trials for left- and right-ward motion for each of motion coherence level were presented. Subjects were asked to indicate the perceived direction of coherent dot motion by pressing a button with the index or middle finger of the right hand, as accurate and quickly as possible. The random dot motion pattern disappeared when subjects made button press or when 2 s elapsed without button press. The response-stimulus interval was varied from 1320 to 1590 ms, and 120 trials x 12 sessions were performed by the subject in the TMS-EEG session. Before the experiment, the subject performed two practice sessions, 120 trials for each, to achieve stable performance in the TMS-EEG session.

MEASUREMENT OF TMS-EPs

In the concurrent TMS-EEG session, we gave a single-pulse TMS on half of the trials in each session of 120 trials using a figure-eight shaped coil (70 mm diameter) and MagStim 200 stimulator (MagStim, UK), while TMS-evoked scalp recorded potentials were recorded using EEG. Position of the TMS coil was adjusted using Brainsight (Rogue Research, UK) based on the structural MRI of the individual subjects' brain. The FEF was determined as the region just below the junction between the superior frontal sulcus and precentral gyrus (Paus, 1996; Blanke et al., 2000; Lobel et al., 2001; Koyama et al., 2004; Grosbras et al., 2005). The PFv was determined as the region located just anterior to the junction of the posterior end of the inferior frontal sulcus and the inferior limb of the precentral sulcus, which has been shown to be active during perceptual decision making in the previous studies (Heekeren et al., 2006; Kayser et al., 2010; Liu and Pleskac, 2011) (**Figure 1B**). Mean coordinate for the FEF stimulation was (38, −3, 50), and that for the PFv stimulation was (53, 13, 30). According to the probabilistic cytoarchitectonic atlas (SPM Anatomy toolbox), the FEF in the present study corresponds to the border between Brodmann's area (BA) 6 and 8, whereas the PFv corresponds to the border between BA44 and 45. For FEF stimulation, TMS coil was oriented 45° from the middle line with its handle pointed posteriorly. For PFv stimulation, TMS coil was oriented parallel to the middle line of the head with its handle pointed posteriorly. The TMS intensity was 35% of the maximum stimulator output, which did not exceed the active motor threshold: The TMS intensity was 69.4% (range: 53–88) and 73.7% (55–92) of the active motor threshold for the FEF and PFv stimulation, respectively. In contrast to other studies of TMS, the low-intensity TMS was used as a means to probe the state of the neural network, rather than as a means to manipulate the underlying neural processes.

TMS was delivered at a variable timing between the stimulus onset and behavioral response. For each subject, we first determined the average RT for each motion coherence level based on the behavioral data in the practice sessions (240 trials in all). During the TMS-EEG experiment, we gave TMS at a variable timing relative to the stimulus onset, with the latest timing determined based on the estimated RT. The estimation of the RT was updated for each experimental session so as to take into account the change in behavior during the experiment. When the response key was pressed earlier than the preprogrammed timing of TMS, the TMS trigger pulse was aborted and no TMS was given. After the experiment, trials were sorted *post-hoc* depending on the time relative to the behavioral response (**Figure 1A**). This was to examine the change in the TMS-EPs according to the relative time to behavioral response.

Throughout the experimental session, we recorded EEG with 60 electrodes placed according to an extended 10/20 system using a TMS-compatible amplifier (BrainAmp, Brain Products, Germany). EEG signals were referenced to the mean of all electrodes, and were low-pass filtered at 1000 Hz, DC-corrected, and sampled at 2500 Hz with 16 bit resolution. Impedance of each electrode was kept below 5 kΩ for all experiments. Eye movements were also recorded by tracking the pupillary position of the left eye at a sampling rate of 60 Hz using ViewPoint eye tracker (Arrington Research, AZ).

EEG data were preprocessed with BrainVision Analyzer (BrainProducts, Germany) and custom programs on MATLAB (Mathworks, MA). We then used the SPM8 (http://www.fil.ion.ucl.ac.uk/spm/) for statistical analysis and data visualization. Artifacts due to TMS were observed on channels around the stimulation site but in the majority of trials they disappeared within 8 ms of the stimulation. Trials with prolonged TMS artifacts were removed: We rejected trials with amplitude larger than 50 μV relative to the baseline during the time window of 8–40 ms after TMS. Trials with muscle activity, blinking artifacts and eye movements were also removed. The mean rejection rate was 31.6% (24.0–39.7) for FEF stimulation and 31.7% (25.1–41.4) for PFv stimulation. The pattern of TMS-induced artifacts did not show a time-dependent change: Trials with large artifacts due to TMS appeared randomly throughout the experimental sessions. This may indicate a subtle change in the coil position, and sometimes the coil may have contacted directly with the electrode leads, causing the artifacts. But the stimulation site monitored by the navigator system was localized within a region of 5 mm in diameter and thus in terms of the stimulated cortical region, the position of the TMS coil was considered to be maintained stably.

After rejection of trials with artifacts, the EEG waveforms on TMS-trials were aligned at the onset of TMS, and were baseline-corrected based on the data within the 4-ms pre-TMS period. In the present study, TMS was given at a variable timing during perceptual decision making, and EEG during the pre-TMS period is not flat and differs across trials even within the same condition. We thus chose to use a time-window of 4 ms as a reference to correct the baseline in order to align the amplitude of EEG at the time of TMS at the zero point. In other words, this duration was arbitrarily chosen to reduce the noise. The problem of using such an extremely short period for baseline correction is the contribution of the phase of oscillatory EEG activity at the time of TMS, and we need to obtain a large number of trials for averaging to cancel out the effect.

ANALYSIS OF TMS-EPs

We focused on two experimental factors that would modulate the TMS-EPs, which are the TMS timing relative to the behavioral response (Time-to-Response) and accuracy of behavioral response (Accuracy). It has been shown that in single unit recording studies in monkeys, activity of neurons in the FEF increases gradually from 200 ms from the stimulus onset until the time of behavioral response (Gold and Shadlen, 2007). Based on these findings, we examined changes in the TMS-EPs according to the TMS timing relative to the behavioral response: In other words, we examined changes in the effective connectivity associated with the amount of accumulated sensory information. The prediction is that the TMS-EPs after FEF stimulation are modulated by the factor of Time-to-Response. By contrast, the previous findings suggest the role of PFv in attentional selection processes (Corbetta and Shulman, 2002; Heekeren et al., 2008). The efficiency in selection of task-relevant information is thought to be associated with accuracy of behavioral performance (Pelli, 1985; Shadlen et al., 1996). Based on these previous studies, we expected that the TMS-EPs after PFv stimulation are modulated by the factor of Accuracy.

During the TMS-EEG experiment, we gave TMS at a variable timing relative to the stimulus onset. After the experiment, trials were sorted *post-hoc* depending on the time relative to the behavioral response. The TMS-EPs data were categorized according to whether the TMS was given early (400–130 ms before response) or late (130–30 ms before response) during the decision process (factor of Time-to-Response, early or late). This categorization of the time windows for analysis was determined based on the time course of firing of FEF neurons obtained from monkeys performing the same motion discrimination task for random dot patterns. It has been shown that when the neuronal firing patterns are aligned to behavioral response, the build-up of FEF neuronal firing starts from around 400 ms before the onset of saccade response and takes a peak value at roughly 30 ms before the saccade response (Ding and Gold, 2012). Although a manual response paradigm was used in the present study instead of a saccade paradigm used in monkey studies, we consider that the FEF neurons show a similar build-up of activity in the manual response paradigm. In fact, a previous imaging study suggests a similar build-up of activity in the FEF between saccade and manual response paradigms (Liu and Pleskac, 2011). Thus, the time window of 30–400 ms before response can be taken to correspond to the build-up phase of neuronal firing, which has been associated with accumulation of decision-related sensory information. We further considered that the FEF neuronal activity in a manual response paradigm may reach a plateau at about 100 ms before the response: Compared to a saccade paradigm, the reaction time in the manual response paradigm is longer by about 100 ms. Thus, the comparison between Early (130–400 ms before response) and Late (30–130 ms before response) epochs can be taken to reflect the difference between the neuronal build-up phase and plateau phase. TMS was given more often during the later period during the decision so as to roughly equate the number of trials between Early and Late. Trials in which TMS was given outside these time windows were excluded from the analysis. The limitation is that these time windows of analysis are based on the single unit firing data obtained from monkeys, which may not be directly applicable to human studies.

We also categorized the TMS-EPs data according to the accuracy of choice response given the sensory information on that trial (factor of Accuracy, correct or error). For the TMS-EPs data thus arranged in a 2-by-2 factorial design, we tested the main effects of Time-to-Response and Accuracy, as well as the interaction between the two factors. We focused on the TMS-EPs within the time window of 8–40 ms after TMS in order to avoid the period that contains artifacts due to the TMS pulse. We also restricted the analysis within the interval of 40 ms after TMS because we were interested in initial spreading patterns of the neural impulse induced by the TMS, which most likely reflects direct impulse transmission from the stimulated region. Using SPM8 for EEG (http://www.fil.ion.ucl.ac.uk/spm/), the TMS-EP data were constructed in a three-dimensional space (x and y for space, and z for time), and the smoothness of the data across space and time was estimated to calculate effective degrees of freedom. To ensure smoothness assumption of the random field theory, we used Gaussian spatial filter with full width half maximum (FWHM) of 48 mm and Gaussian temporal filter with FWHM of 8 ms. Average TMS-EPs for each trial type were calculated for each subject, and the main effects of Accuracy and Time-to-Response and their interaction were tested across subjects. We used a statistical threshold of $p < 0.05$ corrected for multiple comparisons in spatial as well as in time domains.

The effects of the Time-to-Response and Accuracy were also tested on EEG data on no-TMS trials. This was to examine whether or not the effect of Time-to-Response or Accuracy that could be observed on TMS-EPs is due to modulations in the baseline EEG pattern. For this purpose, we extracted epochs of no-TMS trials that match with the time window of analysis for TMS trials. For each TMS trial, we searched a matched no-TMS trial in which a visual stimulus with the same motion coherence was presented as in that particular TMS trial and also in which the RT was within the range of 100 ms relative to the RT of the TMS trial. The TMS trial was excluded from the analysis when we failed to find a matched no-TMS trial. Thus the TMS and no-TMS trials are matched roughly in a pair-wise manner in terms of the motion coherence level of the stimulus and response time. We then extracted an epoch for analysis from the matched no-TMS trial thus selected; the epoch was determined as a 32-ms period with the same time-to-response as the time window of 8–40 ms after TMS in the matched TMS trial. The conventional approach is to subtract the EEG waveforms on no-TMS trials from those on TMS trials so that we can examine the potentials induced by the TMS. In the present study, however, the TMS timing is varied across trials. The time window for ERP analysis is also varied. It can be problematic to subtract waveforms obtained from variable epochs of no-TMS trials in terms of their timing from those obtained from variable epochs of TMS trials. We tried to extract an epoch for no-TMS trial that corresponds to the epoch for a given TMS trial in a pair-wise manner, but the timings of the epochs were not matched exactly. We therefore applied Two-Way ANOVA (with factors of TMS timing and Accuracy) separately for TMS and no-TMS trials.

In a separate model, we also tested the effect of the timing of TMS relative to the visual stimulus onset (factor of Time-from-Stimulus, categorized as early or late depending on whether the TMS was given between 170 and 470 ms or later than 470 ms after stimulus onset). These time windows roughly correspond to the build-up phase of FEF neuronal firing when the neuronal firing is aligned to visual stimulus onset (Ding and Gold, 2012). The division between the Early and Late time windows at 470 ms after visual stimulus onset was to equate the number of trials between Early and Late. Trials analyzed for the effect of Time-to-Response and those analyzed for the effect of Time-to-Stimulus are identical. Of note is that trials categorized as Early in terms of Time-to-Response do not necessarily corresponds to trials categorized as Early in terms of Time-from-Stimulus. The same is true for Late trials.

We also tested the effect of motion coherence level of the stimuli, which was categorized as low (3.2 and 6.4%) or high (12.8, 25.6, and 51.2%). This is to examine if the effect of Accuracy is confounded by the motion coherence (i.e., stimulus strength). In **Table 1**, we report the number of trials composing Early and Late TMS and Correct and Error trials, separately for low and high motion coherence. As shown in the table, the number of trials differs greatly between Correct and Error for high coherence motion trials, but there were at least 25 error trials in high coherence condition, which were enough, though not ideal, for the analysis.

SOURCE ESTIMATION OF SIGNAL TRANSMISSION FROM THE FEF AND PFv

We next identified regions that receive signals from the FEF and PFv using cortical source density analysis based on scalp distribution of TMS-EPs. TMS-EPs were averaged across all trials for each subject and for each stimulation site. We then used sLORETA (Pascual-Marqui, 2002) and estimated the cortical distribution of current source density (CSD) that accounts for the scalp distribution of TMS-EPs during the time window of 20–40 ms after the TMS. This time window was chosen based on the previous studies showing TMS-induced activation in distant regions (Ilmoniemi et al., 1997; Massimini et al., 2005; Morishima et al., 2009; Akaishi et al., 2010) and also based on the results of present study showing significant effect of Time-to-Response and Accuracy on TMS-EPs within this time window. Computations of CSD were performed in a realistic head model, using a template brain of the Montreal Neurological Institute (MNI152), with the three-dimensional solution space restricted to cortical gray matter. The intracerebral volume was partitioned in 6239 voxels at 5 mm spatial resolution. The logarithmically-transformed CSD values for each voxel of the MNI space were compared against zero using one-sample t-test. We used a non-parametric permutation test with a threshold of $p < 0.05$ corrected for multiple voxels based on 5000 randomizations (one-tailed).

Table 1 | Number of trials used for TMS-EP analysis (mean and range).

	Low coherence	High coherence
FEF STIMULATION		
Early	149 (101–173)	206 (136–271)
Late	138 (95–197)	229 (171–263)
Correct	213 (195–264)	386 (320–412)
Error	74 (49–105)	49 (25–65)
PFv STIMULATION		
Early	158 (119–174)	211 (150–271)
Late	143 (106–188)	208 (176–259)
Correct	219 (195–264)	356 (301–417)
Error	82 (43–129)	63 (27–93)

Motion coherence of low coherence trials: 3.2 and 6.4%.
Motion coherence of high coherence trials: 12.8, 25.6, and 51.2%.

RESULTS

TMS EFFECT ON BEHAVIOR

Stimulation of each network had only minimal effects on behavior. Accuracy of task performance decreased slightly after the TMS (mean across subjects: 1.5 and 2.4% decrease for FEF and PFv stimulation, respectively), but the effect did not differ significantly between the two stimulation sites and across motion coherence levels [Three-Way ANOVA on accuracy, Greenhouse-Geisser correction: Main effect of TMS: $F_{(1, 26)} = 11.4$, $p = 0.002$; interaction between TMS and stimulation site: $F_{(1, 26)} = 0.62$; $p = 0.44$; interaction between TMS, stimulation site and coherence: $F_{(2.447, 63.6)} = 0.30$; $p = 0.78$, **Figure 1C** top]. Response time (RT) of the performance was not affected by the stimulation for either site, and the interaction with motion coherence level was not significant [Three-Way ANOVA on RT, Greenhouse-Geisser correction: Main effect of TMS: $F_{(1, 26)} = 0.003$, $p = 0.96$; interaction between TMS and stimulation site: $F_{(1, 26)} = 0.83$; $p = 0.37$; interaction between TMS, stimulation site and coherence: $F_{(3.34, 86.9)} = 1.11$; $p = 0.35$, **Figure 1C** bottom].

MODULATION OF TMS-EPs

We examined the change in the TMS-EPs according to the TMS timing relative to the behavioral response. FEF neuronal activity has been shown to build up during perceptual decision making and reach a plateau just before the behavioral response (Kim and Shadlen, 1999; Ding and Gold, 2012). Based on the finding, we predicted that the TMS-EPs after FEF stimulation are modulated by how close TMS was at the time of behavioral response (Early or Late). By contrast, the previous findings suggest the role of PFv in attentional selection processes (Corbetta and Shulman, 2002; Heekeren et al., 2008). The efficiency in selection of task-relevant information is thought to be associated with accuracy of behavioral performance (Pelli, 1985; Shadlen et al., 1996). Based on these previous studies, we expected that the TMS-EPs after PFv stimulation are modulated by whether the subject select action based on the task relevant sensory information (Correct or Error).

TMS on the FEF produced positive potentials in frontal electrodes and negative potentials in right temporo-parietal electrodes, which after 20 ms of TMS evolved into a pattern of left centro-parietal positive potentials (**Figure 2A** left). By contrast,

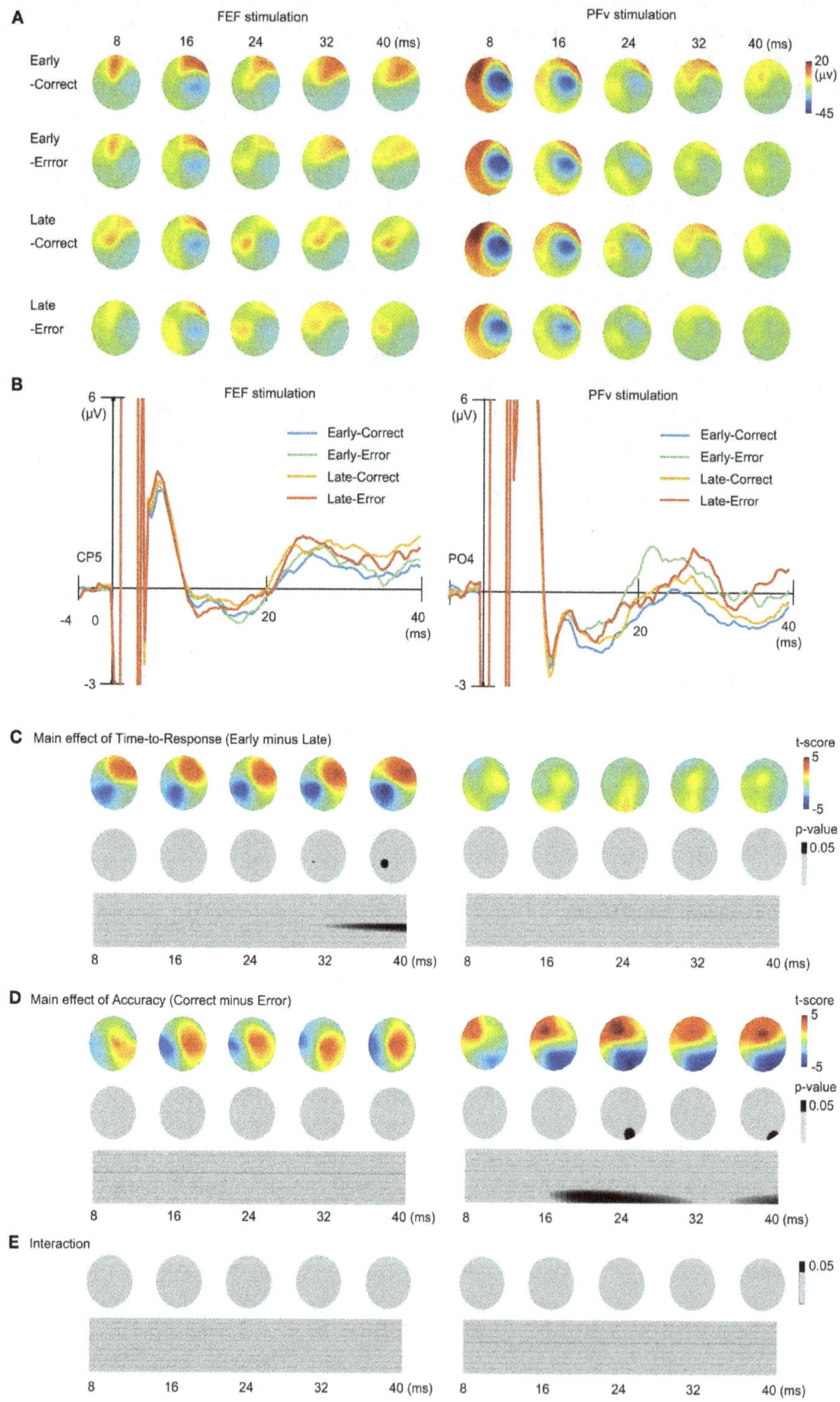

FIGURE 2 | TMS-EEG experiment. (A) Scalp patterns of TMS-EPs shown in time bins of 8 ms after TMS. Data in which TMS was given early or late during the decision process and data in which subjects made correct or erroneous response are shown separately. FEF (left) and PFv stimulation (right). **(B)** Waveform of TMS-EPs from CP5 electrode in FEF stimulation (left) and that from PO4 electrode in PFv stimulation (right). Time bins in which there was a significant main effect of Time-to-Response factor (Early vs. Late) and those in which there was a significant main effect of Accuracy factor (Correct vs. Error) are indicated at the bottom of the trace by red tics. **(C)** Main effect of Time to Response (contrast: Early vs. Late) on TMS-evoked potentials. Scalp distribution of t-scores (upper row) and *p*-values (middle row, threshold: $p = 0.05$, corrected for family-wise error). Bottom row indicates 2-D plot of the continuous time series of *p*-values (abscissa: time from TMS; ordinate: electrode position with left anterior to right posterior electrode shown from top to bottom). Spatial and temporal windows with significant effects are indicated in black. **(D)** Main effect of Accuracy (contrast: Correct vs. Error). Same format as in **(C)**. **(E)** Interaction between Accuracy and Time-to-Response. Only the *p*-value maps are shown.

TMS on PFv produced positive potentials in the left fronto-central electrodes and negative potentials in the right central electrodes, which after 20 ms evolved into a pattern of frontal positive potentials (**Figure 2A** right). As for the data at an electrode level, for FEF stimulation there was a larger positive deflection of the TMS-EP recorded from the CP5 electrode for Late than for Early trials (**Figure 2B** left). For PFv stimulation by contrast, there was a larger positive potential at the PO4 electrode for Error than for Correct trials (**Figure 2B** right).

To overcome the problem of multiple comparisons across electrode space and time, we conducted statistical analysis that took into account the multiple comparisons based on random field theory and smoothness estimate of our own data (in terms of both space and time). We found that TMS-EPs after FEF stimulation were significantly modulated by Time-to-Response especially in the left centro-parietal region, but not by Accuracy, whereas TMS-EPs after PFv stimulation were significantly modulated by Accuracy especially in the right parieto-occipital region, but not by Time-to-Response ($p < 0.05$. corrected for multiple comparisons across space and time; **Figures 2C,D**. Significant effects were observed within the time window of 20–40 ms after the TMS. Importantly, the interaction between Time-to-Response and Accuracy was not significant for either stimulation sites ($p > 0.1$) (**Figure 2E**). This result of double dissociation between FEF and PFv stimulation suggests separation between the processes subserved by the FEF network and those subserved by the PFv network during perceptual decision making. In contrast to the significant effect of Time-to-Response and Accuracy on TMS-EPs in TMS trials, these effects were not significant on the EEG potentials in no-TMS trials ($p > 0.1$). This suggests that the observed modulation of the TMS-EPs cannot be accounted for by the difference in the baseline activity.

The effect of Accuracy in PFv stimulation experiment can be confounded by the motion coherence level of the stimulus because accuracy changes depending on stimulus strength. However, the effect of motion coherence (categorized as low or high) on the TMS-EPs of PFv stimulation was not significant ($p > 0.1$) (**Figure 3A**). The effect of motion coherence on the TMS-EPs of FEF stimulation was not significant, either. On the other hand, the effect of Time-to-Response in the FEF stimulation experiment might also reflect the effect of elapsed time from the stimulus onset. When Time-from-Stimulus was entered as a factor instead of Time-to-Response, a significant effect of Time-from-Stimulus on TMS-EP was observed in the FEF stimulation experiment (**Figure 3B**) although the effect was small and appeared only at a period around 40 ms of TMS. In contrast, a robust effect of the Time-from-Stimulus was observed in the PFv stimulation experiment, despite absence of a significant effect of Time-to-Response in the previous analysis.

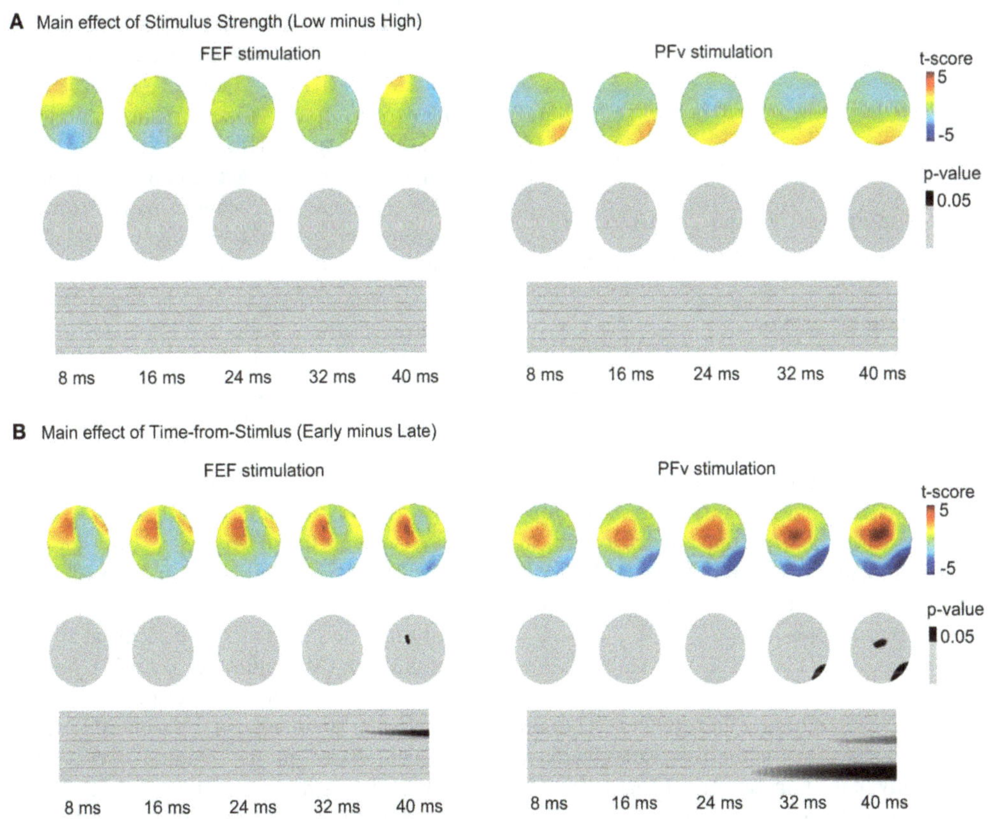

FIGURE 3 | (A) Main effect of motion coherence on TMS-EPs. Same format as in **Figure 2C**. **(B)** Main effect of Time-from-Stimulus on TMS-EPs. Same format as in **Figure 2C**.

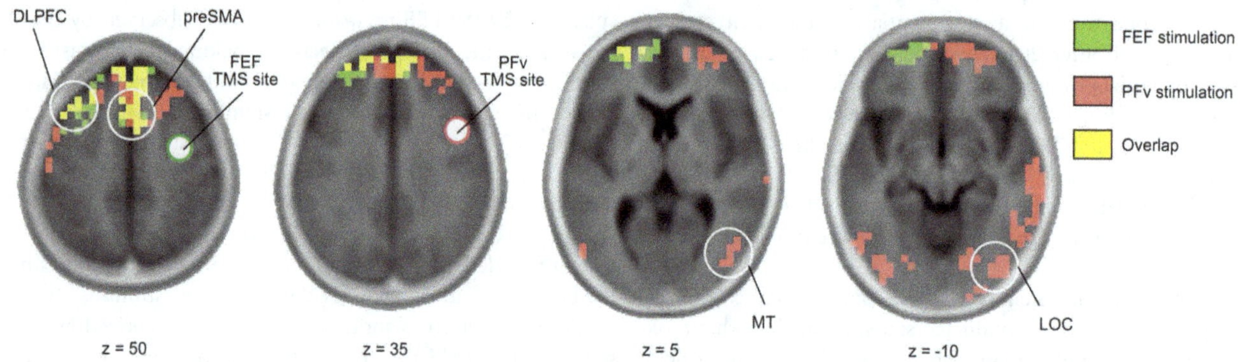

FIGURE 4 | Effective connectivity based on TMS-EEG. Distribution of cortical source density estimated from TMS-evoked potentials during 20–40 ms after stimulation of FEF (green) and PFv (red) (threshold: $p < 0.05$, corrected after 5000 permutation). Overlap is shown in yellow. Clusters with significant cortical source density in pre-SMA, left DLPFC ($z = 50$), MT ($z = 5$), and lateral occipital cortex (LOC) ($z = -10$) are indicated by white circle.

Table 2 | Region and MNI coordinate of the cortical source density peak of TMS-EPs.

Region	Coordinate
FEF STIMULATION	
Rt FPC	5, 65, 20
Rt preSMA	10, 10, 50
Lt DLPFC	−30, 30, 45
PFv STIMULATION	
Rt FPC	10, 60, 30
Rt preSMA	5, 10, 60
Lt DLPFC	−35, 20, 50
Lt MT	−55, −75, 0
Rt MT	50, −75, 5
Rt IT	70, −25, −10
Lt LOC	−45, −80, −10
Rt LOC	45, −80, −10

FPC, fronto-polar cortex; IT, inferior temporal cortex; LOC, lateral occipital cortex.

SPREAD OF SIGNALS FROM THE FEF AND PFv

Short-latency TMS-EPs have been taken to reflect activation induced by direct neural impulse transmission from the stimulated region. Using cortical source density estimation, we found that both FEF and PFv stimulations induced spread of impulse toward common regions in the left dorsolateral prefrontal cortex (DLPFC) and medial frontal region corresponding to the presupplementary motor area (preSMA) and/or supplementary eye field (SEF) at 20–40 ms of stimulation (**Figure 4**, **Table 2**). In addition, PFv stimulation induced activation in posterior visual areas including visual motion-sensitive area MT.

DISCUSSION

Using the concurrent TMS-EEG technique and applying Random Field Theory to the TMS-EPs data for the first time, we have shown that the connectivity of the FEF network changes depending on the timing relative to behavioral response, whereas the connectivity of the PFv network changes depending on the accuracy of perceptual decision. These results are consistent with our hypothesis that the networks of the FEF and PFv are involved in accumulation and selection of information, respectively. We also obtained results suggesting convergence of signals from the FEF and PFv in medial and lateral prefrontal regions.

METHODOLOGICAL ADVANTAGE

We used the TMS-EEG technique to examine task-dependent modulations of neural network connectivity. The idea is that by examining which experimental or behavioral factors modulate the pattern of impulse transmission induced by TMS, we can make inference about the cognitive/computational processes subserved by the network connected with the stimulation site. Compared to fMRI-based effective connectivity analysis such as Granger causality or Dynamic Causal Modeling (Stephan and Roebroeck, 2012), the TMS-EEG technique has three advantages. The first is that by giving TMS on a particular brain region, we are able to examine the state of neural network without a priori assumption about the regions functionally connected to the stimulation site. In fMRI-based effective connectivity analysis, the network connectivity can only be examined within a group of preselected regions, while in TMS-EEG functionally-connected regions can be identified in an exploratory manner.

Secondly, by focusing on short-latency TMS-EPs that occurs in less than 40 ms of the TMS, we can make inference about an early effect of impulse transmission from the stimulated region. It has been shown that inter-regional transmission of neural impulse takes 20–30 ms (Massimini et al., 2005; Morishima et al., 2009; Akaishi et al., 2010; Veniero et al., 2010; Rogasch and Fitzgerald, 2013). Also cortical stimulation and recording studies using subdural electrodes have shown that the induced activation at regions distant from the stimulation site occurs at around 20–30 ms after the stimulation (Matsumoto et al., 2007). It has also been shown that perception of moving phosphene is modulated by TMS on the FEF given 20 ms prior to the MT stimulation (Silvanto et al., 2006). Based on these findings, we consider that the short-latency TMS-EPs that we examined reflect an early effect of the TMS-induced impulse transmission. Our time window of TMS-EP analysis was 20–40 ms after TMS and this seems to be too late if we consider the signal conduction time between bilateral M1s and also between M1 and other regions (SMA, PM, and

IPS), which is thought to be around 10 ms or less. This value of 10 ms is based on the results of experiments using two TMS coils (twin coil study): The inter-stimulus interval with which a conditioning TMS pulse has the largest effect on motor-evoked potentials induced by a test TMS pulse is shown to be around 10 ms. By contrast, when the latency of stimulus-induced activation or stimulus-induced modulation of activation is used, the signal conduction time can be estimated to be around 15–30 ms. We consider that the difference is due to the way to measure the effect of stimulation: Changes in cortical excitability as assessed by response to a test pulse TMS can be observed at an earlier timing, whereas the peak of induced response as measured by EEG or ECoG is observed at a later timing. Had we been able to identify the onset of the stimulus-induced response, the signal transmission time based on TME-EPs can be estimated to be shorter.

Thirdly, the TMS-EEG technique allows us to examine the neural network state at a particular time point during cognitive process, that is, at the time point when TMS is given. By varying the timing of TMS relative to an experimental event, we are able to examine dynamic changes in the network connectivity with high temporal resolution. Because of these advantages, there is a possibility that the TMS-EEG technique is more sensitive to the change in the state of neural network than conventional analysis of regional activation. It could be that temporally- dynamic changes in neural activation may not be reflected in the temporally integrated signals such as BOLD signal of fMRI. The benefit of the high temporal resolution in TMS-EEG can be exploited further by appropriate statistical techniques. A large number of data points in the time domain are associated with an increase in false positive results. In the present study, we overcome this problem using Random Field Theory (Worsley et al., 1996).

METHODOLOGICAL WEAKNESS

The TMS-EEG technique has some weakness as well. First of all, the signal induced by TMS is artificial and we do not know if the physiological neural impulses are transmitted across cortical regions in the same way as the TMS-induced signals. Only when the pattern of TMS-induced activation can be shown to be associated with behavior, we can make an argument that the effective connectivity from the stimulated region to the distant region has functional significance and may be associated with physiological mechanism of the network. The generator mechanism for the TMS-induced signals also remains open. Based on the analysis of D- and I-waves (direct and indirect waves) recorded from the hand muscle or spinal cord elicited by M1 stimulation, it is thought that a low-intensity single-pulse TMS initially excites afferent fibers connected to the neurons in the stimulated region (Ziemann and Rothwell, 2000). A large-scale modeling study has shown a more detailed picture for the effect of TMS on local neural circuits within M1 (Esser et al., 2005). First, a TMS pulse directly activates cortical fiber terminals, and induces spiking activity in both excitatory and inhibitory neurons in all cortical layers. The excitatory and inhibitory currents thus induced results in firing of excitatory neurons in layer 5 via synapses made by neurons from layer 2/3. Layer 5 neurons respond to this net depolarization with one to 3 more spikes, which are timed by their intrinsic neuronal properties. It remains open how such a sequence of physiological events changes according to the properties of neural circuits in regions other than M1. It also remains open how this sequence of events interact with the state of circuit at the time of TMS. The cascade of physiological events within the neural circuit elicited by TMS may change depending on the stage of computational processing within the circuit at which a TMS pulse is given. This results in a change in the pattern of TMS-EPs as we have shown in the present study. The underlying neural mechanisms remain open to future studies.

Second point of the weakness of the TME-EEG technique is low S/N ratio. Especially when we examine task-related modulation of the TMS-EPs, the amount of modulation is around 1 μV and we need to average a sufficient number of trials to recover the signal. In the present study, for example, a better way to test the effect of Time-to-Response is to use the real value of the Time-to-Response as a continuous variable and examine the parametric modulation of the TMS-EPs. We were unable to conduct such analysis because of the low S/N ratio of the TMS-EPs, and instead classified trials into binary category of Early and Late. This issue is also related to the limitation of our analysis time windows based on the single unit firing data obtained from monkeys. The timing of neuronal firing in the human brain may differ from that in monkeys, which could have been examined had we been able to examine the TMS-EP data for a narrower time window at multiple time points during the decision process. In addition, we used unusually short pre-stimulus period of 4 ms as the reference for baseline correction. This was to align the amplitude of EEG at the time of TMS at the zero point, but because this duration was arbitrarily chosen this procedure does not guarantee the reliability of obtained results. We need to establish methods for selecting an appropriate pre-TMS epoch for baseline correction and for selecting corresponding epochs of No-TMS trials for comparison, especially when we examine the time varying nature of the TMS-EPs.

Third problem is the ambiguity in localizing the induced activation. Using EEG as a means to record the TMS-induced activation is advantageous in identifying short-latency responses, but spatial localization of the induced activation needs to be analyzed with several assumptions. In the present study, we were unable to identify specific cortical regions in which the TMS-induced activation is modulated by the experimental factors. Concurrent use of TMS-fMRI could be another option to localize the induced activation, which also allows us to examine induced activation in subcortical structures. We, however, lose temporal resolution with fMRI and we are unable to make inference about the efficacy of signal transmission across regions. EEG, on the other hand, allows us to make inference about an early effect of induced signal transmission, but there might be earlier cortico-cortical signal transmission which cannot be detected using the time window of 20–40 ms after TMS. In the stimulated region, the peak of the activation can be observed at 7–9 ms after the onset of the TMS pulse (Ilmoniemi et al., 1997; Rogasch and Fitzgerald, 2013), and it is likely that neural signals are already transmitted to other cortical regions by that time.

EFFECT OF TIME-TO-RESPONSE AND ACCUMULATION OF INFORMATION

We found significant changes in the TMS-EPs in FEF stimulation depending on the timing of TMS relative to subsequent behavioral response (**Figure 2C** left). Such co-variation with time is consistent with the findings of previous single unit recording studies showing build-up of neural discharge in the FEF, which has been taken to reflect the amount of accumulated sensory evidence used for decision making (Kim and Shadlen, 1999; Ding and Gold, 2012). It is also possible that time-dependent modulation of TMS-EPs of FEF stimulation reflects build-up of motor responses. In contrast to the effect of Time-to-Response, the pattern of TMS-EP after FEF stimulation did not change depending on whether the behavioral response on that trial was correct or error (**Figure 2D** left), which suggests that the state of FEF neural network reflects the amount of accumulated information regardless of whether subsequent action is based on relevant sensory information or not. Importantly, what we have shown here is the time-dependent modulation in the pattern of signal transmission induced by FEF stimulation, which may reflect changes in the influence from the FEF over other cortical regions. In order to examine temporal dynamics in regional activation using fMRI, the behavioral paradigm has to be set up to allow longer time periods for information accumulation (Ploran et al., 2007). In contrast, the ability of TMS-EEG to examine the network state at a specific time point allows us to test the time-varying nature of the network connectivity such as the network dynamics during fast accumulation processes in decision making.

EFFECT OF ACCURACY AND SELECTION OF TASK-RELEVANT INFORMATION

In the PFv stimulation experiment, TMS-EPs changed depending on whether the behavioral response on that trial was correct or error (**Figure 2D** right). Essential for accurate perceptual decision making is the selection of choice-relevant sensory information. It has been shown that in a visual motion discrimination task, signals from different motion directions are used for decision depending on whether the subject performs a coarse or fine motion discrimination task (Jazayeri and Movshon, 2006). It has also been shown that neurons in the PFv show task-dependent changes in firing rate (Zaksas and Pasternak, 2006; Hussar and Pasternak, 2009), suggesting that these neurons may send task-related selection signals to sensory areas. Our result is consistent with the idea that PFv is involved in selection of choice-relevant information because the network state of the PFv reflects whether the task-relevant sensory information drives the action selection or not in a given trial.

We have also shown that stimulation of the PFv induced activation in the MT (**Figure 4**), which is consistent with the idea that the PFv sends selection signals to the region involved in processing of task-relevant sensory information. The connection between the PFv and MT has been verified anatomically (Schall et al., 1995). It has also been reported in a fMRI study that a region in the inferior frontal sulcus, which is close to the PFv in the present study, exert causal influence on MT during motion discrimination task for random dot motion with distracting visual features (Kayser et al., 2010).

Additionally, the TMS-EPs after PFv stimulation was not modulated by Time-to-Response (**Figure 2C** right), but was modulated by Time-from-Stimulus (**Figure 3B**), which suggests that the state of the PFv network is associated with sensory information processing rather than response generation. The main effect of Time-from-Stimulus, however, can be confounded by the build-up of the subjects' expectancy for a TMS pulse. Such expectancy should exist commonly for FEF stimulation and PFv stimulation conditions, and we indeed found a significant effect of Time-from-Stimulus for both conditions. The TMS-EPs after PFv stimulation, however, did not change depending on stimulus strength (**Figure 3A**), suggesting that the PFv does not merely represent the externally-provided sensory information.

DISSOCIATION AND CONVERGENCE BETWEEN THE DORSAL AND VENTRAL NETWORKS

The major finding in the present study is the double dissociation between the FEF and PFv networks. The two networks show significant modulation due to one of the two experimental factors without significant interaction between the two factors (**Figures 2C–E**). This procedure of testing the effects of two independent factors in a 2 × 2 design is comparable to the conventional analysis of fMRI-based regional activation, but here it is the neural network connectivity that has been examined. Segregation in the functional roles between the FEF and PFv networks, however, does not necessarily exclude the possibility of interaction between them. We in fact found that the two prefrontal networks converge at common regions in the medial and lateral prefrontal cortices (**Figure 4**), which can be taken to suggest integration of information processed in the FEF and PFv. The TMS-EEG did not show induced activation in all of the anatomically-connected regions after stimulation of FEF and PFv. For example, the FEF and PFv are shown to be anatomically connected with each other (Stanton et al., 1995; Gerbella et al., 2010), but we failed to identify short-latency signal transmission between the two regions. This is probably because the technique allows us to identify only those regions that are functionally connected with the stimulated region in a given task. Since the TMS-EEG technique allows us to make inference about the efficacy of signal transmission from the stimulated region, the regions we have identified, i.e., MT for PFv stimulation and DLPFC and preSMA/SEF for both stimulations, may be regarded as the target regions that receive efferent signals from the FEF and PFv during perceptual decision making.

It is possible that TMS may have stimulated the head skin and induced different patterns of somatosensory-evoked potentials (SEPs) depending on the stimulation site. The distance between the stimulation sites, however, was less than 5 cm. We do not think that such a small difference in somatotopic representation within the head can account for the distinct patterns of TMS-EPs between FEF and PFv stimulation as reported in **Figure 2A**. Also the activation induced by TMS over FEF and PFv was not observed in somatosensory areas, but rather in regions anatomically connected with the FEF and PFv (**Figure 4**). We thus consider that the dissociation in the patterns of evoked potentials between the FEF and PFv stimulation reflects the difference in the stimulated cortical regions rather than the difference in stimulated head skin regions. We do accept that the TMS-EPs for each stimulation site may contain a component of SEP, but this would not affect our main conclusion about the dissociation.

In sum, the modulation of the TMS-EPs induced by FEF stimulation by the factor of Time-to-Response is consistent with the idea that the FEF is involved in accumulation of information, whereas the modulation of the TMS-EPs induced by PFv stimulation by the factor of Accuracy is consistent with the idea that the PFv is involved in selection of information. Absence of significant interactions between the two factors for both FEF stimulation and PFv stimulation suggests that the processes of accumulation and selection of information work in parallel during decision making. The overlap of cortical regions in which activation is induced by FEF and PFv stimulations may suggest that the two processes are integrated in medial and lateral prefrontal regions to generate behavioral response. The present study also highlights the feasibility of characterizing the computational processes subserved by a network connected with a particular brain region. What remains open is the mechanism of the modulation of neural network connectivity. It has been suggested that low-intensity TMS as we used in the present study primarily activates the afferent fibers that are connected to the neurons in the stimulated region, which then activates those neurons that project to other regions (Esser et al., 2005). Modulation of the TMS-EPs may thus reflect changes in the balance between the excitatory and inhibitory activity of neurons within the stimulated region (Silvanto et al., 2008; Pasley et al., 2009). Another possibility is that the modulation occurs at the regions that receive signals from the stimulated region. More specifically it may be due to the change in the efficacy of synaptic transmission within the target regions that receive inputs from the stimulated region. In either case, the modulation of TMS-EPs can be taken to reflect the state of neural network and its association with experimental or behavioral factors allows us to make inference about the computational processes performed in the neural network connected with a particular region.

AUTHOR CONTRIBUTIONS

Rei Akaishi planned, designed and conducted the experiments. Naoko Ueda helped conducting experiments. Rei Akaishi and Katsuyuki Sakai analyzed the data and wrote the paper.

ACKNOWLEDGMENTS

This study was supported by a Funding Program for Next Generation World-Leading Researchers from the Japan Society for the Promotion of Science (JSPS), and a research grant from Takeda Science Foundation. Rei Akaishi was supported by Research Fellowship of the JSPS.

REFERENCES

Akaishi, R., Morishima, Y., Rajeswaren, V. P., Aoki, S., and Sakai, K. (2010). Stimulation of the frontal eye field reveals persistent effective connectivity after controlled behavior. *J. Neurosci.* 30, 4295–4305. doi: 10.1523/JNEUROSCI.6198-09.2010

Binder, J. R., Liebenthal, E., Possing, E. T., Medler, D. A., and Ward, B. D. (2004). Neural correlates of sensory and decision processes in auditory object identification. *Nat. Neurosci.* 7, 295–301. doi: 10.1038/nn1198

Blanke, O., Spinelli, L., Thut, G., Michel, C. M., Perrig, S., Landis, T., et al. (2000). Location of the human frontal eye field as defined by electrical cortical stimulation: anatomical, functional and electrophysiological characteristics. *Neuroreport* 11, 1907–1913. doi: 10.1097/00001756-200006260-00021

Corbetta, M., and Shulman, G. L. (2002). Control of goal-directed and stimulus-driven attention in the brain. *Nat. Rev. Neurosci.* 3, 201–215. doi: 10.1038/nrn755

Daskalakis, Z. J., Farzan, F., Radhu, N., and Fitzgerald, P. B. (2012). Combined transcranial magnetic stimulation and electroencephalography: its past, present and future. *Brain Res.* 1463, 93–107. doi: 10.1016/j.brainres.2012.04.045

Ding, L., and Gold, J. I. (2012). Neural correlates of perceptual decision making before, during, and after decision commitment in monkey frontal eye field. *Cereb. Cortex* 22, 1052–1067. doi: 10.1093/cercor/bhr178

Driver, J., Blankenburg, F., Bestmann, S., Vanduffel, W., and Ruff, C. C. (2009). Concurrent brain-stimulation and neuroimaging for studies of cognition. *Trends Cogn. Sci.* 13, 319–327. doi: 10.1016/j.tics.2009.04.007

Esser, S. K., Hill, S. L., and Tononi, G. (2005). Modeling the effects of transcranial magnetic stimulation on cortical circuits. *J. Neurophysiol.* 94, 622–639. doi: 10.1152/jn.01230.2004

Esser, S. K., Hill, S., and Tononi, G. (2009). Breakdown of effective connectivity during slow wave sleep: investigating the mechanism underlying a cortical gate using large-scale modeling. *J. Neurophysiol.* 102, 2096–2111. doi: 10.1152/jn.00059.2009

Gerbella, M., Belmalith, A., Borra, E., Rozzi, S., and Luppino, G. (2010). Cortical connections of the macaque caudal ventrolateral prefrontal areas 45A and 45B. *Cereb. Cortex* 20, 141–168. doi: 10.1093/cercor/bhp087

Gold, J. I., and Shadlen, M. N. (2007). The neural basis of decision making. *Annu. Rev. Neurosci.* 30, 535–574. doi: 10.1146/annurev.neuro.29.051605.113038

Grosbras, M.-H., Laird, A., and Paus, T. (2005). Human cortical regions involved in gaze production, attention shifts and gaze perception: a brain imaging meta-analysis. *Hum. Brain Mapp.* 25, 140–154. doi: 10.1002/hbm.20145

Heekeren, H. R., Marrett, S., Ruff, D. A., Bandettini, P. A., and Ungerleider, L. G. (2006). Involvement of human left dorsolateral prefrontal cortex in perceptual decision making is independent of response modality. *Proc. Natl. Acad. Sci. U.S.A.* 103, 10023–10028. doi: 10.1073/pnas.0603949103

Heekeren, H. R., Marrett, S., and Ungerleider, L. G. (2008). The neural systems that mediate human perceptual decision making. *Nat. Rev. Neurosci.* 9, 467–479. doi: 10.1038/nrn2374

Hussar, C. R., and Pasternak, T. (2009) Flexibility of sensory representations in prefrontal cortex depends on cell type. *Neuron* 64, 730–743. doi: 10.1016/j.neuron.2009.11.018

Ilmoniemi, R. J., Virtanen, J., Ruohonen, J., Karhu, J., Aronen, H. J., Näätänen, R., et al. (1997). Neuronal responses to magnetic stimulation reveal cortical reactivity and connectivity. *Neuroreport* 8, 3537–3540. doi: 10.1097/00001756-199711100-00024

Jazayeri, M., and Movshon, J. A. (2006). Optimal representation of sensory information by neural populations. *Nat. Neurosci.* 9, 690–696. doi: 10.1038/nn1691

Kayser, A. S., Erickson, D. T., Buchsbaum, B. R., and D'Esposito, M. (2010). Neural representations of relevant and irrelevant features in perceptual decision making. *J. Neurosci.* 30, 15778–15789. doi: 10.1523/JNEUROSCI.3163-10.2010

Kim, J. N., and Shadlen, M. N. (1999). Neural correlates of a decision in the dorsolateral prefrontal cortex of the macaque. *Nat. Neurosci.* 2, 176–185. doi: 10.1038/5739

Komssi, S., and Kähkönen, S. (2006). The novelty value of the combined use of electroencephalography and transcranial magnetic stimulation for neuroscience research. *Brain Res. Rev.* 52, 183–192. doi: 10.1016/j.brainresrev.2006.01.008

Koyama, M., Hasegawa, I., Osada, T., Adachi, Y., Nakahara, K., and Miyashita, Y. (2004). Functional magnetic resonance imaging of macaque monkeys performing visually guided saccade tasks: comparison of cortical eye fields with humans. *Neuron* 41, 795–807. doi: 10.1016/S0896-6273(04)00047-9

Liu, T., and Pleskac, T. J. (2011). Neural correlates of evidence accumulation in a perceptual decision task. *J. Neurophysiol.* 106, 2383–2398. doi: 10.1152/jn.00413.2011

Lobel, E., Kahane, P., Leonards, U., Grosbras, M., Lehéricy, S., Le Bihan, D., et al. (2001). Localization of human frontal eye fields: anatomical and functional findings of functional magnetic resonance imaging and intracerebral electrical stimulation. *J. Neurosurg.* 95, 804–815. doi: 10.3171/jns.2001.95.5.0804

Massimini, M., Ferrarelli, F., Huber, R., Esser, S. K., Singh, H., and Tononi, G. (2005). Breakdown of cortical effective connectivity during sleep. *Science* 309, 2228–2232. doi: 10.1126/science.1117256

Matsumoto, R., Nair, D. R., LaPresto, E., Bingaman, W., Shibasaki, H., Lüders, H. O. (2007). Functional connectivity in human cortical motor system: a cortico-cortical evoked potential study. *Brain* 130, 181–197. doi: 10.1093/brain/awl257

Miniussi, C., and Thut, G. (2010). Combining TMS and EEG offers new prospects in cognitive neuroscience. *Brain Topogr.* 22, 249–256. doi: 10.1007/s10548-009-0083-8

Morishima, Y., Akaishi, R., Yamada, Y., Okuda, J., Toma, K., Sakai, K. (2009). Task-specific signal transmission from prefrontal cortex in visual selective attention. *Nat. Neurosci.* 12, 85–91. doi: 10.1038/nn.2237

Pascual-Marqui, R. D. (2002). Standardized low-resolution brain electromagnetic tomography (sLORETA): technical details. *Methods Find. Exp. Clin. Pharmacol.* 24(Suppl. D), 5–12.

Pasley, B. N., Allen, E. A., and Freeman, R. D. (2009). State-dependent variability of neuronal responses to transcranial magnetic stimulation of the visual cortex. *Neuron* 62, 291–303. doi: 10.1016/j.neuron.2009.03.012

Paus, T. (1996). Location and function of the human frontal eye-field: a selective review. *Neuropsychologia* 34, 475–483. doi: 10.1016/0028-3932(95)00134-4

Pelli, D. G. (1985). Uncertainty explains many aspects of visual contrast detection and discrimination. *J. Opt. Soc. Am. A* 2, 1508–1532. doi: 10.1364/JOSAA.2.001508

Pessoa, L., and Padmala, S. (2005). Quantitative prediction of perceptual decisions during near-threshold fear detection. *Proc. Natl. Acad. Sci. U.S.A.* 102, 5612–5617. doi: 10.1073/pnas.0500566102

Ploran, E. J., Nelson, S. M., Velanova, K., Donaldson, D. I., Petersen, S. E., and Wheeler, M. E. (2007). Evidence accumulation and the moment of recognition: dissociating perceptual recognition processes using fMRI. *J. Neurosci.* 27, 11912–11924. doi: 10.1523/JNEUROSCI.3522-07.2007

Reithler, J., Peters, J. C., and Sack, A. T. (2011). Multimodal transcranial magnetic stimulation: using concurrent neuroimaging to reveal the neural network dynamics of noninvasive brain stimulation. *Prog. Neurobiol.* 94, 149–165. doi: 10.1016/j.pneurobio.2011.04.004

Rogasch, N. C., and Fitzgerald, P. B. (2013). Assessing cortical network properties using TMS-EEG. *Hum. Brain Mapp.* 34, 1652–1669. doi: 10.1002/hbm.22016

Schall, J. D., Morel, A., King, D. J., and Bullier, J. (1995). Topography of visual cortex connections with frontal eye field in macaque: convergence and segregation of processing streams. *J. Neurosci.* 15, 4464–4467.

Shadlen, M. N., Britten, K. H., Newsome, W. T., and Movshon, J. A. (1996). A computational analysis of the relationship between neuronal and behavioral responses to visual motion. *J. Neurosci.* 16, 1486–1510.

Siebner, H. R., Bergmann, T. O., Bestmann, S., Massimini, M., Johansen-Berg, H., Mochizuki, H., et al. (2009). Consensus paper: combining transcranial stimulation with neuroimaging. *Brain Stimul.* 2, 58–80. doi: 10.1016/j.brs.2008.11.002

Silvanto, J., Lavie, N., and Walsh, V. (2006). Stimulation of the human frontal eye fields modulates sensitivity of extrastriate visual cortex. *J. Neurophysiol.* 96, 941–945. doi: 10.1152/jn.00015.2006

Silvanto, J., Muggleton, N., and Walsh, V. (2008). State-dependency in brain stimulation studies of perception and cognition. *Trends Cogn. Sci.* 12, 447–454. doi: 10.1016/j.tics.2008.09.004

Stanton, G. B., Bruce, C. J., and Goldberg, M. E. (1995). Topography of projections to posterior cortical areas from the macaque frontal eye fields. *J. Comp. Neurol.* 353, 291–305. doi: 10.1002/cne.903530210

Stephan, K. E., and Roebroeck, A. (2012). A short history of causal modeling of fMRI data. *Neuroimage* 62, 856–863. doi: 10.1016/j.neuroimage.2012.01.034

Thielscher, A., and Pessoa, L. (2007). Neural correlates of perceptual choice and decision making during fear disgust discrimination. *J. Neurosci.* 27, 2908–2917. doi: 10.1523/JNEUROSCI.3024-06.2007

Veniero, D., Maioli, C., and Miniussi, C. (2010). Potentiation of short-latency cortical responses by high-frequency repetitive transcranial magnetic stimulation. *J. Neurophysiol.* 104, 1578–1588. doi: 10.1152/jn.00172.2010

Worsley, K. J., Marrett, S., Neelin, P., Vandal, A. C., Friston, K. J., and Evans, A. C. (1996). A unified statistical approach for determining significant signals in images of cerebral activation. *Hum. Brain Mapp.* 4, 58–73.

Zaksas, D., and Pasternak, T. (2006). Directional signals in the prefrontal cortex and in area MT during a working memory for visual motion task. *J. Neurosci.* 26, 11726–11742. doi: 10.1523/JNEUROSCI.3420-06.2006

Ziemann, U., and Rothwell, J. C. (2000). I-waves in motor cortex. *J. Clin. Neurophysiol.* 17, 397–405. doi: 10.1097/00004691-200007000-00005

5

TMS-evoked changes in brain-state dynamics quantified by using EEG data

Tuomas Mutanen[1,2]*, Jaakko O. Nieminen[1,2] and Risto J. Ilmoniemi[1,2]

[1] Department of Biomedical Engineering and Computational Science, Aalto University School of Science, Espoo, Finland
[2] BioMag Laboratory, HUSLAB, Helsinki University Central Hospital, Helsinki, Finland

Correspondence:
Tuomas Mutanen, Department of Biomedical Engineering and Computational Science, Aalto University School of Science, P.O. Box 12200, FI-00076 AALTO, Finland.
e-mail: tuomas.mutanen@aalto.fi

To improve our understanding of the combined transcranial magnetic stimulation (TMS) and electroencephalography (EEG) method in general, it is important to study how the dynamics of the TMS-modulated brain activity differs from the dynamics of spontaneous activity. In this paper, we introduce two quantitative measures based on EEG data, called mean state shift (MSS) and state variance (SV), for evaluating the TMS-evoked changes in the brain-state dynamics. MSS quantifies the immediate TMS-elicited change in the brain state, whereas SV shows whether the rate at which the brain state changes is modulated by TMS. We report a statistically significant increase for a period of 100–200 ms after the TMS pulse in both MSS and SV at the group level. This indicates that the TMS-modulated brain state differs from the spontaneous one. Moreover, the TMS-modulated activity is more vigorous than the natural activity.

Keywords: TMS, EEG, state space, brain dynamics, trajectory, recurrence quantification analysis

1. INTRODUCTION

Combined transcranial magnetic stimulation (TMS) and electroencephalography (EEG) is able to probe the dynamics of the effective connectivity of the brain. Using TMS–EEG it has been possible to show how the activation induced on one hemisphere advances to the contralateral side (Komssi et al., 2002). TMS–EEG can also be used to study the effect of the brain state on the dynamics of excitability: Nikulin et al. (2003) showed that voluntary preparation for hand movement changes the EEG responses evoked by stimulating the primary motor cortex. Massimini et al. (2005) showed that changes in the state of consciousness affect the effective connectivity. Huber et al. (2013) studied the effect of lack of sleep on cortical excitability, demonstrating increased TMS-evoked EEG responses with prolonged wakefulness.

Furthermore, TMS can be used to modulate brain dynamics. Combined TMS–EEG studies have shown that even a single TMS pulse is able to induce changes in the frequency spectrum of brain activity (Paus et al., 2001; Fuggetta et al., 2005; Rosanova et al., 2009). Using preparatory repetitive TMS (rTMS), it has been possible to modulate subsequent single-pulse TMS–EEG responses. Van Der Werf and Paus (2006) showed that facilitatory rTMS at 0.6 Hz on the primary motor cortex had a significant increasing effect on the subsequent N45 deflections. Similarly, Esser et al. (2006) showed that by applying rTMS on the primary motor cortex at 5 Hz, it is possible to significantly potentiate single-pulse deflections with latencies of 15–55 ms. Recently, frequency-tuned rhythmic TMS has been shown to selectively bias perception (Romei et al., 2010) via entrainment of ongoing oscillatory activity (Thut et al., 2011).

However, the differences between pre- and post-TMS activity, i.e., how a single TMS pulse affects concurrent brain dynamics, have not been well characterized. One difficulty in analyzing changes from pre- to post-TMS brain state is that at the trial level the TMS-evoked changes are masked by spontaneous background activity. Furthermore, the spontaneous activity varies from one trial to another.

In this paper, we introduce two quantitative recurrence measures called mean state shift (MSS) and state variance (SV). They can be computed from unaveraged EEG signals and averaged afterwards to show possible changes in the brain dynamics due to TMS. The particular interest of the present work is to study the effects of TMS on the brain state. We use TMS–EEG data to show that TMS, indeed, has a significant effect on both MSS and SV.

2. MATERIALS AND METHODS

2.1. CONNECTION BETWEEN THE BRAIN STATE AND TMS–EEG

The current distribution $\mathbf{J}(\mathbf{r}, t)$ in the brain is often expressed in two parts:

$$\mathbf{J}(\mathbf{r}, t) = \mathbf{J}^{\mathrm{p}}(\mathbf{r}, t) + \mathbf{J}^{\mathrm{v}}(\mathbf{r}, t), \tag{1}$$

where $\mathbf{J}^{\mathrm{p}}$ is the primary current density arising from the bioelectric activation of neurons (e.g., post-synaptic currents), $\mathbf{J}^{\mathrm{v}}$ is the volume current density, $\mathbf{r}$ is the position, and t is the time. $\mathbf{J}^{\mathrm{v}}$ is passive, ohmic current density driven by $\mathbf{J}^{\mathrm{p}}$ (Malmivuo and Plonsey, 1995) (**Figure 1A**).

$\mathbf{J}^{\mathrm{p}}$ can be thought of as the primary source creating all the current density, which in turn affects the charge distribution that defines the electric potential. Hence, the EEG signal, i.e., the voltage, measured by channel j can be expressed as

$$X_j(t) = \int \mathbf{L}_j(\mathbf{r}') \cdot \mathbf{J}^{\mathrm{p}}(\mathbf{r}', t) dv', \tag{2}$$

where $\mathbf{L}_j(\mathbf{r})$ is the lead field determined by the geometry of the measurement set-up and the conductivity of the head (Ilmoniemi

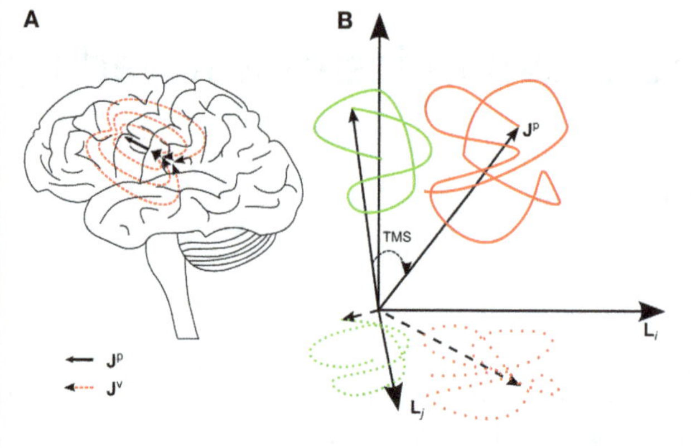

FIGURE 1 | (A) The black arrow represents one primary current source, a flow of ions in synapses in the left primary motor cortex. The dashed red lines represent the returning volume current. $\mathbf{J}^p(\mathbf{r})$ describes the whole primary current distribution in the brain. **(B)** A schematic image of the hypothesis concerning the effect of TMS on the brain state. The green and red curves correspond to pre- and post-TMS brain-state trajectories, respectively. The spontaneous activity draws a trajectory in a certain region. TMS shifts the brain state to a new region in the state space. Furthermore, the brain state fluctuates more after TMS because of the increased free energy until the state gradually returns to the original set of spontaneous states. The projection of these effects can be seen in the EEG signal space, spanned by channels *i* and *j*. In the signal space, the trajectories are measured only at discrete time points, which is emphasized with dotted curves.

and Kičić, 2010). In other words, $\mathbf{L}_j(\mathbf{r})$ describes how efficiently channel *j* detects primary current at $\mathbf{r}$.

Thus, EEG can be considered the measurement of the projection of the primary current density on the signal space, the projection being defined by the lead fields of the channels. Since the primary current density describes accurately the electric state of the brain, the EEG signal can be considered a projection of the electric brain state. As $\mathbf{J}^p(\mathbf{r}, t)$, i.e., the state of the brain, changes, it draws a trajectory in the multidimensional state space. The trajectory is also projected on the EEG signal space (**Figure 1B**).

On the other hand, TMS can be used to modulate $\mathbf{J}^p$. In the brain, the changing magnetic field induces an electric field, which elicits action potentials in the axons. When action potentials reach synapses, post-synaptic currents that are visible in the EEG signal are created.

Our hypothesis is that TMS moves the brain higher in the energy landscape (here the energy landscape describes the tendency of the system to go from low probability to high probability states; from high energy to low energy) reflecting the information processing system. Hence the TMS-modulated activity at the stimulation site is seen in the brain state trajectory as a sudden shift to a new region in the state space (**Figure 1B**), which is spontaneously occupied only with a small probability. We test this hypothesis directly by measuring MSS, which quantifies the mean distance between the brain states from two different time intervals. According to the hypothesis, it is expected that due to TMS there is a transient increase in MSS with respect to the baseline.

If the state of the brain is higher in the energy landscape, it means increased free energy for the brain to act. The brain tends to minimize the free energy and get closer to some local energy minimum leading to enhanced fluctuation after TMS. This fluctuation is quantified using SV, which we expect to be increased until the system is closer to spontaneously probable states.

If the changes in the trajectory due to a single TMS pulse are large enough, they could also be visible in the obtained EEG signal. Since the EEG signal is a low-dimensional projection of the original primary current distribution, any significant difference between the signal vectors also indicates a difference in the original state vectors.

2.2. DATA USED

We used 16 TMS–EEG datasets from our database to characterize TMS-elicited changes in the brain activity. The datasets had been measured from healthy subjects (six males and four females; age varied between 24 and 28 years) who gave their written consent before the experiments. The measurements had been approved by the Ethics Committee of the Hospital District of Helsinki and Uusimaa and they followed the Declaration of Helsinki.

In all datasets, TMS stimuli were given with the same Nexstim eXimia system using a figure-of-eight coil with the outer loop diameter of 70 mm. The stimuli were targeted to the right hand area at the left primary motor cortex. Similarly, the TMS-compatible EEG device (Nexstim eXimia) was the same in all datasets. All the electrodes were prepared so that their impedances were below 5 kΩ. Additionally, two electrodes were attached close to the eyes to record ocular artifacts. The EEG sampling frequency was 1450 Hz.

The datasets were chosen based on the overall signal quality, i.e., low muscle- (Mutanen et al., 2012) and ocular-artifact (Ilmoniemi and Kičić, 2010) levels. The data acquisition and timing paradigms varied slightly across the analyzed datasets which ensures that our findings can be generalized over different measurement set-ups. The details of the measurement paradigms and exceptions are provided in **Table 1**.

To see the possible changes more clearly, only 12 channels close to the stimulus location were used to form the signal subspace under study. Hence, only channels Fc_5, Fc_3, Fc_1, Fc_z, C_5, C_3, C_1, C_z, Cp_5, Cp_3, Cp_1, and Cp_z according to the international 10–20 system were studied.

2.3. COMPUTING MEAN STATE SHIFT AND STATE VARIANCE

Recurrence analysis was introduced by Eckmann et al. (1987) to qualitatively analyze state-space trajectories in order to characterize different dynamical systems. Recurrence analysis describes how often and for how long a certain physical state occurs. The basic idea is simple. An appropriate threshold is first chosen. If the distance between two states is smaller than the threshold value, the state vectors are considered to represent the same state. In EEG studies, recurrence analysis has been used to study, for instance, neurological disorders (e.g., Babloyantz, 1991; Pijn et al., 1997; Ouyang et al., 2008).

To provide quantitative results, several recurrence quantification analysis (RQA) measures, such as recurrence density, determinism, and entropy, have been introduced (Marwan et al., 2007). Strictly speaking, our measures do not fall under RQA category since we do not have any fixed threshold. Instead,

Table 1 | The measurement parameters in different datasets.

Dataset	Stimulation target	Intensity [MT]%	Noise masking	ISI [s]	Number of stimuli	Coil type
1	APB	100	Yes	2–3	100	monophasic
2	APB	100	Yes	2–3	100	monophasic
3	ADM	100	Yes	2–3	259	monophasic
4	APB	100	Yes	2–3	113	monophasic
5	APB	110	No	2–3	100	biphasic
6	APB	110	No	2–3	100	biphasic
7	APB	90	No	1, 3, or 5	376	monophasic
8	APB	90	No	1, 3, or 5	306	monophasic
9	APB	90	No	1, 3, or 5	326	monophasic
10	M1	<100	No	2–3	60	monophasic
11	ADM	100	No	2–3	89	monophasic
12	APB	100	Yes	2–3	115	monophasic
13	ADM	100	Yes	2–3	60	monophasic
14	ADM	100	Yes	2–3	60	monophasic
15	ADM	100	Yes	2–3	60	monophasic
16	APB	100	Yes	2–3	60	monophasic

Stimulation target refers to the cortical area controlling the named muscle (abductor pollicis brevis or abductor digiti minimi). In dataset 10, no hand muscle areas were found and stimulation was given to area usually responsible for controlling the right hand. The stimulus intensities are given with respect to the resting motor threshold (MT) intensity. When noise masking was given, it was adjusted until the subject reported to not hearing the click. Interstimulus interval (ISI) either varied randomly between 2 and 3 s or among 1, 3, and 5 s.

we describe the obtained data by measuring average distances between state vectors. This is sometimes referred to as global recurrence (Marwan et al., 2007) or unthresholded recurrence analysis (Iwanski and Bradley, 1998; Marwan et al., 2007). However, the lack of a threshold value makes our measures more robust since one does not have to choose any arbitrary threshold. To our knowledge, RQA has not been previously applied to TMS–EEG data.

Let us now have a trajectory $\mathscr{X}$ of a system drawn in the state space, or as in our case, drawn in the EEG signal space that is a projection of the original state space. The measured trajectory consists of signal vectors at discrete time points t_l:

$$\mathscr{X} = \{\mathbf{X}(t_l) \mid t_l = t_1, t_2, \ldots, t_n\}. \tag{3}$$

The signal vector at time t_l is defined as

$$\mathbf{X}(t_l) = [X_1(t_l), X_2(t_l), \ldots, X_D(t_l)]^{\mathrm{T}}, \tag{4}$$

where D is the dimension of the signal space, defined by the number of channels, and X_j is the signal measured by channel j, defined in Equation 2.

As the name implies, MSS describes the mean distance between state vectors belonging to two different time intervals:

$$\mathrm{MSS} \equiv \mathrm{MSS}(T_l, T_k) = \frac{1}{N_l N_k} \sum_{t_l \in T_l} \sum_{t_k \in T_k} \|\mathbf{X}(t_l) - \mathbf{X}(t_k)\|, \tag{5}$$

where $\| \bullet \|$ is the Euclidean distance, and T_l and T_k are time intervals consisting of N_l and N_k discrete time points, respectively. Additionally, in this paper, $T_l \cap T_k = \emptyset$ and $N_l = N_k$. The purpose of MSS is to show whether there is a more dramatic average change in the state due to TMS than due to the normal fluctuations in time. Hence, MSS quantifies the immediate effect of TMS on the brain state.

On the other hand, SV measures the rate at which the state changes during a given time interval. It is anticipated that the motion of the state would be more vigorous right after the TMS pulse than before it because of the locally higher free energy which the system tends to minimize. SV is defined as:

$$\mathrm{SV} \equiv \mathrm{SV}(T_l) = \frac{1}{N_l} \sum_{t_l \in T_l} \|\mathbf{X}(t_l) - \bar{\mathbf{X}}(T_l)\|^2, \tag{6}$$

where

$$\bar{\mathbf{X}}(T_l) = \frac{1}{N_l} \sum_{t_l \in T_l} \mathbf{X}(t_l). \tag{7}$$

Conventionally, TMS-evoked potentials are made visible in the EEG by performing several trials and averaging the responses afterwards (e.g., Komssi et al., 2002; Massimini et al., 2005; Lioumis et al., 2009). This is done to suppress the background activity that masks the TMS-evoked potentials. However, it is difficult to design a method to average both the pre- and post-TMS intervals over trials to show the TMS-evoked changes in the activity. Therefore, pre- and post-TMS activity are ideally compared at the trial level. Unfortunately, the changes due to TMS at the trial level are subtle (Mäki and Ilmoniemi, 2010). One benefit of MSS and SV is that they can be computed from trial-level data and averaged later on to highlight the TMS-elicited changes.

2.4. ANALYZING THE EFFECT OF TMS ON MSS AND SV

Before any further data analysis, all the datasets were visually inspected. Bad EEG channels and any trials contaminated by ocular artifacts were removed. The data were also band-pass filtered to 2–80 Hz using a second-order Butterworth filter.

Both MSS and SV were calculated from unaveraged trial-level data. Each accepted trial from each dataset was divided into five different time intervals: $T_1 = [-200, -100]$, $T_2 = [-100, 0]$, $T_3 = [15, 115]$, $T_4 = [115, 215]$, and $T_5 = [215, 315]$, where the times are given in [ms] with respect to the moment of the TMS impulse (minus sign indicating time before the stimulus). Interval T_3 started 15 ms after the stimulus to ensure that the small muscle artifacts (Mutanen et al., 2012) present in some datasets did not affect the results. Additionally, two time intervals, $T_{b1} = [-400, -300]$ and $T_{b2} = [-300, -200]$, were chosen for baseline scaling.

MSS was always calculated with respect to time interval T_1. Hence, for each accepted trial from each dataset, four MSS values were obtained: MSS(T_1, T_2), MSS(T_1, T_3), MSS(T_1, T_4), and MSS(T_1, T_5). These MSS values were then averaged over trials for each dataset. The obtained averages were divided with the subject-dependent average baseline value, MSS(T_{b1}, T_{b2}), to suppress the differences in the subjects and to emphasize the changes due to different time intervals. The effect of time interval on MSS was studied using one-way ANOVA, with different subjects corresponding to different samples. After ANOVA, Bonferroni-corrected *post-hoc* tests were performed to compare the grand averages of the MSS values. To minimize the possibility that auditory artifacts contaminated the results, we performed the same analysis for all the data and only for datasets measured with noise masking.

SV was calculated for each time interval, providing five numerical values for each trial: SV(T_1), SV(T_2), SV(T_3), SV(T_4), and SV(T_5). The same analysis, including averaging, baseline scaling, and statistical testing described above for MSS was also applied to SV. In this case, the baseline division was done using SV(T_{b2}), again for each dataset individually.

3. RESULTS

TMS seemed to have the anticipated effects: Both MSS and SV were increased (**Figure 2**). ANOVA showed that the time interval had a significant effect on SV ($p < 0.001$). Furthermore, *post-hoc* tests revealed a significant increase in SV during time intervals T_3 and T_4 compared to SVs measured at the other time intervals (**Figure 2A**). SV(T_3) and SV(T_4) were 20–25% higher than the baseline value, SV(T_{b2}).

To show that the observed changes were not due to auditory responses, similar analysis was performed over only those datasets measured with auditory masking. ANOVA showed the same significance level for the effect of time interval ($p < 0.001$). Also the *post-hoc* test results were qualitatively very similar (**Figure 2B**). In general, only the significance levels had moderately increased, except that there was no more a statistically significant difference between SV(T_2) and SV(T_4).

Also in the case of MSS, the time interval had an overall significant effect ($p < 0.001$). Furthermore, *post-hoc* tests showed that the MSS value right after the stimulus was significantly increased when compared to MSS(T_1, T_2) and MSS(T_1, T_5) ($p < 0.001$) (**Figure 2C**). With MSS(T_1, T_3) and MSS(T_1, T_4), an increase of 4–6% was observed when compared to the baseline value, MSS(T_{b1}, T_{b2}). With MSS, the only difference between the complete data analysis and the analysis done over auditory-masked data was that in the latter no statistically significant difference between MSS(T_1, T_4) and MSS(T_1, T_5) could be obtained regardless of the large difference in the grand averages. In addition, the significance level for the difference between MSS(T_1,T_2) and MSS(T_1,T_3) had increased ($p < 0.01$) (**Figure 2D**).

The results were not as uniform at the subject level although 13 datasets showed an increase in both SV and MSS due to TMS. However, the durations of the effects differed between subjects. In most cases, the effects lasted 100–200 ms, but in a few cases the measures did not return to the baseline level. Additionally, the sizes of the changes varied significantly: In SV, the increase was 5–50% depending on the dataset, whereas in MSS the increase was 5–15%.

4. DISCUSSION

Our results show that the measures introduced in this work are able to reveal differences in brain dynamics. The grand averages showed a significant increase both in SV and in MSS after TMS until they returned back to the baseline level. However, between the datasets, one could observe some variation even though 13/16 datasets showed an increase in MSS and SV due to TMS.

In the future, the presented measures should be applied to more homogeneous data to see whether the changes at the subject level would be repeatable. However, our hypothesis concerning the effects of TMS on the brain state relates to TMS in general. Thus, the use of datasets with moderate differences is, in this sense, justified.

Both SV and MSS could be easily applied to some other event-related-potential studies where the method to change $\mathbf{J}^p(\mathbf{r})$ would differ from TMS. Furthermore, the connection between the brain state and the EEG signal space is completely analogous to magnetoencephalography (MEG) signal space (Ilmoniemi and Williamson, 1987; Uusitalo and Ilmoniemi, 1997), only the lead field presented in Equation 2 would be different. Thus, SV and MSS would be directly applicable to MEG data. Based on our results, RQA tools seem promising in studying the brain dynamics affected by any stimulation.

The increase in MSS implies that the brain activation following TMS occupies different regions in the brain state space than spontaneous activity. Although numerous empirical results (e.g., Komssi et al., 2002, 2004, 2007; Massimini et al., 2005; Lioumis et al., 2009) lead to expect that TMS changes the primary current distribution, it is far from self-evident that the sudden shift would be measurable from trial-level EEG data, given that EEG is an extremely low-dimensional projection of the original brain state. As discussed earlier, here conventional averaging is not an option. Indeed, the results show that, although the changes in MSS were statistically significant, they were still quite subtle, which is not a surprise, since the primary activation due to TMS is very focal (Hannula et al., 2005). Thus, most of the background activity is likely to stay similar even after the stimulus.

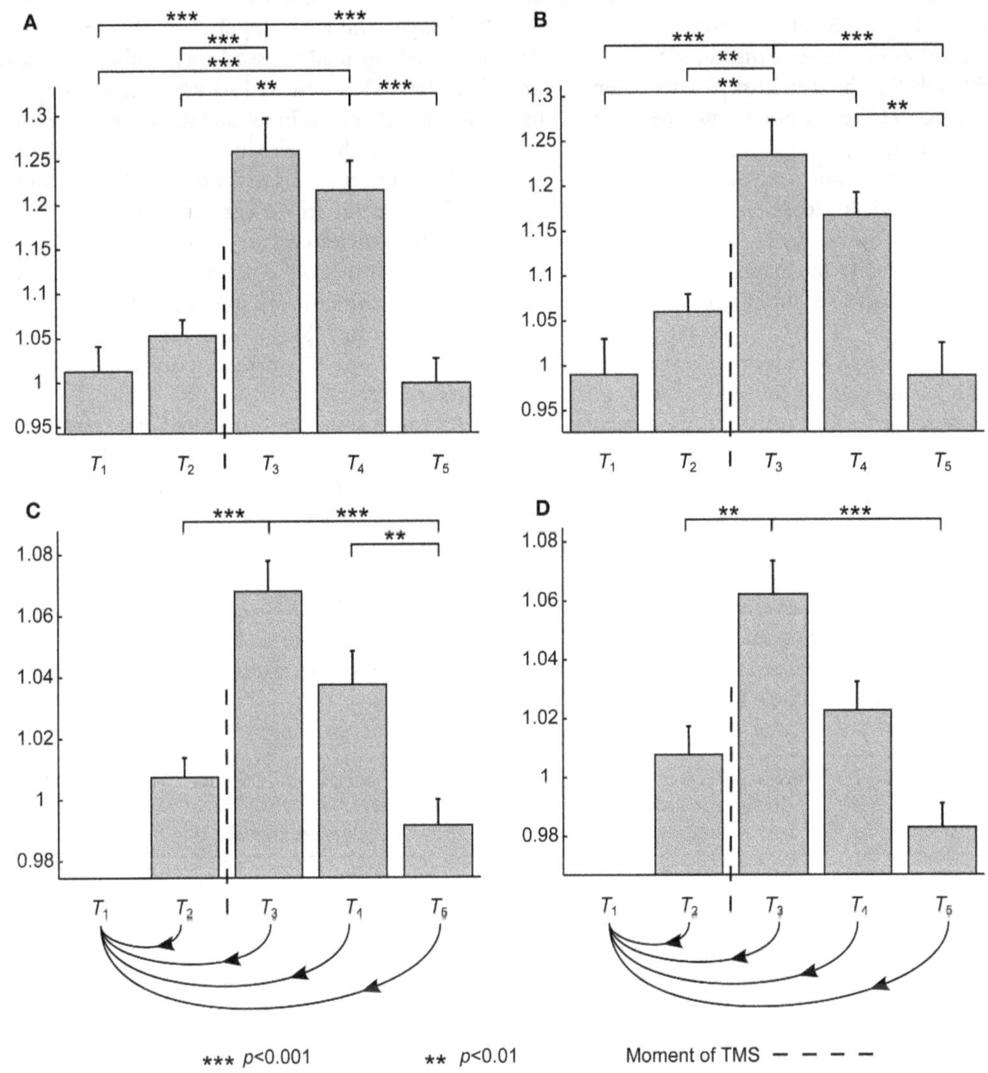

FIGURE 2 | The results averaged over subjects. The asterisks show statistically significant differences between different conditions after the *post-hoc* tests. Error bars show ± standard-error-of-the-means calculated over datasets. Vertical axes are dimensionless and show the differences with respect to the baseline. T_1, T_2, T_3, T_4, and T_5 refer to time intervals (in ms) [−200, −100], [−100, 0], [15, 115], [115, 215], and [215, 315], respectively. **(A,B)** SV at different time intervals averaged over all datasets and averaged over only those with noise masking, respectively. **(C,D)** MSS at different time intervals averaged over all datasets and averaged over only those with noise masking, respectively. The curvy arrow lines indicate that, with MSS, all the time intervals are compared to T_1.

The increase in SV indicates that TMS-modulated activity differs in nature from spontaneous activity. In grand averages, there were differences of up to 25% between pre-TMS SVs and post-TMS SVs, implying that TMS-modulated activity proceeds faster in the state space than the spontaneous one.

Because this study was based on analyzing data measured earlier for other purposes, we lacked sham-TMS data. Hence, we cannot completely exclude the possibility that the increases in SV and MSS are partially due to somatosensory or auditory responses. Indeed, white noise was delivered to the subjects' ears (Paus et al., 2001) to minimize the auditory response at ~100 and ~180 ms in only some of the datasets. Thus, especially the analysis of datasets 5–10 might be affected by the auditory response (Nikouline et al., 1999). The somatosensory response due to scalp nerve activation is likely to have a smaller contribution to the observed changes, since the studied channels were located close to the stimulation site and the somatosensory responses from the scalp are seen on the contralateral hemisphere (Bennett and Jannetta, 1980; Hashimoto, 1988). However, in the future, sham-TMS measurements would be useful to quantify the auditory and somatosensory artifacts in MSS and SV.

Since the stimulation intensity was in all datasets around 100% of the motor threshold, we have to consider the possibility that the motor-evoked-potential (MEP)-related peripheral somatosensory signal might have contributed to the studied measures. Although Nikulin et al. (2003) showed that the MEP-related sensations did not significantly affect the average TMS-evoked EEG responses, it would be advisable to conduct the analysis described in the present work over data measured when TMS has been delivered with sub-threshold intensity or to a non-motor area to ensure that MSS and SV are not affected considerably by the tactile sensation of a MEP.

In the present work, we did not study the dynamical changes in solely spontaneous EEG data. However, we are convinced that the changes in MSS and SV are due to TMS (and indeed possibly due to sensory stimuli elicited by the magnetic impulse) since the increase in SV or MSS is short-lived and returns back to baseline levels.

The effects of TMS on SV and MSS seemed to last 100–200 ms. However, the length of the studied time intervals was 100 ms, limiting the temporal resolution. In principle, the temporal resolution could be improved simply by reducing the length of the time intervals. Unfortunately, this is likely to decrease the signal-to-noise ratio of the measures.

The changes in SV and MSS, in a broad sense, can be explained with the second law of thermodynamics. Although there is a substantial physiological system constantly providing energy and information to the brain, we can approximately consider the brain as an isolated system for the short period of time (~300 ms) that we measure it after the impulse. The spontaneous state before the TMS impulse lies relatively low in the free-energy landscape. The large impulse changes the brain state to a new state that normally has a lower probability meaning increased free energy. The observed activation following the impulse is partially due to the brain settling itself again to a lower energy level. Similar ideas have also been presented earlier (e.g., Hopfield, 1982; Friston et al., 2006; Friston, 2010), although the earlier article discusses the free energy of an artificial neural network and the latter articles deal free energy of a system in a more general level. In short, the results can be interpreted as follows: (1) With TMS, we do work to change the state of the brain, which can be seen in MSS. (2) The brain minimizes the locally high free energy due to work done by TMS, which can be seen as increased SV.

In conclusion, we introduced two novel quantitative tools that were able to characterize dynamic differences between spontaneous and TMS-modulated activity. The results might help us better understand the mechanisms of TMS and combined TMS–EEG method in general.

ACKNOWLEDGMENTS

This study was supported by the Academy of Finland. The authors would like to thank Hanna Mäki for providing the data used in this article.

REFERENCES

Babloyantz, A. (1991). Evidence for slow brain waves: a dynamical approach. *Electroencephalogr. Clin. Neurophysiol.* 78, 402–405.

Bennett, M. H., and Jannetta, P. J. (1980). Trigeminal evoked potentials in humans. *Electroencephalogr. Clin. Neurophysiol.* 48, 517–526.

Eckmann, J. P., Kamphorst, S. O., and Ruelle, D. (1987). Recurrence plots of dynamical systems. *Europhys. Lett.* 4, 973–977.

Esser, S. K., Huber, R., Massimini, M., Peterson, M. J., Ferrarelli, F., and Tononi, G. (2006). A direct demonstration of cortical LTP in humans: a combined TMS/EEG study. *Brain Res. Bull.* 69, 86–94.

Friston, K. (2010). The free-energy principle: a unified brain theory? *Nat. Rev. Neurosci.* 11, 127–138.

Friston, K., Kilner, J., and Harrison, L. (2006). A free energy principle for the brain. *J. Physiol. Paris* 100, 70–87.

Fuggetta, G., Fiaschi, A., and Manganotti, P. (2005). Modulation of cortical oscillatory activities induced by varying single-pulse transcranial magnetic stimulation intensity over the left primary motor area: a combined EEG and TMS study. *Neuroimage* 27, 896–908.

Hannula, H., Ylioja, S., Pertovaara, A., Korvenoja, A., Ruohonen, J., Ilmoniemi, R. J., et al. (2005). Somatotopic blocking of sensation with navigated transcranial magnetic stimulation of the primary somatosensory cortex. *Hum. Brain Mapp.* 26, 100–109.

Hashimoto, I. (1988). Trigeminal evoked potentials following brief air puff: enhanced signal-to-noise ratio. *Ann. Neurol.* 23, 332–338.

Hopfield, J. J. (1982). Neural networks and physical systems with emergent collective computational abilities. *Proc. Natl. Acad. Sci. U.S.A.* 79, 2554–2558.

Huber, R., Mäki, H., Rosanova, M., Casarotto, S., Canali, P., Casali, A. G., et al. (2013). Human cortical excitability increases with time awake. *Cereb. Cortex* 23, 1–7.

Ilmoniemi, R. J., and Kičić, D. (2010). Methodology for combined TMS and EEG. *Brain Topogr.* 22, 233–248.

Ilmoniemi, R. J., and Williamson, S. J. (1987). Analysis for the magnetic alpha rhythm in signal space. *Soc. Neurosci. Abstr.* 13, 46.

Iwanski, J. S., and Bradley, E. (1998). Recurrence plots of experimental data: to embed or not to embed? *Chaos* 8, 861–871.

Komssi, S., Aronen, H. J., Huttunen, J., Kesäniemi, M., Soinne, L., Nikouline, V. V., et al. (2002). Ipsi- and contralateral EEG reactions to transcranial magnetic stimulation. *Clin. Neurophysiol.* 113, 175–184.

Komssi, S., Kähkönen, S., and Ilmoniemi, R. J. (2004). The effect of stimulus intensity on brain responses evoked by transcranial magnetic stimulation. *Hum. Brain Mapp.* 21, 154–164.

Komssi, S., Savolainen, P., Heiskala, J., and Kähkönen, S. (2007). Excitation threshold of the motor cortex estimated with transcranial magnetic stimulation electroencephalography. *Neuroreport* 18, 13–16.

Lioumis, P., Kičić, D., Savolainen, P., Mäkelä, J. P., and Kähkönen, S. (2009). Reproducibility of TMS—Evoked EEG responses. *Hum. Brain Mapp.* 30, 1387–1396.

Mäki, H., and Ilmoniemi, R. J. (2010). The relationship between peripheral and early cortical activation induced by transcranial magnetic stimulation. *Neurosci. Lett.* 478, 24–28.

Malmivuo, J., and Plonsey, R. (1995). *Bioelectromagnetism: Principles and Applications of Bioelectric and Biomagnetic Fields*. New York, NY: Oxford University Press.

Marwan, N., Carmen Romano, M., Thiel, M., and Kurths, J. (2007). Recurrence plots for the analysis of complex systems. *Phys. Rep.* 438, 237–329.

Massimini, M., Ferrarelli, F., Huber, R., Esser, S. K., Singh, H., and Tononi, G. (2005). Breakdown of cortical effective connectivity during sleep. *Science* 309, 2228–2232.

Mutanen, T., Mäki, H., and Ilmoniemi, R. J. (2012). The effect of stimulus parameters on TMS–EEG muscle artifacts. *Brain Stimul.* doi: 10.1016/j.brs.2012.07.005. [Epub ahead of print].

Nikouline, V., Ruohonen, J., and Ilmoniemi, R. J. (1999). The role of the coil click in TMS assessed with simultaneous EEG. *Clin. Neurophysiol.* 110, 1325–1328.

Nikulin, V. V., Kičić, D., Kähkönen, S., and Ilmoniemi, R. J. (2003). Modulation of electroencephalographic responses to transcranial magnetic stimulation: evidence for changes in cortical excitability related to movement. *Eur. J. Neurosci.* 18, 1206–1212.

Ouyang, G., Li, X., Dang, C., and Richards, D. A. (2008). Using recurrence plot for determinism analysis of EEG recordings in genetic absence epilepsy rats. *Clin. Neurophysiol.* 119, 1747–1755.

Paus, T., Sipila, P. K., and Strafella, A. P. (2001). Synchronization of neuronal activity in the human primary motor cortex by transcranial magnetic stimulation: an EEG study. *J. Neurophysiol.* 86, 1983–1990.

Pijn, J. P. M., Velis, D. N., van der Heyden, M. J., DeGoede, J., van Veelen, C. W. M., and Lopes da Silva, F. H. (1997). Nonlinear dynamics of epileptic seizures on basis of intracranial EEG recordings. *Brain Topogr.* 9, 249–270.

Romei, V., Gross, J., and Thut, G. (2010). On the role of prestimulus alpha rhythms over occipito-parietal areas in visual input regulation: correlation or causation? *J. Neurosci.* 30, 8692–8697.

Rosanova, M., Casali, A., Bellina, V., Resta, F., Mariotti, M., and Massimini, M. (2009). Natural frequencies of human corticothalamic circuits. *J. Neurosci.* 29, 7679–7685.

Thut, G., Veniero, D., Romei, V., Miniussi, C., Schyns, P., and Gross, J. (2011). Rhythmic TMS causes local entrainment of natural oscillatory signatures. *Curr. Biol.* 21, 1176–1185.

Uusitalo, M. A., and Ilmoniemi, R. J. (1997). Signal-space projection method for separating MEG or EEG into components. *Med. Biol. Eng. Comput.* 35, 135–140.

Van Der Werf, Y. D., and Paus, T. (2006). The neural response to transcranial magnetic stimulation of the human motor cortex. I. Intracortical and cortico-cortical contributions. *Exp. Brain Res.* 175, 231–245.

6

Transcranial magnetic stimulation-induced global propagation of transient phase resetting associated with directional information flow

Masahiro Kawasaki[1,2,3]*, Yutaka Uno[2], Jumpei Mori[2,4], Kenji Kobata[2,4] and Keiichi Kitajo[2,3]*

[1] Department of Intelligent Interaction Technology, Graduate School of Systems and Information Engineering, University of Tsukuba, Tsukuba, Japan
[2] Rhythm-based Brain Information Processing Unit, RIKEN BSI-TOYOTA Collaboration Center, Wako, Japan
[3] Laboratory for Advanced Brain Signal Processing, RIKEN Brain Science Institute, Wako, Japan
[4] School of Fundamental Science and Technology, Graduate School of Science and Technology, Keio University, Yokohama, Japan

***Correspondence:**
Masahiro Kawasaki, Department of Intelligent Interaction Technology, Graduate School of Systems and Information Engineering, University of Tsukuba, 1-1-1, Tennodai, Tsukuba-shi, Ibaraki 305-8573, Japan
e-mail: kawasaki@iit.tsukuba.ac.jp;
Keiichi Kitajo, Laboratory for Advanced Brain Signal Processing, RIKEN Brain Science Institute, 2-1, Hirosawa, Wako-shi, Saitama 351-0198, Japan
e-mail: kkitajo@brain.riken.jp

Electroencephalogram (EEG) phase synchronization analyses can reveal large-scale communication between distant brain areas. However, it is not possible to identify the directional information flow between distant areas using conventional phase synchronization analyses. In the present study, we applied transcranial magnetic stimulation (TMS) to the occipital area in subjects who were resting with their eyes closed, and analyzed the spatial propagation of transient TMS-induced phase resetting by using the transfer entropy (TE), to quantify the causal and directional flow of information. The time-frequency EEG analysis indicated that the theta (5 Hz) phase locking factor (PLF) reached its highest value at the distant area (the motor area in this study), with a time lag that followed the peak of the transient PLF enhancements of the TMS-targeted area at the TMS onset. Phase-preservation index (PPI) analyses demonstrated significant phase resetting at the TMS-targeted area and distant area. Moreover, the TE from the TMS-targeted area to the distant area increased clearly during the delay that followed TMS onset. Interestingly, the time lags were almost coincident between the PLF and TE results (152 vs. 165 ms), which provides strong evidence that the emergence of the delayed PLF reflects the causal information flow. Such tendencies were observed only in the higher-intensity TMS condition, and not in the lower-intensity or sham TMS conditions. Thus, TMS may manipulate large-scale causal relationships between brain areas in an intensity-dependent manner. We demonstrated that single-pulse TMS modulated global phase dynamics and directional information flow among synchronized brain networks. Therefore, our results suggest that single-pulse TMS can manipulate both incoming and outgoing information in the TMS-targeted area associated with functional changes.

Keywords: transcranial magnetic stimulation, electroencephalogram, synchronization, transfer entropy, information flow, transient phase resetting, oscillations

INTRODUCTION

Increasing evidence indicates that synchronous neural oscillations play an important role in linking multiple brain regions dynamically and in establishing information transfer among these regions (Engel and Singer, 2001; Varela et al., 2001; Ward, 2003). In general, the stable and constant electroencephalogram (EEG) oscillatory phase differences among distant brain regions reveal global synchronization, whereas EEG amplitude typically reveals the extent of task involvement for a local neural ensemble (i.e., local synchronization) (Fries, 2005; Klimesch et al., 2008). It has been demonstrated in humans that such large-scale phase synchronizations lead to dynamic brain networks that mediate cognitive functions, such as visual awareness (Rodriguez et al., 1999; Cosmelli et al., 2004; Kitajo et al., 2007; Melloni et al., 2007), working memory (Mizuhara and Yamaguchi, 2007; Kawasaki et al., 2010; Kawasaki and Yamaguchi, 2013), and attention (Womelsdorf and Fries, 2007; Doesburg et al., 2008). Although phase synchronization analyses can evaluate the interaction or communication among brain areas, it is difficult to identify the causal relationship, or the directional information flow, among these brain areas. Considering that neurons are typically directional cells, the information flow among brain areas should also be directional.

Transcranial magnetic stimulation (TMS) is an ideal method to examine this issue, as it allows a non-invasive stimulation of the human brain that can perturb EEG oscillations (Massimini et al., 2005; Thut et al., 2005). It has been suggested that single-pulse TMS can induce transient neural oscillations in several frequency bands in different cortical areas of the human brain (Paus et al., 2001; Fuggetta et al., 2005; Van Der Werf and Paus, 2006; Taylor et al., 2008; Rosanova et al., 2009; Thut and Miniussi, 2009; Veniero et al., 2011). Furthermore, some of the aforementioned studies have suggested that TMS-induced oscillations reflect phase resetting in ongoing cortical oscillations. To our knowledge, however, almost no study has estimated quantitatively TMS-induced phase resetting, although a recent study has addressed the signal transmission of TMS-modulated EEG phase dynamics (Casali et al., 2010). Moreover, previous studies using event-related brain potential (ERP) analyses have reported that TMS-induced responses propagate globally among distant brain areas (Ilmoniemi et al., 1997; Massimini et al., 2005; Morishima et al., 2009). These findings indicate that it is possible to investigate global frequency-specific phase dynamics by applying TMS while recording EEG activity. We investigated transient phase resetting in the TMS-targeted area and distant areas, their time-course relationships, and directional information flow among the brain areas.

Here, we used an information theoretic approach to test our working hypothesis. Transfer entropy (TE), which is an information theory measure that evaluates directional information transfer between 2 systems (Schreiber, 2000; Kaiser and Schreiber, 2002; Vicente et al., 2011), was used to evaluate the causal information flow between non-linear oscillators in the brain. TE was selected for this analysis because it does not require a model of interaction, and it is not limited to linearity and stationarity, unlike structural equation modeling (Bullmore et al., 2000), dynamic causal modeling (Friston et al., 2003), and Granger causality (Brovelli et al., 2004; Roebroeck et al., 2005) in functional magnetic resonance imaging (fMRI) analyses. In fact, TE was used to show causalities between non-linear biological signals, such as heart and respiration rates (Schreiber, 2000), and auditory cortical neurons (Gourevitch and Eggermont, 2007). We examined TMS-induced global propagations of phase resetting and used TE to quantify the causal and directional information flow among human brain regions. By calculating the TE from the TMS-targeted visual area to another distant area (i.e., motor area), we estimated directional information flow successfully.

MATERIALS AND METHODS

SUBJECTS

Ten healthy right-handed volunteers (2 females and 8 males; mean age, 25.8 ± 2.1 years) participated in this experiment. The subjects reported via subjective questionnaires on having normal visual acuity (with or without correction), hearing, and motor abilities. All subjects gave written informed consent prior to participation in this study. The study was approved by the RIKEN Ethics Committee (in accordance with the Declaration of Helsinki). The data obtained from 1 female subject were excluded from the statistical analysis because of the insufficient amount of significant EEG data.

TMS

While subjects sat in a relaxed position and rested with their eyes closed, single-pulse TMS was delivered to the visual cortex at intervals ranging between 2.5 and 3.5 s. TMS was delivered through a figure-of-eight coil with a 70-mm wing diameter that was connected to a biphasic stimulator (Magstim Rapid, Magstim Company Ltd., UK). To fix the coil at the same position and direction throughout each session, we used the flexible arm of a camera stand. Prior to performing the experiments, we determined the motor threshold (MT) of each subject by applying single TMS pulses over the left motor cortex and recording the intensity at which a single pulse evoked a minimally perceptible movement of the right index finger. When delivering TMS stimulation during the experiment, we fixed the TMS coil over the occipital pole with the handle oriented upward. Under the sham TMS condition, TMS pulses were delivered at a location 15 cm from the top of the head.

EXPERIMENTAL PROCEDURE

Subjects completed 3 sessions in a counter-balanced order. In 2 sessions, TMS targeting the visual cortex (Oz) was delivered at either 95% MT (higher-intensity TMS) or 50% MT (lower-intensity TMS), and in 1 session, subjects underwent a sham-TMS condition at 50% MT. Each session consisted of 50 TMS applications. Throughout each session (duration, 2.5 min), subjects were required to sit in a chair, keep their eyes closed, and maintain their head position within a chin rest. TMS sessions were conducted in a dim electronic- and sound-shielded room. Subjects wore earplugs to help attenuate the effects of TMS-related auditory noises. Furthermore, to confirm the arousal, subjects were asked to respond by pressing a keyboard button by their right index finger when they sensed a white flashed square (visual angle, $1° \times 1°$; color, [r, g, b] = [255, 255, 255]; luminance, 60 cd/m^2) that was presented intermittently on a 24 in computer display (ProLite E2410HDS, Iiyama, Japan) between TMS intervals.

EEG RECORDINGS AND ANALYSES

EEG was recorded continuously from 67 scalp electrodes (Ag/AgCl) embedded in a TMS-compatible electrode cap (EasyCap; EASYCAP Gmbh, Germany), and in accordance with the placement of the international 10/10 system. EEG signals were referenced digitally to the averaged recordings from the right and left earlobes. Electrode impedance was maintained below 10 kΩ. Electrooculography (EOG) was recorded from electrodes that were placed above and below the left eye, to monitor eye blinks or vertical eye movements. EOG electrodes placed 1 cm lateral from the right and left eyes monitored horizontal eye movements. The EEG and EOG signals were amplified using a BrainAmp MR+ apparatus (Brain Products, Germany). The sampling rate was 1000 Hz. In accordance with a previous study (Sekiguchi et al., 2011), we rearranged the lead wires relative to the coil orientation, to reduce TMS-induced artifacts.

EEG data were preprocessed by first segmenting the EEG data into 5-s epochs (with 3-s pre-TMS and 2-s post-TMS periods; 5000 time points in total). We removed the EEG data points that were affected by TMS artifacts (from −1 to 7 ms from TMS onset) using linear interpolation. The duration of artifacts was consistent with a previous study (Veniero et al., 2009). The EEG data were 0.1 Hz high-pass filtered. Next, epochs containing artifacts caused by blinks or eye movements were detected from the EOG and EEG data using an amplitude criterion (±150 μV) and were excluded from further analysis. Finally, after the 47 Hz low-pass filter, to identify the cortical activity with reduced effects of volume conduction, we applied current source density transformation to the voltage distribution on the surface of the scalp using the spherical Laplace operator (Perrin et al., 1989; Kayser and Tenke, 2006).

To identify the time-frequency phases, we applied wavelet transforms using Morlet's wavelet function (Tallon-Baudry et al., 1996). We used Morlet's wavelets for the high time and frequency resolutions, which allowed us to observe transitions in both the low and high frequency oscillations better (Herrmann et al., 2005). The phase for each time point in each TMS application was the arctangent of the results of the convolution of the original EEG signal $s(t)$ with a complex Morlet's wavelet function $w(t, f)$:

$$w(t,f) = \sqrt{f}\exp\left(-\frac{t^2}{2\sigma_t^2}\right)\exp(i2\pi ft)$$

where σ_t is a standard deviation of the Gaussian window. The wavelet used here was roughly characterized by the number of cycles n_{co} within a $6\sigma_t$ interval (Lachaux et al., 2000), which contains about 99.7% of the power of the Gaussian window. We chose $n_{co} = 3(= 6f\sigma_t)$, with f ranging from 2 to 40 Hz in 1-Hz steps.

PLF

TMS-evoked phase resetting was calculated using phase locking factors (PLF; (Tallon-Baudry et al., 1996)) at each electrode (ch), time point (t), and frequency (f) as follows.

$$PLF(t,f,ch) = \frac{1}{N}\left|\sum_{n=1}^{N}\exp\left(i\varphi(t,f,ch,n)\right)\right|$$

where φ is the instantaneous phase of EEG data and N is the total number of epochs included in the calculation. Using the averaged baseline PLF (PLF_b; -1000 to -500 ms from TMS onset), a standardized PLF (PLF_z) was calculated to reduce the formula's sampling number bias for epochs:

$$PLF_z(t,f,ch) = \frac{\mathrm{PLF}(t,f,ch) - \overline{\mathrm{PLF}_b(t,f,ch)}}{\sigma(\mathrm{PLF}_b(t,f,ch))}.$$

We tested the statistical significance of the difference between PLFz around the TMS application and pre-TMS periods averaged across subjects. Specifically, we obtained a pre-TMS PLF_z distribution in which we computed PLF_z from 200 time points selected randomly in pre-TMS periods (-1700 to -500 ms). Subsequently, we tested whether the mean PLF_z around TMS was higher (or smaller) than the upper (or lower) limit of the 99% confidence interval of the pre-TMS PLF_z distributions.

ZPPI

To confirm the PLFz results, we also analyzed another phase resetting measure, the phase-preservation index (PPI) (Mazaheri and Jensen, 2006). The PPI quantifies the consistency in phase stability as a function of time over epochs taking a value between 0 and 1 for each time point (t), frequency (f), reference time point (t_{ref}), and electrode (ch) as follows.

$$\mathrm{PPI}(t,f,t_{ref},ch) = \frac{1}{N}\left|\sum_{n=1}^{N}\exp\left\{i\left(\varphi(t,f,ch,n) - \varphi(t_{ref},f,ch,n)\right)\right\}\right|$$

We tested the statistical significance of the difference between the decay time of PPI around TMS application and pre-TMS periods averaged across subjects. The averaged PPI is more strongly biased by the results of subjects whose number of trials is small (i.e., bad signal/noise ratio) because PPI increases as the number of trials decreases. To decrease the effect of this bias, the PPI was transformed to Rayleigh's Z-value using the formula $\mathrm{ZPPI} = n \times \mathrm{PPI}^2$, where n is the number of trials for each subject. Then we averaged ZPPI across subjects (Fisher, 1993; Mazaheri and Jensen, 2006).

First, we obtained 3000 ZPPI for the phase data that were shuffled randomly in time from pre-TMS periods (-1700 to -1000 ms). This procedure provides a ZPPI estimate with no temporal correlations for each subject. We computed the critical value as the upper 5% limit of the null distribution. Next, we assessed the decay time defined as the interval from a reference point to the time point where ZPPI became lower than the critical value.

To detect TMS-induced phase resetting by the ZPPI, the reference time point has to be close enough to TMS onset because ZPPI decays to the critical value around 300 ms even in the pre-TMS baseline periods. If it is too close, however, TMS causes a biased phase distribution at the reference point, which renders it hard to detect TMS-induced phase resetting by the ZPPI. Therefore, we set the reference time point at -300 and -200 ms for electrodes Oz and C3, respectively. Indeed, the phase distributions were not biased because PLFz were not significantly high at the reference points (**Figures 2A–C**).

Finally, we assessed if the decay time of ZPPI around TMS application was faster than the decay time of pre-TMS ZPPI. Specifically, we estimated the 95% confidence intervals of 200 pre-TMS ZPPI curves (and decay time) averaged across subjects, which were computed for pre-TMS periods by setting the reference points randomly between -1700 and -1000 ms (non-shuffled data), and compared them with the subject-averaged ZPPI curve (and decay time) around TMS application.

TRANSFER ENTROPY

To estimate directional information flow among brain regions, we used TE, which is an information theory measure developed by Schreiber (2000). TE can quantify the directional information flow between 2 systems X and Y by quantifying how the future state of X is determined by the current states of X and Y.

To compute TE, entropy rate (h_1) was first calculated using the current observation values x_t and y_t and the time-shifted (τ) observation value $x_{t+\tau}$ as follows.

$$h_1 = -\sum_{x_{t+\tau},x_t,y_t} p(x_{t+\tau},x_t,y_t)\log_2 p(x_{t+\tau}|x_t,y_t),$$

where $p(x|y)$ denotes the conditional probability and $p(x, y)$ denotes the joint probability. If we assume that the 2 systems are independent, the time-shifted observation value ($x_{t+\tau}$) of system X is independent of the current observation value of the other electrode, y_t. Therefore, the entropy rate (h_2) is defined as:

$$h_2 = -\sum_{x_{t+\tau},x_t,y_t} p(x_{t+\tau},x_t,y_t)\log_2 p(x_{t+\tau}|x_t).$$

The TE (TE) from system Y to X is defined as the difference between h_1 and h_2, as follows.

$$TE_{Y\to X} = h_2 - h_1 = \sum_{x_{t+\tau},x_t,y_t} p(x_{t+\tau}, x_t, y_t) \log_2 \left(\frac{p(x_{t+\tau}|x_t, y_t)}{p(x_{t+\tau}|x_t)} \right)$$

Since the formula is not symmetric, we can estimate the information flow between the 2 systems separately for both directions. More specifically, the *TE* from system *X* to *Y* is obtained by,

$$TE_{X\to Y} = \sum_{y_{t+\tau},y_t,x_t} p(y_{t+\tau}, y_t, x_t) \log_2 \left(\frac{p(y_{t+\tau}|x_t, y_t)}{p(y_{t+\tau}|y_t)} \right).$$

We used the instantaneous phases of CSD signals from 2 electrodes (i.e., the C3 electrode as the left motor area and the Oz electrode as the visual area) as the observation values of 2 systems, and then estimated the TE between the 2 signals.

A straightforward approach for estimating TE is to divide the state space into bins of a given width and construct multidimensional histograms from the data, to evaluate the probability density (Schreiber, 2000; Vicente et al., 2011). However, the arbitrary bin size often biases the estimate when there is a limited number of data points, which are too sparse in the state space. Non-parametric estimation using kernel techniques is a useful alternative to binning a distribution (Silverman, 1981, 1986; Kaiser and Schreiber, 2002). Therefore, we estimated multidimensional probability density functions using the kernel density estimation method (Silverman, 1981, 1986), rather than using probabilities estimated by empirical histograms. As phase is a circular (i.e., $\pi = -\pi$) measure, we used a von Mises distribution, which is a continuous probability distribution on the circle, as a kernel density function. The kernel bandwidth ($\kappa = 8$) was optimized using the least-squares cross-validation method (Sain et al., 1994).

Next, we used the estimated multidimensional probability density function to compute TE, as follows.

$$TE_{Y\to X} = \iiint p(x_{t+\tau}, x_t, y_t) \log_2 \left(\frac{p(x_{t+\tau}|x_t, y_t)}{p(x_{t+\tau}|x_t)} \right) dx_t dx_{t+\tau} dy_t.$$

The integral was numerically estimated via a 20-point Gauss–Legendre quadrature.

We used phase data extracted in a 200-ms period around the time of a TMS pulse (pre-100 ms, post-100 ms) as the current observation values x_t, y_t, and phase data from a time-lagged 200-ms period as the corresponding observation values $x_{t+\tau}$. We estimated the TE for each subject as the function of the time lag (τ) ranging from 0 to 600 ms, in 5-ms steps. We tested the statistical significance of the difference between TE around the TMS application and pre-TMS periods averaged across subjects. We obtained a 200-ms pre-TMS TE distribution in which we computed TE from 200 sets of randomly selected consecutive 200-ms pre-TMS periods (−1700 to −500 ms). More specifically, we tested whether the mean TE around TMS was higher (or smaller) than the upper (or lower) limit of the 99% confidence interval of the pre-TMS TE distributions.

ADDITIONAL EXPERIMENTS

We conducted additional experiments to address (1) the effects of the TMS click sound on the EEG (Nikouline et al., 1999), (2) the influences of the sham TMS intensity (50% MT), and (3) the signal/noise ratio (i.e., effects of the number of trials).

We included 12 healthy right-handed volunteers (6 females and 6 males; mean age, 26.3 ± 6.1 years) in this experiment and used the same subjective questionnaires used in the previous study. The additional experiments were approved by the institutional ethics committee. The data obtained from 2 subjects were excluded from the statistical analysis because the TMS intensities were not large enough to evoke responses.

The additional experiments included 1 visual TMS condition and 2 sham TMS conditions. The experimental paradigm, environment, and equipment were similar to those for the previous experiments, except for the following points. First, subjects wore in-ear headphones with earmuffs and listened to a masking white noise. The noise was adjusted so that the subjects could not hear the TMS coil click during the TMS experiments (Paus et al., 2001; Fuggetta et al., 2005; Massimini et al., 2005). Second, the TMS intensity was set to 95% or 50% MT in all 3 conditions. Third, we placed a thin layer of plastic foam between the scalp and the coil when the coil was positioned over the visual area to attenuate conduction of the TMS click through the bone (Paus et al., 2001; Massimini et al., 2005; Van Der Werf and Paus, 2006; Rosanova et al., 2009; Casali et al., 2010; Mäki and Ilmoniemi, 2010; Ter Braack et al., 2013). Fourth, 100 trials were completed in all conditions.

The sham TMS condition was divided into 2 types. In the first type (sham1), the TMS coil handle was oriented rightward with the handle axis rotated 90 degrees so that only one wing of the figure-of-eight coil was oriented to the scalp. A 3.6-cm plastic cube with a thin layer of plastic form was used as a spacer that was placed between the occipital pole and the coil wing (Esser et al., 2006). In the second type (sham2), the TMS pulses were delivered at a location 15 cm from the top of head.

The statistical analyses were similar to those performed in the previous experiments, except that the reference time point in the PPI analyses was −300 ms from the TMS onset for electrode C3, whereas the previous experiments used −200 ms. We added 100 ms because the rise time of the C3 PLF_z in the additional experiments was faster than that in the previous experiments. Representative EEG signals and averaged TMS evoked potentials for the main and additional experiments are shown in **Figures S1** and **S2**.

RESULTS

PLF_z AND ZPPI RESULTS

The time-frequency EEG results showed transient enhancements of PLF_z ranging from 2 to 40 Hz at the TMS-targeted electrode at the times at which TMS was delivered under the higher-intensity (95% MT) TMS condition (**Figure 1A**). These enhancements were observed ahead of the TMS onsets because of the wavelet time resolution. In particular, the low frequency PLF_z, especially theta (4–8 Hz) oscillations, increased from the TMS onset at both the TMS target locations (i.e., Oz) and the distant brain areas (e.g., C3; the electrode showing the maximum PLF_z). The instant

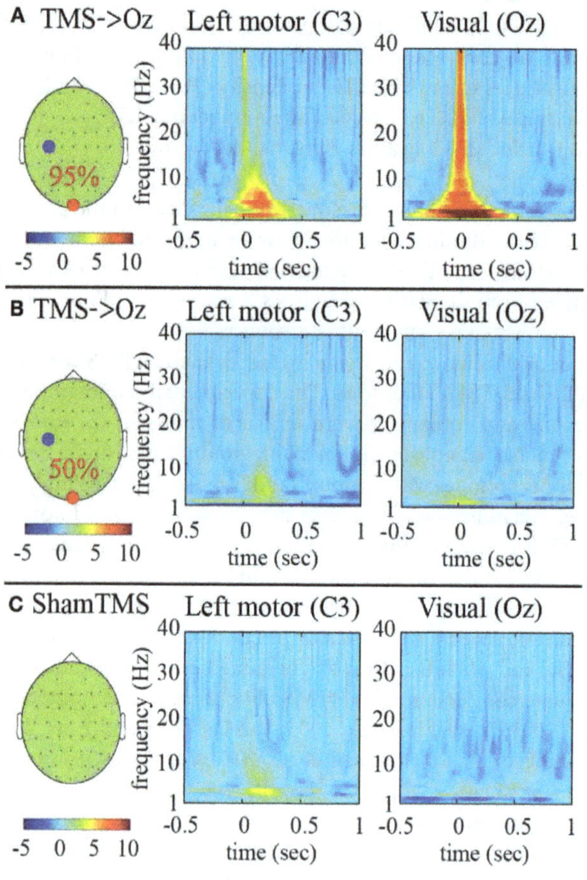

FIGURE 1 | Subject-averaged ($N = 9$) time-frequency *PLFz* of the C3 (left) and Oz (right) electrodes at the onset of TMS applications under the 95% MT TMS (A), 50% MT TMS (B), and sham-TMS (C) conditions. The left topographies show the C3 (blue) and Oz (red) electrodes on the recording montage.

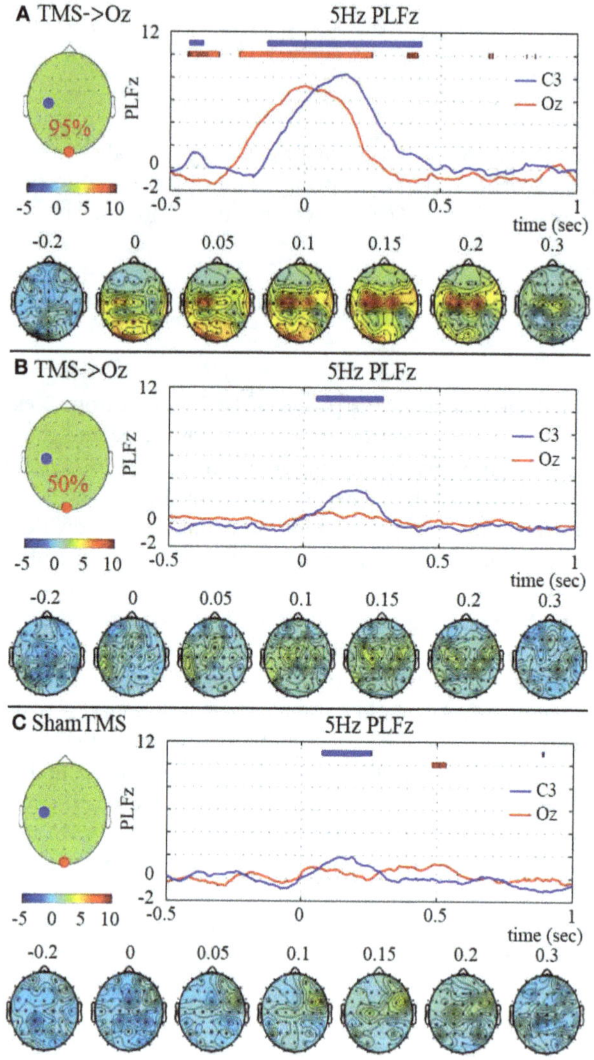

FIGURE 2 | Subject-averaged ($N = 9$) time course of 5 Hz *PLFz* (top) and their topographies (bottom) of the C3 (blue) and Oz (red) electrodes at the onset of TMS applications under the 95% MT TMS (A), 50% MT TMS (B), and sham-TMS (C) conditions. The thick lines in the upper part of line graphs indicate the time periods in which *PLFz* was significantly higher than the pre-TMS periods at the C3 (blue) and Oz (red) electrodes ($P < 0.01$). The left topographies show the C3 (blue) and Oz (red) electrodes on the recording montage.

amplifications of PLF_z at the TMS target electrodes increased significantly as TMS increased from lower (50% MT) to higher intensities (**Figures 1A,B**; false-discovery rate corrected $P < 0.01$; Wilcoxon sign rank test).

We observed global phase resetting in the distant brain regions. With higher-intensity TMS, transient phase resetting of the theta (frequency-measuring peak PLF_z; 5 Hz) oscillations was transmitted from the visual areas to the motor areas (in particular the left motor area) (**Figure 2A**). The TMS-enhanced theta PLF_z was significantly higher than those of the pre-TMS periods in both the visual and motor areas. In addition, the left motor electrode showed the highest theta PLF_z from approximately 152 ms after TMS onset, whereas PLF_z at the visual electrode reached peak factors at the time TMS was applied. Such observation of phase resets at the distant electrode decreased and disappeared with lower-intensity TMS and with sham TMS (**Figures 2B,C**).

Next, we analyzed if the TMS-induced increase in PLF_z was associated with changes in another phase-resetting measure, ZPPI. **Figure 3** shows the ZPPI computed for 5-Hz phase at the TMS target locations (Oz) (**Figure 3A**) and the distant brain area (C3) (**Figure 3B**) averaged across subjects under the higher-intensity (95% MT) TMS condition. ZPPI around TMS application (thick black line), which was computed using the reference time point of −300 ms, showed a significantly shorter decay time ($P < 0.05$) to the critical value (red line) than did the pre-TMS ZPPI curves (−1700 to −500 ms) (95% confidence intervals, greenish areas in **Figure 3**) for the Oz electrode. ZPPI around TMS application, which was computed using the reference time point of −200 ms for the C3 electrode, was significantly shorter ($P < 0.05$) in decay time to the critical value (red line), than was the pre-TMS ZPPI. **Figures 3C,D** show the results obtained for the lower-intensity TMS (50% MT) condition. ZPPI around TMS application was not significantly different from ZPPI of pre-TMS periods for both the Oz and C3 electrodes. In the sham condition, we did not observe any significant changes in

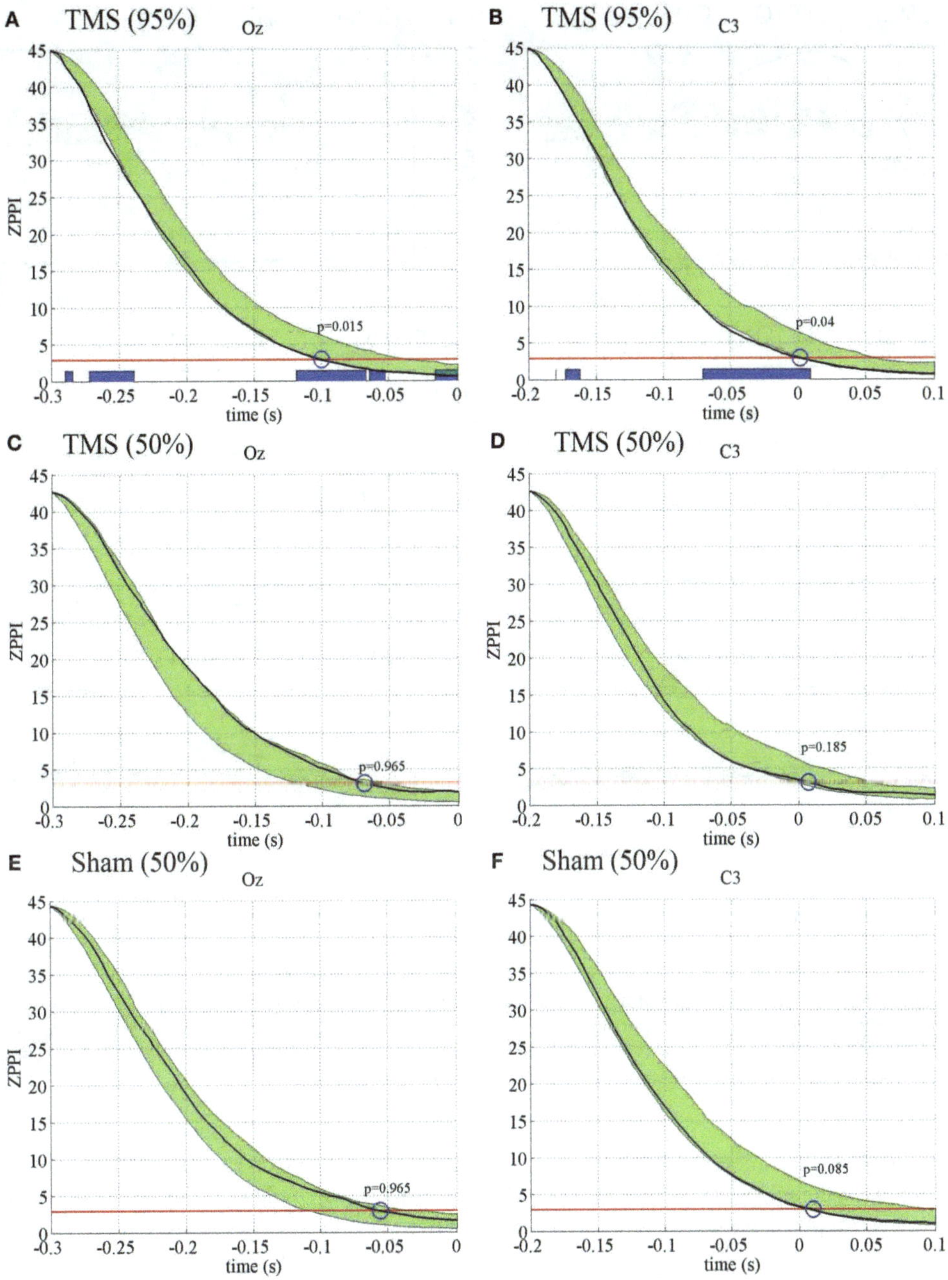

FIGURE 3 | Subject-averaged ($N = 9$) PPI for the electrodes Oz and C3 under the 95% MT TMS (A,B), 50% MT TMS (C,D), and Sham-TMS conditions (E,F). The black thick lines indicate PPI around TMS applications (reference time point at −300 and −200 ms for the electrodes Oz and C3, respectively). The red lines indicate the critical values defined as the upper 5% limit of the null distribution. The greenish areas indicate the 95% confidence intervals of pre-TMS PPI. Using the 95% confidence intervals, we assessed if the decay time of PPI to the critical value around TMS application was significantly shorter than the decay time of pre-TMS PPI (blue circles and *P*-values). The blue thick lines in the lower part of graphs indicate the time periods in which PPI decayed significantly faster than pre-TMS PPI.

ZPPI around sham TMS application for both the Oz and C3 electrodes compared with pre-TMS periods (**Figures 3E,F**).

These results indicate that the TMS-induced increase in PLF_Z is accompanied by a significantly shorter decay time in ZPPI compared with pre-TMS periods more prominently in the higher-intensity TMS (95% MT) condition.

TRANSFER ENTROPY RESULTS

Considering that we found the most prominent time-delayed TMS-induced phase resetting from Oz to C3 at 5 Hz, we evaluated the information transfer between electrodes Oz and C3 by computing TE for 5-Hz phase signals. **Figure 4A** demonstrates mean TE (Oz to C3) as a function of TE time lag with the

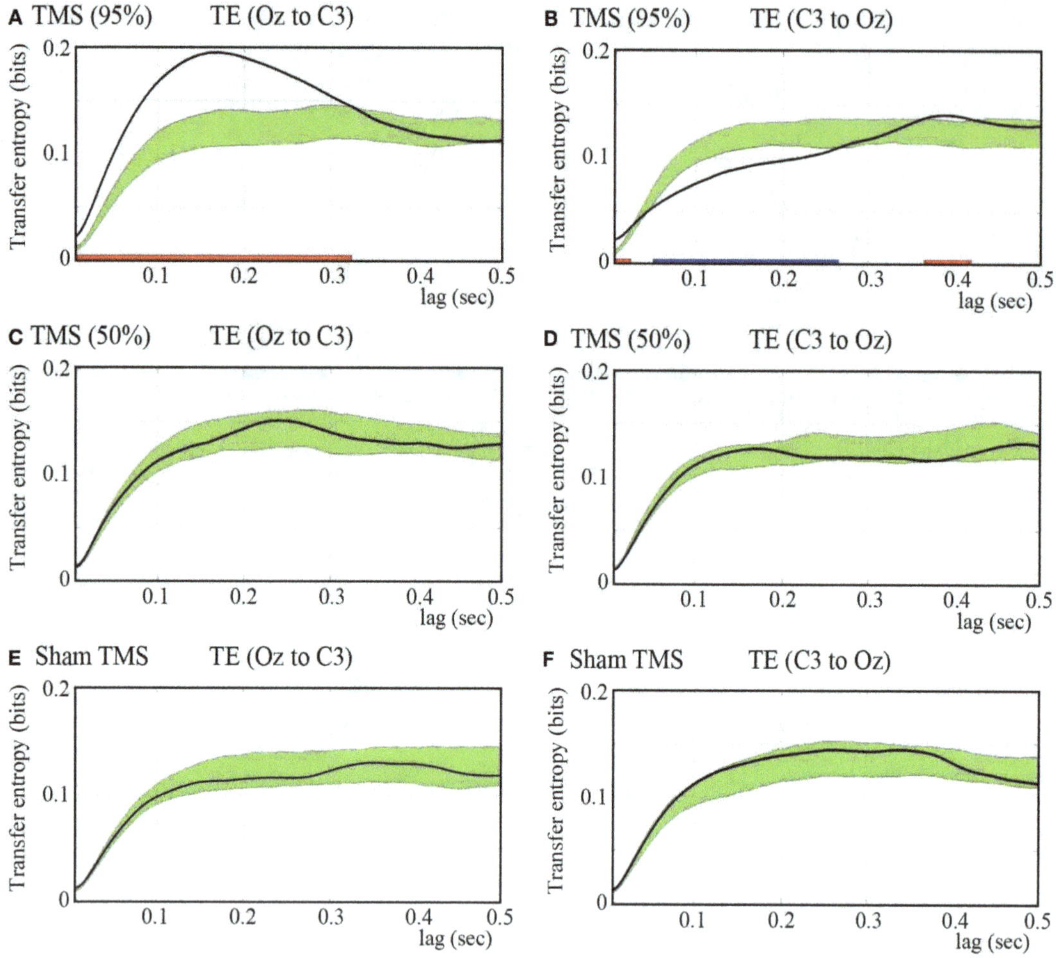

FIGURE 4 | Subject-averaged ($N = 9$) TE as a function of time lag. TE (Oz to C3) **(A)** and TE (C3 to Oz) **(B)** under the 95% MT TMS conditions. Greenish areas indicate the 99% confidence intervals calculated using these pre-TMS periods. The red and blue thick lines in the lower part of line graphs indicate the time periods in which TE was significantly higher than the pre-TMS TE ($P < 0.01$). **(C,D)** TE (Oz to C3) and TE (C3 to Oz) under the 50% MT TMS condition. **(E,F)** TE (Oz to C3) and TE (C3 to Oz) under the sham-TMS condition.

higher-intensity TMS. In the higher-intensity TMS condition, we observed a prominent peak in the subject-averaged TE (Oz to C3) at a 165-ms lag. We also computed pre-TMS TE from 200-ms periods selected randomly between −1700 and −500 ms pre-TMS, which is a stable period that precedes TMS. Using these pre-TMS periods, we computed the 99% confidence intervals (greenish areas in **Figure 4**). We observed that the pre-TMS periods were not affected by the previous TMS (i.e., the minimum time interval was 2500 ms) or the PLF_z enhancements preceding the TMS in that epoch (see **Figure 1**). TE around TMS application (Oz to C3) was significantly higher than the pre-TMS TE (Oz to C3) with a time lag between 5 and 325 ms in the higher-intensity TMS condition. In addition, we observed a baseline information flow between Oz and C3 in pre-TMS data. These results suggest the existence of information flow from TMS-targeted visual areas (Oz) to motor areas (C3), which was enhanced by single-pulse TMS maximized at a 165-ms lag.

In contrast, we found a significantly lower TE around the time of TMS application (C3 to Oz) compared with the pre-TMS TE with a lag (C3 to Oz) between 50 and 265 ms in the higher-intensity TMS condition. These results indicate that the information flow from C3 to Oz around the time of TMS application was suppressed within this time-lag range. Moreover, TE (C3 to Oz) showed a later peak at a time lag of approximately 400 ms (**Figure 4B**). The peak of TE around the time of TMS application was significantly different from TE for the pre-TMS periods.

Figures 4C,D show the results obtained for the lower-intensity TMS (50% MT) condition. We observed a less prominent and later peak for TE (Oz to C3) compared with what was observed for higher-intensity TMS. TE (Oz to C3) around the time of TMS application was not significantly different from pre-TMS TE (Oz to C3). Moreover, TE (C3 to Oz) was not significantly different from TE (C3 to Oz) of the pre-TMS periods. In the sham condition, we did not observe any significant changes in TE around TMS application for either direction (i.e., Oz to C3 and C3 to Oz) from pre-TMS periods (**Figures 4E,F**).

The TE results showed that TMS can enhance directional information flow from the TMS-targeted visual area to motor areas with higher-intensity TMS, which is consistent with the PLF_Z and ZPPI results that indicated prominent propagation of transient phase resetting from the TMS-targeted visual areas to the motor areas.

ZPPI RESULTS OF THE ADDITIONAL EXPERIMENTS: PLF_Z, ZPPI, AND TE

Figures 5–7 presents the results of the additional experiments. These results include the PLF_Z, ZPPI, and TE results in the 5-Hz phases under the visual TMS, as well as the sham1 and sham2 TMS conditions (all TMS intensities were 95% MT).

The PLFz results from the additional experiments replicated those from the previous experiments (**Figure 5**). In the visual condition (95% MT), the TMS-enhanced 5-Hz PLF_Z was significantly higher than those in the pre-TMS periods for both the visual (Oz) and motor areas (C3). Moreover, the C3 electrode showed the highest theta PLF_Z from 116 ms after TMS onset, whereas the Oz electrode PLF_Z peaked at the time TMS was applied. Such prominent increases in PLFz were not observed in the 2 sham conditions at 95% MT or any condition at 50% MT.

The ZPPI results for the additional experiments also were similar to those for the previous experiments (**Figure 6**). The ZPPI measured around the time of the TMS application for the Oz and C3 electrodes showed a significantly shorter decay time ($P < 0.05$) to the critical value than did the pre-TMS ZPPI curves in the visual TMS condition at 95% MT. In contrast, the ZPPI measured around the time of the TMS application was not significantly different from the ZPPI of the pre-TMS periods for either the Oz or C3 electrodes in the sham2 condition at 95% MT. However, the ZPPI for the C3 electrode showed a significantly shorter decay time in the sham1 condition at 95% MT. Such a decay in ZPPI was not observed in any condition at 50% MT.

The TE results for the additional experiments also were similar to those for the main experiments. In the visual TMS condition, we observed a prominent peak in the subject-averaged TE (Oz to C3) at 175 ms. The *TE*-values were significantly higher than those for the pre-TMS TE. The TE modulations appearing around the TMS application for the opposite direction (C3 to Oz) in the visual TMS condition and for either direction (i.e., Oz to C3 and C3 to Oz) in the 2 sham conditions were partially significant (see **Figure 7**).

These results indicate that any artifact produced by the TMS click or a low number of trials should not have affected our finding that TMS can enhance directional information flow from the TMS-targeted visual area to motor areas.

DISCUSSION

The present study demonstrated that single-pulse TMS can induce a large-scale propagation of transient phase resetting that is accompanied by causal information flow from the TMS-targeted area to distant areas via bottom-up synchrony networks during TMS-induced brain states. Previous TMS–EEG studies have shown either TMS-induced oscillations within local areas (Paus et al., 2001; Fuggetta et al., 2005; Van Der Werf and Paus, 2006; Taylor et al., 2008; Rosanova et al., 2009; Thut and Miniussi, 2009; Veniero et al., 2011) or global propagation of averaged responses (Ilmoniemi et al., 1997; Massimini et al., 2005; Morishima et al., 2009). In addition, the present study revealed several important findings. First, the time-frequency EEG analysis showed that the PLF_Z reached the highest factor at the distant area with a time lag that followed the peak PLF_Z enhancements of the TMS-targeted area. Second, the TMS-induced increase in PLF_Z was accompanied by a significantly shorter decay time in ZPPI compared with pre-TMS periods more prominently in the higher-intensity TMS (95% MT) condition. Third, the TE from the TMS-targeted area to the distant area clearly increased with a time lag from the TMS onset. Interestingly, the averaged time lags were almost coincident between the PLF_Z (152 ms) and TE (165 ms) results. This finding provides strong evidence that the emergence of the delayed phase resetting, which was indicated by the delayed PLF_Z peaks, is associated with the incoming causal information flow from the TMS-targeted visual area to the non-target motor area, as was indicated by TE.

TMS appears to manipulate the oscillatory phase dynamics and causal information flow among large-scale brain networks in a TMS-intensity-dependent manner, as such TMS-induced

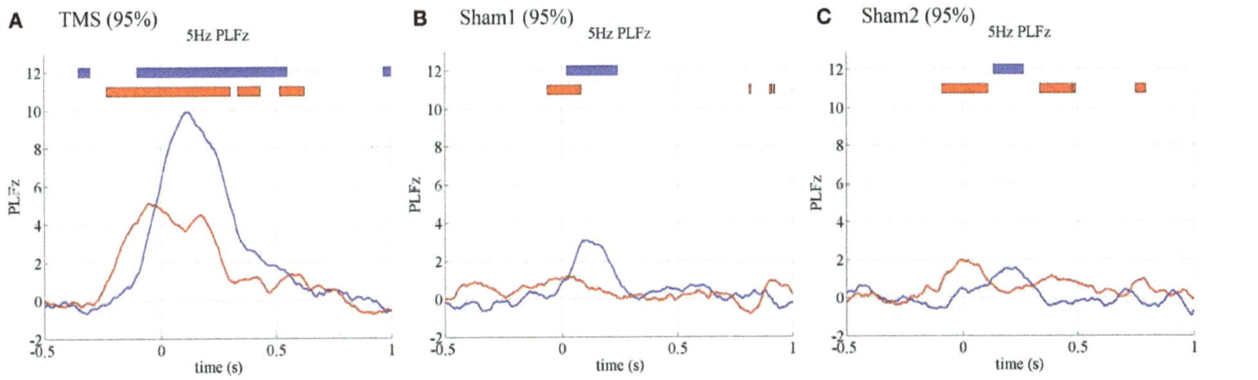

FIGURE 5 | Subject-averaged ($N = 10$) time course of 5 Hz *PLFz* at the onset of TMS applications under the 95% MT TMS (A), 95% MT sham1 TMS (B), and 95% MT sham2 TMS (C) conditions in the additional experiments. The thick lines in the upper part of line graphs indicate the time periods in which *PLFz* was significantly higher than the pre-TMS periods at the C3 (blue) and Oz (red) electrodes ($P < 0.01$).

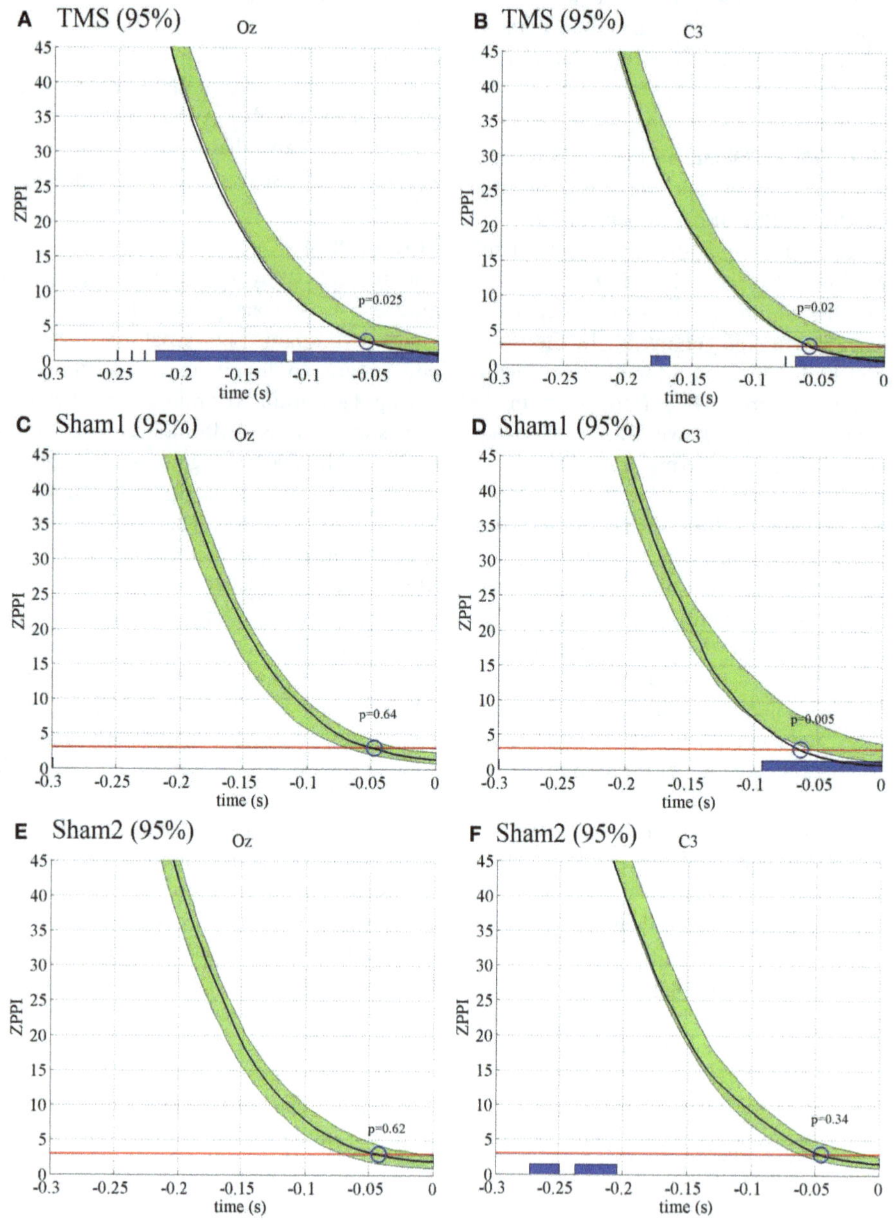

FIGURE 6 | Subject-averaged (*N* = 10) ZPPI for the electrodes Oz and C3 under the 95% MT TMS (A,B), 95% MT sham1 TMS (C,D), and 95% MT sham2 TMS (E,F) conditions in the additional experiments. The black thick lines indicate ZPPI around TMS applications (reference time point at −300 and −200 ms for the electrodes Oz and C3, respectively). The red lines indicate the critical values defined as the upper 5% limit of the null distribution. The greenish areas indicate the 95% confidence intervals of pre-TMS ZPPI. Using the 95% confidence intervals, we assessed if the decay time of ZPPI to the critical value around TMS application was significantly shorter than the decay time of pre-TMS ZPPI (blue circles and *P*-values). The blue thick lines in the lower part of graphs indicate the time periods in which ZPPI decayed significantly faster than pre-TMS ZPPI.

modulations were observed only in the higher-intensity TMS condition. The slightly increased PLF_Z observed under the sham and low-intensity TMS conditions in the main experiment might not be due to the information transfer from the visual area to the motor area, because the TE was not significantly different from TE observed in the pre-TMS periods. Global oscillatory modulations were found in the theta range (peak frequency, 5 Hz), although TMS consistently induces frequency-specific oscillations in each brain area, such as alpha oscillations in the occipital areas and beta oscillations in the motor areas (Rosanova et al., 2009). Previous findings indicate that the slow-oscillatory (i.e., theta) synchronization plays an important role in linking dynamically brain areas within the resting-state networks (Von Stein and Sarnthein, 2000; Buzsaki and Draguhn, 2004; Jensen and Colgin, 2007). Slow-oscillatory (i.e., theta) synchronization is similar to the global theta phase synchronization observed for several

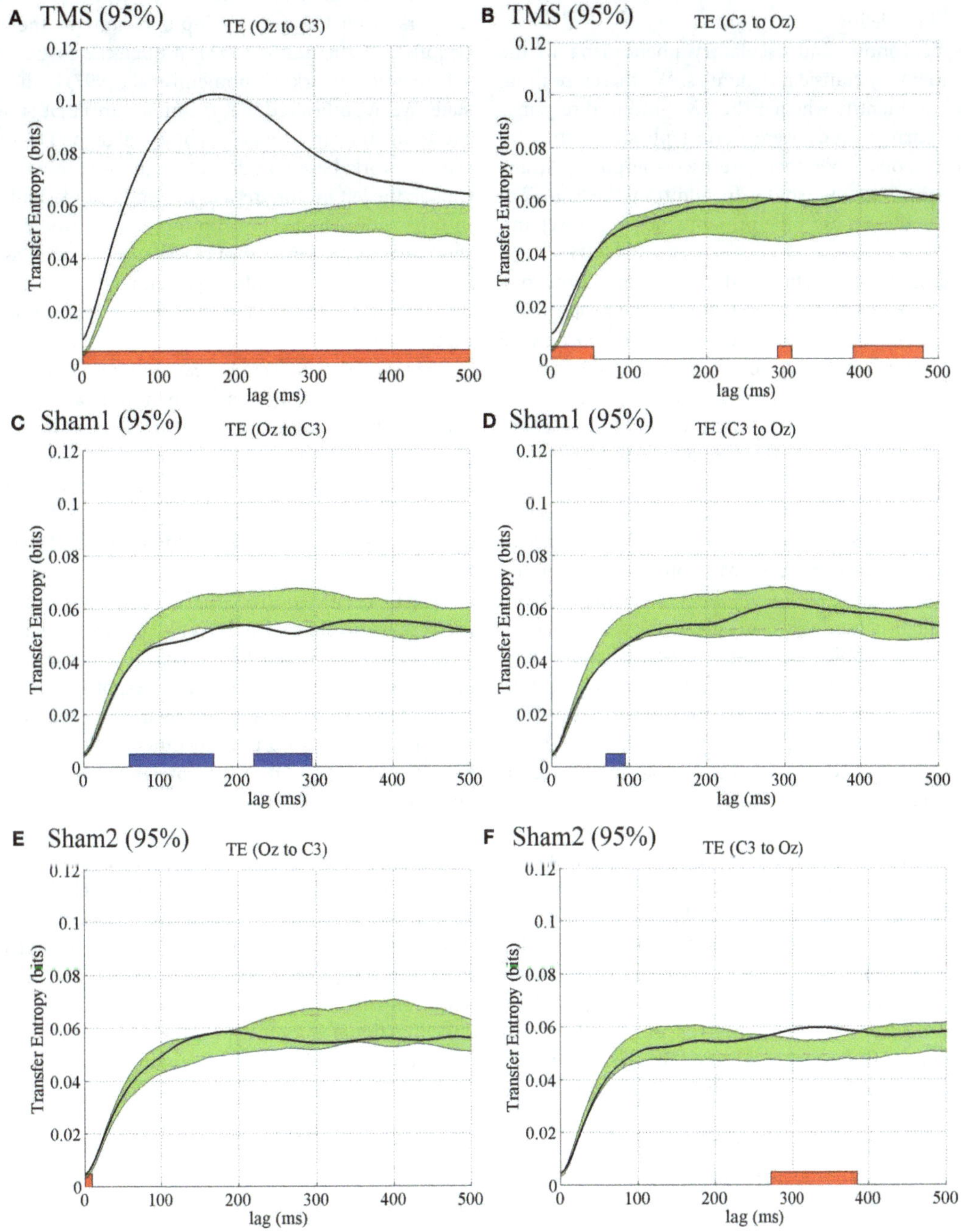

FIGURE 7 | Subject-averaged ($N = 9$) TE as a function of time lag. TE (Oz to C3) **(A)** and TE (C3 to Oz) **(B)** under the 95% MT TMS conditions. Greenish areas indicate the 99% confidence intervals calculated using these pre-TMS periods. The red and blue thick lines in the lower part of line graphs indicate the time periods in which TE was significantly higher than the pre-TMS TE ($P < 0.01$). **(C,D)** TE (Oz to C3) and TE (C3 to Oz) under the 95% MT sham1 TMS, and **(E,F)** TE (Oz to C3) and TE (C3 to Oz) under the 95% MT sham2 TMS conditions in the additional experiments.

cognitive functions, including working memory (Sauseng et al., 2005; Mizuhara and Yamaguchi, 2007; Klimesch et al., 2008; Kawasaki et al., 2010). Therefore, the PLF_z patterns of different frequency oscillations in different brain regions, and the relationships between resting and cognitive functions, should be clarified in future studies.

Although the PLF and ZPPI results possibly suggest the macroscopic phase resetting at the EEG level, the findings are not direct evidence for the microscopic phase resetting at the single neuron level. Previous studies argued that such phase modulations could be either related to additive evoked responses or phase resetting (Sauseng et al., 2007; Becker et al., 2008). Moreover, it is not clear whether the macroscopic phase resetting of EEG oscillations reflects the microscopic phase resetting or additive evoked responses at the single neuron level (Telenczuk et al., 2010). Therefore, it is necessary to examine the issues by combining experimental data at different spatial scales using several indices and mathematical modeling.

Moreover, synchronous and oscillatory phenomena in the brain actually show very transient dynamics. We therefore think it is very difficult to identify whether the TMS-induced response observed in the current study were perfect phase resetting or additive evoked responses. We therefore used the phrase "transient phase resetting" in our study. In addition the transient TMS-evoked phase dynamics in the present study are novel and important.

Moreover, it should be noted that artifacts such as volume conduction of TMS-evoked activity do not explain the propagation of transient phase resetting and directional information flow, as there was a time lag between PLF_Z peaks that matched the optimal lag at which the TE from Oz to C3 was maximized. If the global propagation of transient phase resetting and information transfer was a spurious phenomenon caused by volume conduction, then there should be no time lag.

Furthermore, it is possible that the EEG data was slightly affected by indirect TMS effects, such as the air- and bone-conducted sound produced by the TMS coil click (Nikouline et al., 1999) in the main experiments. To reduce such effects, we applied TMS slightly (about 0.5 cm) above the scalp over the occipital area and asked subjects to wear earplugs. Unfortunately, the method did not prevent auditory effects perfectly, because a weak increase in PLFz was observed under the sham-TMS condition, which does not have direct TMS effects on brain activity (**Figure 2C**). Moreover, the main experiments lacked higher-intensity sham-TMS data (95% MT).

To address these issues, we conducted additional experiments in which the subjects listened to a masking white noise sound with headphones. In addition, we included two sham conditions in which the TMS intensity was 95% MT or the TMS was applied near the visual area. The PLF_Z, ZPPI, and TE results for the additional experiments were similar to those for the previous experiments. The increased PLFz, faster ZPPI decay, and TE enhancements from Oz to C3 were observed in only the visual TMS condition but not the sham2 condition (i.e., the TMS pulses were delivered at a location 15 cm from the top of head). These results suggest that our findings were not influenced by auditory evoked potentials evoked by the associated TMS click sound or by the TMS intensity and location in the sham conditions.

Note that the enhancement of the ZPPI decay in the motor area was significant only in the sham1 condition (i.e., with placing a cube with thin layer of plastic foam between the scalp and the rotated coil) in the additional experiment, whereas the enhanced ZPPI decay was not observed in the visual area. Such results might be due to somatosensory stimulation by bone-conducted vibration from the TMS click but not by auditory effects of the TMS click. It is because that the phase resetting was not found in the sham2 condition, although the auditory masking was same between the sham1 and sham2 conditions. However, this possibility did not influence our findings regarding phase resetting in the motor area in the 95% MT visual TMS condition because the phenomenon was commonly found in both the main experiments (without the somatosensory effects) and additional experiments (without the auditory effects).

Our findings suggest the existence of a potential bottom-up network from the sensory input regions to the motor output regions (i.e., the motor areas) through the corticocortical and/or subcortical networks (Ilmoniemi et al., 1997) in the TMS-induced state. We hypothesized that the motor area that is contralateral to the dominant hand appears to be a goal of the TMS-induced brain state network, based on the convergence of transient phase resetting on the left motor areas in the right-handed subjects included in this study. The bottom-up mechanism would be related to a spontaneous preparation of reaction series, such as the task used in this study. For example, we can imagine seeing a visual stimulus, making a decision, and then responding via output from the motor areas.

We asked the subjects to respond to a visual flash (with their eyes-closed), to monitor and keep the arousal level. Thereafter, the visual flashes possibly influence the arousal level and indirectly affect the excitability of the visual cortex, although the visual flashes are assumed to be temporally far from the TMS timing, not to be presented in every TMS interval (10 flashes and 50 TMS applications in each session), and not to affect the TMS-induced response directly.

It has been reported that TMS induces rapid (<50 ms) increases in firing rates in the cat V1 cortex (Moliadze et al., 2003). This should be related to the transient phase resetting of local oscillations in the targeted area. In response to the TMS-induced increase in spike rate, the targeted area can subsequently increase the strength of its outputs to other areas. This might account for the enhanced bottom-up information flow observed in the current study.

TE is a model-free measure of information flow without the assumption of linearity and stationarity (Schreiber, 2000; Kaiser and Schreiber, 2002; Vicente et al., 2011). TE would be an appropriate information theoretical measure for an exploratory investigation of information flow in complex networks, such as the brain. Our results provide evidence that TE is an appropriate information theoretical measure that evaluates the causal and directional information flow in the brain. Interestingly, it has been shown that Ganger causality and TE are equivalent to Gaussian variables (Barnett et al., 2009). As phase is a circular measure, however, we cannot use Granger causality, which assumes a Gaussian distribution in predicting signals, for detecting causal information flow in phase signals. Therefore, we propose that TE is useful to detect information flow in phase signals, as it evaluates the causal and directional information flow between specific brain areas in synchronous networks. Although we focused our analyses on information transfer between 2 specific brain areas in the current study, future work should analyze information flow more extensively across the entire brain. In fact, TE has been used to detect information flow in complex systems, such as social information flow on the web (Oka and Ikegami, 2012).

The results of the current study indicate the possibility that TE is a quantifiable index of causal information flow among brain networks. Our experimental paradigm had the explicit consequence of information flow by virtue of TMS. In fact, TE indicates that TMS can modulate large-scale causal information flow in the brain, particularly in the case of higher-intensity TMS.

Therefore, future studies should examine whether TE reflects causality among brain areas without TMS application.

In conclusion, we demonstrated that single-pulse TMS modulated global phase dynamics and information flow among synchronous networks in the human brain. Our results suggest that single-pulse TMS modulates both incoming and outgoing information flow in the TMS-targeted areas associated with functional changes.

ACKNOWLEDGMENTS

The research was supported by a Grant-in-Aid for Scientific Research on Innovative Areas (21120005) to Masahiro Kawasaki and Keiichi Kitajo, a Grant-in-Aid for Young Scientists (B) (23700328) to Masahiro Kawasaki, and JST PRESTO to Keiichi Kitajo. The authors would like to thank Tadashi Kitahara, Yohei Yamada, and Yuji Mizuno for their support in the data analyses and Hiroshi Endo and Yuka Okazaki for their support in developing experimental settings.

SUPPLEMENTARY MATERIAL

Figure S1 | Representative EEG data from 1 subject in the main experiments under the 95% MT TMS, 50% MT TMS, and 50% sham-TMS conditions. Upper panels: 20 single-trial EEG signals (dashed lines) for the C3 and Oz electrodes randomly selected from all trials for each TMS condition. 0 ms indicates TMS onset. EEG signals were low cut filtered (30 Hz) by a Butterworth filter. Lower panels: Corresponding averaged TMS evoked potentials (solid lines) for each condition in each subject.

Figure S2 | Representative EEG data from 1 subject in additional experiments under the 95% MT TMS, sham1, and sham2 conditions. Upper panels: 20 single-trial EEG signals (dashed lines) for the C3 and Oz electrodes randomly selected from all trials for each TMS condition. 0 ms indicates TMS onset. EEG signals were low cut filtered (30 Hz) by a Butterworth filter. Lower panels: Corresponding averaged TMS evoked responses (solid lines) for each condition in each subject.

REFERENCES

Barnett, L., Barrett, A. B., and Seth, A. K. (2009). Granger causality and transfer entropy are equivalent for Gaussian variables. Phys. Rev. Lett. 103, 238701-1-4. doi: 10.1103/PhysRevLett.103.238701

Becker, R., Ritter, P., and Villringer, A. (2008). Influence of ongoing alpha rhythm on the visual evoked potential. Neuroimage 39, 707 716. doi: 10.1016/j.neuroimage.2007.09.016

Brovelli, A., Ding, M., Ledberg, A., Chen, Y., Nakamura, R., and Bressler, S. L. (2004). Beta oscillations in a large-scale sensorimotor cortical network: direc- tional influences revealed by Granger causality. Proc. Natl. Acad. Sci. U.S.A. 101, 9849–9854. doi: 10.1073/pnas.0308538101

Bullmore, E., Horwitz, B., Honey, G., Brammer, M., Williams, S., and Sharma, T. (2000). How good is good enough in path analysis of fMRI data? Neuroimage 11, 289–301. doi: 10.1006/nimg.2000.0544

Buzsaki, G., and Draguhn, A. (2004). Neuronal oscillations in cortical networks.

Science 304, 1926–1929. doi: 10.1126/science.1099745

Casali, A. G., Casarotto, S., Rosanova, M., Mariotti, M., and Massimini, M. (2010). General indices to characterize the electrical response of the cerebral cortex to TMS. Neuroimage 49, 1459–1468. doi: 10.1016/j.neuroimage.2009.09.026

Cosmelli, D., David, O., Lachaux, J. P., Martinerie, J., Garnero, L., Renault, B., et al. (2004). Waves of consciousness: ongoing cortical patterns during binocular rivalry. Neuroimage 23, 128–140. doi: 10.1016/j.neuroimage.2004.05.008

Doesburg, S. M., Roggeveen, A. B., Kitajo, K., and Ward, L. M. (2008). Large-scale gamma-band phase synchronization and selective attention. Cereb. Cortex 18, 386–396. doi: 10.1093/cercor/bhm073

Engel, A., and Singer, W. (2001). Temporal binding and the neural correlates of sen- sory awareness. Trends Cogn. Sci. 5, 16–25. doi: 10.1016/S1364-6613(00)01568-0 Esser, S. K., Huber, R., Massimini, M., Peterson, M. J., Ferrarelli, F., and Tononi, G. (2006). A direct demonstration of cortical LTP in humans: a combined TMS/EEG study. Brain Res. Bull. 69, 86–94. doi: 10.1016/j.brainresbull.2005.11.003

Fisher, N. I. (1993). Statistical Analysis of Circular Data. Cambridge, UK: Cambridge University Press. doi: 10.1017/CBO9780511564345

Fries, P. (2005). A mechanism for cognitive dynamics: neuronal communi- cation through neuronal coherence. Trends Cogn. Sci. 9, 474–480. doi: 10.1016/j.tics.2005.08.011

Friston, K. J., Harrison, L., and Penny, W. (2003). Dynamic causal modelling.

Neuroimage 19, 1273–1302. doi: 10.1016/S1053-8119(03)00202-7

Fuggetta, G., Fiaschi, A., and Manganotti, P. (2005). Modulation of cortical oscil- latory activities induced by varying single-pulse transcranial magnetic stimula- tion intensity over the left primary motor area: a combined EEG and TMS study. Neuroimage 27, 896–908. doi: 10.1016/j.neuroimage.2005.05.013

Gourevitch, B., and Eggermont, J. J. (2007). Evaluating information transfer between auditory cortical neurons. J. Neurophysiol. 97, 2533–2543. doi: 10.1152/jn.01106.2006

Herrmann, C. S., Grigutsch, M., and Busch, N. A. (2005). "EEG oscillations and wavelet analysis" in Event-Related Potentials: A Methods Handbook, ed T. C. Handy (Cambridge, MA: MIT Press), 229–259.

Ilmoniemi, R. J., Virtanen, J., Ruohonen, J., Jari, K., Aronen, H. J., Näätänen, R., et al. (1997). Neuronal responses to magnetic stimulation reveal cortical reactivity and connectivity. Neuroreport 8, 3537–3540. doi: 10.1097/00001756- 199711100-00024

Jensen, O., and Colgin, L. L. (2007). Cross-frequency coupling between neuronal oscillations. Trends Cogn. Sci. 11, 267–269. doi: 10.1016/j.tics.2007.05.003

Kaiser, A., and Schreiber, T. (2002). Information transfer in continuous processes. Phys. D 166, 43–62. doi: 10.1016/S0167-2789(02)00432-3

Kawasaki, M., Kitajo, K., and Yamaguchi, Y. (2010). Dynamic links between theta executive functions and alpha storage buffers in auditory and visual working memory. Eur. J. Neurol. 31, 1683–1689. doi: 10.1111/j.1460-9568.2010.07217.x

Kawasaki, M., and Yamaguchi, Y. (2013). Frontal theta and beta synchronizations for monetary reward increase visual working memory capacity. Soc. Affect. Cogn. Neurosci. 8, 523–530. doi: 10.1093/scan/nss027

Kayser, J., and Tenke, C. E. (2006). Principal components analysis of Laplacian waveforms as a generic method for identifying ERP generator patterns: I.

Evaluation with auditory oddball tasks. Clin. Neurophysiol. 117, 348–368. doi: 10.1016/j.clinph.2005.08.034

Kitajo, K., Doesburg, S. M., Yamanaka, K., Nozaki, D., Ward, L. M., and Yamamoto, Y. (2007). Noise-induced large-scale phase synchronization of human brain activity associated with behavioural stochastic resonance. Europhys. Lett. 80, 40009. doi: 10.1209/0295-5075/80/40009

Klimesch, W., Freunberger, R., Sauseng, P., and Gruber, W. (2008). A short review of slow phase synchronization and memory: evidence for con- trol processes in different memory systems? Brain Res. 1235, 31–44. doi: 10.1016/j.brainres.2008.06.049

Lachaux, J. P., Rodriguez, E., Le Van Quyen, M., Lutz, A., Martinerie, J., and Varela, F. J. (2000). Studying single-trials of phase synchronous activity in the brain. Int. J. Bifurcat. Chaos 10, 2429–2439. doi: 10.1142/S0218127400001560

Mäki, H., and Ilmoniemi, R. J. (2010). The relationship between peripheral and early cortical activation induced by transcranial magnetic stimulation. Neurosci. Lett. 478, 24–28. doi: 10.1016/j.neulet.2010.04.059

Massimini, M., Ferrarelli, F., Huber, R., Esser, S. K., Singh, H., and Tononi, G.

(2005). Breakdown of cortical effective connectivity during sleep. Science 309, 2228–2232. doi: 10.1126/science.1117256

Mazaheri, A., and Jensen, O. (2006). Posterior alpha activity is not phase- reset by visual stimuli. Proc. Natl. Acad. Sci. U.S.A. 103, 2948–2952. doi: 10.1073/pnas.0505785103

Melloni, L., Molina, C., Pena, M., Torresm, D., Singer, W., and Rodriguez, E. (2007). Synchronization of neural activity across cortical areas correlates with con- scious perception. J. Neurosci. 27, 2858–2865. doi: 10.1523/JNEUROSCI.4623-06.2007

Mizuhara, H., and Yamaguchi, Y. (2007). Human cortical circuits for central execu- tive function emerge by theta phase synchronization. Neuroimage 36, 232–244. doi: 10.1016/j.neuroimage.2007.02.026

Moliadze, V., Zhao, Y., Eysel, Y., and Funke, K. (2003). Effect of tran- scranial magnetic stimulation on single-unit activity in the cat pri- mary visual cortex. J. Physiol. 553, 665–679. doi: 10.1113/jphysiol.2003.0 50153

Morishima, Y., Akaishi, R., Yamada, Y., Okuda, J., Toma, K., and Sakai, K. (2009).

Task-specific signal transmission from prefrontal cortex in visual selective attention. Nat. Neurosci. 12, 85–91. doi: 10.1038/nn.2237

Nikouline, V., Ruohonen, J., and Ilmoniemi, R. J. (1999). The role of the coil click in TMS assessed with simultaneous EEG. Clin. Neurophysiol. 110, 1325–1328. doi: 10.1016/S1388-2457(99)00070-X

Oka, M., and Ikegami, T. (2012). Characterizing autonomy in the web via transfer entropy network. Artif. Life 13, 234–242. doi: 10.7551/978-0-262-31050-5-ch032

Paus, T., Sipila, P. K., and Strafella, P. (2001). Synchronization of neuronal activity in the human primary motor cortex by transcranial magnetic stimulation: an EEG study. J. Neurophysiol. 86, 1983–1990.

Perrin, F., Pernier, J., Bertrand, O., and Echallier, J. F. (1989). Spherical splines for scalp potential and current density mapping. Electroencephalogr. Clin. Neurophysiol. 72, 184–187. doi: 10.1016/0013-4694(89) 90180-6

Rodriguez, E., George, N., Lachaux, J. P., Martinerie, J., Renault, B., and Varela, F.

J. (1999). Perception's shadow: long-distance synchronization of human brain activity. Nature 397, 430–433. doi: 10.1038/17120

Roebroeck, A., Formisano, E., and Goebel, R. (2005). Mapping directed influence over the brain using Granger causality and fMRI. Neuroimage 25, 230–242. doi: 10.1016/j.neuroimage.2004.11.017

Rosanova, M., Casali, A., Valentina, B., Resta, F., Mariotti, M., and Massimini, M. (2009). Natural frequencies of human corticothalamic circuits. J. Neurosci. 29, 7679–7685. doi: 10.1523/JNEUROSCI.0445-09.2009

Sain, S. R., Baggerly, K. A., and Scott, D. W. (1994). Cross-validation of multi- variate densities. J. Am. Stat. Assoc. 89, 807–817. doi: 10.1080/01621459.1994.10 476814

Sauseng, P., Klimesch, W., Gruber, W. R., Hanslmayr, S., Freunberger, R., and Doppelmayr, M. (2007). Are event-related potential components generated by phase resetting of brain oscillations? A critical discussion. Neuroscience 146, 1435–1444. doi: 10.1016/j.neuroscience.2007.03.014

Sauseng, P., Klimesch, W., Schabus, M., and Doppelmayr, M. (2005). Frontoparietal EEG coherence in theta and upper alpha reflect central executive functions of working memory. Int. J. Psychophysiol. 57, 97–103. doi: 10.1016/j.ijpsycho.2005.03.018

Schreiber, T. (2000). Measuring information transfer. Phys. Rev. Lett. 85, 461–464. doi: 10.1103/PhysRevLett.85.461

Sekiguchi, H., Takeuchi, S., Kadota, H., Kohno, Y., and Nakajima, Y. (2011). TMS-induced artifacts on EEG can be reduced by rearrangement of the elec- trode's lead wire before recording. Clin. Neurophysiol. 122, 984–990. doi: 10.1016/j.clinph.2010.09.004

Silverman, B. W. (1981). Using kernel density estimates to investigate multimodal- ity. J. R. Stat. Soc. Series B Stat. Methodol. 43, 97–99.

Silverman, B. W. (1986). Density Estimation for Statistics and Data Analysis, Monographs on Statistics and Applied Probability. Vol. 26. London: Chapman and Hall. doi: 10.1007/978-1-4899-3324-9

Tallon-Baudry, C., Bertrand, O., Delpuech, C., and Pernier, J. (1996). Stimulus specificity of phase-locked and non-phase-locked 40 Hz visual responses in human. J. Neurosci. 16, 4240–4249.

Taylor, P., Walsh, V., and Eimer, M. (2008). Combining TMS and EEG to study cog- nitive function and cortico-cortico interactions. Behav. Brain Res. 191, 141–147. doi: 10.1016/j.bbr.2008.03.033

Telenczuk, B., Nikulin, V. V., and Curio, G. (2010). Role of neuronal synchrony in the generation of evoked EEG/MEG responses. J. Neurophysiol. 104, 3557–3567. doi: 10.1152/jn.00138.2010

Ter Braack, E. M., de Vos, C. C., and van Putten, J. A. M. (2013). Masking the audi- tory evoked potential in TMS-EEG: a comparison of various methods. Brain Topogr. doi: 10.1007/s10548-013-0312-z. [Epub ahead of print].

Thut, G., Ives, J. R., Kampmann, F., Pastor, M., and Pascual-Leone, A. (2005). A new device and protocol for combining TMS and online recordings of EEG and evoked potentials. J. Neurosci. Methods 141, 207–217. doi: 10.1016/j.jneumeth.2004.06.016

Thut, G., and Miniussi, C. (2009). New insights into rhythmic brain activity from TMS-EEG studies. Trends Cogn. Sci. 13, 182–189. doi: 10.1016/j.tics.2009.01.004

Van Der Werf, Y. D., and Paus, T. (2006). The neural response to transcranial magnetic stimulation of the human motor cortex. I. Intracortical and cortico- cortical contributions. Exp. Brain Res. 175, 231–245. doi: 10.1007/s00221-006- 0551-2

Varela, F., Lachaux, J. P., Rodriguez, E., and Martinerie, J. (2001). The brain- web: phase synchronization and large-scale integration. Nat. Rev. Neurosci. 2, 229–239. doi: 10.1038/35067550

Veniero, D., Bortoletto, M., and Miniussi, C. (2009). TMS-EEG co-registration: on TMS-induced artifact. Clin. Neurophysiol. 120, 1392–1399. doi: 10.1016/j.clinph.2009.04.023

Veniero, D., Brignani, D., Thut, G., and Miniussi, C. (2011). Alpha-generation as basic response-signature to transcranial magnetic stimulation (TMS) tar- geting the human resting motor cortex: a TMS/EEG co-registration study. Psychophysiology 48, 1381–1389. doi: 10.1111/j.1469-8986.2011.01218.x

Vicente, R., Wibral, M., Lindner, M., and Gordon, P. J. (2011). Transfer entropy— a model-free measure of effective connectivity for the neurosciences. Comput. Neurosci. 30, 45–67. doi: 10.1007/s10827-010-0262-3

Von Stein, A., and Sarnthein, J. (2000). Different frequencies for different scales of cortical integration: from local gamma to long range alpha/theta synchroniza- tion. Int. J. Psychophysiol. 38, 301–313. doi: 10.1016/S0167-8760(00)00172-0

Ward, L. M. (2003). Synchronous neural oscillations and cognitive processes.

Trends Cogn. Sci. 7, 553–559. doi: 10.1016/j.tics.2003.10.012

Womelsdorf, T., and Fries, P. (2007). The role of neuronal synchroniza- tion in selective attention. Curr. Opin. Neurobiol. 17, 154–160. doi: 10.1016/j.conb.2007.02.002

7

Movement and afferent representations in human motor areas: a simultaneous neuroimaging and transcranial magnetic/peripheral nerve-stimulation study

H. Shitara[1,2], T. Shinozaki[3], K. Takagishi[2], M. Honda[1] and T. Hanakawa[1,4,5]*

[1] Department of Functional Brain Research, National Center of Neurology and Psychiatry, National Institute of Neuroscience, Kodaira, Japan
[2] Department of Orthopedic Surgery, Gunma University Graduate School of Medicine, Maebashi, Japan
[3] Department of Orthopedic Surgery, Maki Hospital, Takasaki, Japan
[4] Department of Advanced Neuroimaging, Integrative Brain Imaging Center, National Center of Neurology and Psychiatry, Kodaira, Japan
[5] PRESTO, Japan Science and Technology Agency, Kawaguchi, Japan

***Correspondence:**
T. Hanakawa, Department of Advanced Neuroimaging, Integrative Brain Imaging Center, National Center of Neurology and Psychiatry, 4-1-1 Ogawahigashi, Kodaira 187-8551, Japan
e-mail: hanakawa@ncnp.go.jp

Neuroimaging combined with transcranial magnetic stimulation (TMS) to primary motor cortex (M1) is an emerging technique that can examine motor-system functionality through evoked activity. However, because sensory afferents from twitching muscles are widely represented in motor areas the amount of evoked activity directly resulting from TMS remains unclear. We delivered suprathreshold TMS to left M1 or gave electrical right median nerve stimulation (MNS) in 18 healthy volunteers while simultaneously conducting functional magnetic resonance imaging and monitoring with electromyography (EMG). We examined in detail the localization of TMS-, muscle afferent- and superficial afferent-induced activity in M1 subdivisions. Muscle afferent- and TMS-evoked activity occurred mainly in rostral M1, while superficial afferents generated a slightly different activation distribution. In 12 participants who yielded quantifiable EMG, differences in brain activity ascribed to differences in movement-size were adjusted using integrated information from the EMGs. Sensory components only explained 10–20% of the suprathreshold TMS-induced activity, indicating that locally and remotely evoked activity in motor areas mostly resulted from the recruitment of neural and synaptic activity. The present study appears to justify the use of fMRI combined with suprathreshold TMS to M1 for evoked motor network imaging.

Keywords: connectivity, motor cortex, multimodal neuroimaging, proprioceptive afferents

INTRODUCTION

For online control of movement, the status of muscles controlling the target effector needs to be properly monitored and integrated with a motor plan. Somatosensory afferents from the effector carry critical information for this somatosensory-motor integration. Such integration likely occurs at multiple levels in the central nervous system, from the spinal cord up through cortical motor areas. In primates, both superficial and proprioceptive sensations reach cortical motor areas including the primary motor cortex (M1) (Strick and Preston, 1978; Fetz et al., 1980; Lemon, 1981) presumably via the thalamus (Horne and Tracey, 1979) and primary somatosensory cortex (S1) (Pons and Kaas, 1986). We can therefore expect afferent-induced neural activity in motor areas during overt movement. Indeed, previous studies in humans have reported motor-area activity during peripheral nerve stimulation that elicits muscle-twitching (Korvenoja et al., 1999; Spiegel et al., 1999; Del Gratta et al., 2000; Shitara et al., 2011) and during vibrotactile stimulation to muscles (Naito et al., 2002; Gizewski et al., 2005; Bardouille and Ross, 2008). In contrast, few human neuroimaging studies have addressed the issue of motor-area activity ascribed to sensory afferents. This omission likely results from difficulty controlling the effects of sensory afferents during voluntary movement accompanying a complicated temporal pattern of muscle activity.

Neuroimaging combined with transcranial magnetic stimulation (TMS) to M1 is an emerging technique for non-invasively studying the organization of motor-control neural networks in humans. Suprathreshold TMS to M1 consistently induces increased brain metabolism or hemodynamic responses in the stimulated area as well as remote motor areas (Bestmann et al., 2003; Speer et al., 2003; Komssi et al., 2004; Fox et al., 2006; Hanakawa et al., 2009; Shitara et al., 2011). However, because suprathreshold TMS induces motor evoked potentials (MEPs) visible on surface electromyography (EMG), we must consider the effects of proprioceptive afferents from the twitching muscles when interpreting such motor-area activity.

Technical advances now allow us to measure MEPs with surface EMG in a simultaneous TMS-fMRI (functional magnetic resonance imaging) environment (Bestmann et al., 2004; Hanakawa et al., 2009; Shitara et al., 2011). An MEP is composed of a brief oligophasic potential similar in shape to a compound muscle action potential (CMAP) evoked by peripheral nerve stimulation. Motor-area activity during peripheral nerve stimulation, if any, should reflect processing of sensory afferents without preceding motor commands. Given the similarity of MEPs and CMAPs, using peripheral nerve stimulation as a control condition for muscle afferents during suprathreshold M1 stimulation seems reasonable. However, MEPs are always smaller than CMAPs because of phase cancellation of action potentials at the corticospinal and spinal neuron levels (Magistris et al., 1998). Still, CMAPs and MEPs should provide rough yet comparable estimates of proprioceptive afferent size because the phase cancellation occurs at the motor efferent level, not at the muscular or afferent level. Additionally, peripheral nerve stimulation between the motor and sensory thresholds can provide a condition akin to superficial sensory stimulation.

Based on these assumptions, here we conducted a multimodal imaging study to differentiate neural activity in the motor network that generates movement from those used for afferent information processing resulting from the movements. The main goal was to compare local and remote brain activity resulting from suprathreshold single-pulse TMS to M1 with those resulting from electrical median nerve stimulation (MNS) above the motor threshold. In particular, we were interested in assessing TMS-evoked and sensory-evoked activity in M1 subdivisions (M1a and M1p) that are reported to have a differential distribution of proprioceptive and superficial afferent information (Strick and Preston, 1982; Geyer et al., 1996).

MATERIALS AND METHODS

SUBJECTS

We analyzed data from 18 healthy adults (female, 15; male, 3; mean age, 29.3 years; range, 20-46 years) in our previous study (Shitara et al., 2011). From this previous study, we selected participants who underwent both the TMS and MNS conditions in the same experimental session. All participants were right handed. None reported any history of neuropsychiatric disorders, including epilepsy. The Institutional Review Board of the National Center of Neurology and Psychiatry approved the study protocol. The participants were fully informed about the experimental procedure, and all gave written informed consent prior to the participation.

STIMULATION AND ELECTROMYOGRAPHY MONITORING

We used a 3-Tesla whole-body MRI scanner equipped with a circular polarization head coil (Siemens Magnetom Trio; Erlangen, Germany). The "motor hot spot" at which TMS evoked a maximal motor response in the right abductor pollicis brevis (APB) muscle was identified for each participant while lying supine on the scanner bed. The APB was the primary muscle of interest in this experiment, as with our previous TMS-fMRI experiments (Hanakawa et al., 2009; Shitara et al., 2011). An MRI-compatible figure-eight TMS coil with an outer-wing diameter of 70 mm (MR coil, Magstim, Witland, Wales, UK) was positioned tangentially to the scalp at the "motor hot-spot." TMS-coil orientation was ~45° from the medial-lateral axis. The TMS coil was connected to a stimulator (SuperRapid, Magstim, Witland, Wales, UK) via a 7-m cable running through a wave-guide tube appropriate for radiofrequency wave filtering. The TMS stimulator produced a biphasic electrical lasting ~250 μs with a rise time of 50 μs.

For the MNS-fMRI experiment, electrical stimulation was delivered through a pair of MRI-compatible silver/silver chloride electrodes (Nihon Kohden, Tokyo, Japan). The electrodes were connected to an electric current stimulator (Nihon Kohden, Tokyo, Japan) placed outside the scanner room. The maximum stimulator output was 50 mV. Constant-voltage square waves with pulse duration of 0.3 ms were applied to the right median nerve at the wrist. The sensory threshold was determined by each participant's verbal report of sensation in the first three fingers without muscle twitching. A motor threshold for eliciting APB activity was defined according to the recommendations of the IFCN Committee (Rossini et al., 1994a) as the minimum stimulus intensity that produced a liminal EMG response (more than 50 mV in 50% of trials). No participants reported a sensation of pain. The stimulation procedure did not cause any artifacts in the functional MR images.

MEPs were recorded from the APB and abductor digiti minimi (ADM) muscles bilaterally, using BrainAmp ExG MR (Brain Products, Gilching, Germany). The amplifier and MRI scanner were synchronized using SyncBox (Brain Products, Gilching, Germany). Surface electrodes were placed over the bilateral APB and ADM muscles with an inter-electrode distance of ~2 cm. EMG signals were fed into a battery-driven amplifier placed on the scanner bed. EMG data were sampled at a digitization rate of 5 kHz with an amplitude resolution of 0.5 μV/bit and a dynamic range of 16 mV.

To minimize joint movements and reflexive antagonistic muscle contraction, both upper limbs were tightly fixed onto custom-made, non-magnetic splints (covering the hand, wrist, and elbow joints) with elastic bandages. Hence, both TMS- and MNS-evoked movements were primarily isometric contractions. Fixing the hand position also helped minimize EMG changes and imaging artifacts throughout the experiment. The position of the TMS coil was adjusted while stimulation was delivered every 5 s until MEPs were consistently recorded from the right APB muscle. The TMS coil was then fixed immobile to the scanner bed with a custom-made holder made from polyetheretherketone plastic. Foam pads and vacuum cushions were used to minimize head motion during scanning. After participants' heads were fixed, the resting motor threshold (RMT) was defined individually as the percentage of stimulator output that elicited MEPs of greater than 50 μV peak-to-peak amplitude in the APB at rest in more than 5 of 10 successive trials (Rossini et al., 1994a). The active motor threshold (AMT) was similarly determined during weak isometric contraction of the APB muscle at ~20% of the maximum contraction under EMG monitoring.

EXPERIMENTAL TASKS

During the fMRI experiments, participants were instructed to relax and remain awake. Vision was not constrained. In each fMRI run, 42 single-pulse TMS or MNS were given during 110-ms inter-volume acquisition delay periods. Stimulus onset asynchrony (SOA) was semi-randomized between 7.98 and 13.97 s (stimulus frequency, 0.072-0.125 Hz). All participants underwent the TMS-fMRI and MNS experiment. The experimental conditions were composed of suprathreshold TMS at an intensity of 120% of the RMT (supra-TMS), MNS above the motor threshold (motor-MNS), and MNS between the sensory and the motor thresholds (sensory-MNS). The sensory-MNS condition was included to account for the sensory-component stimulation of the MNS condition and to map representations of non-muscular afferents to motor areas. Stimulus intensity during motor-MNS varied semi-randomly between the motor threshold and 120% of the motor threshold to yield variability similar in evoked movement size as in the supra-TMS condition. Intensity of sensory-MNS was kept between the motor and the sensory thresholds for all participants and was not varied.

Stimulation timing was controlled by Presentation software (Neurobehavioral systems, Albany, CA, USA) on a personal computer synchronized with the MRI scanner via transistor-transistor logic pulses converted from the default optic signals of the scanner. To avoid image degradation, TMS pulses were delivered during the inter-volume delay periods. The same stimulation timing was used for all conditions.

IMAGE ACQUISITION

We measured hemodynamic signals with echo planar imaging (EPI) as follows: repetition time (TR) = 998 ms, inter-volume acquisition delay = 110 ms, echo time (TE) = 25 ms, flip angle (FA) = 60°, 64 × 64 matrix, 12 slices, 500 volumes, field of view (FOV) = 192 mm, and 3 × 3 × 4-mm voxel size. Bilateral cortical motor and somatosensory areas, basal ganglia, and thalami were covered with approximately coronal acquisition. Most of the cerebellum was outside the search volume. A short TR was employed originally to investigate the signal time-course of TMS-evoked activity with fine temporal resolution (Shitara et al., 2011). The timing of gradient pulses was carefully designed and the MRI scanner and amplifier were synchronized so that EMG signals could be constantly sampled at 1 kHz without being disturbed by gradient pulses (Anami et al., 2003). The inter-volume acquisition delay allowed us to acquire EPI without interference from induced electromagnetic fields or vibration of the TMS coil.

For anatomic registration, T1-weighted three-dimensional structural images were also acquired with a magnetization-prepared, rapid-gradient echo sequence (TR = 2000 ms, TE = 4.38 ms, FA = 8°, FOV = 192 mm, matrix = 176 × 192, voxel size = 1 × 1 × 1 mm). For correcting distortion of functional images, field-map imagers were obtained in the same space as the functional image (TR = 511 ms, TE = 5.19 and 7.65 ms, FA = 60°, FOV = 192 mm, matrix = 64 × 64, voxel size = 3 × 3 × 4 mm).

EMG AND IMAGE DATA ANALYSIS

To remove gradient artifacts, we pre-processed all EMG data using an averaged subtraction method implemented in Analyzer 2 (Brain Products, Gilching, Germany). A band-pass filter of 20-200 Hz was applied. We visually checked the quality of artifact-removed EMG data from the target (right APB) for quantitative assessment of right APB activity and those of non-target (left APB and bilateral ADM) muscles to confirm the absence of EMG. The artifact-free EMG data from the right APB were rectified and integrated to produce an integral EMG value (iEMG) as a parameter of movement size. iEMG is adequate for quantifying total muscle activity with surface EMG (Hermens et al., 1991; Shitara et al., 2011) especially because we aimed to estimate the amount of muscle afferents in two types of evoked movements (MEP and CMAP) with slightly different temporal profiles. These different temporal profiles result from larger temporal jittering in TMS-evoked descending volleys than MNS-induced peripheral nerve excitation. Thus, it would be difficult to estimate the size of efferent signals by comparing iEMG between different modalities. However, iEMG can still serve as a surrogate marker for the quantity of afferent signals from the twitched APB. For computing the iEMG, time windows for the integration were modified to extract EMG signals specific to experimental conditions as purely as possible. Time for integration was between 20-40 ms for TMS and between 5–25 ms for the MNS (Shitara et al., 2011).

Two parameters were computed from the iEMG. First, mean iEMG was defined as the average of raw iEMG values divided by the EMG-evoking events in an fMRI run for the supra-TMS and the motor-MNS conditions. Mean iEMG data were compared across conditions with a paired t-test. Second, the minimum and maximum iEMG values across all EMG-evoking events were determined for each individual. Then, normalized iEMG was computed individually for each EMG-evoking event as follows: (iEMG - minimum iEMG)/(maximum iEMG - minimum iEMG). Normalized iEMG represented the variation of iEMG values across all the EMG-evoking events and served a parametric modulator in the first-level general linear model (GLM) analysis.

Imaging data were pre-processed with SPM5 (Wellcome Department of Imaging Neuroscience, UCL, London, UK) using Matlab (MathWorks, Inc., Natick, MA, USA) and FSL (FMRIB, Oxford University, Oxford, UK) using VMware player (VMware, Palo Alto, CA, USA). The first 10 volumes in each experimental run were discarded to allow for T1 equilibrium effects. The remaining functional images were corrected for differences in slice acquisition timing. The non-linear distortion of EPI data resulting from inhomogeneity of the magnetic field was corrected using FUGUE (FSL) by referencing to the field map image acquired for each participant before the fMRI experiment. The functional images were motion-corrected, and residual noise was detected with an independent component-analysis filter (MELODIC, FSL). We removed ICA components with time-course that showed abrupt spikes and those with maps showing alternating patterns of signal variation for every other slice (corresponding to motion during interleaved MRI data acquisition) (Tohka et al., 2008). The motion-corrected and artifact-removed images were then spatially normalized to fit to the Montreal Neurological Institute (MNI) template based on the standard stereotaxic coordinate system. Subsequently, all images were smoothed with an isotropic Gaussian kernel of 8-mm full-width at half-maximum.

Statistical analysis was performed using SPM5. A train of delta functions representing stimulus onsets was convolved with the canonical hemodynamic response function (HRF) and its temporal derivative, and these served as regressors for each condition (supra-TMS, motor-MNS, and sensory-MNS) in the first-level GLM analysis. Although neural events associated with these conditions may differ in the range of several tens of milliseconds, our previous study investigating fine temporal time-course of fMRI responses has clearly showed that we can estimate size of brain activity using the same HRF function for the three conditions (Shitara et al., 2011). We built two types of first-level design matrix: one with the normalized iEMG regressor as a parametric modulator of the EMG-evoking events and the other without. The latter design was used for analysis that included the sensory-MNS condition, which did not evoke muscle activity. Six parameters representing the head motion were included in the design matrix as covariates. Global signal normalization was performed only between runs. Low frequency noise was removed with a 128-s high-pass filter, and serial correlations were adjusted using an auto-regression model. We computed summary images reflecting the effects of interest on fMRI signals by applying linear contrasts to the parameter estimates. These summary images were fed into the subsequent second-level random-effect model analysis.

First, group-level statistical parametric maps (SPMs) were generated by performing one-sample t-tests on the summary images representing the effects of each experimental condition relative to the implicit baseline. Second, we defined proprioceptive and superficial sensory-evoked brain activity using the motor-MNS and sensory-MNS conditions. Muscle proprioception-evoked activity was defined by the difference in activation between the motor-MNS and sensory-MNS conditions (motor-MNS minus sensory-MNS). To define areas related to superficial afferent processing, a conjunction analysis was performed between the motor-MNS and sensory-MNS conditions since both types of stimulation should involve superficial afferents. Furthermore, we explored variation of brain activity explained by the size variation of the normalized iEMG regressor.

In the group-level SPM, the threshold was initially set at a voxel-wise height-level of $P < 0.05$ corrected for multiple comparisons (family-wise error; FWE). Clusters exceeding a height threshold of uncorrected $P < 0.005$ were reported as a trend. The cytoarchitectonic nomenclature of significant brain activity was identified according to the SPM5 anatomy toolbox when applicable.

DISTRIBUTION OF TMS- AND AFFERENT-INDUCED BRAIN ACTIVITY IN M1 SUBDIVISIONS

Previous animal and human studies have indicated differences in proprioceptive and superficial afferent information coded in M1 (Strick and Preston, 1982; Geyer et al., 1996). We therefore assessed the difference in spatial distribution between TMS- and two afferent-induced activities in M1 subdivisions (M1a and M1p). We created M1a and M1p mask-images (SPM5 anatomy toolbox) according to the MNI coordinates. The transformed M1a and M1p images were thresholded at 40% of their probabilistic distributions, and were then transformed into binary mask images (M1a and M1p masks). Brain activity obtained from the conjunction analysis of motor-MNS and sensory-MNS conditions was defined as the activity coding superficial afferents. Muscle afferent-related activity was defined as the contrast motor-MNS minus sensory-MNS (as described above). The "pure" TMS-induced activity was defined as the contrast supra-TMS minus muscle afferent-related activity to exclude the contribution of sensory components. In this particular analysis, we will report significant activities thresholded at $P < 0.05$ (FWE-corrected) after small volume correction according to our previous reports (Hanakawa et al., 2009; Shitara et al., 2011).

We also used small-volume correction (svc) analysis with spherical volumes of interest (VOIs). We applied a 5-mm radius to left M1 ($x, y, z = -36, -24, 52$), right M1 ($x, y, z = 34, -30, 64$), left dorsal premotor cortex ($x, y, z = -32, -10, 60$), left S1 ($x, y, z = -32, -32, 68$), left supplementary motor area (SMA) ($x, y, z = -6, -12, 48$), left putamen ($x, y, z = -30, -10, 0$), and left thalamus ($x, y, z = -14, -22, 4$), and a 3-mm radius to the left subthalamic nucleus ($x, y, z = -12, -18, -4$) (Hanakawa et al., 2009; Shitara et al., 2011). We also report trends toward activation thresholded at uncorrected $P < 0.005$.

DISTRIBUTION OF TMS-INDUCED AND AFFERENT-INDUCED ACTIVITY IN M1SUBDIVISIONS

We evaluated the spatial distribution of afferent-related activity and "purely" TMS-evoked activity represented in M1 subdivisions. We measured the total number of suprathreshold voxels at uncorrected $P < 0.005$ for "purely" TMS-evoked activity, muscle afferent-related activity, and superficial afferent-related activity within the M1a and M1p masks. To semi-quantify the differences in muscle- and superficial-afferent representations within the M1 subdivisions, an M1 divisional index (M1-DI) was calculated as follows: $DI = (V_{\mathrm{M1a}} - V_{\mathrm{M1p}})/(V_{\mathrm{M1a}} + V_{\mathrm{M1p}})$, where $\mathrm{V_{M1a}}$ and $\mathrm{V_{M1p}}$ refer to the number of activated voxels within the M1a and M1p masks, respectively. DI ranged from -1.0 to 1.0. A positive DI value indicates that the activity is distributed disproportionately in M1a and a negative DI means that the activity is distributed disproportionately in M1p. Additionally, we computed DI for supra-TMS induced activity to test its distribution in the M1 subdivisions. A non-parametric statistic was applied to assess differences in DI for muscle afferents and superficial afferents. To gain knowledge about spatial distribution of TMS-induced activity within M1 subdivisions, we also computed DI for voxels related to the "pure" TMS.

REMOVAL OF MUSCLE AFFERENT-INDUCED ACTIVITY CORRECTED FOR MOVEMENT SIZE FROM TMS-INDUCED ACTIVITY IN MOTOR AREAS

By controlling differences in muscle activity across conditions, we were able to explore supra-TMS-evoked activity that could not be explained by sensory afferent responses to twitching movements. Supra-TMS and motor-MNS induced activities were corrected using iEMG size as a parametric modulator. The corrected activities are referred to as supra-$\mathrm{TMS_{iEMG\_corr}}$. and motor-$\mathrm{MNS_{iEMG\_corr}}$., respectively. Data from 12 participants were available for this comparison of motor MNS- and TMS-evoked brain activities. fMRI signals (beta values) were extracted from the motor area VOIs (as described above; left M1a mask, left M1p mask, left premotor cortex, and left SMA) using MarsBaR (Brett et al., 2002) for the contrast that compared motor MNS- and TMS- induced brain activity with and without iEMG correction. We then calculated how much of the activity during the supra-TMS condition could be ascribed to responses induced by the muscle afferents and how much could be explained purely by TMS with and without correction for iEMG differences. For this purpose, muscle afferent-induced activity was defined as motor-MNS minus sensory-MNS as above. "Pure" TMS-induced activity was defined as supra-TMS activity minus muscle afferent-induced activity. We computed these values with and without correction for iEMG size during the supra-TMS and motor-MNS conditions.

RESULTS

TMS INTENSITY AND MEAN IEMG VALUES

The mean RMT was 80.6% (*SD* = 8.7) of the machine output within the MRI scanner. Accordingly, the mean stimulus-intensity for the supra-TMS condition was 96.7% (10.4). For participants who required stimulation above 100% of the machine output to reach the 120% RMT stimulation, the maximum machine output of the TMS stimulator was reset to 110% of the default machine output (enhanced mode), which was within the safety guidelines of the manufacturer and its distributor in Japan (Magstim and Miyuki Giken). All participants completed the planned experimental conditions, and none experienced significant adverse events.

We visually checked artifact-removed EMG data to confirm sufficient data quality for quantitative analysis. As reported previously (Shitara et al., 2011), muscle activity was only observed in the right APB muscle in both supra-TMS and motor-MNS conditions. We did not find any muscle activity in the bilateral ADM or the left APB muscle(s). This finding indicated that TMS-evoked muscle activity did not spread to neighboring muscles. However, EMG data from six subjects were excluded from the iEMG analysis in the motor-MNS condition because artifacts substantially overlapped with CMAP. Hence, only data from 12 participants were available for the comparison between the motor MNS- and TMS-evoked brain activities that used iEMG as a parametric modulator. The mean iEMG expressed in mV × ms was 5.0 (*SEM* = 1.2) in the supra-TMS condition, and 34.7 (6.8) in the motor-MNS condition. A paired *t*-test showed a significant difference in iEMG across conditions ($P < 0.0001$).

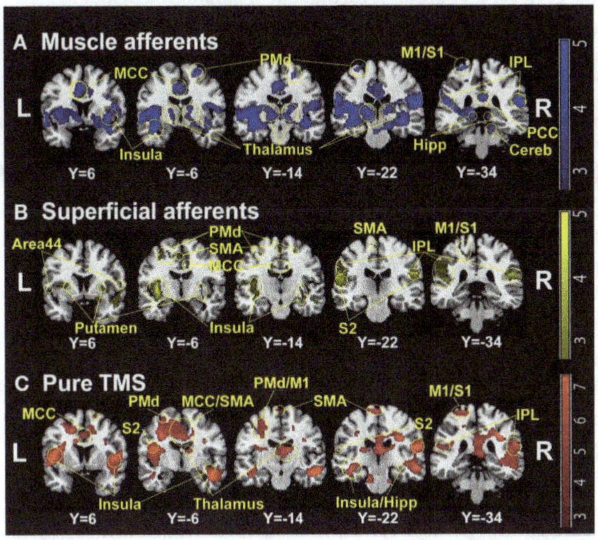

FIGURE 1 | Group-level statistical parametric maps ($n = 18$) showing the categorical comparison of conditions (thresholded at $P < 0.005$ uncorrected for display purpose). (A) Muscle afferent-related activity (contrast, motor-MNS minus sensory-MNS). Brain activation was observed in bilateral insula, middle and posterior cingulate cortices, bilateral thalami, bilateral dorsal premotor cortices, bilateral hippocampi, bilateral inferior parietal cortices, right cerebellum, left M1, and left S1. **(B)** Superficial afferent-related activity (conjunction, motor-MNS and sensory MNS). Brain activation was observed in bilateral Area 44, bilateral putamen, bilateral insula, middle cingulate cortex, bilateral dorsal premotor cortices, SMA, bilateral S2, bilateral inferior parietal cortices, left M1, and left S1. **(C)** Supra-TMS-induced activity after removing the effects of muscle afferent-induced activity [contrast, (supra-TMS minus implicit baseline) minus (motor-MNS minus sensory-MNS)]. Brain activation was observed in bilateral insula, middle cingulate cortex, SMA, bilateral thalami, bilateral hippocampi, bilateral S2, bilateral inferior parietal cortices, left dorsal premotor cortex, left M1, and left S1. *MCC*, middle cingulate cortex; *PCC*, posterior cingulate cortex; *SMA*, supplementary motor cortex; *PMd*, dorsal premotor cortex; *M1*, primary motor cortex; *S1*, primary somatosensory cortex; *S2*, secondary somatosensory cortex; *IPL*, inferior parietal lobule; *Hipp*, hippocampus; *Cereb*, cerebellum.

MUSCLE AFFERENT-RELATED ACTIVITY: COMPARISON BETWEEN MOTOR-MNS AND SENSORY-MNS

Whole-brain analysis revealed significant activation related to muscle afferents in bilateral superior temporal gyri, bilateral insula, left middle cingulate cortex, left postcentral gyrus, and right supramarginal gyrus at the formal threshold ($P < 0.05$, FWE-corrected). After small volume correction, significant activation was observed in left precentral gyrus, left SMA, left putamen, left thalamus, and the subthamamic nucleus at a threshold of $P < 0.05$, FWE-corrected. Trends were found in the right inferior frontal gyrus, right inferior temporal gyrus, and left inferior parietal lobule ($P < 0.005$ uncorrected) (**Figure 1A; Table 1A**).

BRAIN AREAS RELATED TO SUPERFICIAL AFFERENTS

Significant activation related to superficial afferents was found in left insula, bilateral superior temporal gyri, right Rolandic operculum, right temporal pole, and inferior frontal gyrus at the formal threshold ($P < 0.05$, FWE-corrected). After small volume correction, significant activation was observed in left precentral gyrus, left SMA, and left putamen at the threshold of $P < 0.05$, FWE-corrected. Trends toward activation ($P < 0.005$ uncorrected) were found in the left postcentral gyrus, right precentral gyrus, left paracentral lobule, bilateral middle cingulate cortices, left supraparietal lobule, right middle frontal gyrus, and right thalamus (**Figure 1B; Table 1B**).

COMPARISON BETWEEN SUPRA-TMS AND MUSCLE AFFERENT-INDUCED ACTIVITY WITHOUT CORRECTION FOR IEMG SIZE

Because iEMG during motor-MNS was significantly larger than that during supra-TMS, a simple subtraction of muscle afferent-related activity from supra-TMS-induced activity would overcorrect the muscle afferent-related components in the supra-TMS-induced activity. Hence, although the components evoked by supra-TMS should be underestimated, the contrast supra-TMS > motor-MNS minus sensory-MNS revealed significant activation in the bilateral insula, right inferior frontal gyrus, right supraparietal lobule, and right middle temporal gyrus ($P < 0.05$ FWE-corrected). After small volume correction, significant activation was observed in the left pre/post central gyrus, left SMA, and left putamen at the threshold of

Table 1 | Results of group-level statistical parametric mapping analysis.

N = 18	Coordinates (mm)			Z-values
Activity clusters (functional anatomy)	x	y	z	
(A) MOTOR-MNS MINUS SENSORY-MNS (UNCORRECTED $P < 0.005$)				
Left superior temporal gyrus (Insula)	−40	−6	−12	5.06*
Right superior temporal gyrus (IPL)	58	−34	20	4.71*
Right supramarginal gyrus (OP1, IPL)	62	−22	22	4.55*
Left middle cingulate cortex	−6	10	34	3.84*
Left postcentral gyrus (S1)	−30	−34	72	3.81*
Right superior frontal gyrus (SMA)	20	−10	60	3.82
Left subthalamic nucleus	−12	−20	−2	3.63#
Left thalamus	−12	−22	0	3.59#
Left SMA	−4	−10	44	3.51#
Left putamen	−34	−12	−2	3.33#
Left precentral gyrus (M1)	−32	−32	68	3.29#
Right inferior frontal gyrus (Area 44)	40	10	30	2.89
Left precentral gyrus (M1)	−22	−28	54	2.87
Left precentral gyrus (S1, M1)	−24	−36	50	2.77
Right inferior temporal gyrus	44	−12	−28	2.67
Left inferior parietal lobule (S1)	−50	−38	56	2.62
(B) CONJUNCTION OF MOTOR-MNS AND SENSORY-MNS (UNCORRECTED $P < 0.005$)				
Left insula (OP3)	−38	−8	2	5.71*
Left superior temporal gyrus (OP1)	−64	−28	16	5.14*
Right superior temporal gyrus	52	−36	22	5.03*
Left putamen	−34	−8	−2	5.03#
Right rolandic operculum (OP1)	56	−22	22	4.39*
Right temporal pole-Insula	46	2	−18	4.27*
Right inferior frontal gyrus (Area 44)	50	14	14	4.11*
Right temporal pole	50	10	−22	3.90*
Left postcentral gyrus (M1/S1)	−28	−36	64	3.58
Left postcentral gyrus (S1)	−16	−34	50	2.96
Left middle cingulate cortex	−12	−14	34	3.48
Right middle cingulate cortex	10	−6	38	3.27
Left precentral gyrus (PMd)	−30	−8	54	3.25
Left precentral gyrus (PMd/M1)	−40	−14	52	2.84
Left SMA	−2	−6	52	3.08
Left paracentral lobule (SMA)	−6	−22	66	2.97
Right precentral gyrus (PMd/Area 44)	52	10	40	3.09
Right PMd	20	−12	56	3.00
Right middle frontal gyrus	28	10	50	3.00
Left SMA	−4	−8	50	3.00#
Left SPL	−20	−40	40	2.70
Right thalamus	4	−20	−6	2.59
Left precentral gyrus (M1)	−38	−20	54	2.47#
(C) (SUPRA-TMS GREATER THAN MOTOR-MNS) MINUS SENSORY-MNS (UNCORRECTED $P < 0.005$)				
Right middle temporal gyrus	52	−14	−16	5.27*
Right insula	46	−4	−22	4.88*
Right inferior frontal gyrus (Area 44)	48	14	4	4.87*
Right SPL	34	−32	34	4.89*
Left insula	−46	4	6	4.85*
Right PMd	34	−24	32	4.66*

(Continued)

Table 1 | Continued

N = 18	Coordinates (mm)			Z-values
Activity clusters (functional anatomy)	x	y	z	
Right cerebellum	18	−24	−30	3.86
Left paracentral lobule (M1)	−16	−32	72	3.83
Left paracentral lobule (SMA/M1)	−4	−22	72	3.50
Left PMd	−30	−10	58	3.16
Left M1	−18	−30	52	3.14
Left Hippocampus	−42	−24	−14	3.77
Left middle temporal gyrus	−46	−8	−22	3.39
Left S1	−28	−32	70	3.33#
Left superior temporal gyrus (OP1)	−60	−30	14	3.70
Left IPL	−40	−38	22	3.18
Left M1	−32	−32	68	3.03#
Right middle frontal gyrus	38	4	58	2.76
Left SMA	−4	−8	46	2.73#
Left putamen	−34	−8	2	2.41#
Left M1	−34	−20	50	2.35#
Right parahippocampal gyrus (Hippocampus)	22	−38	−10	2.65
Right superior frontal gyrus (SMA)	18	6	66	2.64
Right hippocampus	32	−20	−10	2.61

**FWE $P < 0.05$.*

#$P < 0.05$ (FWE-corrected) after small volume correction.

M1, primary motor cortex; S1, primary somatosensory cortex; SPL, superior parietal lobe; hIP, intraparietal sulcus; OP, parietal operculum/secondary somatosensory cortex; IPL, inferior parietal lobule; TE, auditory cortex; Area 44, 45, Broca's areas.

$P < 0.05$ FWE-corrected. Trends toward activation were found in the left paracentral lobule (M1 and SMA), left middle-superior temporal gyrus, right middle-superior frontal gyrus, bilateral hippocampi, and right cerebellum (**Figure 1C**; **Table 1C**).

COMPARISON BETWEEN SUPRA-TMS AND MUSCLE AFFERENT-INDUCED ACTIVITY WITH CORRECTION FOR IEMG

Because motor-MNS produced larger muscle activity than supra-TMS, simple subtraction of muscle afferent-induced activity from supra-TMS-induced activity should overcorrect the effects of muscle afferents included in the supra-TMS-induced activity. We therefore reanalyzed data from the twelve participants for whom iEMG values were available for both supra-TMS and motor-MNS conditions. Specifically, to correct for differences in iEMG sizes, we used iEMG values as a parametric modulator of stimulation events for supra-TMS and motor-MNS. The contrast supra-TMS minus motor-MNS-corrected-for-iEMG revealed significant activity in left M1, left SMA, and left PMd ($P < 0.05$ FWE-corrected for small volume within VOIs) according to our previous reports (Hanakawa et al., 2009; Shitara et al., 2011) (**Table 2**). Trends toward activation were found in left postcentral gyrus (S1), middle frontal gyrus, bilateral precentral gyri (PMd), bilateral Rolandic operculum, bilateral insula, bilateral inferior temporal gyri, right thalamus, right SMA, left paracentral lobule, bilateral superior temporal gyri, left middle temporal

Table 2 | Supra-TMS compared with motor-MNS (Uncorrected *P* < 0.005).

N = 12	Functional anatomy	Coordinates (mm)			iEMG correction	
Activity clusters		***x***	***y***	***z***	**(+)**	**(−)**
					***Z*-values**	***Z*-values**
Left middle frontal gyrus	PMd	−24	−6	48	3.75	NA
Left precentral gyrus	PMd	−32	−8	58	3.43#	NA
Left rolandic operculum		−44	−2	16	3.44	NA
Left insular lobe	Insula	−34	2	14	3.11	NA
Right inferior temporal gyrus		52	−4	−34	3.38	3.19
Left inferior temporal gyrus		−44	0	−32	3.23	NA
Right thalamus		24	−28	12	3.15	NA
Right SMA		10	8	52	3.05	NA
Left postcentral gyrus	S1	−18	−32	74	3.05	3.00
Left paracentral lobule	M1a, S1, SMA	−10	−32	72	2.82	2.80
Right superior temporal gyrus	IPL, OP1	60	−34	10	2.91	NA
Left middle temporal gyrus		−56	4	−18	2.83	NA
Right precentral gyrus	PMd	42	−2	38	2.82	NA
Left paracentral lobule	M1a, SMA	−8	−28	74	2.79	2.66
Left inferior parietal lobule	SPL	−36	−34	38	2.76	NA
Right insula lobe	Insula	36	−20	6	2.68	NA
Left superior temporal gyrus	TE1	−50	−24	10	2.62	NA
Right rolandic operculum	Area44	54	10	0	2.60	2.64
Right middle cingulate cortex	SMA	8	−12	44	2.60	NA
Left precentral gyrus	M1a	−34	−20	52	2.51#	NA
Left SMA		−8	−14	48	2.49#	NA

#*P* < 0.05 *(FWE-corrected) after small volume correction, NA: voxels not available within 5-mm sphere VOIs with sphere center at the coordinate in the iEMG corrected analysis.*

gyrus, left inferior parietal lobule, and right MCC. Less prominent activity compared to a similar analysis without iEMG correction (described above) resulted from a lower degree of freedom. In fact, when the data from the same twelve participants were reanalyzed without using the iEMG parameter (**Table 2**), the iEMG-corrected analysis tended to yield greater Z values than the non-iEMG-corrected version. This finding supports the notion that a simple comparison between supra-TMS and motor-MNS would have underestimated "pure" TMS-induced activity. Therefore, the non-iEMG corrected analysis above is conservative in claiming that muscle afferents alone cannot explain motor-area activity during supra-TMS delivered to M1 (**Figure 2; Table 2**).

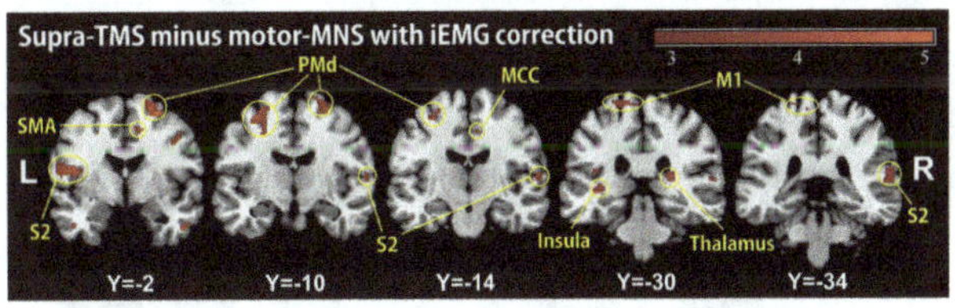

FIGURE 2 | A group-level statistical parametric map categorically comparing hemodynamic changes of the supra-TMS- and motor-MNS-induced activity after iEMG correction (*P* < 0.005 uncorrected for display purpose), corresponding to "pure" TMS-evoked activity. This activity was observed in bilateral insula, bilateral secondary somatosensory area (S2), bilateral thalami, left primary motor cortex (M1), bilateral dorsal premotor cortex (PMd), supplementary motor cortex (SMA) and middle cingulate cortex (MCC).

LOCALIZATION OF TMS-, MUSCLE AFFERENT- AND SUPERFICIAL AFFERENT-INDUCED BRAIN ACTIVITY WITHIN M1 SUBDIVISIONS

We assessed the spatial distribution of activated voxels representing "pure" TMS-, muscle afferent-, and superficial afferent-induced activity in the two subdivisions of M1, M1a and M1p (**Figure 3**). Visual inspection showed muscle afferent-related activity primarily in M1a and superficial afferent-related activity in M1p. To semi-quantify any biased distribution across the two MNS conditions, we calculated the M1-DI for the suprathreshold voxels representing muscle afferent- and superficial afferent-induced activity. The M1-DI for muscle afferent-induced activity (mean ± SEM, 0.30 ± 0.26) was significantly larger than that for superficial afferent-induced activity (0.01 ± 0.24) ($P = 0.043$ by Mann-Whitney U test). This indicates that muscle afferents were mainly represented in the M1a subdivision, while superficial afferents were distributed evenly across the two divisions. Similar DI analysis showed that "pure" TMS-evoked activity was predominantly distributed in M1a (0.32 ± 0.21).

AMOUNT OF MUSCLE AFFERENT-INDUCED ACTIVITY INCLUDED IN SUPRA-TMS-INDUCED ACTIVITY WITH AND WITHOUT CORRECTION FOR MOVEMENT SIZE

The muscle afferent-related responses included in the pure TMS-evoked responses without iEMG correction were around

40% in motor-related areas (**Figure 4**). When adjusted with the iEMG, motor-MNS-induced fMRI signals within supra-TMS-induced signals were 0, 10.0, 22.9, and 8.5% in left M1a, left M1p, left PMd, and left SMA, respectively. Thus, the present analysis indicates that "pure" supra-TMS components can explain approximately 80–90% of activity in motor areas during supra-TMS (120% RMT) delivered to M1.

DISCUSSION

The present study evaluated motor-area activity ascribed to deep and superficial sensory afferents in an effort to understand the properties of motor-area activity evoked by suprathreshold TMS delivered to M1. The present study used standard HRF to compare the size of TMS- and MNS-induced activities because previous evidence supported the use of standard HRF for detecting single-pulse TMS-induced and MNS-induced activities (Shitara et al., 2011). Distribution of cortico-cortico evoked activity in the motor network agreed with previous findings from simultaneous fMRI/PET studies (Bestmann et al., 2003; Fox et al., 2006; Hanakawa et al., 2009) and simultaneous EEG studies (Nikulin et al., 2003; Komssi et al., 2004; Fuggetta et al., 2005; Bonato et al., 2006) during TMS applied to M1. Additionally, the present MNS-induced brain activity was consistent with previous studies (Davis et al., 1995; Manganotti et al., 2009). Key novel findings here were: (1) muscle afferent-induced activity was mainly located in the rostral sector (M1a) of M1 also in humans and (2) "pure" TMS-induced activity in motor areas remained significant after removal of muscle afferent-induced activity and was located in both M1a and M1p.

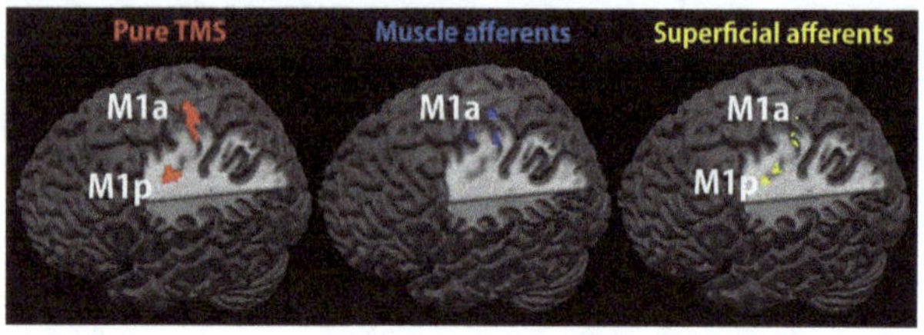

FIGURE 3 | Representations of TMS-, muscle afferent- and superficial afferent-induced brain activity within M1 subdivisions. Muscle afferent-related brain activity was predominantly distributed in M1a while superficial afferent-related activity was seen in both M1a and M1p. Pure TMS-evoked activity was mainly distributed in M1a. *Red*, pure TMS-related brain activity [(supra-TMS minus implicit baseline) minus (motor-MNS minus sensory-MNS)]. *Dark blue*, muscle afferent-related brain activity (motor-MNS minus sensory-MNS). *Yellow*, superficial afferent-related brain activity (conjunction of motor-MNS and sensory-MNS). Activity was thresholded at $P < 0.005$ uncorrected for display purpose.

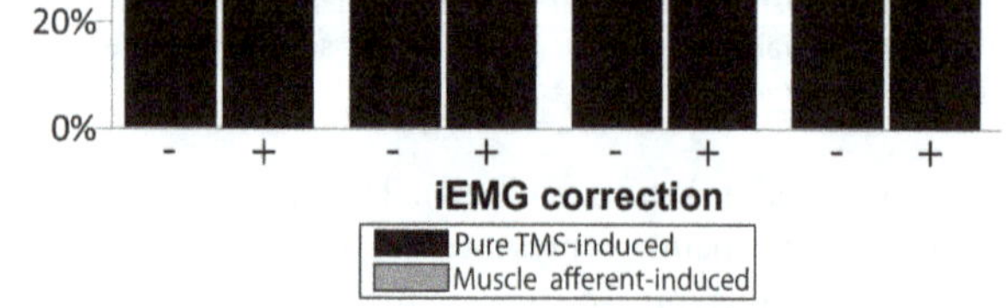

FIGURE 4 | Percentage of fMRI signals ascribed to the "pure" TMS- and muscle afferent-induced activity within supra-TMS-induced activity. Data are shown for representative motor areas. *Black*, percentage of the contrast Supra-TMS minus Motor-MNS. *Gray*, percentage of the contrast Motor-MNS minus implicit baseline. (−), without iEMG correction. (+), with iEMG correction. *L*, left; *M1a* and *M1p*, anterior and posterior subdivisions of primary motor cortex; *PMd*, dorsal premotor cortex; *SMA*, supplementary motor area.

TMS INTENSITY

In the present study, for participants who required stimulation above 100% of the machine output to reach the 120% RMT stimulation, the maximum machine output of the TMS stimulator was reset to 110% of the default machine output, within the safety guidelines of the manufacturer. No adverse effects were reported by the participants or observed by the investigators during or after the stimulation.

The mean RMT of 80.6% of machine output may seem high, considering TMS to M1 in standard, outside-MRI environments. There are a couple of reasons for this. First, we placed the TMS-coil orientation ~45° from the medial-lateral axis, but the handle of the TMS coil had to be placed toward the back because of the interference between the TMS coil and MRI head coil. This set-up induces currents in the posterior-to-anterior direction. With the bisphasic stimulation (Magstim Rapid), the RMT for the posterior-to-anterior current is higher than that for the anterior-to-posterior current (Kammer et al., 2001). Moreover, since we connected the MRI-compatible TMS coil to the TMS stimulator outside the radiofrequency shielded cabin via an 8-m cable, the TMS output intensities were supposed to be reduced by ~20% (Bestmann et al., 2003). We consider that these two factors primarily make RMT seemingly high in this simultaneous TMS-fMRI experiment. In fact, the mean RMT was 79.6 and 85.4% of the default machine output, respectively, in our previous TMS-fMRI studies (Hanakawa et al., 2009; Shitara et al., 2011). Hence, 80.6% of the machine output was not particularly high as for RMT in the simultaneous fMRI environment. In consistent, we observed MEP only in the right APB muscle although we recorded MEPs also from non-target muscles (right ADM and left hand). This finding indicated that TMS-evoked muscle activity did not spread to neighboring motor representations.

TMS- OR MNS-INDUCED NEURAL ACTIVITIES AND fMRI SIGNALS

We are able to capture fMRI signal changes associated with short-lasting transient neural activity because fMRI measures slow haemodynamic changes (lasting several seconds after brief neuronal activations) as a surrogate marker of neural/synaptic activities (Friston et al., 1994). A proposed model to describe the temporal relationship between the neural/synaptic activities and vascular signals is called neurovascular coupling or HRFs.

Because of the delays in hemodynamic responses, fMRI signal changes following neural/synaptic activities, which would last for only tens to hundreds of milliseconds after TMS- or MNS-stimulation, last over several seconds. To account for hemodynamic delay, convolution of modeled neural/synaptic activity changes with HRF is widely used to create regressors for fMRI data analyses. As we sampled such fMRI signals every 1 s, we were able to detect fMRI signal change correlated with neural/synaptic activity.

One may wonder if there are correlations in activity size between brief neuronal/synaptic activities and fMRI signals. Logothetis and colleagues have pioneered the simultaneous acquisition of electrophysiological and fMRI signal acquisition in primates. This work has shown that the fMRI signals are tightly coupled with electrophysiological activity, particularly local field potentials that represent synchronized synaptic inputs to a given neural population (Logothetis et al., 2001). This agrees with data showing a significant correlation between fMRI responses and evoked potentials in humans (Arthurs et al., 2000). Moreover, ample evidence from animal studies indicates correlations between short-lasting evoked field potentials and slow hemodynamic changes (Tsubokawa et al., 1980; Mathiesen et al., 1998; Brinker et al., 1999; Ngai et al., 1999; Nielsen et al., 2000; Ogawa et al., 2000). This justifies the "cognitive subtraction" method in which one may assume that motor-MNS condition would induce additional activity ascribed to muscle afferents on top of superficial sensory activity evoked by sensory-MNS.

EFFECT OF MUSCLE AFFERENTS ON SUPRA-TMS-INDUCED BRAIN ACTIVITY

Many simultaneous TMS-imaging studies have reported that stimulated M1 shows increased activity only with suprathreshold TMS (Bestmann et al., 2003; Fox et al., 2006; Hanakawa et al., 2009; Shitara et al., 2011). When different TMS intensities are applied, non-linear responses emerge in M1 around the motor threshold (Hanakawa et al., 2009), meaning that only supra-TMS accompanying MEPs induces activity in the region of M1 that is directly stimulated. One natural interpretation of these observations is that M1 activity during suprathreshold TMS may at least partially reflect proprioceptive afferents from twitched muscles, as discussed in previous reports (Bestmann et al., 2003; Komssi et al., 2004; Fox et al., 2006; Hanakawa et al., 2009). Previous evidence supports this "muscle afferent" hypothesis. Magnetoencephalography (MEG), intracranial electrical recording, and fMRI studies have consistently revealed M1 activity during MNS-induced muscle twitching (Spiegel et al., 1999; Huang et al., 2000; Balzamo et al., 2004). Furthermore, M1 plays essential roles in motor perception based on the processing of muscle-afferent information (Naito et al., 2002). Here, results partially support the idea that muscle afferents affect motor-area activity during supra-TMS applied to M1. We found widespread muscle afferent-induced activity in motor areas even though the experimental setup should have minimized their effects. In M1, moderate activity was observed during motor-MNS after removing the effects of sensory-MNS that induced only superficial sensory perception. Because motor-MNS induced activation in remote motor areas other than M1, muscle afferent-induced activity may even explain activity in the remote motor network during supra-M1 stimulation. Previous research has shown that MNS above the motor threshold can evoke long-latency cortical potentials, but not short-latency potentials, in motor-related areas such as the SMA (Allison et al., 1991). Although a wide representation of muscle-afferent information in motor-related areas is already recognized, previous neuroimaging studies have largely neglected the contribution of muscle afferents to motor-area activity during movement.

Here, we carefully examined the effect of muscle afferents on motor-area activity during supra-TMS. A simple comparison of activity between supra-TMS and motor-MNS revealed motor-area activity, strongly indicating that neither local nor remote activity induced by supra-TMS could be explained solely by muscle afferents. However, this finding was difficult to interpret, especially quantitatively, because of the significant differences in the amount of muscle activity (iEMG) across conditions. We therefore re-analyzed the data correcting for muscle afferent-induced activity using iEMG. The effects of muscle afferents on supra-TMS-induced activity can never be neglected. In M1, ~10% of activity during supra-TMS was ascribed to muscle afferents. Nevertheless, the analysis of supra-TMS-induced activity after removal of muscle afferent-related activity supports the claim that supra-TMS evoked neuronal and/or synaptic activity. Surplus activity during supra-TMS that is greater than the muscle-afferent component would include M1 neural activity involving both inter-neurons and pyramidal neurons to produce a significant number of descending volleys to the spinal motoneuron pools (Barker et al., 1985; Hallett, 2007). Although the small contribution of muscle afferent-induced activity to supra-TMS induced activity is not surprising, previous TMS-fMRI studies only discussed this possibility. To our knowledge, the present study was the first to quantify contribution of muscle afferent-induced activity to supra-TMS induced activity. Since the muscle afferent contribution to supra-TMS-evoked motor network activity was relatively modest, we considered that it would be reasonable to use PET/fMRI with supra-TMS to M1 as a technique for evoked motor network imaging.

LOCALIZATION OF THE TMS-, MUSCLE AFFERENT- AND SUPERFICIAL AFFERENT-INDUCED BRAIN ACTIVITY WITHIN M1 SUBDIVISIONS

The findings here support the existence of two M1 subdivisions (M1a and M1p) in humans. Human thumb movements have been shown to be dually represented within these two subdivisions, each with a specific though not exclusive function (Geyer et al., 1996). M1a is considered to be "executive" and its activity directly results in actual movement. In contrast, M1p appears to be involved in a number of cognitive tasks and non-executive functions. M1p is activated by sensory inputs, modulated by attention (Binkofski et al., 2002; Johansen-Berg and Matthews, 2002), and affected by ageing (Ward and Frackowiak, 2003).

The rostral region of M1 (M1a) in squirrel monkeys primarily receives deep sensations from muscles and tendons, while the caudal region (M1p) receives superficial sensations from the skin (Strick and Preston, 1982). Consistently in other single-unit recording studies in non-human primates, the rostral M1 (M1a) predominantly receives non-cutaneous inputs while the cutaneous input is primarily confined to the caudal part of M1 (M1p) (Tanji and Wise, 1981; Picard and Smith, 1992). To our knowledge, no studies have shown detailed localization of TMS-, muscle afferent- and superficial afferent-induced brain activity within M1 subdivisions. The present results support the notion that in humans, muscle afferent-induced activity is localized primarily in M1a, although superficial afferent-induced activity is located in both M1a and M1p, despite being modest in intensity. Wide representations of superficial sensory inputs in humans could be related to dexterity of hand movements. Here, the supra-TMS condition did not include cognitive or attentional components and it should not evoke much activity in M1p. Another simple explanation for the M1a-predominant supra-TMS induced activity may be that M1a is closer to the scalp than M1p, and thus is more susceptible to TMS.

By capitalizing on superior temporal resolution, previous single-pulse TMS-EEG studies identified temporal evolution of TMS-evoked cortical activities. In addition to early activation of the stimulated and contralateral motor cortex (Komssi et al., 2002, 2004), several TMS-EEG studies have reported subsequent activation of frontal regions that likely coincide with ipsilateral supplementary/premotor areas (Paus et al., 2001; Komssi et al., 2004; Bonato et al., 2006; Litvak et al., 2007). It is not entirely clear if these late frontal activations reflect direct cortico-cortical evoked activity only or include effects of somatosensory afferents.

Suprathreshold TMS to the motor cortex results in muscle activations measured as MEP, accompanying muscle contraction and possibly joint movement. Such peripheral reactions should yield somatosensory afferents especially from muscles and joints and may generate somatosensory-evoked potentials detectable with EEG (Paus et al., 2001; Schürmann et al., 2001; Komssi et al., 2002; Nikulin et al., 2003). The early components of the TMS-evoked potential (<40 ms) are unlikely to be affected by somatosensory-evoked potentials, taking into account the conduction time from the cortex to the muscle and back again (Paus et al., 2001; Komssi et al., 2002). Evidence is available to argue for an idea that later components such as N45 and N100 may also be independent of sensory afferents as their peak amplitudes do not correlate with MEP size and they even occur at subthreshold intensities (Paus et al., 2001; Nikulin et al., 2003; Komssi et al., 2004, 2007). Although these studies can obviously claim the presence of cortico-cortical potentials evoked by TMS, possible somatosensory components in the suprathreshold TMS-evoked EEG potentials have not been well specified.

Esser and colleagues reported that the early peaks of the global mean field power (<40 ms after suprathreshold TMS to M1) corresponded to activity in the ipsilateral M1-premotor cortex and that the later peaks (>40 ms after stimulation) corresponded to activity in the ipsilateral M1-S1 (Esser et al., 2006). They interpreted that later peaks included somatosensory components of MEP, and suggested the location of "pure" TMS-evoked activity was located more anteriorly than that of the sensory afferents induced activity. Ferreri and colleagues described that, in addition to N7 that likely reflected cortico-cortical TMS-evoked potentials in the premotor cortex, N44 might be related to somatosensory evoked potentials generated by TMS-induced muscles twitches (Ferreri et al., 2011). N44 showed a diffuse spatial distribution with antero-posterior amplitude gradient. This study indicated that "pure" TMS-evoked activity was distributed in M1 and premotor cortex and muscle/superficial afferent induced activities were diffusely located. These two TMS-EEG studies indicate that the comparison with somatosensory-evoked components can better characterize "pure" TMS evoked potentials. In reference to these TMS-EEG findings, we consider that the present study has advanced understanding of TMS-evoked motor network activity. By taking advantage of superior spatial localization, we showed precise localization of "pure" TMS-evoked activity in comparison with superficial/deep sensory mapping of motor areas. This information cannot be obtained with TMS-EEG only. We propose that TMS-EEG and TMS-fMRI are complementary methods, which together propel the understanding of motor network.

To interpret the relation between the superficial afferent and the muscle afferent, we referred to previous reports using cutaneous anaesthesia. Intriguingly, anesthesia of fingers induces short-term enlargement and spatial shifts of the cortical representation of the unanesthetized fingers (Rossini et al., 1994b). When the target muscle was totally "enveloped" within the anesthetized area but was still dispatching a normal proprioceptive feedback by temporal cutaneous block, the cortical representation of the target muscle was significantly reduced (Rossi et al., 1998). Moreover, variability in MEP and F-wave significantly decreased in the target muscle. Thus, those anesthesia studies have shown that the disruptions of superficial afferents induce modifications of the corticospinal pathways and somatotopical representations, suggesting complex interactions among superficial and deep sensory inputs, and motor representations. However, it should be noted that these complex processes most likely result from short-term neuroplasticity after anesthesia interventions. Although these plasticity issues are interesting, we should also possess basic knowledge of superficial and deep sensory representations in motor cortex without influence of plastic changes. For example, although we had previously measured fMRI activity induced by suprathreshold TMS (Hanakawa et al., 2009; Shitara et al., 2011), contribution of muscle twitch-induced sensory activity to the induced fMRI activity was unknown. Presence of plastic changes would make the interpretation of the findings difficult. We hence employed a simple approach by comparing fMRI activities across supra-TMS, motor-MNS and superficial-MNS conditions. This approach should provide a fundamental knowledge about sensory representations in the motor areas, without ongoing interactions between the motor commands and sensory afferents as seen in object manipulation or by short-term plasticity after anesthesia.

STUDY LIMITATIONS

In the present study, we contrasted the supra-TMS condition with the two MNS conditions, not with other TMS conditions. The effects of TMS to M1 could be non-specific such as eye blinking, tactile sensation on the scalp and loud auditory clicks (Jahanshahi and Rothwell, 2000; Anand and Hotson, 2002). Sounds induced by TMS may influence M1 since large sounds temporary suppress M1 excitability (Furubayashi et al., 2000). However, it is disputable if the TMS-induced click sounds significantly activates M1 during TMS-fMRI experiments. Hart et al. reported that activity in motor areas did not change in relation to sound levels (Hart et al., 2003). In contrast to the auditory cortex showing activity in proportion to sound levels, M1 activity changes abruptly at around the RMT (Hanakawa et al., 2009). Thus, it seems less likely that motor area activity in the present experiment was significantly affected by the levels of click sound produced by TMS. Similarly, we cannot completely exclude the possibility that tapping sensation of the scalp associated with TMS since it is exaggerated in the MRI environment even with careful fixation of the coil. The overlapping of the supra-TMS-induced activity with the MNS-induced activity strongly supports that the present supra-TMS-induced activity was localized to hand representation of the M1. However, the non-specific effects of TMS in the concurrent TMS-fMRI set-up need to be addressed formally in the future studies.

Finally, we applied peripheral nerve stimulation as control conditions for muscle afferents during supra-TMS stimulation to M1 and for superficial afferents. Since they are not natural somatosensory stimuli, it is uncertain if we can extend the present observations to the case of somatosensory stimuli associated with natural movements on one hand. On the other, we consider the MNS conditions have best served as control conditions to address somatosensory effects associated with supra-TMS as addressed here.

CONCLUSION

Using simultaneous measurements from fMRI, TMS/peripheral nerve electrical stimulation, and EMG, our results provide the first evidence for detailed localization of TMS-, muscle afferent- and superficial afferent-induced brain activity within human M1 subdivisions. Muscle afferent-induced activity was mainly located in the rostral M1. Moreover, the present study demonstrated relatively limited effects of muscle afferents on supra-TMS-evoked local and remote activity in the motor network. Considering this, the present findings favor the interpretation that recruitment of neural populations contributes to motor-area activity during supra-TMS applied to M1. Based on these and previous findings (Hanakawa et al., 2009), we propose that the non-linear emergence of brain activity at the stimulated site might be a useful marker for threshold-level TMS.

FUNDING

This research was partly supported by grants from PRESTO, KAKENHI (20033030 and 20019041) and the Takeda Science Foundation to T. Hanakawa and by grants from Grant-in-Aid for Young Scientists (B) (12813501) to H. Shitara.

REFERENCES

Allison, T., McCarthy, G., Wood, C. C., and Jones, S. J. (1991). Potentials evoked in human and monkey cerebral cortex by stimulation of the median nerve. A review of scalp and intracranial recordings. *Brain* 114(Pt 6), 2465–2503. doi: 10.1093/brain/114.6.2465

Anami, K., Mori, T., Tanaka, F., Kawagoe, Y., Okamoto, J., Yarita, M., et al. (2003). Stepping stone sampling for retrieving artifact-free electroencephalogram during functional magnetic resonance imaging. *Neuroimage* 19, 281–295. doi: 10.1016/S1053-8119(03)00048-X

Anand, S., and Hotson, J. (2002). Transcranial magnetic stimulation: neurophysiological applications and safety. *Brain Cogn.* 50, 366–386. doi: 10.1016/S0278-2626(02)00512-2

Arthurs, O. J., Williams, E. J., Carpenter, T. A., Pickard, J. D., and Boniface, S. J. (2000). Linear coupling between functional magnetic resonance imaging and evoked potential amplitude in human somatosensory cortex. *Neuroscience* 101, 803–806. doi: 10.1016/S0306-4522(00)00511-X

Balzamo, E., Marquis, P., Chauvel, P., and Regis, J. (2004). Short-latency components of evoked potentials to median nerve stimulation recorded by intracerebral electrodes in the human pre- and postcentral areas. *Clin. Neurophysiol.* 115, 1616–1623. doi: 10.1016/j.clinph.2004.02.012

Bardouille, T., and Ross, B. (2008). MEG imaging of sensorimotor areas using inter-trial coherence in vibrotactile steady-state responses. *Neuroimage* 42, 323–331. doi: 10.1016/j.neuroimage.2008.04.176

Barker, A. T., Jalinous, R., and Freeston, I. L. (1985). Non-invasive magnetic stimulation of human motor cortex. *Lancet* 1, 1106–1107. doi: 10.1016/S0140-6736(85)92413-4

Bestmann, S., Baudewig, J., Siebner, H. R., Rothwell, J. C., and Frahm, J. (2003). Subthreshold high-frequency TMS of human primary motor cortex modulates inter-connected frontal motor areas as detected by interleaved fMRI-TMS. *Neuroimage* 20, 1685–1696. doi: 10.1016/j.neuroimage.2003.07.028

Bestmann, S., Baudewig, J., Siebner, H. R., Rothwell, J. C., and Frahm, J. (2004). Functional MRI of the immediate impact of transcranial magnetic stimulation on cortical and subcortical motor circuits. *Eur. J. Neurosci.* 19, 1950–1962. doi: 10.1111/j.1460-9568.2004.03277.x

Binkofski, F., Fink, G. R., Geyer, S., Buccino, G., Gruber, O., Shah, N. J., et al. (2002). Neural activity in human primary motor cortex areas 4a and 4p is modulated differentially by attention to action. *J. Neurophysiol.* 88, 514–519.

Bonato, C., Miniussi, C., and Rossini, P. M. (2006). Transcranial magnetic stimulation and cortical evoked potentials: a TMS/EEG co-registration study. *Clin. Neurophysiol.* 117, 1699–1707. doi: 10.1016/j.clinph.2006.05.006

Brett, M., Anton, J., Valabregue, R., and Poline, J. (2002). "Region of interest analysis using an SPM toolbox," in *The 8th International Conference on Functional Mapping of the Human Brain* (Sendai: Available on CD-ROM in NeuroImage), 497.

Brinker, G., Bock, C., Busch, E., Krep, H., Hossmann, K. A., and Hoehn-Berlage, M. (1999). Simultaneous recording of evoked potentials and T2*-weighted MR images during somatosensory stimulation of rat. *Magn. Reson. Med.* 41, 469–473. doi: 10.1002/(SICI)1522-2594(199903)41:3<469::AID-MRM7>3.3.CO;2-0

Davis, K. D., Wood, M. L., Crawley, A. P., and Mikulis, D. J. (1995). fMRI of human somatosensory and cingulate cortex during painful electrical nerve stimulation. *Neuroreport* 7, 321–325.

Del Gratta, C., Della Penna, S., Tartaro, A., Ferretti, A., Torquati, K., Bonomo, L., et al. (2000). Topographic organization of the human primary and secondary somatosensory areas: an fMRI study. *Neuroreport* 11, 2035–2043. doi: 10.1097/00001756-200006260-00046

Esser, S. K., Huber, R., Massimini, M., Peterson, M. J., Ferrarelli, F., and Tononi, G. (2006). A direct demonstration of cortical LTP in humans: a combined TMS/EEG study. *Brain Res. Bull.* 69, 86–94. doi: 10.1016/j.brainresbull.2005.11.003

Ferreri, F., Pasqualetti, P., Määttä, S., Ponzo, D., Ferrarelli, F., Tononi, G., et al. (2011). Human brain connectivity during single and paired pulse transcranial magnetic stimulation. *Neuroimage* 54, 90–102. doi: 10.1016/j.neuroimage.2010.07.056

Fetz, E. E., Finocchio, D. V., Baker, M. A., and Soso, M. J. (1980). Sensory and motor responses of precentral cortex cells during comparable passive and active joint movements. *J. Neurophysiol.* 43, 1070–1089.

Fox, P. T., Narayana, S., Tandon, N., Fox, S. P., Sandoval, H., Kochunov, P., et al. (2006). Intensity modulation of TMS-induced cortical excitation: primary motor cortex. *Hum. Brain Mapp.* 27, 478–487. doi: 10.1002/hbm.20192

Friston, K. J., Tononi, G., Reeke, G. N., Sporns, O., and Edelman, G. M. (1994). Value-dependent selection in the brain: simulation in a synthetic neural model. *Neuroscience* 59, 229–243. doi: 10.1016/0306-4522(94)90592-4

Fuggetta, G., Fiaschi, A., and Manganotti, P. (2005). Modulation of cortical oscillatory activities induced by varying single-pulse transcranial magnetic stimulation intensity over the left primary motor area: a combined EEG and TMS study. *Neuroimage* 27, 896–908. doi: 10.1016/j.neuroimage.2005.05.013

Furubayashi, T., Ugawa, Y., Terao, Y., Hanajima, R., Sakai, K., Machii, K., et al. (2000). The human hand motor area is transiently suppressed by an unexpected auditory stimulus. *Clin. Neurophysiol.* 111, 178–183. doi: 10.1016/S1388-2457(99)00200-X

Geyer, S., Ledberg, A., Schleicher, A., Kinomura, S., Schormann, T., Burgel, U., et al. (1996). Two different areas within the primary motor cortex of man. *Nature* 382, 805–807. doi: 10.1038/382805a0

Gizewski, E. R., Koeze, O., Uffmann, K., de Greiff, A., Ladd, M. E., and Forsting, M. (2005). Cerebral activation using a MR-compatible piezoelectric actuator with adjustable vibration frequencies and *in vivo* wave propagation control. *Neuroimage* 24, 723–730. doi: 10.1016/j.neuroimage.2004.09.015

Hallett, M. (2007). Transcranial magnetic stimulation: a primer. *Neuron* 55, 187–199. doi: 10.1016/j.neuron.2007.06.026

Hanakawa, T., Mima, T., Matsumoto, R., Abe, M., Inouchi, M., Urayama, S., et al. (2009). Stimulus-response profile during single-pulse transcranial magnetic stimulation to the primary motor cortex. *Cereb. Cortex* 19, 2605–2615. doi: 10.1093/cercor/bhp013

Hart, H. C., Hall, D. A., and Palmer, A. R. (2003). The sound-level-dependent growth in the extent of fMRI activation in Heschl's gyrus is different for low- and high-frequency tones. *Hear. Res.* 179, 104–112. doi: 10.1016/S0378-5955(03)00100-X

Hermens, H. J., Freriks, B., Merletti, R., Hägg, G., Stegeman, D., Blok, J., et al. (1991). *European Recommendations for Surface Electromyography.* Enschede: Roessingh Research and Development b.v.

Horne, M. K., and Tracey, D. J. (1979). The afferents and projections of the ventroposterolateral thalamus in the monkey. *Exp. Brain Res.* 36, 129–141.

Huang, M. X., Aine, C., Davis, L., Butman, J., Christner, R., Weisend, M., et al. (2000). Sources on the anterior and posterior banks of the central sulcus identified from magnetic somatosensory evoked responses using multistart spatio-temporal localization. *Hum. Brain Mapp.* 11, 59–76. doi: 10.1002/1097-0193(200010)11:2<59::AID-HBMIO>3.0.CO;2-5

Jahanshahi, M., and Rothwell, J. (2000). Transcranial magnetic stimulation studies of cognition: an emerging field. *Exp. Brain Res.* 131, 1–9. doi: 10.1007/s002219900224

Johansen-Berg, H., and Matthews, P. M. (2002). Attention to movement modulates activity in sensori-motor areas, including primary motor cortex. *Exp. Brain Res.* 142, 13–24. doi: 10.1007/s00221-001-0905-8

Kammer, T., Beck, S., Erb, M., and Grodd, W. (2001). The influence of current direction on phosphene thresholds evoked by transcranial magnetic stimulation. *Clin. Neurophysiol.* 112, 2015–2021. doi: 10.1016/S1388-2457(01)00673-3

Komssi, S., Aronen, H. J., Huttunen, J., Kesäniemi, M., Soinne, L., Nikouline, V. V., et al. (2002). Ipsi- and contralateral EEG reactions to transcranial magnetic stimulation. *Clin. Neurophysiol.* 113, 175–184. doi: 10.1016/S1388-2457(01)00721-0

Komssi, S., Kahkonen, S., and Ilmoniemi, R. J. (2004). The effect of stimulus intensity on brain responses evoked by transcranial magnetic stimulation. *Hum. Brain Mapp.* 21, 154–164. doi: 10.1002/hbm.10159

Komssi, S., Savolainen, P., Heiskala, J., and Kähkönen, S. (2007). Excitation threshold of the motor cortex estimated with transcranial magnetic stimulation electroencephalography. *Neuroreport* 18, 13–16. doi: 10.1097/WNR.0b013e328011b89a

Korvenoja, A., Huttunen, J., Salli, E., Pohjonen, H., Martinkauppi, S., Palva, J. M., et al. (1999). Activation of multiple cortical areas in response to somatosensory stimulation: combined magnetoencephalographic and functional magnetic resonance imaging. *Hum. Brain Mapp.* 8, 13–27. doi: 10.1002/(SICI)1097-0193(1999)8:1<13::AID-HBM2>3.0.CO;2-B

Lemon, R. N. (1981). Functional properties of monkey motor cortex neurones receiving afferent input from the hand and fingers. *J. Physiol.* 311, 497–519.

Litvak, V., Komssi, S., Scherg, M., Hoechstetter, K., Classen, J., Zaaroor, M., et al. (2007). Artifact correction and source analysis of early electroencephalographic responses evoked by transcranial magnetic stimulation over primary motor cortex. *Neuroimage* 37, 56–70. doi: 10.1016/j.neuroimage.2007.05.015

Logothetis, N. K., Pauls, J., Augath, M., Trinath, T., and Oeltermann, A. (2001). Neurophysiological investigation of the basis of the fMRI signal. *Nature* 412, 150–157. doi: 10.1038/35084005

Magistris, M. R., Rosler, K. M., Truffert, A., and Myers, J. P. (1998). Transcranial stimulation excites virtually all motor neurons supplying the target muscle. A demonstration and a method improving the study of motor evoked potentials. *Brain* 121(Pt 3), 437–450. doi: 10.1093/brain/121.3.437

Manganotti, P., Formaggio, E., Storti, S. F., Avesani, M., Acler, M., Sala, F., et al. (2009). Steady-state activation in somatosensory cortex after changes in stimulus rate during median nerve stimulation. *Magn. Reson. Imaging* 27, 1175–1186. doi: 10.1016/j.mri.2009.05.009

Mathiesen, C., Caesar, K., Akgören, N., and Lauritzen, M. (1998). Modification of activity-dependent increases of cerebral blood flow by excitatory synaptic activity and spikes in rat cerebellar cortex. *J. Physiol.* 512(Pt 2), 555–566. doi: 10.1111/j.1469-7793.1998.555be.x

Naito, E., Roland, P. E., and Ehrsson, H. H. (2002). I feel my hand moving: a new role of the primary motor cortex in somatic perception of limb movement. *Neuron* 36, 979–988. doi: 10.1016/S0896-6273(02)00980-7

Ngai, A. C., Jolley, M. A., D'Ambrosio, R., Meno, J. R., and Winn, H. R. (1999). Frequency-dependent changes in cerebral blood flow and evoked potentials during somatosensory stimulation in the rat. *Brain Res.* 837, 221–228. doi: 10.1016/S0006-8993(99)01649-2

Nielsen, A. N., Fabricius, M., and Lauritzen, M. (2000). Scanning laser-Doppler flowmetry of rat cerebral circulation during cortical spreading depression. *J. Vasc. Res.* 37, 513–522. doi: 10.1159/000054084

Nikulin, V. V., Kiciæ, D., Kähkönen, S., and Ilmoniemi, R. J. (2003). Modulation of electroencephalographic responses to transcranial magnetic stimulation: evidence for changes in cortical excitability related to movement. *Eur. J. Neurosci.* 18, 1206–1212. doi: 10.1046/j.1460-9568.2003.02858.x

Ogawa, S., Lee, T., Stepnoski, R., Chen, W., Zhu, X., and Ugurbil, K. (2000). An approach to probe some neural systems interaction by functional MRI at neural time scale down to milliseconds. *Proc. Natl. Acad. Sci. U.S.A.* 97, 11026–11031. doi: 10.1073/pnas.97.20.11026

Paus, T., Sipila, P. K., and Strafella, A. P. (2001). Synchronization of neuronal activity in the human primary motor cortex by transcranial magnetic stimulation: an EEG study. *J. Neurophysiol.* 86, 1983–1990.

Picard, N., and Smith, A. M. (1992). Primary motor cortical activity related to the weight and texture of grasped objects in the monkey. *J. Neurophysiol.* 68, 1867–1881.

Pons, T. P., and Kaas, J. H. (1986). Corticocortical connections of area 2 of somatosensory cortex in macaque monkeys: a correlative anatomical and electrophysiological study. *J. Comp. Neurol.* 248, 313–335. doi: 10.1002/cne.902480303

Rossi, S., Pasqualetti, P., Tecchio, F., Sabato, A., and Rossini, P. M. (1998). Modulation of corticospinal output to human hand muscles following deprivation of sensory feedback. *Neuroimage* 8, 163–175. doi: 10.1006/nimg.1998.0352

Rossini, P. M., Barker, A. T., Berardelli, A., Caramia, M. D., Caruso, G., Cracco, R. Q., et al. (1994a). Non-invasive electrical and magnetic stimulation of the brain, spinal cord and roots: basic principles and procedures for routine clinical application. Report of an IFCN committee. *Electroencephalogr. Clin. Neurophysiol.* 91, 79–92. doi: 10.1016/0013-4694(94)90029-9

Rossini, P. M., Martino, G., Narici, L., Pasquarelli, A., Peresson, M., Pizzella, V., et al. (1994b). Short-term brain 'plasticity' in humans: transient finger representation changes in sensory cortex somatotopy following ischemic anesthesia. *Brain Res.* 642, 169–177. doi: 10.1016/0006-8993(94)90919-9

Schürmann, M., Nikouline, V. V., Soljanlahti, S., Ollikainen, M., Basar, E., and Ilmoniemi, R. J. (2001). EEG responses to combined somatosensory and transcranial magnetic stimulation. *Clin. Neurophysiol.* 112, 19–24. doi: 10.1016/S1388-2457(00)00509-5

Shitara, H., Shinozaki, T., Takagishi, K., Honda, M., and Hanakawa, T. (2011). Time course and spatial distribution of fMRI signal changes during single-pulse transcranial magnetic stimulation to the primary motor cortex.

Neuroimage 56, 1469–1479. doi: 10.1016/j.neuroimage.2011.03.011

Speer, A. M., Willis, M. W., Herscovitch, P., Daube-Witherspoon, M., Shelton, J. R., Benson, B. E., et al. (2003). Intensity-dependent regional cerebral blood flow during 1-Hz repetitive transcranial magnetic stimulation (rTMS) in healthy volunteers studied with H215O positron emission tomography: I. Effects of primary motor cortex rTMS. *Biol. Psychiatry* 54, 818–825. doi: 10.1016/S0006-3223(03)00002-7

Spiegel, J., Tintera, J., Gawehn, J., Stoeter, P., and Treede, R. D. (1999). Functional MRI of human primary somatosensory and motor cortex during median nerve stimulation. *Clin. Neurophysiol.* 110, 47–52. doi: 10.1016/S0168-5597(98)00043-4

Strick, P. L., and Preston, J. B. (1978). Sorting of somatosensory afferent information in primate motor cortex. *Brain Res.* 156, 364–368. doi: 10.1016/0006-8993(78)90520-6

Strick, P. L., and Preston, J. B. (1982). Two representations of the hand in area 4 of a primate. II. Somatosensory input organization. *J. Neurophysiol.* 48, 150–159.

Tanji, J., and Wise, S. P. (1981). Submodality distribution in sensorimotor cortex of the unanesthetized monkey. *J. Neurophysiol.* 45, 467–481.

Tohka, J., Foerde, K., Aron, A. R., Tom, S. M., Toga, A. W., and Poldrack, R. A. (2008). Automatic independent component labeling for artifact removal in fMRI. *Neuroimage* 39, 1227–1245. doi: 10.1016/j.neuroimage.2007.10.013

Tsubokawa, T., Katayama, Y., Kondo, T., Ueno, Y., Hayashi, N., and Moriyasu, N. (1980). Changes in local cerebral blood flow and neuronal activity during sensory stimulation in normal and sympathectomized cats. *Brain Res.* 190, 51–64. doi: 10.1016/0006-8993(80)91159-2

Ward, N. S., and Frackowiak, R. S. (2003). Age-related changes in the neural correlates of motor performance. *Brain* 126, 873–888. doi: 10.1093/brain/awg071

8

Cortical modulation of short-latency TMS-evoked potentials

Domenica Veniero[1,2†], Marta Bortoletto[2†] and Carlo Miniussi[1,2*]

[1] *Neuroscience Section, Department of Clinical and Experimental Sciences, University of Brescia, Brescia, Italy*
[2] *Cognitive Neuroscience Section, IRCCS Centro San Giovanni di Dio Fatebenefratelli, Brescia, Italy*

Correspondence:
Carlo Miniussi, Neuroscience Section, Department of Clinical and Experimental Sciences, University of Brescia, Viale Europa 11, 25123 Brescia, Italy.
e-mail: carlo.miniussi@cognitiveneuroscience.it

†These authors equally contributed to this work.

Transcranial magnetic stimulation–electroencephalogram (TMS–EEG) co-registration offers the opportunity to test reactivity of brain areas across distinct conditions through TMS-evoked potentials (TEPs). Several TEPs have been described, their functional meaning being largely unknown. In particular, short-latency potentials peaking at 5 (P5) and 8 (N8) ms after the TMS pulse have been recently described, but because of their large amplitude, the problem of whether their origin is cortical or not has been opened. To gain information about these components, we employed a protocol that modulates primary motor cortex excitability (MI): low frequency stimulation of premotor area (PMC). TMS was applied simultaneously with EEG recording from 70 electrodes. Amplitude of TEPs evoked by 200 single-pulses TMS delivered over MI at 110% of resting motor threshold (rMT) was measured before and after applying 900 TMS conditioning stimuli to left PMC with 1 Hz repetition rate. Single subject analyses showed reduction in TEPs amplitude after PMC conditioning in a sample of participants and increase in TEPs amplitude in two subjects. No effects were found on corticospinal excitability as recorded by motor-evoked potentials (MEPs). Furthermore, correlation analysis showed an inverse relation between the effects of the conditioning protocol on P5-N8 complex amplitude and MEPs amplitude. Because the effects of the used protocol have been ascribed to a cortical interaction between premotor area and MI, we suggest that despite the sign of P5-N8 amplitude modulation is not consistent across participant; this modulation could indicate, at least in part, their cortical origin. We conclude that with an accurate experimental procedure early latency components can be used to evaluate the reactivity of the stimulated cortex.

Keywords: transcranial magnetic stimulation, electroencephalography, TMS–EEG, premotor cortex, non-invasive brain stimulation, NIBS, motor-evoked potentials, motor cortex

INTRODUCTION

Combining transcranial magnetic stimulation (TMS) with electroencephalogram (EEG) recording makes possible to test the reactivity of brain areas, i.e., the cortical response to the magnetic pulse (Ilmoniemi et al., 1997), by means of TMS-evoked potentials (TEPs), which are directly generated by the cortex and provide a marker of the brain state (for a review, see Komssi and Kähkönen, 2006; Miniussi and Thut, 2010).

Despite their reproducibility across different studies (Komssi et al., 2002, 2004; Kähkönen et al., 2004; Bonato et al., 2006; Lioumis et al., 2009; Ferreri et al., 2011; Busan et al., 2012), TEP components are still not completely understood, and both their functional meaning and cortical origin are highly debated. Moreover, EEG analyses have often been restricted to several ms after the TMS pulse, i.e., starting from 10 ms (Komssi et al., 2002; Litvak et al., 2007), or even longer intervals. Recently, short-latency TEPs peaking at 5 and 8 ms after TMS pulse (P5 and N8, respectively) have been described (Bonato et al., 2006; Esser et al., 2006; Veniero et al., 2010; Ferreri et al., 2011). In particular, Veniero et al. (2010) showed that when TMS is applied over primary motor cortex (MI), P5, and N8 components reach their peak over motor areas and can be modulated by the frequency of stimulation, suggesting that they might represent the direct response of the stimulated motor cortex. Because P5 and N8 are large signal deflections, their cortical origin has remained uncertain. However, data suggest that P5 and N8 are not residual magnetic artifacts and that they cannot be fully explained by spurious muscle activation (Veniero et al., 2010; but see Mäki and Ilmoniemi, 2011). To gain further information about these components, we designed a protocol to modulate MI excitability by means of premotor cortex (PMC) stimulation. The effects induced by this type of protocol have been ascribed to a cortical phenomenon, i.e., a change in excitability of the circuits within MI after PMC stimulation (Gerschlager et al., 2001; Munchau et al., 2002; Rizzo et al., 2004; Suppa et al., 2008). Therefore, a modulation of P5 and N8 components would support their cortical origin.

MATERIALS AND METHODS

PARTICIPANTS

Fifteen right-handed healthy volunteers participated in the study. Two participants were excluded from the final analysis due to excessive noise in the EEG recording. The remaining 13 participants (8 males and 5 females) aged between 18 and 30 years. None had a history of psychiatric, neurological or other relevant medical disease or any contraindication for TMS (Rossi et al.,

2009). The protocol was performed in accordance with ethical standards and approved by the CEIOC Ethics Committee of IRCCS Centro San Giovanni di Dio Fatebenefratelli, Brescia, Italy. Informed consent was obtained from participants prior to the beginning of the experiment.

PROCEDURE

Participants were comfortably seated on an armchair with the right arm in a resting position, looking at a fixation cross in front of them. TMS was delivered using a Super Rapid transcranial magnetic stimulator connected to four booster modules and a double 50-mm figure-eight custom coil (Magstim Company, Whitland, UK). The coil was placed tangentially to the scalp, with the longer axes perpendicular to the central sulcus. The hot-spot was defined as the point at which the TMS induced the maximum motor-evoked potentials (MEPs) from the relaxed right first dorsal interosseous (FDI), and the resting motor threshold (rMT) was defined as the TMS intensity eliciting MEPs of at least 50 μV in 5 out of 10 trials (Rossini et al., 1994).

Each session started with TMS over the left MI (pre-conditioning block), followed by a 10-min rest period as displayed in **Figure 1**. The conditioning stimulation was then applied. Finally, TMS was delivered over the left MI (post-conditioning block). During the pre- and post-conditioning blocks, 200 single TMS pulses were delivered at random intervals (0.2–0.7 Hz) at 110% of the rMT, which ensured a high signal to noise ratio. During the conditioning stimulation, 1 Hz TMS was delivered in three blocks of 300 stimuli at 70% of the rMT, interspersed with 1-min periods of no TMS (for a total of 900 stimuli). Two sites were conditioned: the PMC and the MI (as a control site). For PMC stimulation, the coil was moved 8% of the nasion-inion distance anteriorly from the MI hot-spot (Munchau et al., 2002). When stimulating MI the closest electrodes to the hot-spot were C3 and C1 in all subjects. During the conditioning block over PMC, 10 subjects had the stimulated area close to FC3 and FC1, and three subjects had the spot over a site located among FC3-FC1-F3. The position of the coil was controlled with a TMS neuronavigation system (SofTaxic, E.M.S., Bologna, Italy) via a graphic user interface and a 3D optical digitiser (NDI, Polaris Vicra, Ontario, Canada) to keep a high degree of reproducibility and accuracy throughout the experimental sessions (Cincotta et al., 2010; Carducci and Brusco, 2012). Two sessions at least 1 week apart were run for PMC and MI conditioning in counterbalanced order across participants. To reduce auditory contamination of EEG induced by coil clicks, subjects wore earplugs during the entire experiment.

TEP AND MEP RECORDINGS

During the pre- and post-conditioning blocks, EEG, electrooculogram (EOG), and electromyogram (EMG) were acquired (BrainAmp, Brain Products GmbH, Munich, Germany). EEG was recorded from 70 scalp electrodes using electrodes mounted on an elastic cap following the International 10-10 system of EEG sensor placement. The ground electrode was positioned in Fpz, while referenced to TP10. Horizontal and vertical eye movements were detected by EOG. The voltage between two electrodes located to the left and right of the external canthi recorded horizontal eye movements. The voltage difference between reference electrodes and electrodes located beneath the right eye recorded vertical eye movements and blinks. MEPs were recorded from the right FDI via surface electrodes in the belly tendon-montage. Skin/electrode impedance was maintained below 5 kΩ. Data were digitized at 5000 Hz and bandpass filtered between 0.01 and 1000 Hz (for recording details see Veniero et al., 2009).

EEG was re-referenced offline to the average signal of TP10 and TP9. For the analysis of cortical and peripheral responses to TMS, the continuous EEG, EOG, and EMG signals were

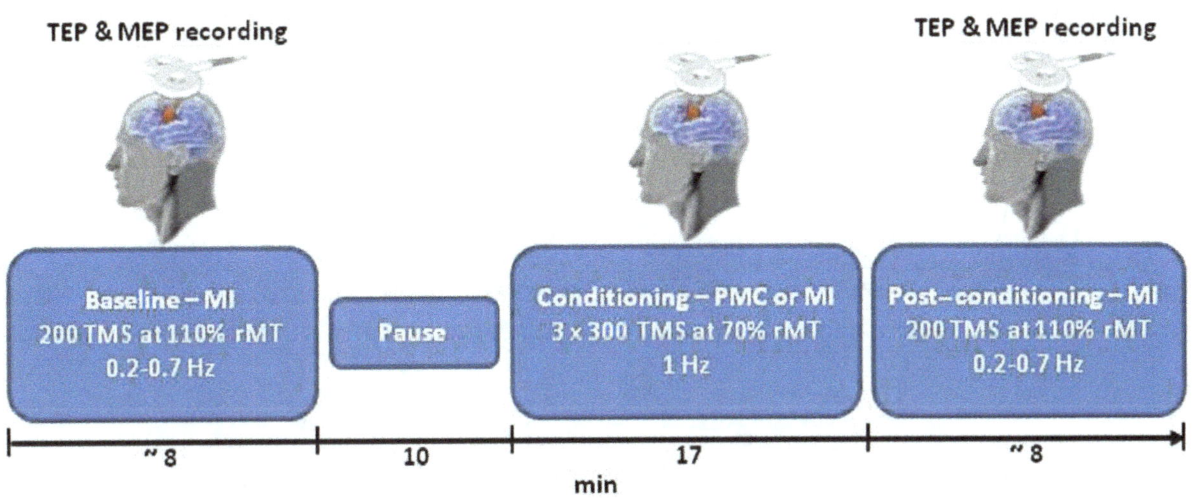

FIGURE 1 | A schematic representation of the experimental procedure. TEPs and MEPs evoked by single pulse TMS over MI were collected for each participant before (baseline) and after (post-conditioning) TMS at 1 Hz (conditioning). In the main condition TMS was applied over PMC; MI was chosen as control site. PMC and MI conditioning were performed in two separate days. TMS, transcranial magnetic stimulation; MEP, motor-evoked potentials; MI, primary motor cortex; PMC, premotor cortex; TEP, TMS-evoked potentials; and the rMT, resting motor threshold.

divided off-line into epochs from 100 ms before the TMS pulse (baseline) to 500 ms after, and were baseline corrected. Before averaging, all epochs were visually inspected to exclude excessively noisy EEG, eye-movement artifacts in the EOG or muscle artifacts in the EEG and EMG. To obtain the cortical evoked responses to TMS (i.e., TEPs) the epochs were averaged for each subject and condition. P5 and N8 showed the same topography with opposite polarity (see **Figure 2**) and were similarly modulated by our protocol; therefore we considered that they may represent a unique TEP complex, i.e., P5-N8 complex.

DATA ANALYSIS

P5 and N8 components were calculated as the average signal of five electrodes (F3, FC5, FC3, FC1, and C3) and defined as positive peak between 5 and 7 ms and negative peak between 7 and 10 ms, respectively. MEPs were measured on the same trials as peak-to-peak amplitude in the EMG signal.

To test for cortical modulation of short-latency TEPs induced by PMC or MI conditioning, a 2 by 2 repeated-measures ANOVA was performed, considering the peak to peak amplitude of P5-N8 complex. We tested for significant effects for the factors Conditioning (MI and PMC) and Time (pre-and post-conditioning). The same analysis was run to test for MEP modulation. Additionally, we performed a factorial ANOVA on each subject's data to test for significant modulations of P5-N8. The normal distribution of P5-N8 amplitude was tested using the Kolmogorov–Smirnov test (for all $p > 0.20$). When appropriate, the Greenhouse-Geisser correction was used, and *post-hoc* comparisons were Bonferroni corrected. We verified that the intensity of stimulation did not change between sessions through a paired t-test.

Moreover, we investigated whether PMC conditioning effects on the P5-N8 complex correlated with the effects on the MEP amplitude. We calculated the difference in P5-N8 amplitude between pre- and post-PMC conditioning and divided the result by the mean P5-N8 complex amplitude in the pre- and post-conditions. We applied the same procedure to the MEPs and submitted the data to a Pearson correlation analysis. Considering the high between-subjects variability of TEPs and MEPs, we applied this procedure to ensure that the effects of the conditioning protocol were not influenced by the absolute amplitude of P5-N8 in a single participant. With this analysis we are able to investigate if cortical components and peripheral measures of cortical reactivity, i.e., MEPs, are linearly related so that the participants who show the biggest PMC conditioning effects on

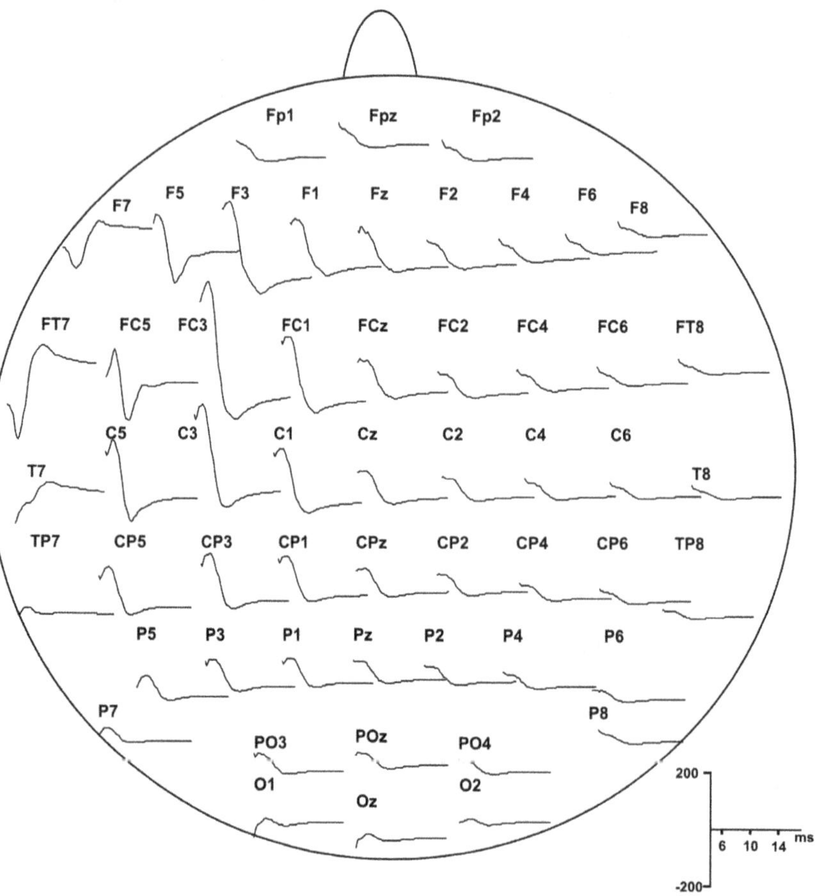

FIGURE 2 | Grand average of the TEPs responses recorded from all subjects showing scalp distribution of P5 and N8 components, starting from 5 ms after the pulse delivery.

the TEPs are also the participants who show the biggest effects on the MEPs.

RESULTS

Mean TMS intensity during conditioning was 63.3 ± 7.6% in the PMC session and 63.8 ± 7.1% in the MI session [no difference between sessions: $t_{(12)} = 1.05, p = 0.32$].

The group analyses did not reveal any significant effect of the TMS conditioning paradigm on MEPs and on P5-N8 amplitude. Baseline values for MEPs and TEPs were not different across conditions [MEPs: $t_{(12)} = 0.35$, $p > 0.05$; P5-N8: $t_{(12)} = 0.20$, $p > 0.05$]. No significant main effect of Conditioning [$F_{(1, 12)} = 0.16$, $p > 0.05$] or significant Conditioning by Time interaction [$F_{(1, 12)} < 0.01$, $p > 0.05$] emerged for MEPs (pre-MI: 896.60; post-MI: 905.78; pre-PMC: 832.67 post-PMC: 841.76). P5-N8 showed a decrease in amplitude after PMC conditioning (pre-PMC: 365.98; post-PMC: 276.90) but not after MI conditioning (pre-MI: 340.21 post-MI: 347.31). However this result was not statistically significant—nor as main effect of Conditioning [$F_{(1, 12)} = 0.06, p > 0.05$] neither as Conditioning by Time interaction [$F_{(1, 12)} < 0.81, p > 0.05$], suggesting that the TMS conditioning protocol may have induced subtle or inconsistent effects across subjects. Accordingly, single subject analyses showed that the PMC conditioning was effective, by significantly modulating TEPs (P5-N8), in 8 out of 13 participants: TEPs amplitude was reduced in six participants (**Figure 3**) [Conditioning by Time interaction, s01: $F_{(1, 667)} = 1887.28$, $p < 0.05$; s02: $F_{(1, 702)} = 2941.29$, $p < 0.05$; s04: $F_{(1, 467)} = 281.93, p < 0.05$; s05: $F_{(1, 420)} = 71.47$, $p < 0.05$; s13: $F_{(1, 305)} = 122.58, p < 0.05$; Main effect Time: s11: $F_{(1, 493)} = 19.81$, $p < 0.05$; all *post-hoc* $p < 0.05$] and increased in two participants [Conditioning by Time interaction, s03: $F_{(1, 553)} = 9.22$, $p < 0.05$; s09: $F_{(1, 558)} = 287.10$, $p < 0.05$; all *post-hoc* $p < 0.05$] after PMC conditioning. Opposite or null results in different subjects suggest that the TMS conditioning did not have a consistent effect across subjects and may have been ineffective in some participants. Noteworthy, the P5-N8 modulation after PMC conditioning was significantly stronger than the effect of MI conditioning, as indicated by significant interactions Conditioning by Time in seven subjects, therefore suggesting that such modulations were related to the specific stimulation of PMC.

Moreover, to address the question on the cortical origin of early TEPs, we took an additional approach by investigating the correlation between P5-N8 and the MEPs amplitude. Importantly, we found that the modulation of P5-N8 complex after PMC conditioning correlated with the modulation of MEPs ($r = -0.60, p < 0.05$) so that the stronger the decrease of P5-N8 complex amplitude, the higher the increase of MEPs. In other words, the participants showing reduced P5-N8 amplitude after PMC conditioning, showed increased MEP amplitude, and vice versa, participants showing increased P5-N8 amplitude showed decreased MEP amplitude (**Figure 4**). The correlation between the modulation of P5-N8 complex after MI conditioning and the modulation of MEPs was not significant ($r = 0.41, p > 0.05$).

DISCUSSION

The aim of the present study was to provide new information about two short-latency TEPs, namely P5-N8, by indirectly manipulating MI excitability. Although applying an inhibitory

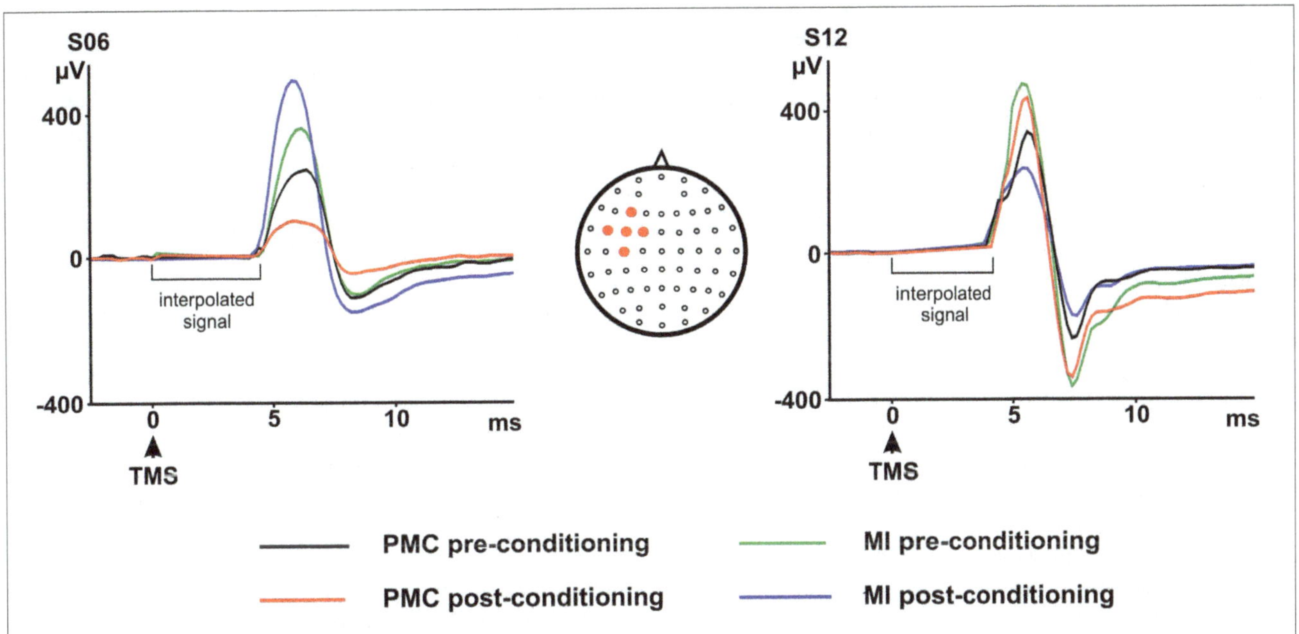

FIGURE 3 | P5 and N8 pre- and post-primary motor cortex (MI) or premotor cortex (PMC) conditioning as recorded from the marked electrodes. On the left a representative participant showing a decrease in P5 and N8 amplitudes after PMC conditioning and an increase in P5 and N8 amplitudes after MI conditioning. On the right a representative participant showing an increase in P5 and N8 after PMC conditioning and the opposite result after MI conditioning. Electrodes montage is also shown on the upper right side of the figure. Filled circles indicate five electrodes from which the P5-N8 average signal was calculated.

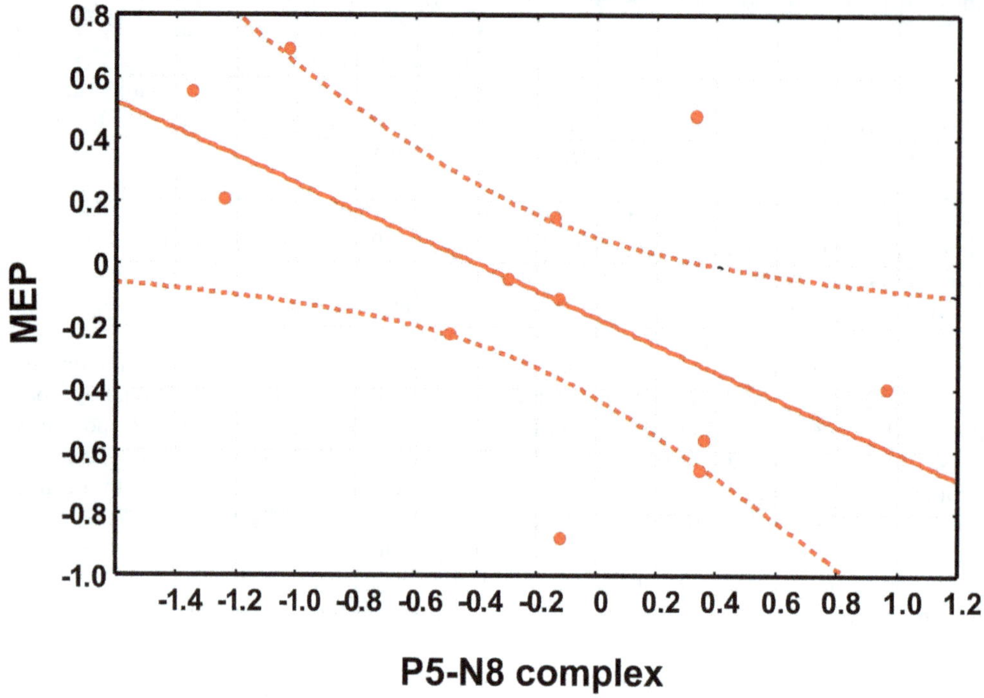

FIGURE 4 | The scatter plot shows the significant negative correlation between the changes in motor-evoked potentials (MEPs) amplitude, on the x-axis and the changes in P5-N8 complex amplitude. Note that negative values indicate a reduced amplitude of P5-N8 complex or a reduction of MEPs amplitude after the conditioning session (see main text for details about data analysis).

protocol to PMC did not consistently change MI activation across all subjects, we were able to study the relationship between P5-N8 and peripheral measures of cortical excitability with two specific analyses: single subject analyses and correlation between P5-N8 and MEPs.

Results from the single subjects analysis indicated a significant modulation of P5-N8 complex when conditioning session was performed over PMC, but not over MI. Given that both sites of stimulation are close to the facial muscles it is highly unlikely that we were stimulating facial muscles in PMC condition and not in the MI, thus we can exclude that we are simply manipulating the responses of the facial muscles. Moreover, it is unlikely that results are influenced by those artifact generated by the stimulation of the scalp, because pre- and post-conditioning session have been performed in the same way, so the artifactual activity in all session is likely to be the same. Last, additional somatosensory activation generated by the muscle twitch should be very unlikely to be involved in the generation of the early TEPs because the afferent response takes about 20 ms to reach the cortex.

By correlating the modulation of P5-N8 with the MEPs modulation, we were able to show that the P5-N8 complex shares an inverse linear relationship with the MEPs, i.e., the peripheral measure of cortical reactivity. Therefore, P5-N8 complex may represent an inhibitory process initiated by the premotor area. Indeed, our data show that the bigger was the conditioning effect on these early components, the stronger was the inhibition over MI. Accordingly, some recent TMS–EEG studies (Esser et al., 2006; Ferreri et al., 2011) localized the cortical source of both P5 and N8 in the PMC. Moreover, it has been shown that a magnetic pulse delivered over the ipsilateral PMC at 2–15 ms prior to a second stimulus over MI can reduce the MEPs amplitude, with the biggest effect at 6 ms (Civardi et al., 2001).

In contrast with previous studies, the effect of the PMC conditioning on MEP was not significant over all subjects, as indicated by no change in MEPs and TEPs amplitude in the group analyses. These results may depend on the TMS intensity (70% rMT) set during conditioning. Such a low intensity was chosen to avoid MI stimulation during the PMC conditioning and was comparable to intensities used in previous studies (Gerschlager et al., 2001; Munchau et al., 2002). Moreover, because of the PMC localization method used, it might be that the same area was not precisely targeted in all subjects. The spatial precision of the optical TMS neuronavigation system in the localization of the target area is generally a few millimetres (Herwig et al., 2001; Julkunen et al., 2008; Cincotta et al., 2010). Nevertheless this spatial precision is dependent on the resolution of the MRI data. In this case, the coil was moved 8% of the nasion-inion distance anteriorly from the MI hot-spot and it is likely that the actual TMS target site differed across subjects (Sack et al., 2009). For these reasons, the conditioning stimulation may have been ineffective in some participants, in turn leading to opposite or null results in different subjects.

The present study shows that P5 and N8 can be modulated by cortical phenomena such as the PMC conditioning at least at single subject level. Therefore, according to previous studies reporting an early TEPs modulation after paired pulse TMS

(Ferreri et al., 2011) and 20 Hz rTMS (Veniero et al., 2010), it is possible to conclude that different protocols classically designed to modulate MI excitability have an impact over P5-N8 amplitude. Importantly, despite not consistently manipulated by the protocol, the amplitude of the early components was correlated to MEPs amplitude. Therefore, in our view these results points to a cortical involvement in P5 and N8 generation. However, some studies (Julkunen et al., 2008; Mutanen et al., 2012) have linked the large responses recorded after few ms from the stimulus to an exclusively artifactual phenomenon. In the present study we cannot totally exclude an involvement of muscular activity, indeed non-cortical phenomena induced by our protocol, e.g., the repeated stimulation of facial muscles, should also be considered because they can affect early TEPs. Moreover, the modulation of P5-N8 appears to have a significant inter-individual variability that should be further explored. A possible parsimonious explanation is that the P5-N8 complex may represent a cortical response together with muscular activation and that the influence of this second component on the recorded signal may vary across individuals. This would be in line with recent findings by Mutanen et al. (2012) showing that the amplitude of muscular artifact recorded during EEG-TMS experiment depends on coil rotation, tilt angles and stimulation intensities. These parameters are not constant across subjects because when MI is stimulated the final coil position is chosen with the aim to evoke a reliable MEP with the lowest intensity. Possibly more sophisticated analyses, e.g., independent component analyses (ICA) and principal component analyses (PCA), can isolate the cortical component and provide a better index of cortical activity. It has however to be noted that the muscular and the cortical activation could theoretically overlap in time and it is also possible that these different components share similar brain topography. Mäki and Ilmoniemi (2011) applied PCA to TMS–EEG data to remove muscular activation, by subtracting some components according to their frequency, amplitude and topography. This procedure however resulted in a flattening of signals covering the stimulated area. More successful approach for removing large muscle artifacts from TEPs, after stimulation of lateral areas of the scalp, have been recently applied by Korhonen et al. (2011) with the enhanced deflation method.

It has to be noted that previous studies found a correlation between late TEP components and MEPs amplitude (Mäki and Ilmoniemi, 2010; Ferreri et al., 2011). However the latency of these late components, about 30 ms, is not compatible with the generation of the descending output responsible for the targeted muscle activation. On the other hand it appears more plausible that early component could reflect those activations responsible for MEPs typically recorded after 20–25 ms from the magnetic pulse.

In conclusion, we report important results about the nature of two short-latency TEPs. Because our conditioning protocol is considered to induce cortical effects (Munchau et al., 2002), the changes in P5 and N8 amplitude and their correlation with MEPs amplitude suggest that these early TEPs have a cortical component and that they can be used to evaluate the reactivity of the stimulated cortex. Despite the possibility of a residual muscular activation, our study suggests that with careful study design, namely keeping the experimental conditions comparable and considering that a muscular activation can as well be involved, these early TEP components can be informative on the reactivity of the targeted area.

ACKNOWLEDGMENTS

This work was supported by a grant from the Italian Ministry of Health.

REFERENCES

Bonato, C., Miniussi, C., and Rossini, P. M. (2006). Transcranial magnetic stimulation and cortical evoked potentials: a TMS/EEG co-registration study. *Clin. Neurophysiol.* 117, 1699–1707.

Busan, P., Zanon, M., Vinciati, F., Monti, F., Pizzolato, G., and Battaglini, P. P. (2012). Transcranial magnetic stimulation and preparation of visually-guided reaching movements. *Front. Neuroeng.* 5:18. doi: 10.3389/fneng.2012.00018

Carducci, F., and Brusco, R. (2012). Accuracy of an individualized MR-based head model for navigated brain stimulation. *Psychiatry Res.* 203, 105–108.

Cincotta, M., Giovannelli, F., Borgheresi, A., Balestrieri, F., Toscani, L., Zaccara, G., et al. (2010). Optically tracked neuronavigation increases the stability of hand-held focal coil positioning: evidence from "transcranial" magnetic stimulation-induced electrical field measurements. *Brain Stimul.* 3, 119–123.

Civardi, C., Cantello, R., Asselman, P., and Rothwel, J. C. (2001). Transcranial magnetic stimulation can be used to test connections to primary motor areas from frontal and medial cortex in humans. *Neuroimage* 14, 1444–1453.

Esser, S. K., Huber, R., Massimini, M., Peterson, M. J., Ferrarelli, F., and Tononi, G. (2006). A direct demonstration of cortical LTP in humans: a combined TMS/EEG study. *Brain Res. Bull.* 69, 86–94.

Ferreri, F., Pasqualetti, P., Maatta, S., Ponzo, D., Ferrarelli, F., Tononi, G., et al. (2011). Human brain connectivity during single and paired pulse transcranial magnetic stimulation. *Neuroimage* 54, 90–102.

Gerschlager, W., Siebner, H. R., and Rothwell, J. C. (2001). Decreased corticospinal excitability after subthreshold 1 Hz rTMS over lateral premotor cortex. *Neurology* 57, 449–455.

Herwig, U., Padberg, F., Unger, J., Spitzer, M., and Schonfeldt-Lecuona, C. (2001). Transcranial magnetic stimulation in therapy studies: examination of the reliability of "standard" coil positioning by neuronavigation. *Biol. Psychiatry* 50, 58–61.

Ilmoniemi, R. J., Virtanen, J., Ruohonen, J., Karhu, J., Aronen, H. J., Naatanen, R., et al. (1997). Neuronal responses to magnetic stimulation reveal cortical reactivity and connectivity. *Neuroreport* 8, 3537–3540.

Julkunen, P., Pääkkönen, A., Hukkanen, T., Könönen, M., Tiihonen, P., Vanhatalo, S., et al. (2008). Efficient reduction of stimulus artefact in TMS-EEG by epithelial short-circuiting by mini-punctures. *Clin. Neurophysiol.* 119, 475–481.

Kähkönen, S., Wilenius, J., Komssi, S., and Ilmoniemi, R. J. (2004). Distinct differences in cortical reactivity of motor and prefrontal cortices to magnetic stimulation. *Clin. Neurophysiol.* 115, 583–588.

Komssi, S., Aronen, H. J., Huttunen, J., Kesäniemi, M., Soinne, L., Nikouline, V. V., et al. (2002). Ipsi- and contralateral EEG reactions to transcranial magnetic stimulation. *Clin. Neurophysiol.* 113, 175–184.

Komssi, S., and Kähkönen, S. (2006). The novelty value of the combined use of electroencephalography and transcranial magnetic stimulation for neuroscience research. *Brain Res. Rev.* 52, 183–192.

Komssi, S., Kähkönen, S., and Ilmoniemi, R. J. (2004). The effect of stimulus intensity on brain responses evoked by transcranial magnetic stimulation. *Hum. Brain Mapp.* 21, 154–164.

Korhonen, R. J., Hernandez-Pavon, J. C., Metsomaa, J., Mäki, H., Ilmoniemi, R. J., and Sarvas, J. (2011). Removal of large muscle artifacts from transcranial magnetic stimulation-evoked EEG by independent component analysis. *Med. Biol. Eng. Comput.* 49, 397–407.

Lioumis, P., Kicic, D., Savolainen, P., Makela, J. P., and Kähkönen, S. (2009). Reproducibility of TMS-Evoked EEG responses. *Hum. Brain Mapp.* 30, 1387–1396.

Litvak, V., Komssi, S., Scherg, M., Hoechstetter, K., Classen, J., Zaaroor, M., et al. (2007). Artifact correction and source analysis of early electroencephalographic responses evoked by transcranial magnetic stimulation over primary motor cortex. *Neuroimage* 37, 56–70.

Mäki, H., and Ilmoniemi, R. J. (2010). The relationship between peripheral and early cortical activation induced by transcranial magnetic stimulation. *Neurosci. Lett.* 478, 24–28.

Mäki, H., and Ilmoniemi, R. J. (2011). Projecting out muscle artifacts from TMS-evoked EEG. *Neuroimage* 54, 2706–2710.

Miniussi, C., and Thut, G. (2010). Combining TMS and EEG offers new prospects in cognitive neuroscience. *Brain Topogr.* 22, 249–256.

Munchau, A., Bloem, B. R., Irlbacher, K., Trimble, M. R., and Rothwell, J. C. (2002). Functional connectivity of human premotor and motor cortex explored with repetitive transcranial magnetic stimulation. *J. Neurosci.* 22, 554–561.

Mutanen, T., Mäki, H., and Ilmoniemi, R. J. (2012). The effect of stimulus parameters on TMS-EEG muscle artifacts. *Brain Stimul.* doi: 10.1016/j.brs.2012.07.005. [Epub ahead of print].

Rizzo, V., Siebner, H. R., Modugno, N., Pesenti, A., Munchau, A., Gerschlager, W., et al. (2004). Shaping the excitability of human motor cortex with premotor rTMS. *J. Physiol.* 554(Pt 2), 483–495.

Rossi, S., Hallett, M., Rossini, P. M., Pascual-Leone, A., and the "Safety of TMS Consensus Group." (2009). Safety, ethical considerations, and application guidelines for the use of transcranial magnetic stimulation in clinical practice and research. *Clin. Neurophysiol.* 120, 2008–2039.

Rossini, P. M., Barker, A. T., Berardelli, A., Caramia, M. D., Caruso, G., Cracco, R. Q., et al. (1994). Non-invasive electrical and magnetic stimulation of the brain, spinal cord and roots: basic principles and procedures for routine clinical application. Report of an IFCN committee. *Electroencephalogr. Clin. Neurophysiol.* 91, 79–92.

Sack, A. T., Cohen Kadosh, R., Schuhmann, T., Moerel, M., Walsh, V., and Goebel, R. (2009). Optimizing functional accuracy of TMS in cognitive studies: a comparison of methods. *J. Cogn. Neurosci.* 21, 207–221.

Suppa, A., Bologna, M., Gilio, F., Lorenzano, C., Rothwell, J. C., and Berardelli, A. (2008). Preconditioning repetitive transcranial magnetic stimulation of premotor cortex can reduce but not enhance short-term facilitation of primary motor cortex. *J. Neurophysiol.* 99, 564–570.

Veniero, D., Bortoletto, M., and Miniussi, C. (2009). TMS-EEG co-registration: on TMS-induced artifact. *Clin. Neurophysiol.* 120, 1392–1399.

Veniero, D., Maioli, C., and Miniussi, C. (2010). Potentiation of short-latency cortical responses by high-frequency repetitive transcranial magnetic stimulation. *J. Neurophysiol.* 104, 1578–1588.

9

Covert oculo-manual coupling induced by visually guided saccades

Luca Falciati, Tiziana Gianesini and Claudio Maioli*

Department of Clinical and Experimental Sciences and National Institute of Neuroscience, University of Brescia, Brescia, Italy

Correspondence:
Claudio Maioli, Dipartimento di Scienze Cliniche e Sperimentali, Università di Brescia, V.le Europa 11, 25123 Brescia, Italy
e-mail: maioli@med.unibs.it

Hand pointing to objects under visual guidance is one of the most common motor behaviors in everyday life. In natural conditions, gaze and arm movements are commonly aimed at the same target and the accuracy of both systems is considerably enhanced if eye and hand move together. Evidence supports the viewpoint that gaze and limb control systems are not independent but at least partially share a common neural controller. The aim of the present study was to verify whether a saccade execution induces excitability changes in the upper-limb corticospinal system (CSS), even in the absence of a manual response. This effect would provide evidence for the existence of a common drive for ocular and arm motor systems during fast aiming movements. Single-pulse TMS was applied to the left motor cortex of 19 subjects during a task involving visually guided saccades, and motor evoked potentials (MEPs) induced in hand and wrist muscles of the contralateral relaxed arm were recorded. Subjects had to make visually guided saccades to one of 6 positions along the horizontal meridian (±5°, ±10°, or ±15°). During each trial, TMS was randomly delivered at one of 3 different time delays: shortly after the end of the saccade or 300 or 540 ms after saccade onset. Fast eye movements toward a peripheral target were accompanied by changes in upper-limb CSS excitability. MEP amplitude was highest immediately after the end of the saccade and gradually decreased at longer TMS delays. In addition to the change in overall CSS excitability, MEPs were specifically modulated in different muscles, depending on the target position and the TMS delay. By applying a simple model of a manual pointing movement, we demonstrated that the observed changes in CSS excitability are compatible with the facilitation of an arm motor program for a movement aimed at the same target of the gaze. These results provide evidence in favor of the existence of a common drive for both eye and arm motor systems.

Keywords: eye-hand coupling, saccade, transcranial magnetic stimulation, motor evoked potentials, motor excitability

INTRODUCTION

Reaching and manipulating objects under visual guidance is one of the most common motor behaviors in everyday life. Converging evidence from a large number of studies indicates that a tight coordination of gaze and arm movements is of paramount importance for the accurate execution of visually guided aiming tasks.

Typically, a saccade is made shortly before a hand movement is initiated (Prablanc et al., 1979; Lünenburger et al., 2000; Dean et al., 2011), thereby bringing the target into the fovea. If foveation of the target is prevented, pointing accuracy decreases considerably (Vercher et al., 1994; Henriques et al., 1998; Neggers and Bekkering, 1999; van Donkelaar and Staub, 2000; Medendorp and Crawford, 2002; Horstmann and Hoffmann, 2005). Moreover, subjects cannot fixate to a new target before the hand reach is completed, indicating that the gaze is anchored to the target during the entire pointing movement (Neggers and Bekkering, 2000, 2002). Finally, a high correlation between hand position and gaze error has been reported in pointing tasks to remembered visual targets (Flanders et al., 1999; Admiraal et al., 2003, 2004) or during an illusion in which the perceived direction of target motion is altered by a moving background (Soechting et al., 2001). Experimental evidence strongly supports the viewpoint that extraretinal gaze signals are required for precise pointing and reaching movements and that eye and arm motor control systems are mutually coupled (van Donkelaar and Staub, 2000; Engel and Soechting, 2003; Dean et al., 2011).

Some clinical observations also support the existence of a tight coupling between arm and eye control systems for fast aiming movements. Patients suffering from bilateral parietal lobe atrophy sometimes show a slavish dependence of reach on gaze (Buxbaum and Coslett, 1997; Carey et al., 1997). In fact, these patients are incapable of reaching objects they do not look at and inevitably move their hand to the place their eyes are fixating on ("magnetic misreaching"). A possible interpretation of these data is that whenever the eyes move, a motor plan is formed that carries the arm to the same target. Normally, eye or hand motor responses can be separately inhibited, depending on the ongoing behavioral goal. However, neurological disorders can induce a pathological incapacity to disjoin eye and upper-limb movements to the same visual target.

In a previous transcranial magnetic stimulation (TMS) study, we showed that smooth pursuit eye movements are linked to a modulation of corticospinal system (CSS) excitability of the resting arm (Maioli et al., 2007). Excitability changes were found to be compatible with a motor plan encoding an aiming movement of the hand toward the same target tracked by the eyes. In the presence of a common drive to ocular and arm motor systems, we expect that the execution of an eye saccade would also induce excitability changes in the upper-limb CSS in a pure oculomotor task. In this paper, we demonstrate that similar to smooth pursuit eye movements, highly specific changes in the upper-limb CSS excitability also occur in a strict temporal relationship with eye saccades, even if the task does not demand a manual response.

MATERIALS AND METHODS

SUBJECTS

Nineteen adult volunteers (10 males and 9 females, mean age: 20.7 years, range: 20–23 years) with no history of head trauma or neurological disease participated in the study. All subjects were right-handed (as measured by the Edinburgh handedness inventory) and naïve to the purpose of the experiment. This study was conducted in accordance with the ethical guidelines set forth by the Declaration of Helsinki. Written informed consent was obtained from all participants.

EYE MOVEMENT AND EMG RECORDING

Horizontal and vertical eye movements were recorded (DC-200 Hz low-pass filtered) by means of electrooculography (EOG). Ag-AgCl electrodes were placed at the external canthi and above and below the right eye. EOG calibration was frequently repeated during the experimental session. Drift of DC offset was compensated within each trial by making the subject look at a central fixation cross before the presentation of the saccade target. Surface electromyograms (EMG) were recorded on the right hand side from the *first dorsal interosseous* (FDI), *abductor digiti minimi* (ADM), *extensor carpi radialis* (ECR), and *flexor carpi ulnaris* (FCU) muscles (1000× amplification; 0.2 Hz −1 kHz bandwidth). EOG and EMG signals were digitally converted at a sampling rate of 5 kHz (National Instruments PCI-MIO-16E-4) and analyzed off-line using custom-written Labview software (National Instruments, Austin, TX).

TRANSCRANIAL MAGNETIC STIMULATION

A 70 mm figure-of-eight double coil connected to a MagStim Super Rapid magnetic stimulator (Mag-1450-00, MagStim Co. Ltd Whitland, UK) was positioned over the left motor cortex, contralateral to the EMG recorded muscles. The coil was placed tangentially to the scalp with the handle pointing backwards and laterally at a 45° angle to the sagittal plane. This orientation was chosen because the lowest motor threshold is achieved when the induced electrical current in the brain flows approximately perpendicular to the central sulcus (Mills and Nithi, 1997).

The scalp site at which motor evoked potentials (MEPs) were elicited at the lowest stimulus strength in the FDI muscle was determined. Once the optimal scalp site was found, the coil was securely fixed in place with an appropriate mechanical device. The response threshold was defined as the stimulus intensity at which 5 out of 10 consecutive stimuli at the optimal site evoked an MEP with a peak-to-peak amplitude of at least 100 μV in the relaxed muscle. Stimulus intensity during the entire stimulation paradigm was set at 1.2 times the FDI motor threshold. The mean stimulation intensity across subjects was equal to 71.5% of the maximum power of the magnetic stimulator. This stimulation intensity at the optimal scalp site for FDI also evoked MEPs in the ADM, ECR, and FCU muscles in almost all experimental sessions, although these MEPs generally occurred at a considerably lower amplitude. In order to ensure that excitability changes were measured against a reliable baseline for each muscle, subjects were included in the analysis only if the evoked responses were larger than the above defined threshold amplitude. This acceptance criterion was fulfilled in 15, 18, and 18 subjects for the ADM, ECR, and FCU muscles, respectively. Furthermore, 2 subjects had to be excluded from the analysis of the ADM muscle due to technical issues in recording.

EXPERIMENTAL PROTOCOL

Subjects sat comfortably, with their right upper-limb resting in a relaxed position on a horizontal support. The support was formed by a polystyrene-bead vacuum splint and molded on the hand palm and forearm of the subject. This device enabled the limb to be loosely restrained in order to maintain the longitudinal axis of the pronated hand horizontally aligned with the forearm and pointing toward the central vertical meridian (**Figure 1A**). The head was stabilized using a combination chin-rest and head-support device. White visual stimuli were rear-projected on a wide tangent black screen (160 cm in width and 120 cm in height) that was placed 1 m in front of the subject. Participants had to fixate on a central cross for 3 s. One second after a warning tone, the fixation cross turned off, and a new target (a square subtending 0.6° of visual angle) randomly appeared for 3 s at one of 6 peripheral positions along the horizontal meridian, at eccentricities of 5°, 10°, or 15°, in the left or right visual field. Subjects were instructed to quickly respond by moving their gaze to the peripheral stimulus, and to fixate it as accurately as possible. After the target turned off, the central fixation cross was presented again, marking the beginning of a new trial.

Particular attention was paid during task explanation to avoid drawing the subject's attention to the possibility of making an aiming arm movement toward the target. In addition, the lack of any imagery of manual pointing movements was assessed through a subject interview after the experimental session. In order for a trial to be included in the analysis, the following criteria had to be fulfilled: (1) subjects had to keep their muscles completely relaxed, as defined by the absence of any detectable EMG activity for the entire task duration; (2) the latency of the saccadic response had to be shorter than 300 ms in order to ensure the presence of a high and constant arousal level in the subject; and (3) the saccadic responses could not be anticipatory. To this end, trials with a saccadic latency shorter than 90 ms were discarded.

During each trial, single-pulse TMS was triggered by the EOG signal at one of 3 different time delays, with respect to the saccade onset (**Figure 1B**). Labview software controlling the experiment

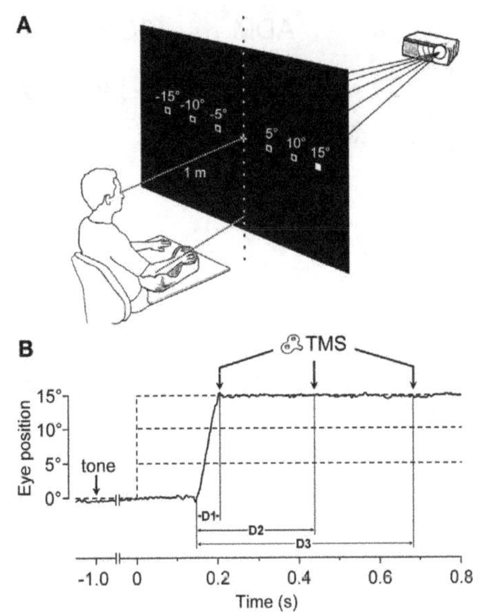

FIGURE 1 | Experimental Setup and Protocol. (A) The target stimulus was projected at one of six possible spatial locations. The filled square represents the actual visual target, while empty squares indicate the other possible positions. The head was immobilized using a chin-rest and a head-support device (not shown). Notice the arm-hand posture imposed on the subject with respect to the central vertical meridian (see text). **(B)** An EOG recording (solid line) during a representative saccadic eye movement executed toward a 15° eccentric target. Dashed lines indicate the onset (vertical) and the possible eccentricities (horizontal) of the visual target, which was presented 1000 ms after a warning tone. TMS pulses were randomly delivered at 60 ms (D1), 300 ms (D2), or 540 ms (D3) after the beginning of the saccade.

was programmed in order to randomly deliver TMS pulses at 0, 250, or 500 ms after saccade onset, as identified by a real-time analysis of the EOG signal. However, the buffered data acquisition (with buffer time epochs of 40 ms) imposed a certain degree of uncertainty to the recognition of saccadic occurrence. Therefore, actual TMS delays with respect to the precise saccade onset were computed off-line, trial-by-trial, using a semi-automatic computer-based analysis. The mean values (±SD) of TMS latencies with respect to saccade onset for the 3 delay conditions were as follows: 56 ± 15 ms (shortly after the end of saccade execution), 296 ± 19 ms, and 537 ± 23 ms. For the remainder of this report, these 3 delay conditions will be conventionally referred to as $D1 = 60$ ms, $D2 = 300$ ms, and $D3 = 540$ ms.

Each experimental session comprised 5 blocks of 36 trials (with 3 min intervals between blocks), yielding an overall number of 180 trials (10 trials for each of the 18 target-eccentricity × TMS-delay conditions).

STATISTICAL ANALYSIS

MEP amplitudes are continuous variates characterized by a very large variability among subjects in the mean and standard deviation of their statistical distribution. Therefore, in order to compare data from different subjects and apply statistical significance tests, data transformation was required. Details on the adopted statistical procedures have been previously described (Maioli et al., 2007). Briefly, for each subject, raw data were transformed as follows:

$$X = \frac{x - \mu_s}{\sigma_s}$$

where X is the standardized measure and x is the original experimental value having a distribution with μ_s mean and σ_s standard deviation. This transformation normalized the experimental variability and permitted direct data comparison among subjects because MEP amplitude became a standard variate with zero mean and unitary standard deviation. For each subject, μ_s was obtained by averaging peak-to-peak MEP amplitudes across all experimental conditions. The standard deviation σ_s was computed as the square-root of the residual variance within each subject, i.e., the variance within groups defined by all combinations of target-eccentricity and TMS-delay conditions. Using this procedure, the intra-subject variability of experimental data was normalized without cancelling the effects that might result from the application of the different experimental conditions.

In order to test the statistical significance of the effects of target position on MEP amplitude, a Two-Way ANOVA for repeated measurements was performed on the average MEP amplitudes computed for each subject for a given experimental condition. The factors were "*side*" (left vs. right visual hemifield) and "*eccentricity*" (5°, 10°, 15°). Separate analyses were run for each muscle and TMS delay.

RESULTS

OVERALL CHANGES OF CSS EXCITABILITY IN UPPER-LIMB MUSCLES

Making a saccadic eye movement to a peripheral target induced clear-cut excitability changes in the CSS of the resting arm, which were strictly time-locked to saccade execution. The mean saccadic latency across subjects recorded within our experimental condition was 158 ± 34 ms. **Figure 2** shows the mean MEPs recorded from the 4 investigated muscles in a representative subject as a function of the TMS delay from saccadic onset and irrespective of the target position. Each trace represents the average MEP of 54–59 TMS stimuli delivered in a single experimental session. Trials with different TMS delay values were presented in a random order so that subjects were completely unaware of the timing of the TMS occurrence. It is clear that MEP amplitude is largest at *D1* (~60 ms after saccade onset) and gradually decreases at longer TMS delays.

Figure 3 depicts the average variation across subjects in peak-to-peak MEP amplitude as a function of the TMS delay and irrespective of the target position. The CSS excitability decays linearly in all muscles. On average, mean MEP amplitude at TMS delay *D3* is ~20% smaller than shortly after saccade onset.

Our experimental protocol did not allow a direct measurement of resting MEP amplitudes, i.e., during fixation before the saccade onset. Therefore, we cannot determine whether this decay is the result of a sudden transient increase of excitability occurring before or in correspondence to the execution of a saccade or whether it reflects a progressive CSS depression lasting for several hundreds of milliseconds following the onset of a saccadic eye movement.

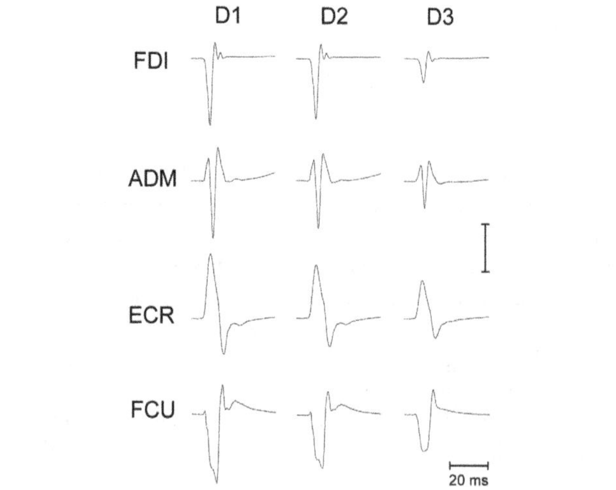

FIGURE 2 | Average EMG recordings from relaxed FDI, ADM, ECR, and FCU muscles in a representative subject. All muscles show a progressive decay of MEP amplitude as a function of the TMS delay (D1, D2, and D3) from saccade onset. The amplitude calibration mark represents 1.0, 0.2, 0.35, and 0.2 mV for the FDI, ADM, ECR, and FCU muscles, respectively.

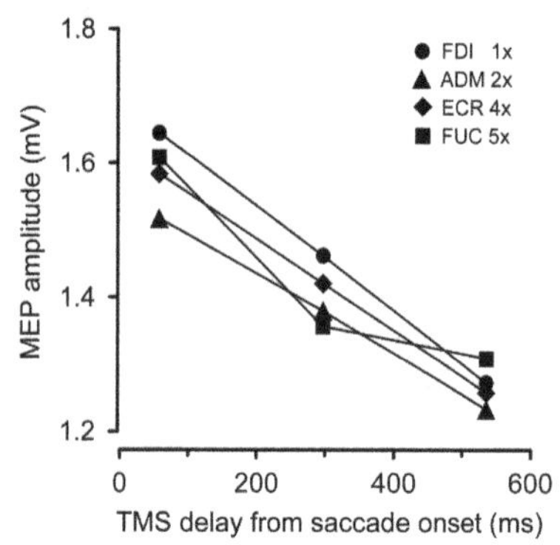

FIGURE 3 | Changes in mean MEP amplitudes as a function of TMS delay from saccade onset for each recorded muscle. Depicted MEP amplitudes represent the grand mean across subjects and target positions. MEP amplitudes for different muscles have been scaled according to the values shown in the legend.

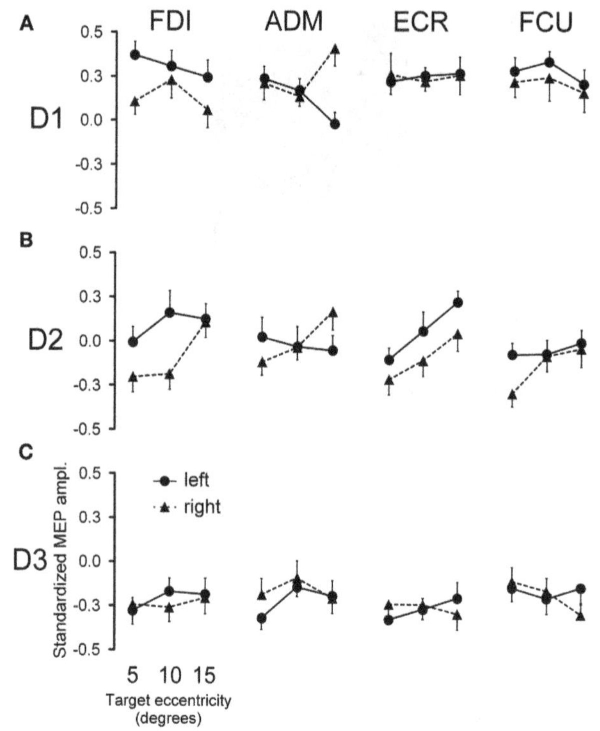

FIGURE 4 | Effects of saccadic target position on MEP amplitude. The modulation of mean MEP amplitude across all subjects following saccade execution is shown for each muscle. Points represent the mean standardized MEP amplitudes as a function of target eccentricity and visual hemi-field of presentation for TMS delay D1 **(A)**, D2 **(B)**, and D3 **(C)**. Error bars represent the standard error of the mean.

EFFECTS OF SIDE AND ECCENTRICITY OF THE SACCADIC TARGET ON EXCITABILITY CHANGES

In addition to the decay in overall CSS excitability, MEP amplitudes are modulated in a highly specific manner in different muscles, depending on the target position of the visually guided saccade and on the timing of TMS stimulation with respect to saccade onset. **Figure 4** shows the average values across subjects of standardized MEP amplitudes for all recorded muscles as a function of TMS delay, visual hemi-field of target appearance and target eccentricity.

No changes in mean MEP amplitude occurred at TMS delay *D3* as a function of target position (**Figure 4C**). By contrast, quite large MEP modulations were observed in some muscles at *D1* and *D2*, depending on both the direction and eccentricity of the visually guided saccade (**Figures 4A,B**).

In order to test the statistical significance of the observed changes in motor excitability, a Two-Way repeated measures ANOVA (**Table 1**) was performed for each muscle and TMS delay on the mean MEP amplitudes of each subject, with the target side and eccentricity as grouping factors. The analysis at delay *D1* demonstrates that the direction of the saccadic movement ("*side*" factor) had a significant principal effect on MEP amplitude only for the FDI and ADM muscles. Furthermore, in the ADM muscle, a significant "*eccentricity* × *side*" interaction was also present. **Figure 4A** shows that the "*side*" principal effect in the FDI muscle was determined by the fact that MEP amplitude after leftward saccades was considerably larger than after rightward saccades, independently of the target eccentricity. By contrast, an opposite modulation of MEP amplitude as a function of saccade direction was observed in the ADM muscle, which increased in size at the most eccentric target position of 15° [$F_{(1,\,14)} = 11.667$, $P = 0.004$]. Conversely, no significant changes in MEP amplitude were observed as a function of either side or eccentricity of the target in the more proximal ECR and FCU muscles.

A different picture emerges from the analysis of the data at the intermediate TMS delay *D2*. Both "*eccentricity*" and "*side*" of the saccadic target induced a clear-cut modulation of MEP amplitude in the ECR muscle. By contrast, only a "*side*" principal effect was found in the FDI muscle. No statistically significant effects were detected on MEPs recorded in the ADM and FCU muscles.

Table 1 | Two-Way repeated measures ANOVAs of MEP amplitudes.

Muscle (N)	Eccentricity		Side		Ecc. × Side	
	$F_{2,(N-1)\times 5}$	P	$F_{1,(N-1)\times 5}$	P	$F_{2,(N-1)\times 5}$	P
D1 60 ms						
FDI (19)	1.148	0.322	**7.158**	**0.009****	0.677	0.510
ADM (15)	0.528	0.592	**4.589**	**0.036****	**7.159**	**0.001****
ECR (18)	0.051	0.950	0.000	0.994	0.098	0.907
FCU (18)	0.703	0.498	0.831	0.364	0.027	0.973
D2 300 ms						
FDI (19)	2.732	0.071	**5.771**	**0.018****	1.507	0.227
ADM (15)	0.672	0.514	0.095	0.758	1.722	0.186
ECR (18)	**5.998**	**0.004****	**4.815**	**0.031****	0.087	0.917
FCU (18)	1.999	0.142	1.740	0.191	0.970	0.383
D3 540 ms						
FDI (19)	0.332	0.719	0.146	0.704	0.290	0.749
ADM (15)	1.429	0.246	0.773	0.382	0.413	0.663
ECR (18)	0.121	0.886	0.018	0.892	0.709	0.495
FCU (18)	0.809	0.449	0.160	0.690	1.138	0.325

*N is the number of subjects. ** denotes statistical significance ($P < 0.05$).*

It should also be noted that in all muscles, "*eccentricity*" and "*side*" factors did not have a statistically significant interaction.

Finally, at the longest delay of TMS pulse delivery (~540 ms after saccade onset), the target position of visually guided saccades was completely ineffective at inducing changes of motor excitability in all muscles (delay *D3* in **Table 1** and **Figure 4C**). This last finding supports the conclusion that the above described target-dependent modulations of CSS excitability in upper-limb muscles are highly specific and strictly time-locked to saccade execution.

The time course of the effects of target position on CSS excitability can be better appreciated in **Figures 5, 6**, where the influences of target eccentricity and side on the mean MEP amplitude are separately plotted for each muscle. This procedure is justified by the lack of a significant "*eccentricity × side*" interaction in the ANOVAs (except at delay *D1* in the ADM muscle). **Figure 5** illustrates the changes in motor excitability induced by target eccentricity. Filled symbols indicate that the differences in MEP amplitude at a given TMS delay were statistically significant. The graphs demonstrate that, on top of the overall decay in MEP amplitude, a time-locked specific modulation of motor excitability as a function of saccade amplitude occurred in the ECR muscle (**Figure 5B**) ~300 ms after saccade onset. A similar trend can also be observed for the FDI muscle (**Figure 5A**), but this effect did not reach statistical significance. By contrast, the excitability of the ADM and FCU muscles (**Figures 5C,D**) steadily decreased after saccadic execution but did not show any sign of a specific modulation as a function of saccade amplitude. The excitability decay also appeared somewhat faster in the FCU muscle than in the other muscles (**Figure 5D**).

Figure 6 shows the changes in motor excitability related to the side of target appearance (same conventions as in **Figure 5**). Here too, a specific modulation of MEP amplitude depending on the direction of the eye movement occurred in a precise time window after saccade onset; this effect was absent at TMS delay *D3*. In contrast to the target eccentricity, a side-specific modulation of MEP amplitude was present, although on the opposite sign in both the FDI and ADM muscles; this modulation occurred early after saccade onset at TMS delay *D1* (**Figures 6A,C**). Furthermore, a statistically significant difference in motor excitability was also observed in the FDI and ECR muscles at delay *D2* (**Figures 6A,B**), with MEP amplitudes larger in both muscles after leftward compared to rightward saccades.

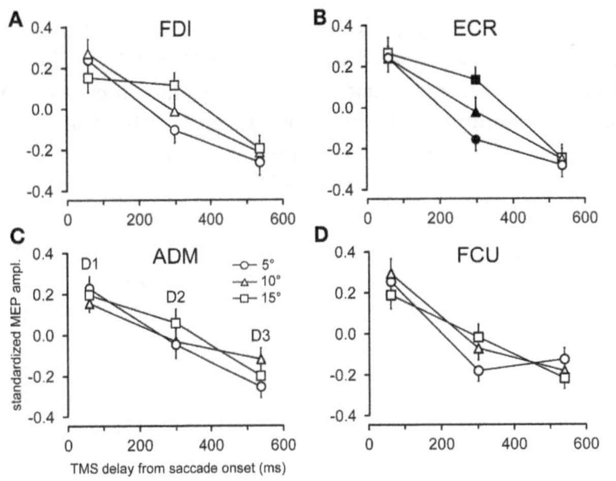

FIGURE 5 | Effects of target eccentricity on MEP amplitude. Mean MEP amplitudes across subjects are shown as a function of TMS delay for target eccentricities of 5°, 10°, and 15°, irrespective of the visual hemi-field of stimulus presentation, in the FDI **(A)**, ECR **(B)**, ADM **(C)**, and FCU **(D)** muscles. Filled symbols denote a statistically significant difference between MEP amplitudes at a given TMS delay. Error bars represent the standard error of the mean.

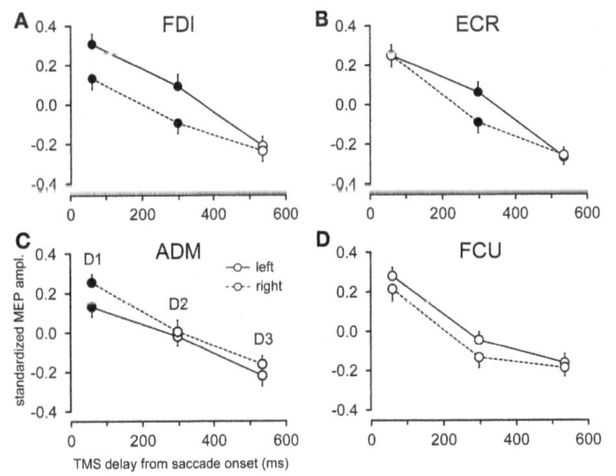

FIGURE 6 | Effects of target side on MEP amplitude. Mean MEP amplitudes across subjects are shown as a function of TMS delay for leftward and rightward saccades, irrespective of target eccentricity, in the FDI **(A)**, ECR **(B)**, ADM **(C)**, and FCU **(D)** muscles. Filled symbols denote a statistically significant difference between MEP amplitudes at a given TMS delay. Error bars represent the standard error of the mean.

DISCUSSION

The hand rarely moves without being coupled to an eye saccade. Although saccades can be performed without any accompanying limb movement, they are often functional as a means to gather visuospatial information for motor coordination while reaching or manipulating objects. Our results clearly demonstrate that the execution of visually guided saccades involves excitability changes in the motor control system of the arm, in the absence of any overt upper-limb movement or sign of EMG activation. These changes last for at least 300 ms after eye movement onset and reveal an overall decay in excitability of the upper-limb CSS, which is modulated in a highly specific manner in hand and wrist muscles, depending on saccade direction and target eccentricity. Therefore, this effect cannot be generically ascribed to arousal level or to a non-specific variation of cortical excitability resulting from task execution. Similar to what was previously described in a smooth pursuit task (Maioli et al., 2007), we believe that the observed changes in CSS excitability are compatible with the facilitation of a motor program for an upper-limb movement aiming at the same target of the gaze. One may argue that the changes in excitability of the motor cortex in this study could be caused by mental imagery of the pointing arm movement by the subject. However, this explanation seems unlikely because we carefully avoided drawing participants' attention to the possibility of making an aiming arm movement. Moreover, interviews after the experimental session confirmed the absolute absence of any imagery of manual pointing.

Specific modulations in MEP amplitude are inscribed on a global linear decay in CSS excitability, whereby responses in all muscles are smallest at the longest tested TMS delay after saccade onset. Our paradigm does not allow us to ascertain whether this excitability decay is the result of an initial facilitation that slowly decreases toward baseline values or represents a progressive CSS inhibition following saccade execution. However, it is interesting to notice that in a previous smooth pursuit study (Maioli et al., 2007), gaze movements were linked to an overall decrease in excitability of the motor control system of the resting arm. This finding was interpreted as a mechanism to prevent muscle contraction in an eye tracking task that engages the upper-limb motor system but does not require an overt manual response.

On top of the decay in overall excitability, changes in MEP amplitude present a complex time-dependent modulation as a function of the direction and/or amplitude of the saccadic movement, whose interpretation requires a separate discussion for each TMS delay. Data show that the modulation of MEP amplitudes in relation to target position extinguishes at TMS delay *D3*, i.e., ~540 ms after saccadic onset. It is interesting to compare this finding with the temporal coupling between eye and hand movements in an oculo-manual pointing task. Sailer et al. (2000), using visual stimuli presented with a procedure almost identical to our experimental method, reported that the hand arrives at the target in less than 500 ms after the beginning of the eye movement, with a saccade latency very similar to that found in our study. Under the hypothesis that the observed modulations in MEP amplitude reflected the activation of a sub-threshold motor program for an aiming hand movement, we should expect that TMS at delay *D3* would test upper-limb CSS excitability beyond the time interval within which a hand pointing movement is normally executed. Accordingly, no changes in MEP amplitude are observed as a function of target position. Furthermore, eye-hand coordination studies in aiming manual tasks have repeatedly reported that saccadic movement starts between 70 and 90 ms before the initiation of the hand movement (Carnahan and Marteniuk, 1994; Helsen et al., 1998; Lünenburger et al., 2000; Sailer et al., 2000). This means that at delay *D1* (60 ms), TMS is delivered shortly before the expected time of the hand movement onset during an eye-hand coordination task.

At TMS delay *D1*, when the overall CSS excitability is at its highest level, MEP amplitude modulation related to saccade direction is only limited to the most distal muscles. The FDI muscle (abductor of the index finger) on the right-hand side shows higher MEP amplitudes after leftward compared to rightward saccades. The activation of this muscle with a pronated hand posture would indeed produce a leftward deviation of the index finger, i.e., in the same direction of the saccadic eye movement. Therefore, this MEP modulation is compatible with a coarse sub-threshold finger motor program coupled with gaze direction, as CSS excitability modulation does not scale with saccade amplitude. Similarly, the ADM muscle shows a side-specific modulation, which becomes more evident at the largest saccade amplitudes (15°). Interestingly, the excitability changes are opposite to that observed in the FDI muscle, i.e., MEP amplitudes are largest following rightward saccades. ADM muscle activation in a pronated hand would then induce a rightward deviation of the little finger. Therefore, also in this case we observe a facilitation of a finger movement that is congruent with the direction of the preceding eye saccade.

MEP amplitude modulations are much more difficult to interpret at TMS delay *D2*, which corresponds to ~300 ms after saccade onset. Here, CSS excitability varies with target position only in the FDI and ECR muscles. However, the relationship cannot be interpreted in a straightforward manner. **Figure 7** shows the mean amplitudes of MEPs recorded in the FDI (squares) and ECR (dots) muscles as a function of saccadic target position. Negative values in the abscissa indicate a target location in the left

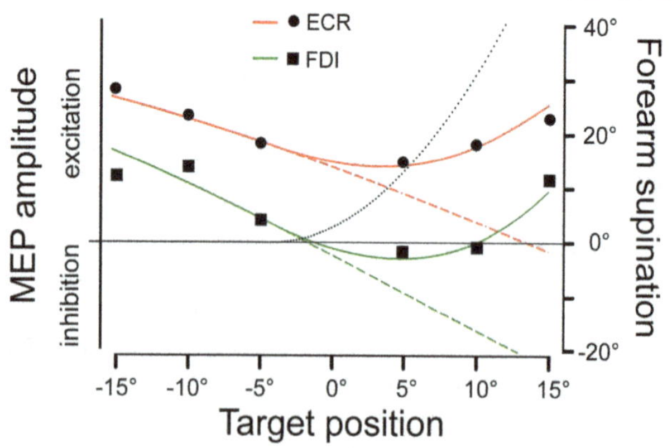

FIGURE 7 | Model predictions of changes in MEP amplitude in the ECR and FDI muscles as a function of saccadic target position. Experimental mean MEP amplitudes in arbitrary units are depicted by dots and squares for the ECR and FDI muscles, respectively. Model predictions are shown by red (ECR) and green (FDI) traces and by varying (continuous lines) or maintaining constant (dashed lines) the angle of forearm supination. The black dotted line illustrates the changes in the forearm supination angle, which predicted the best fitting of the experimental data.

visual field. Plotted data are those of **Figure 4B** but were scaled to arbitrary units in order to provide the best-fit with the predictions of the model, as presented in the next section. For both muscles, CSS excitability decreases from –15° to +5° target positions, but thereafter it increases again at the most eccentric positions in the right visual field. In fact, at a target eccentricity of 15°, mean MEP amplitudes did not show a statistically significant difference between the two visual hemi-fields.

MODELING SACCADE-RELATED MODULATION OF MEP AMPLITUDE

In an attempt to find a functional interpretation of these modulations in CSS excitability, we tried to model the observed changes in MEP amplitude under the assumption that they reflect a facilitation of an aiming movement of the upper-limb toward the same target of the eye saccade. Furthermore, the model was construed by taking into account the undeniable fact that, if the hand begins to move from a fully pronated posture (**Figure 1A**), a natural pointing movement of the right limb toward a target in the right visual field involves a certain degree of forearm supination.

The angular motion of the wrist and of the 2nd metacarpo-phalangeal joints (MPJ) can be vectorially represented in polar plots, as depicted in **Figures 8A,B** respectively. Each joint has two degrees-of-freedom, corresponding to flexion/extension and radial/ulnar deviations for the wrist and to flexion/extension and abduction/adduction for the 2nd MPJ. The pulling directions of the ECR and FDI muscles in the respective joint angular space are shown by the bold oriented axes. The ECR pulling direction (**Figure 8A**) was computed by vectorial summation of the maximal isometric force vectors reported by Bawa et al. (2000) for the *longus* and *brevis* heads of the muscle. It should be noticed that the ECR muscle is not a pure extensor, but its action is even stronger in producing a radial deviation of the wrist. By contrast, the FDI muscle can be considered as a pure abductor of the index finger (**Figure 8B**).

Filled dots connected by a continuous line in the polar plots represent the angular deviation that should be made in a single-joint movement to direct the hand (**Figure 8A**) or the index finger (**Figure 8B**) toward the visual target of the eye saccade. Of course, a real manual aiming movement would involve several joints of the upper-limb at the same time. Therefore, the actual activation of each muscle would be determined in a complex manner by the multi-jointed movement of the whole limb. However, as a rough approximation, it is fair to assume that a motor program for an aiming movement would activate the ECR and FDI muscles by an amount proportional to the orthogonal projection (dotted lines in **Figures 8A,B**) of the movement vector in the single-joint angular space onto the oriented axis representing the muscle pulling direction. If the projection vector has the same sense as the pulling direction vector, we should expect facilitation in muscle excitability; if the two vectors have an opposite sense, the muscle should be inhibited. This theoretical muscle activation as a function of target position is represented by dashed lines in **Figure 7** for the ECR (red) and FDI (green) muscles. Clearly, the experimental data points diverge from this prediction. In fact, when visually guided saccades are directed to the right hemi-field, MEP amplitudes of both the ECR and FDI muscles are expected to decrease monotonically with target eccentricity, while experimentally they start to increase again at eccentricities larger than 5°.

As mentioned above, a more realistic model should, however, take into account that if the forearm starts in a fully pronated posture, an aiming movement to a visual target on the right hemi-field would involve a certain degree of hand supination. If the forearm rotates about its long axis, then the movement vector in the intrinsic joint angular space rotates to the opposite direction, as shown by the dashed trajectories and empty dots in the

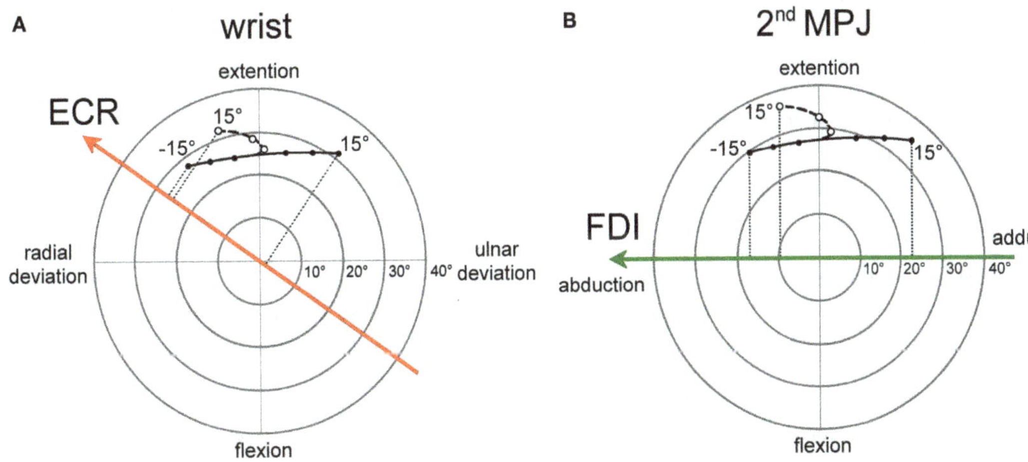

FIGURE 8 | Polar plot representations of the angular motion of wrist (A) and 2nd metacarpo-phalangeal (B) joints that were utilized for computing model predictions. Bold vectors represent the pulling directions of the ECR (red) and FDI (green) muscles in the respective joint angular space. The ECR **(A)** and FDI **(B)** muscles are activated in a single-joint pointing movement by an amount proportional to the orthogonal projection of the movement representation in the joint angular space onto the muscle pulling vector. Filled dots connected by a continuous line describe single-joint pointing movements in the absence of changes in forearm supination. Empty dots connected by a dashed line describe pointing movements occurring in the presence of a variable amount of forearm supination computed by the model-fitting procedure.

polar plots of **Figure 8** for both the wrist (**A**) and 2nd MPJ (**B**). The black dotted line in **Figure 7** shows the forearm supination angle that should be associated with the aiming movement to provide the best least-squares fit with experimental MEP data from both muscles. For sake of simplicity, the fitted function describing the change in the supination angle was a second-order parametric curve. The only constraint imposed to the fitting algorithm was that a fully pronated position (0°) of the forearm had to be maintained at the most eccentric target positions on the left visual hemifield. The parameters of the second-order curve and the target position at which hand supination began to develop were computed by the non-linear fitting procedure. Fitted parameters reasonably predicted that the supination of the forearm from its initial pronated posture would begin with a target position at a few degrees to the left of the central fixation point and would increase to approximately 50° for a target eccentricity of 15° in the right hemi-field. When a certain degree of supination is taken into account, model predictions fit very well with the experimentally observed changes of MEP amplitude in both the ECR and FDI muscles. It should also be stressed that the proposed model does not intend to describe the entire motor program of a hand pointing movement coupled with the eye saccade. Instead, the model attempts to predict muscle activation during a possible manual pointing movement toward the gaze target, coherent with the changes in CSS excitability photographed by TMS in a narrow time interval at about 300 ms after saccadic onset.

In summary, this very simplistic model with few reasonable assumptions demonstrates that the experimentally observed changes in MEP amplitude are compatible with the facilitation of a motor program, whose goal is to direct the hand toward the same target as that of the gaze movement. Although other functional interpretations of the experimental data can be conceived, our model provides a suitable conceptual framework for the clear fact that within a narrow time window after the occurrence of a visually guided saccade, the excitability of the CSS controlling upper-limb musculature undergoes highly specific modulations, which are tightly correlated with the target position of the preceding gaze movement.

BEHAVIORAL AND NEUROPHYSIOLOGIC EVIDENCE OF A COMMON DRIVE FOR EYE AND HAND MOVEMENTS

In natural tasks, eye and arm movements are tightly linked (Neggers and Bekkering, 2000, 2002). It is well-known that eyes begin to move and arrive at the target before the hand (Prablanc et al., 1979; Lünenburger et al., 2000; Sailer et al., 2000; Dean et al., 2011), resulting in more accurate manual pointing compared with when the hand moves alone (Vercher et al., 1994; Henriques et al., 1998; Neggers and Bekkering, 1999; van Donkelaar and Staub, 2000; Medendorp and Crawford, 2002; Horstmann and Hoffmann, 2005). It should also be noted that short-term adaptation of saccadic gaze amplitude induces congruent changes also in the amplitude of goal-directed limb movements (Kröller et al., 1999), indicating that plastic changes must occur in a common neural substrate. Moreover, studying eye movements in task-oriented behaviors has demonstrated that saccades are not normally directed to the most visually salient points of the visual scene, but rather to objects or locations that are relevant for the task to be executed (Land et al., 1999; Hayhoe et al., 2003; Hayhoe and Ballard, 2005). In particular, gaze is most often directed toward the point of contact of objects that will subsequently be the target of a reach or toward critical points that are highly relevant for guiding the ongoing motor act (Johansson et al., 2001; Hayhoe et al., 2003).

The large amount of behavioral evidence in favor of a tight eye-hand coupling has stimulated the proposal of several models capable of simulating temporal and spatial properties of oculomanual coordination. Two main approaches have been used to explain eye-hand coupling: (1) synchronization as a consequence of a common command to separate control systems for the two effectors (e.g., Howard, 1971; Bock, 1987) and (2) mutually coupled controllers exchanging information during movement, whereby coordination is ultimately achieved (e.g., Lazzari et al., 1997; Dean et al., 2011). Model predictions of reaction time correlations during eye-hand coordination in monkeys have been shown to be compatible only with a mutual excitation between two effector-specific controllers, but not with the common input hypothesis (Dean et al., 2011).

The existence of a saccade-related modulation of upper-limb CSS excitability, which is compatible with a sub-threshold motor plan for an aiming hand movement even in a pure oculomotor task, strongly supports the hypothesis that saccadic and manual control systems share a common input signal. This conclusion is corroborated by a similar modulation of upper-limb CSS excitability described during smooth pursuit eye movements (Maioli et al., 2007). This viewpoint is also supported by the finding of a shared internal representation of end position for both eye and arm movements and by the fact that both effectors always move to the same target when multiple targets are present (Gielen et al., 1984). Spatial coupling and our TMS data can hardly be accounted for without assuming the presence of a common command signal, at least at the early stages of sensorimotor integration and/or at the level of the visual signal processing mechanism. It should also be noted that common command signals and information exchange between effector-specific controllers are not mutually exclusive mechanisms for explaining eye-hand coordination.

The idea that eye movements are linked to a plan for an aiming movement of the arm to the same target also is supported by a particular form of optic ataxia, in which misreaching occurs only when targets are presented in non-foveal vision. Some patients with a lesion in the posterior parietal lobe show a slavish dependence of reach on gaze ("magnetic misreaching," Buxbaum and Coslett, 1997; Carey et al., 1997). In fact, they inevitably move their hand to the spatial target they are fixating on, being incapable of reaching objects that they are not looking at. However, their performance is normal when allowed to foveate on the target. Because we found that a motor plan for the hand is normally associated with saccadic eye movements, this neurological defect could be interpreted as an incapacity to suppress the arm motor program when a hand movement is not required. This neurological defect may be due to a misfunctioning of the parietofrontal cortical network that underlies the control of visually guided reaching behavior.

A common control mechanism at the early stages of sensorimotor integration for pointing and saccades is also supported by the neurophysiologic finding of a lack of strictly effector-specific visuospatial maps in frontal and parietal cortical areas. In fact, various fMRI studies in humans (Hagler et al., 2007; Levy et al., 2007; Beurze et al., 2009) have shown a large overlap in the neural circuitry involved in the preparation of saccades and hand pointing movements, including the frontal eye fields and regions around the intraparietal sulcus [corresponding to the parietal reach region (PRR) and lateral intraparietal (LIP) area in the monkey]. The interpretation of these investigations is that cortical modules encoding pointing-specific maps are largely effector independent.

This conclusion is also supported by neurophysiologic data from monkeys. The classically held view that the LIP area is essentially involved in the generation of saccadic eye movements, while the PRR is dedicated primarily to the generation of aiming arm movements, has been challenged by the finding that the LIP area and PRR contain neurons that are either responsive to both effectors or even specific for the "wrong" effector (Snyder et al., 1997; Colby and Goldberg, 1999; Gottlieb and Goldberg, 1999). One can then surmise that whenever a visual stimulus activates the saliency map in the posterior parietal cortex (PPC) and elicits an orienting eye movement, a covert coarse motor plan for the arm is also formed, even if a hand pointing movement is not required.

Furthermore, the superior colliculus (SC) deep layers contain reach-related neurons (Werner, 1993; Kutz et al., 1997; Stuphorn et al., 2000), a finding that is particularly relevant in our context considering the pivotal role of the SC in the generation of reflexive saccades, such as the ones elicited in this study. It has been demonstrated that SC reach-related neurons fire shortly before and during arm reaches with a specific movement vector, i.e., with a particular direction and amplitude (Werner, 1993; Stuphorn et al., 2000); these neurons present a high correlation between their firing and the EMG activity pattern of shoulder muscles (Werner et al., 1997; Stuphorn et al., 1999). For 40% of SC reach-related neurons, the movement vector is coded in a retinal reference frame, i.e., they are locked to a gaze-related coordinate system (Stuphorn et al., 2000). These data have been interpreted as demonstrating a role of the SC in eye-hand coordination (Lünenburger et al., 2001). Consistent with these electrophysiological studies in the monkey, recent neuroimaging investigations provide evidence for reach-related neurons also in the human SC, both in deep and superficial layers (Linzenbold and Himmelbach, 2012; Himmelbach et al., 2013).

The PPC and the SC are heavily connected by anatomical projections and are well-known to play a crucial role in the generation of reflexive saccades. The current study demonstrated that visually guided saccades are accompanied by changes in CSS excitability compatible with a pointing hand movement toward the gaze target. Therefore, the presence of reach-related neurons in both neuronal maps, in register with gaze-related neurons, constitutes an important neurophysiological correlate for interpreting the main finding of this paper.

REFERENCES

Admiraal, M. A., Keijsers, N. L. W., and Gielen, C. C. A. M. (2003). Interaction between gaze and pointing towards remembered visual targets. *J. Neurophysiol.* 90, 2136–2148. doi: 10.1152/jn.00429.2003

Admiraal, M. A., Keijsers, N. L. W., and Gielen, C. C. A. M. (2004). Gaze affects pointing toward remembered visual targets after a self-initiated step. *J. Neurophysiol.* 92, 2380–2393. doi: 10.1152/jn.01046.2003

Bawa, P., Chalmers, G. R., Jones, K. E., Søgaard, K., and Walsh, M. L. (2000). Control of the wrist joint in humans. *Eur. J. Appl. Physiol.* 83, 116–127. doi: 10.1007/s004210000270

Beurze, S. M., de Lange, F. P., Toni, I., and Medendorp, W. P. (2009). Spatial and effector processing in the human parietofrontal network for reaches and saccades. *J. Neurophysiol.* 101, 3052–3062. doi: 10.1152/jn.91194.2008

Bock, O. (1987). Coordination of arm and eye movements in tracking of sinusoidally moving targets. *Behav. Brain Res.* 24, 93–100. doi: 10.1016/0166-4328(87)90247-6

Buxbaum, L. J., and Coslett, H. B. (1997). Subtypes of optic ataxia: reframing the disconnection account. *Neurocase* 3, 159–166. doi: 10.1080/13554799708404050

Carey, D. P., Coleman, R. J., and Della Sala, S. (1997). Magnetic misreaching. *Cortex* 33, 639–652. doi: 10.1016/S0010-9452(08)70722-6

Carnahan, H., and Marteniuk, R. G. (1994). Hand, eye, and head coordination while pointing to perturbed targets. *J. Mot. Behav.* 26, 135–146. doi: 10.1080/00222895.1994.9941668

Colby, C. L., and Goldberg, M. E. (1999). Space and attention in parietal cortex. *Annu. Rev. Neurosci.* 22, 319–349. doi: 10.1146/annurev.neuro.22.1.319

Dean, H. L., Martì, D., Tsui, E., Rinzel, J., and Pesaran, B. (2011). Reaction time correlations during eye-hand coordination: behavior and modeling. *J. Neurosci.* 31, 2399–2412. doi: 10.1523/JNEUROSCI.4591-10.2011

Engel, K. C., and Soechting, J. F. (2003). Interactions between ocular motor and manual responses during two-dimensional tracking. *Prog. Brain Res.* 142, 141–153. doi: 10.1016/S0079-6123(03)42011-6

Flanders, M., Daghestani, L., and Berthoz, A. (1999). Reaching beyond reach. *Exp. Brain Res.* 126, 19–30. doi: 10.1007/s002210050713

Gielen, C. C., van den Heuvel, P. J., and van Gisbergen, J. A. (1984). Coordination of fast eye and arm movements in a tracking task. *Exp. Brain Res.* 56, 154–61. doi: 10.1007/BF00237452

Gottlieb, J., and Goldberg, M. E. (1999). Activity of neurons in the lateral intraparietal area of the monkey during an antisaccade task. *Nat. Neurosci.* 2, 906–912. doi: 10.1038/13209

Hagler, D. J., Riecke, L., and Sereno, M. I. (2007). Parietal and superior frontal visuospatial maps activated by pointing and saccades. *Neuroimage* 35, 1562–1577. doi: 10.1016/j.neuroimage.2007.01.033

Hayhoe, M., and Ballard, D. (2005). Eye movements in natural behavior. *Trends Cogn. Sci.* 9, 188–194. doi: 10.1016/j.tics.2005.02.009

Hayhoe, M. M., Shrivastava, A., Mruczek, R., and Pelz, J. B. (2003). Visual memory and motor planning in a natural task. *J. Vis.* 3, 49–63. doi: 10.1167/3.1.6

Helsen, W. F., Elliott, D., Starkes, J. L., and Ricker, K. L. (1998). Temporal and spatial coupling of point of gaze and hand movements in aiming. *J. Mot. Behav.* 30, 249–259. doi: 10.1080/00222899809601340

Henriques, D. Y. P., Klier, E. M., Smith, M. A., Lowey, D., and Crawford, J. D. (1998). Gaze-centered remapping of remembered visual space in an open-loop pointing task. *J. Neurosci.* 18, 1583–1594.

Himmelbach, M., Linzenbold, W., and Ilg, U. J. (2013). Dissociation of reach-related and visual signals in the human superior colliculus. *Neuroimage* 82, 61–67. doi: 10.1016/j.neuroimage.2013.05.101

Horstmann, A., and Hoffmann, K. P. (2005). Target selection in eye-hand coordination: do we reach to where we look or do we look to where we reach? *Exp. Brain Res.* 167, 187–95. doi: 10.1007/s00221-005-0038-6

Howard, I. P. (1971). Perceptual learning and adaptation. *Br. Med. Bull.* 27, 248–252.

Johansson, R., Westling, G., Backstrom, A., and Flanagan, J. R. (2001). Eye-hand coordination in object manipulation. *J. Neurosci.* 21, 6917–6932.

Kröller, J., De Graaf, J. B., Prablanc, C., and Pélisson, D. (1999).

Effects of short-term adaptation of saccadic gaze amplitude on hand-pointing movements. *Exp. Brain Res.* 124, 351–362. doi: 10.1007/s002210050632

Kutz, D. F., Dannenberg, S., Werner, W., and Hoffmann, K. P. (1997). Population coding of arm-movement-related neurons in and below the superior colliculus of Macaca mulatta. *Biol. Cybern.* 76, 331–337. doi: 10.1007/s004220050346

Land, M., Mennie, N., and Rusted, J. (1999). The roles of vision and eye movements in the control of activities of daily living. *Perception* 28, 1311–1328. doi: 10.1068/p2935

Lazzari, S., Vercher, J. L., and Buizza, A. (1997). Manuo-ocular coordination in target tracking. I. A model simulating human performance. *Biol. Cybern.* 77, 257–266. doi: 10.1007/s004220050386

Levy, I., Schluppeck, D., Heeger, D. J., and Glimcher, P. W. (2007). Specificity of human cortical areas for reaches and saccades. *J. Neurosci.* 27, 4687–4696. doi: 10.1523/JNEUROSCI.0459-07.2007

Linzenbold, W., and Himmelbach, M. (2012). Signals from the deep: reach-related activity in the human superior colliculus. *J. Neurosci.* 32, 13881–13888. doi: 10.1523/JNEUROSCI.0619-12.2012

Lünenburger, L., Kleiser, R., Stuphorn, V., Miller, L. E., and Hoffmann, K. P. (2001). A possible role of the superior colliculus in eye–hand coordination. *Prog. Brain Res.* 134, 109–125. doi: 10.1016/S0079-6123(01)34009-8

Lünenburger, L., Kutz, D. F., and Hoffmann, K. P. (2000). Influence of arm movements on saccades in humans. *Eur. J. Neurosci.* 12, 4107–4116. doi: 10.1046/j.1460-9568.2000.00298.x

Maioli, C., Falciati, L., and Gianesini, T. (2007). Pursuit eye movements involve a covert motor plan for manual tracking. *J. Neurosci.* 27, 7168–7173. doi: 10.1523/JNEUROSCI.1832-07.2007

Medendorp, W. P., and Crawford, J. D. (2002). Visuospatial updating of reaching target in near and far space. *Neuroreport* 13, 633–636. doi: 10.1097/00001756-200204160-00019

Mills, K. R., and Nithi, K. A. (1997). Corticomotor threshold to magnetic stimulation: normal values and repeatability. *Muscle Nerve* 20, 570–576. doi: 10.1002/(SICI)1097-4598(199705)20:5<570::AID-MUS5>3.3.CO;2-F

Neggers, S. F. W., and Bekkering, H. (1999). Integration of visual and somatosensory target information in goal-directed eye and arm movements. *Exp. Brain Res.* 125, 97–107. doi: 10.1007/s002210050663

Neggers, S. F. W., and Bekkering, H. (2000). Ocular gaze is anchored to the target of an ongoing pointing movement. *J. Neurophysiol.* 83, 639–651.

Neggers, S. F. W., and Bekkering, H. (2002). Coordinated control of eye and hand movements in dynamic reaching. *Hum. Mov. Sci.* 21, 349–76. doi: 10.1016/S0167-9457(02)00120-3

Prablanc, C., Echallier, J. F., Komilis, E., and Jeannerod, M. (1979). Optimal response of eye and hand motor systems in pointing at a visual target. *Biol. Cybern.* 35, 113–124. doi: 10.1007/BF00337436

Sailer, U., Eggert, T., Ditterich, T., and Straube, A. (2000). Spatial and temporal aspects of eye-hand coordination across different tasks. *Exp. Brain Res.* 134, 163–173. doi: 10.1007/s002210000457

Snyder, L. H., Batista, A. P., and Andersen, R. A. (1997). Coding of intention in the posterior parietal cortex. *Nature* 386, 167–170. doi: 10.1038/386167a0

Soechting, J. F., Engel, K. C., and Flanders, M. (2001). The Dunker illusion and eye-hand coordination. *J. Neurophysiol.* 85, 843–854.

Stuphorn, V., Bauswein, E., and Hoffmann, K. P. (2000). Neurons in the primate superior colliculus coding for arm movements in gaze-related coordinates. *J. Neurophysiol.* 83, 1283–1299.

Stuphorn, V., Hoffmann, K. P., and Miller, L. E. (1999). Correlation of primate superior colliculus and reticular formation discharge with proximal limb muscle activity. *J. Neurophysiol.* 81, 1978–1982.

van Donkelaar, P., and Staub, J. (2000). Eye-hand coordination to visual versus remembered targets. *Exp. Brain Res.* 133, 414–418. doi: 10.1007/s002210000422

Vercher, J. L., Magenes, G., Prablanc, C., and Gauthier, G. M. (1994). Eye-head-hand coordination in pointing at visual targets: spatial and temporal analysis. *Exp. Brain Res.* 99, 507–523. doi: 10.1007/BF00228987

Werner, W. (1993). Neurons in the primate superior colliculus are active before and during arm movements to visual targets. *Eur. J. Neurosci.* 5, 335–40. doi: 10.1111/j.1460-9568.1993.tb00501.x

Werner, W., Dannenberg, S., and Hoffmann, K. P. (1997). Arm-movement-related neurons in the primate superior colliculus and underlying reticular formation: comparison of neuronal activity with EMGs of muscles of the shoulder, arm and trunk during reaching. *Exp. Brain Res.* 115, 191–205. doi: 10.1007/PL00005690

10

Time-frequency analysis of short-lasting modulation of EEG induced by TMS during wake, sleep deprivation and sleep

Paolo Manganotti[1,2] *, Emanuela Formaggio[2], Alessandra Del Felice[1], Silvia F. Storti[1], Alessandro Zamboni[3], Alessandra Bertoldo[3], Antonio Fiaschi[1,2] and Gianna M. Toffolo[3]

[1] *Clinical Neurophysiology and Functional Neuroimaging Unit, Section of Neurology, Department of Neurological and Movement Sciences, University of Verona, Verona, Italy*
[2] *Department of Neurophysiology, Foundation IRCCS San Camillo Hospital, Venice, Italy*
[3] *Department of Information Engineering, University of Padova, Padova, Italy*

Correspondence:
Paolo Manganotti, Clinical Neurophysiology and Functional Neuroimaging Unit, Section of Neurology, Department of Neurological and Movement Sciences, University of Verona, Policlinico G. B. Rossi – P.le L.A. Scuro 10, 37134 Verona, Italy
e-mail: paolo.manganotti@univr.it

The occurrence of dynamic changes in spontaneous electroencephalogram (EEG) rhythms in the awake state or sleep is highly variable. These rhythms can be externally modulated during transcranial magnetic stimulation (TMS) with a perturbation method to trigger oscillatory brain activity. EEG-TMS co-registration was performed during standard wake, during wake after sleep deprivation and in sleep in six healthy subjects. Dynamic changes in the regional neural oscillatory activity of the cortical areas were characterized using time-frequency analysis based on the wavelet method, and the modulation of induced oscillations were related to different vigilance states. A reciprocal synchronizing/desynchronizing effect on slow and fast oscillatory activity was observed in response to focal TMS after sleep deprivation and sleep. We observed a sleep-related slight desynchronization of alpha mainly over the frontal areas, and a widespread increase in theta synchronization. These findings could be interpreted as proof of the interference external brain stimulation can exert on the cortex, and how this could be modulated by the vigilance state. Potential clinical applications may include evaluation of hyperexcitable states such as epilepsy or disturbed states of consciousness such as minimal consciousness.

Keywords: EEG, TMS, cortical excitability, wavelet analysis, vigilance state

INTRODUCTION

Oscillatory human brain activity occurs at different frequencies (Niedermeyer, 1999) and can be rapidly modulated over the occipital regions by eyes opening and over the central parietal regions by movement and sensory stimulation. The occurrence of dynamic changes in spontaneous electroencephalogram (EEG) rhythms in the awake state or sleep is highly variable. These rhythms can be externally modulated with a perturbation method to trigger oscillatory brain activity. The method involves delivering an external stimulus by transcranial magnetic stimulation (TMS) and recording its effects on cortical activity by EEG. Advanced EEG systems compatible with TMS (EEG-TMS co-registration) offer the ability to study EEG reactivity in humans in the awake state.

Most studies to date have focused on slow EEG responses evoked by a single magnetic stimulus in the time domain (Ilmoniemi et al., 1997; Izumi et al., 1997; Paus et al., 1998, 2001; Komssi et al., 2002; Thut et al., 2003; Bonato et al., 2006; Thut and Pascual-Leone, 2010; Del Felice et al., 2011) by investigating more complex and widespread brain oscillatory activity induced by external stimulation (Thut and Miniussi, 2009). The application of EEG-TMS co-registration to high frequencies instead of low frequencies (i.e., cortical evoked potentials) has opened new and intriguing lines of research, yielding a wealth of data on rhythmic brain activities (Fuggetta et al., 2008; Thut and Miniussi, 2009; Manganotti et al., 2012) and on the connectivity of brain areas during the wake state or sleep (Massimini et al., 2005, 2007, 2009). Indeed, single-pulse TMS (Paus et al., 2001; Fuggetta et al., 2005; Van Der Werf et al., 2006; Rosanova et al., 2009; Manganotti et al., 2012) or a TMS pulse train (Brignani et al., 2008; Fuggetta et al., 2008; Plewnia et al., 2008; Noh et al., 2012) induce synchronous rhythmic rapid brain activity that preferably oscillates in the natural frequency of the target site. Such an experimental paradigm was proposed by Johnson et al. as a way to clarify the behavioral effects of TMS, e.g., by studying TMS-induced oscillatory activity modifications (Johnson et al., 2010).

Although the real meaning and site of rapid oscillatory synchronization evoked by TMS remain to be elucidated, cortical and subcortical sources have been suggested (Van Der Werf et al., 2006; Rosanova et al., 2009). In a previous work (Manganotti et al., 2012), we documented the different and dynamic time course of all frequencies, defined as slow (delta and theta) and fast (alpha and beta) activities, after single, paired and transcallosal TMS using wavelet time-frequency analysis, where we suggested possible inhibitory network activation by brain stimulation in the rest awake state for these synchronized evoked rhythms. This method is appealing for studying different states of the brain and it is feasible with different EEG systems.

Recent research into the effects of sleep and sleep deprivation has largely focused on standard TMS parameters, so-called transcranial evoked potentials (TEPs), which are the slow, early components recorded on EEG after a TMS pulse. Standard TMS studies have shown decreased motor excitability in normal subjects during sleep (Manganotti et al., 2001; Grosse et al., 2002; Avesani et al., 2008), while a discordant effect on motor evoked potentials

(MEPs), with a mild amplitude decrease according to Manganotti et al. (2001) or an increase according to Civardi et al. (2001), was described in normal subjects after sleep deprivation. Conversely, sleep deprivation in epileptic patients results in a marked increase in cortical excitability (Manganotti et al., 2006). TEP modulation by vigilance states appears to be more nuanced. While the reproducible slow components evoked by TMS during wake and sleep have been identified (Komssi et al., 2004; Bonato et al., 2006; Massimini et al., 2007), the main difference with standard TMS parameters lies in the marked increase in the amplitude of evoked potentials during NREM sleep (Massimini et al., 2009; Del Felice et al., 2011) and during anesthesia (Ferrarelli et al., 2010), with a pronounced increase seen after sleep deprivation (Del Felice et al., 2011). Indeed, Huber et al. (2013) observed that the excitability of the human frontal cortex, measured as the immediate (0–20 ms) EEG reaction to TMS, progressively increases with time awake, from morning to evening and after one night of total sleep deprivation, and that it decreases after recovery sleep. Finally, in an altered hyperexcitable cortex, as in epilepsy, TEPs reflect this state, showing an impressive augmentation in amplitude during sleep and particularly after sleep deprivation (Del Felice et al., 2011).

The aim of this study was to investigate slow and fast oscillatory activities synchronized by single-pulse TMS delivered over the primary motor area (M1) in the time-frequency domain during wake, NREM sleep, and sleep deprivation. The time-frequency approach was applied to detect dynamic changes in the regional neural oscillatory activity of cortical areas and to relate the modulation of these induced oscillations to the different brain states.

MATERIALS AND METHODS

SUBJECTS

The study sample was 6 healthy subjects (3 men and 3 women; mean age, 28.6 years ± standard deviation 4.7 years), right-handed as assessed by the Edinburgh Handedness Inventory (Oldfield, 1971). None of the subjects had a medical history of neurological disease or was taking any medications. Basal EEG was normal in all subjects. Sleep was scored according to American Academy of Sleep Medicine (AASM) guidelines on monopolar montage, considering frontal, central and occipital leads, with additional electro-oculogram and electromyogram derivations on a 30 s basis (Silber et al., 2007). Continuous EEG recordings showed unmistakable N1 and N2 sleep stages in all subjects. Only brief lapses of N3 sleep stage were scored in the majority subjects. None of the EEG recordings showed REM sleep (see **Table 1** for polysomnographic data). All subjects initially experienced difficulty in falling asleep owing to the effect of TMS before entering a distinct sleep stage. In accordance with the Declaration of Helsinki, written informed consent to participate in the study was obtained. The study design and protocol were approved by the Local Ethics Committee of the Verona University Department and Hospital.

EEG RECORDINGS

Electroencephalogram data were acquired using a magnetic resonance (MR)-compatible EEG amplifier (BrainAmp 32MRplus, BrainProducts GmbH, Munich, Germany) and a cap providing 30 TMS-compatible coated-electrodes positioned according to a 10/20 system. Additional electrodes were used as ground (AFz) and reference (FCz). The EEG data were bandpass-filtered at 0.1–500 Hz and digitized at a sampling rate of 5 KHz.

TMS STIMULATION

Transcranial magnetic stimulation was performed using a Magstim-Rapid Stimulator in biphasic pulse configuration (Magstim Company Ltd, London, UK) which generates a maximum magnetic field of 1.5 T. TMS was delivered through a figure-of-eight focal coil oriented so that the induced electric current flowed in a posterior-anterior direction over the left M1. MEPs were recorded from the right thenar eminence (TE) muscle with Ag/AgCl surface electrodes fixed to the skin with a belly tendon montage. The coil was placed tangentially to the scalp, with the handle pointing backwards and laterally at a 45° angle away from the midline. The stimulation coil was positioned with the handle pointing backwards and over the optimal scalp position to obtain the highest MEP, corresponding approximately to between C3 and P3 in all subjects. Induced currents were directed postero-anteriorly. Stimulus intensity was set at 110% of motor threshold (MT) intensity. MT intensity was approached from individual suprathreshold levels by reducing the stimulus intensity in 1% steps. MT intensity was defined as the lowest stimulator output intensity capable of inducing MEPs of at least 50 μV peak-to-peak amplitude in relaxed right TE muscles in at least half of 10 trials over the optimal scalp position (Rossini et al., 1994). Stimulus intensities are expressed as a percentage of maximum stimulator output.

The click associated with the coil discharge propagates through air and bone and can elicit an auditory N1–P2 complex at latencies of 100–200 ms (Nikouline et al., 1999; Tiitinen et al., 1999). In this study, we inserted earphones to mask the coil-generated click in all subjects to avoid any effect of clicks in the modulation of cortical oscillatory activities. A white noise (90 dB) was played through the inserted earphones to mask the coil-generated click (Fuggetta et al., 2005). All subjects confirmed that the white noise was sufficient to mask the auditory input.

Table 1 | Polysomnographic parameters. Mean and standard deviation.

PSG parameters	
Total sleep time	53.4 (±10.7) min
Total recording time	103 (±18.8) min
Sleep onset latency	27.2 (±10.8) min
WASO	12.4 (±9.6) min
NREM	100%
REM	0%
N1	37 (±4.1) min
N2	49 (±6.5) min
N3	14 (±3.2) min

WASO, wakefulness after sleep onset, NREM, non-rapid eye movement, REM, rapid eye movement, N1, N2, N3, NREM sleep stages.

EXPERIMENTAL DESIGN

The subjects were asked to maintain a regular sleep schedule for at least 5 days prior to the beginning of the study. The first TMS recording was performed between 1 p.m. and 3 p.m. in basal conditions (T_0), and the second TMS recording from 1 p.m. to 3 p.m. the day after partial sleep deprivation (T_1). Partial sleep deprivation was achieved by having the subject stay awake from 3 a.m. until morning; no napping was permitted. Sleep was recorded in the same session as the sleep deprivation recording, immediately after the latter (T_2). Subjects were asked to refrain from taking any stimulating substances (e.g., coffee, cola, smoking). The EEG recording was performed before, during and after each TMS stimulation. An EEG baseline acquisition in resting state condition was also performed before the beginning of each stimulation (before T_0, T_1, and T_2), with eyes open at T_0 and T_1 and with eyes closed at T_2. Although the eyes open condition produced a higher number of trials that had to be discarded due to blinking artifacts, it ensured the subjects did not fall asleep during the experiment. During the awake and sleep deprivation recordings, the subjects were seated in an armchair with the elbow semi-flexed; the forearm was pronated, fully relaxed and supported by the arm of the chair. During the sleep recordings, the subjects lay in bed in a dark, sound proof laboratory room; the head was reclined over an *ad hoc* tailored foam-rubber pillow to allow correct positioning of the coil over the scalp (Del Felice et al., 2011). To ensure that masking would be effective, the subjects had the earphones inserted with the white noise turned on for the entire duration of the experiment.

Transcranial magnetic stimulation single-pulse stimuli were delivered at random, with a minimum inter-trial interval (ITI) of 0.8 s and a maximum of 3 s (**Figure 1**). During the awake and sleep deprivation sessions, at least 150 stimuli were administered; during the sleep session, stimulation continued throughout the entire sleep period.

WAVELET ANALYSIS

The EEG data were analyzed using a time-frequency procedure to characterize TMS-induced oscillations (Manganotti et al., 2012). The EEG data were downsampled to 250 Hz and all recordings were visually inspected; trials with artifacts produced by environmental noise, muscle activity or eye movement were rejected. Only trials recorded during N1–N2 stages were included in the analysis, whereas trials recorded during N3 stage were excluded in order to ensure the maximum possible homogeneity. Epochs with interstimulus interval greater than 2.2 s were selected for the analysis, to ensure the results were comparable with the previous study (Manganotti et al., 2012). Since magnetic artifacts were contained in the first 130 ms, the EEG traces were analyzed 130 ms after magnetic stimulation. In this way the early, slow TEP was excluded from the analysis, focusing on the time-course of the power of all frequency ranges during the relative long-term. Trials of 2 s were selected from 130 to 2130 ms after the stimulus by visual inspection.

Time-frequency analysis was performed on the most representative channels (F3, Fz, F4, C3, Cz, C4, P3, Pz, and P4) with continuous Morlet wavelet transform, which provides a time course after magnetic stimulation of the relative power in the main frequency bands: delta (1–4 Hz), theta (4–8 Hz), alpha (7–12 Hz), and beta (15–22 Hz). A family of Morlet wavelets was constructed at 1 Hz frequency intervals ranging from 1 to 30 Hz. Each wavelet function has a Gaussian distribution in the time (SD: σ_t) and frequency domains (SD: σ_f) around the center frequency f_0 and it depends on a parameter, the number of oscillations (f_0/σ_f), which has to be chosen by the user. The number of oscillations in each data window can be critical. There is no rule for determining this parameter. After several attempts, we choose these parameters because we could best investigate power changes as the optimal compromise in time-frequency using a 1–30 Hz frequency range and a temporal window of 2 s. Our wavelet family was computed using a ratio of 4 oscillations for delta, 8 for theta, 12 for alpha and 22 for beta bands (coinciding with the highest frequency). 20 epochs of 2 s of basal EEG devoid of artifacts were selected for each subject and for each condition. The reference baseline spectra was calculated by averaging wavelet spectra across time and frequency, obtaining one value for each band. The mean and the standard deviation of relative power for each

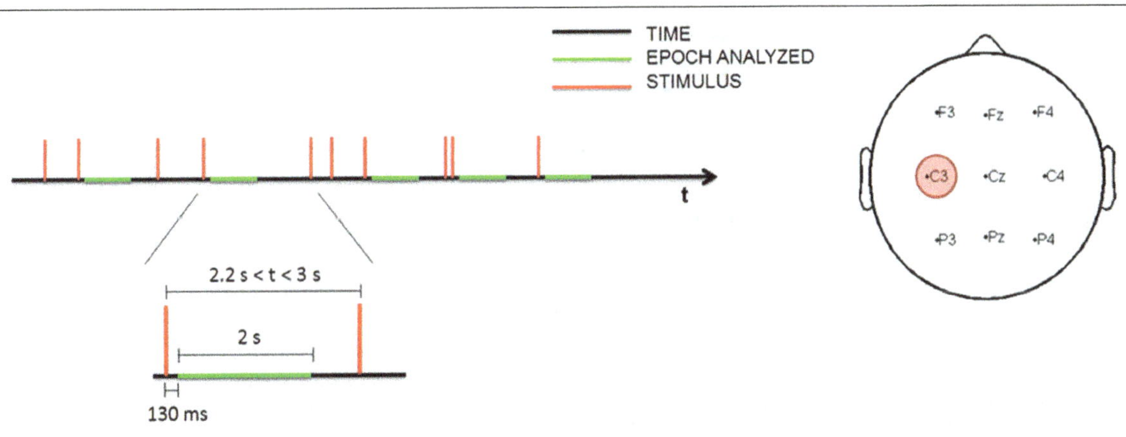

FIGURE 1 | Time schedule for measuring EEG data during the stimulation (left). Topographic distribution of the nine electrodes analyzed with the site of stimulation (in red; right)

channel were computed. Profiles for each subject were averaged from the post-stimulus trials (a mean of 86 epochs of 2 s at T_0, 94 at T_1 and 455 at T_2; **Figure 2**) and normalized to the baseline value (expressed as 1) after the grand-average. The EEG baseline acquisition was performed in a resting state condition, differently from TEP study paradigms, where the evoked high amplitude EEG deflections are compared to a very short epoch of some ms preceding the stimulus. Nevertheless, our aim was to compare changes of oscillatory activity induced on EEG by a series of stimulation during the three vigilance states to a reference value, devoid of any pre-planned external perturbation, in a 2 s interval, thus evaluating the long term effect of the stimulation and not the early short-lasting TEP.

ANOVA for repeated measures was applied to relative powers with the factors "condition" (T_0, T_1, T_2) and "time point" (number of time point in 2 s: 500). *Post-hoc* paired *t*-test adjusted for multiple comparisons with Bonferroni method was used. Statistical significance was set at $p < 0.05$. In order to check whether post-stimulus activity differed significantly from the basal level, a paired samples *t*-test was performed at each sampling time ($p < 0.05$) to evidence the intervals during which the relative power differed significantly from baseline.

RESULTS

The times/latencies below mentioned, in which EEG modifications were observed, refer to the time in the processed epochs and not latency with respect to TMS. Trials of 2 s were indeed selected from 130 to 2130 ms after the stimulus.

ALPHA BAND

In the alpha band, TMS induced a decrease of power in proximity of the stimulation site, followed by progressive synchronization in time, especially over the frontal and central electrodes. Basal conditions returned about 1 s or more after the stimulation (**Figure 3**).

The power of the *frontal electrodes* (F3-Fz-F4) decreased (by about 20%) in the 1-s period during the wake state and sleep deprivation (time limited significant decrease in F4 at T_0, T_1, and T_2), followed by a more evident increase lasting from 1 to 2 s; the decrease was less clear over Fz. During sleep, the power decrease was more evident (significant decrease in F3) (40% in F3 and F4). An asterisk above the bars indicates a statistically significant difference between the post-stimulus activity and the basal value. A similar pattern was observed over the *central electrodes* (C3-Cz-C4): during the wake state and after sleep deprivation, the power decreased (by 50% at T_0 and 30% at T_1 in C3) over baseline during the first 1-s period, followed by an increase lasting from 1 to 2 s, which was clearly visible over C3. The power during sleep decreased significantly by about 30% only in C3. This pattern, though also observable over the *parietal electrodes* (P3-Pz-P4), was not significant.

ANOVA testing the alpha power for each electrode disclosed a significant main effect for the factor "condition" (T_0, T_1, and T_2)

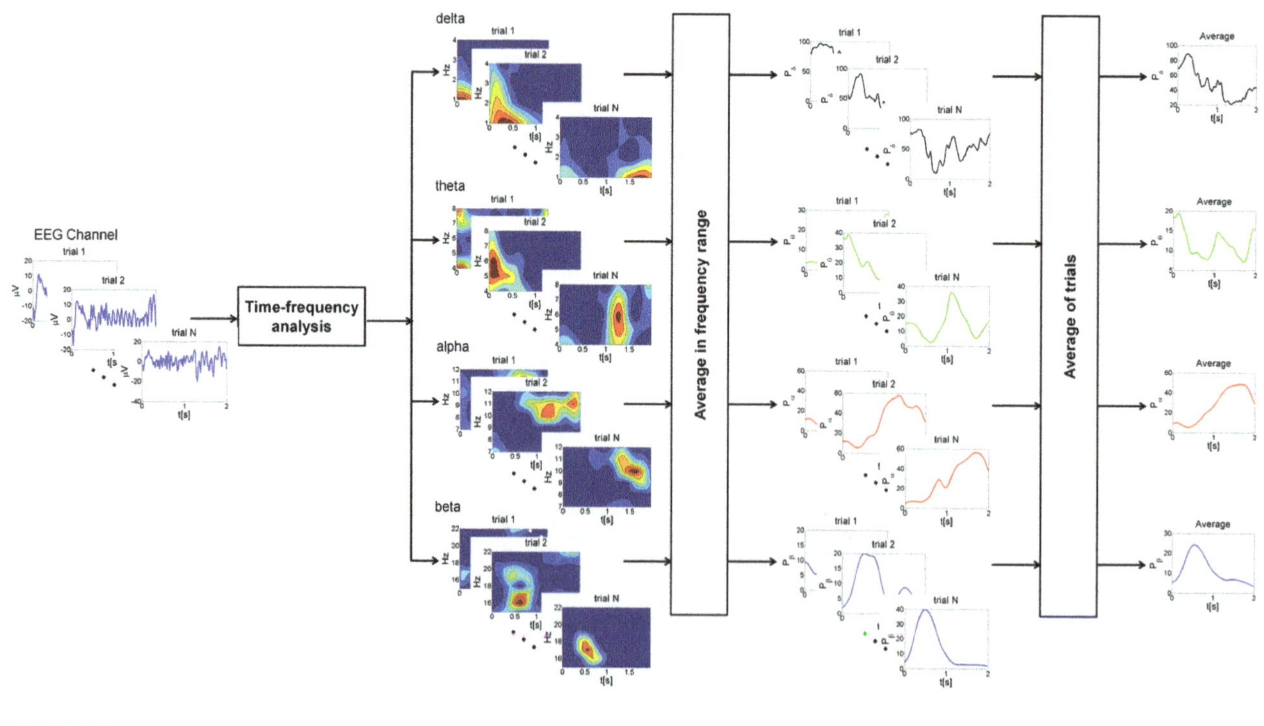

FIGURE 2 | Schematic representation of the different steps of the analysis at single subject level. For each EEG channel trials with intervals greater than 2.2 s were selected for the analysis. Time-frequency analysis was performed on each trial with continuous Morlet wavelet transform in the main frequency bands: delta (1–4 Hz), theta (4–8 Hz), alpha (7–12 Hz), and beta (15–22 Hz). The power was then averaged in the frequency ranges of interest, producing a power time course for each trial. Finally, profiles for each trial were averaged and normalized to the baseline value. This procedure was applied for each condition (wake state, sleep deprivation and sleep).

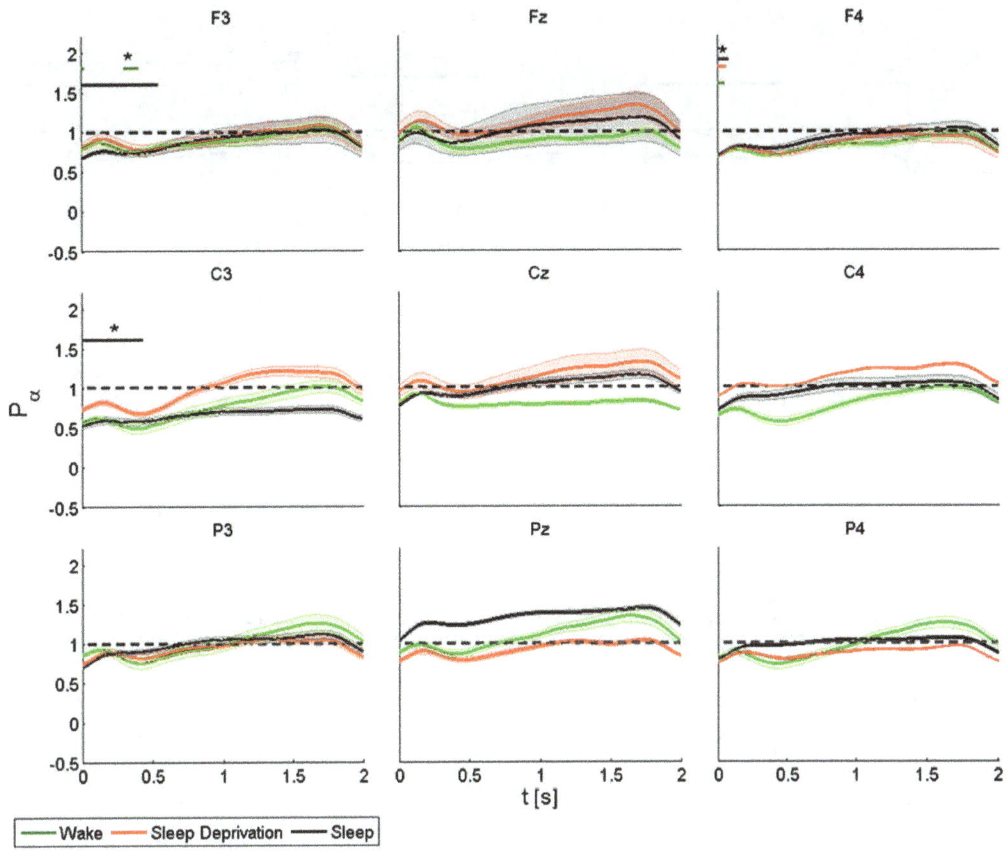

FIGURE 3 | Average ($N = 6$) relative wavelet power and standard error in alpha range (7–12 Hz), after single-pulse TMS, during wake (green), sleep deprivation (red), and sleep (black). Asterisk (*) above the bars indicates values significantly different from basal level. Data are analyzed from 130 to 2130 ms after the stimulus onset.

in Fz ($F(2,10) = 4.192$, $p < 0.05$). No significant differences were observed between the conditions.

BETA BAND

We observed a more rapid initial decrease in power in the beta band than in the alpha band, followed by an increase in power again more marked in proximity of the stimulation site and the homolateral frontal regions, but also over the parietal areas (**Figure 4**).

The power of the *frontal electrodes* (F3-Fz-F4) decreased significantly in F3 and F4 by about 40% after sleep and by more than 40% during all three conditions in F4. The power over the F4 electrode remained below the baseline value during the entire post-stimulus interval. An increase lasting from 1 to 2 s was observed in the three frontal electrodes during all the conditions. During sleep, the power of the *central electrodes* (C3-Cz-C4) decreased (significant decrease of 50% in C3 and C4) from the baseline value and lasted 0.3 s, followed by an evident rebound. In Cz the power at T_0 and T_2 remained below the baseline value during the entire post-stimulus interval, even if no significant change was noted. After stimulation, the power of the *parietal electrodes* (P3-Pz-P4) decreased significantly from the baseline value in Pz and in P4 at T_1. A significant power modification from the baseline was also observed in Pz during sleep from 0.2 to 0.7 s.

ANOVA testing the beta power for each electrode disclosed a significant main effect for the factor "condition" (T_0, T_1, and T_2) only in Cz ($F(2,10) = 6.778$, $p < 0.05$). No significant differences were observed between conditions.

THETA BAND

An increase in amplitude of theta relative power was observed in the first 0.3 s (**Figure 5**).

During the wake state and after sleep deprivation, the power of the *frontal electrodes* (F3-Fz-F4) increased markedly but not significantly from the baseline value, with a maximum at 0.2 s and lasting 0.5 s; while the power increased significantly during sleep in F3 and F4. A significant decrease was also observed in F3 from 0.5 to 2 s at T_0, from 0.5 to 1 at T_1 and from 0.7 to 1 s at T_2; in Fz from 0.5 to 1.5 s at T_2; in F4 from 0.5 to 1 s at T_2 and from 1.3 to 1.5 s at T_1. A similar pattern was observed in the *central electrodes* (C3-Cz-C4), but the increase was significant only after sleep deprivation in Cz and C4 and during sleep in C4. During the wake state, the power remained below the baseline value for the entire interval of 2 s, and this trend was significant for C3 and C4. The same pattern was also observed in the *parietal electrodes*

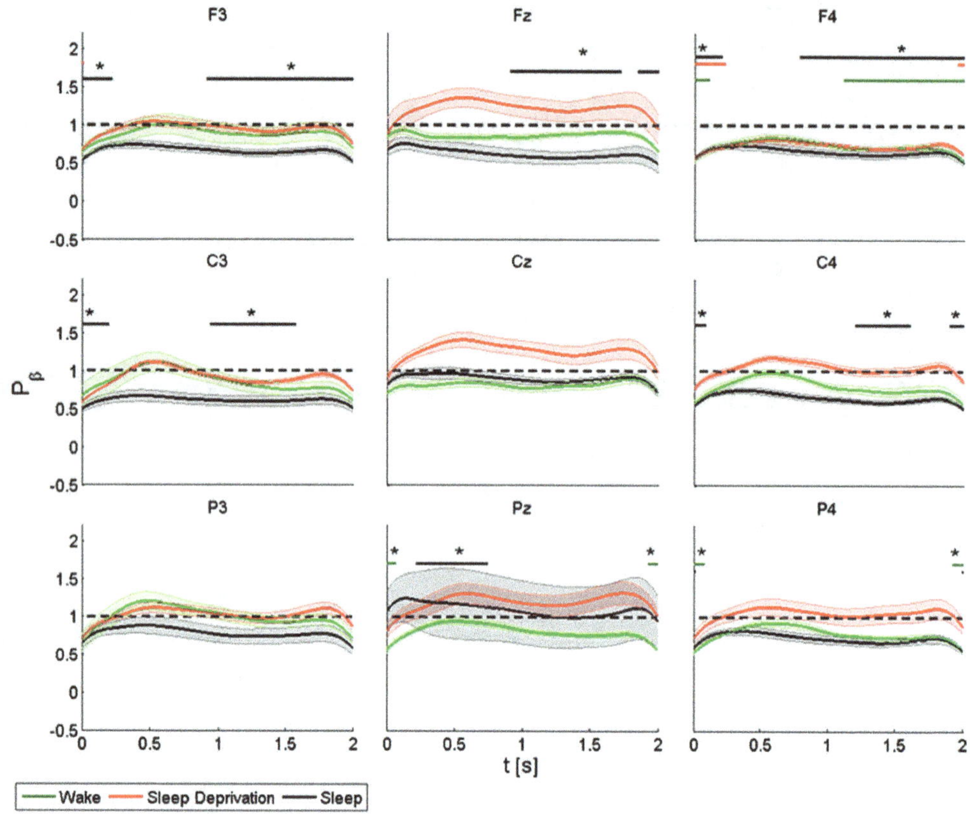

FIGURE 4 | Average ($N = 6$) relative wavelet power and standard error in beta range (15–22 Hz), after single-pulse TMS, during wake (green), sleep deprivation (red), and sleep (black). Asterisk (*) above the bars indicates values significantly different from basal level. Data are analyzed from 130 to 2130 ms after the stimulus onset.

(P3-Pz-P4), but the power increased significantly (by about 40%) only in P3 and in P4 during sleep deprivation and in Pz and in P4 during sleep. The decrease in power after 0.5 s was significant in P3 during sleep, and in P4 during the wake state.

ANOVA testing the theta power for each electrode disclosed a significant main effect for the factor "condition" (T_0, T_1 and T_2) in P4 ($F(2,10) = 3.956$, $p < 0.05$). A t-test disclosed a significant difference between wake state and sleep ($p < 0.05$) from 0 to 0.08 s and between sleep deprivation and sleep ($p < 0.05$) from 1.6 to 2 s.

DELTA BAND

The delta rhythm was characterized by synchronization, with a peak at about 0.3 s, followed by a gradual reduction in power until returning to the basal condition (**Figure 6**).

During the wake state and after sleep deprivation, the power of the *frontal electrodes* (F3-Fz-F4) increased significantly by about 40% in F4 over the baseline value, with a maximum at 0.3 s and lasting 1 s. This pattern was also observed in F3 and Fz. During sleep, the power increased significantly in F3, Fz and F4, peaking after 0.3 s. In Fz a significant difference from the baseline value was observed from 1.8 to 2 s during T_1. During T_0, T_1 and T_2, the power of the *central electrodes* (C3-Cz-C4) increased from the baseline value, with a maximum at 0.3 s and lasting less than 1 s. There was a significant increase only in C3 during sleep. After sleep deprivation, the power remained below the baseline value in Cz and C4. The pattern, though also observable in the *parietal electrodes* (P3-Pz-P4), was significant only in P3, where the power increased from the baseline with a maximum at 0.3 s during sleep, and in Pz where the power remained below the baseline from 1.8 to 2 s during sleep.

ANOVA testing the delta power for each electrode disclosed a significant main effect for the factor "condition" (T_0, T_1, and T_2) in F3 ($F(2,10) = 34.626$, $p < 0.05$) and in C4 ($F(2,10) = 3.849$, $p < 0.05$). A t-test disclosed a significant difference only in F3 between wake state and sleep from 0.8 to 1.2 s ($p < 0.05$).

DISCUSSION

This study investigated the time course of different patterns of the main brain oscillatory activities after brain stimulation during different states of vigilance: wake, sleep deprivation and sleep. Insight on externally modulated brain rhythm patterns can be gained from the effects of single-pulse TMS on brain oscillations. Single-pulse TMS can induce synchronization of rapid brain rhythms (Paus et al., 2001; Fuggetta et al., 2005; Van Der Werf et al., 2006; Rosanova et al., 2009; Manganotti et al., 2012), and the behavioral correlates of such oscillatory modulations have

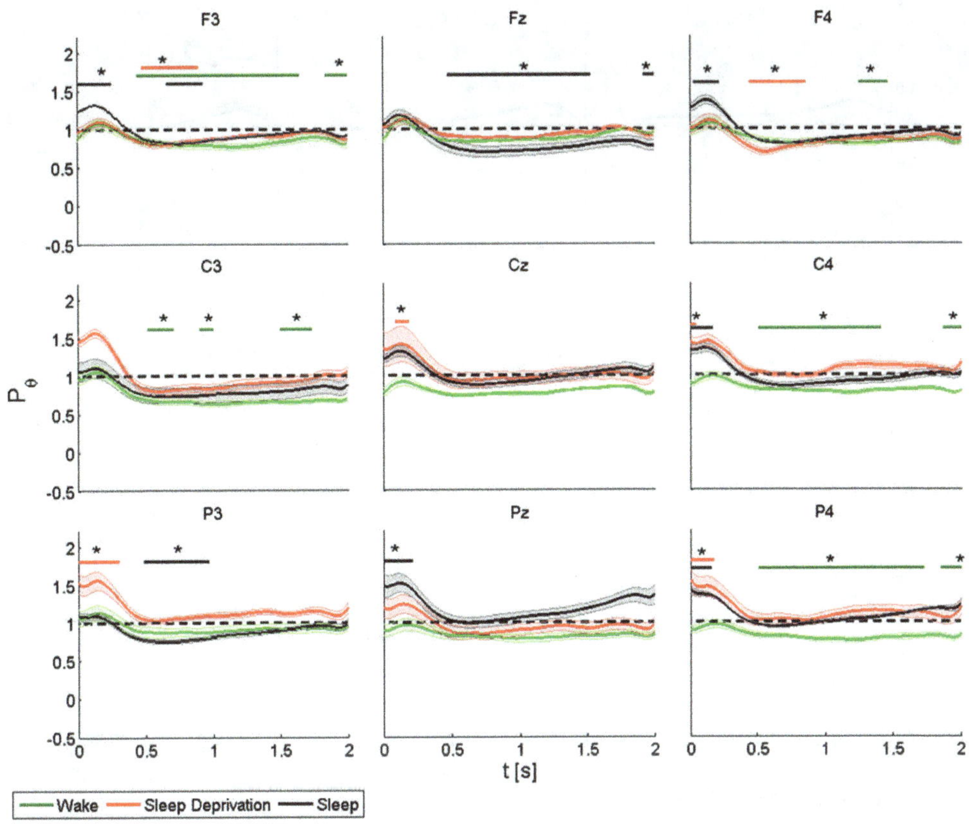

FIGURE 5 | Average ($N = 6$) relative wavelet power and standard error in theta range (4–8 Hz), after single-pulse TMS, during wake (green), sleep deprivation (red), and sleep (black). Asterisk (*) above the bars indicates values significantly different from basal level. Data are analyzed from 130 to 2130 ms after the stimulus onset.

been identified in the phase locking of ongoing brain oscillations (Dugué et al., 2011), the encoding of different aspects of the stimulus by different frequencies ("multiplexing;" Siegel et al., 2009; Panzeri et al., 2010), or by aligning two oscillatory neural populations to their high excitability phase ("communication-through-coherence" Fries, 2005). The novelty of the present method stands in the application of a time-frequency analysis to the time course of different rapid and slow brain oscillations induced by TMS not only in an awake state, but also in sleep deprivation and sleep.

The dynamic and short-time modulation of brain activity is confirmed by the fact that low-intensity single-pulse TMS, applied on the sensorimotor areas in the awake state, induces early desynchronization over the frontal and central-parietal electrodes, followed by a rebound of synchronization in the alpha and beta bands, paralleled by early synchronization in delta and theta activities and subsequent desynchronization. This pattern reveals the distinct behavior of oscillations after an external perturbation, (TMS), and suggests the possibility to differentiate each brain rhythm solely on the basis of a single shock of depolarization by TMS (Manganotti et al., 2012). In the awake state, this pattern of EEG reactivity to TMS was consistent in our group of subjects.

The main study finding was that this pattern can be also slightly affected by brain intrinsic states: during light NREM sleep (N1 and N2) there was slight precocious desynchronization of alpha over the stimulated areas, with a minimal contralateral effect, as well as a similar desynchronization of beta band rhythms over the antero-central cortex, whereas an early, not well localized increase in theta synchronization, and a more anterior and site-related synchronization of delta emerged again in sleep. Given that the stimulation site was over the primary motor area, this peculiar localization of rhythms responses bears an important physiological meaning that will be discussed below. Indeed, these results are of interest also because they seem to be maintained throughout the trials, where a potential bias could have been generated by the very short ITI intervals. The very short ITI might influence the findings, since we reported results obtained analyzing epochs with ITI greater than 2.2 s, discarding the epochs shorter. Differences found in oscillatory activity could possibly not completely depend on stimulation itself, but also to some spurious state-dependent differences between the two EEG states (resting state/baseline condition and stimulation conditions). Indeed, the reproducibility of the results throughout states and subjects hints to the major effect of TMS, that could nonetheless be endowed with endogenous processes, the course of which were beyond the aim of our study. Since not all stimulations were delivered in exactly the same condition, the persistence of analogous responses adds robustness to our data and possibly points to a strong modulating effect of vigilance states,

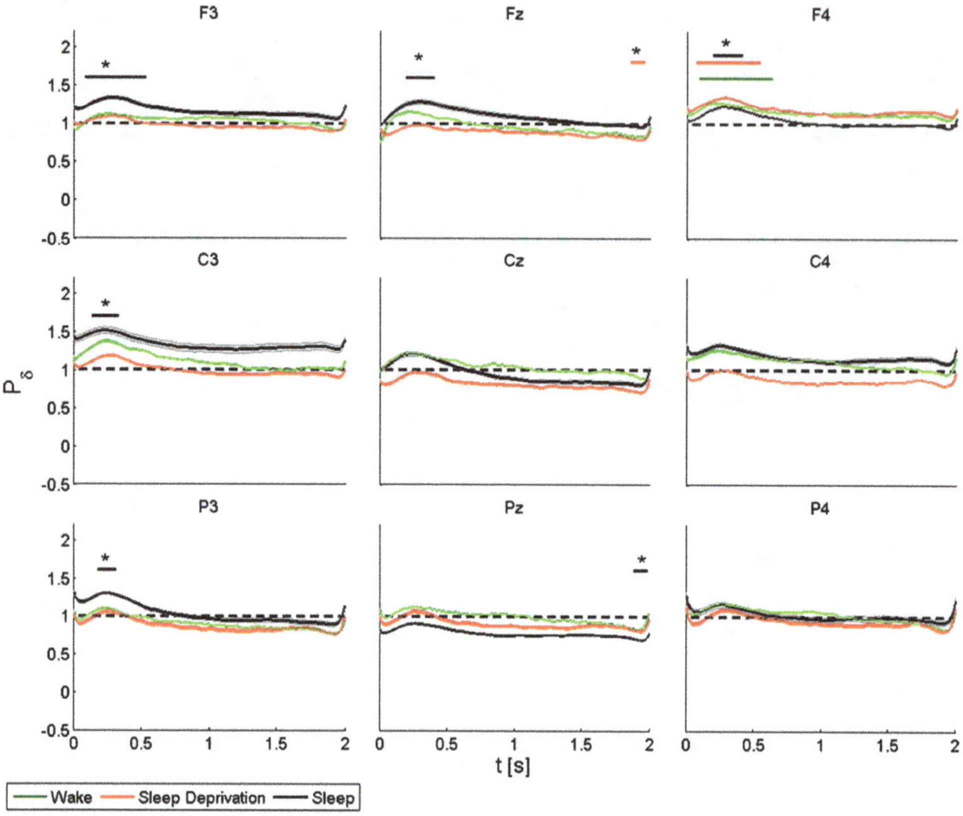

FIGURE 6 | Average ($N = 6$) relative wavelet power and standard error in delta range (1–4 Hz), after single-pulse TMS, during wake (green), sleep deprivation (red), and sleep (black). Asterisk (*) above the bars indicates values significantly different from basal level. Data are analyzed from 130 to 2130 ms after the stimulus onset.

in which the neurotransmitters balance is distinct in each condition, on brain rhythms. Interestingly, partial sleep deprivation was not responsible for any clear-cut modulating effect, except for a minor desynchronization of theta over the frontal bilateral leads and a precocious synchronization over the posterior areas, in contrast with our previous data (Del Felice et al., 2011) on the massive impact of sleep deprivation on cortical excitability.

WAKE OSCILLATORY ACTIVITY

Early research on EEG-TMS co-registration reported only synchronization in beta activity after single magnetic stimulation and linked it to a sort of resetting or disruption of the ongoing oscillatory activity of M1 produced by external magnetic stimulation of the brain (Paus et al., 2001). Fuggetta et al. observed that single-pulse TMS produces an increase in power in both the beta and alpha bands, unlike the self motor finger movement which produces a well-known decrease in alpha and beta powers. Also, using MT and minimal intensity stimulation, they noted a significant effect on brain modifications, which suggests an effect of magnetic stimulation on the cortical sources (Fuggetta et al., 2005).

An increase in beta power has been observed by other authors (Van Der Werf et al., 2006; Rosanova et al., 2009). However, in most of these studies, spectral estimation was performed using fast Fourier transform which does not detect dynamic changes. To overcome this limitation, methods that can monitor the temporal variation of EEG power are needed. In this study we used a wavelet-based method to detect the temporal modulation of brain oscillations in the main frequency bands. This approach has already been applied to experiments with single, paired-pulse and transcallosal TMS (Manganotti et al., 2012). Single pulse, paired-pulse and transcallosal TMS, which investigate intra- and transcortical inhibition, induce similar patterns. Specifically, single pulse TMS provokes an initial mainly anterior decrease of power in the alpha and beta bands, followed by a more prominent increase of power in beta activity over the ipsilateral and contralateral M1. Similar results are observed also on our data, although the significance is not robust as in our previous study, with a minimal precocious desynchronization of the anterior alpha and a slow desynchronization of beta mainly over the contralateral motor area, as well as the late desynchronization of theta over the frontal and central areas, mainly on the stimulated site. These results, in line with the previous ones (Manganotti et al., 2012), differ from other literature data on the basis of the innovative analysis approach that defines the time course of the oscillation and does not rely on an averaged analysis.

Finally, the spontaneous EEG signal is the indistinguishable summation of the activation of both fast and slow excitatory postsynaptic potentials (fEPSPs and sEPSPs, respectively) as well as fast and slow inhibitory postsynaptic potentials (fIPSPs and sIPSPs, respectively) (Rosenthal et al., 1967). fIPSPs are mediated by γ-aminobutyric acid ($GABA_A$) postsynaptic receptors lasting approximately 20–30 ms (Davies et al., 1990). TMS can explore the inhibitory system of motor areas. Short intracortical inhibition ([SICI] as evaluated by means of MEP amplitude modulation at ISI 3 ms) is thought to explore the net effect of the activation of inhibitory $GABA_A$ circuits in M1. We can hypothetically exclude that single TMS, which induces patterns similar to paired TMS on brain oscillations, can investigate similar inhibitory circuits in sleep and sleep deprivation.

SLEEP DEPRIVATION, BRAIN EXCITABILITY AND OSCILLATORY RHYTHMS

The homeostatic process regulates the propensity to sleep in relation to the length of prior wakefulness (Borbély and Achermann, 1999), and the amount slow-wave sleep (SWS) during subsequent NREM sleep has been proposed as a measurement for sleep homeostasis, equated to sleep intensity or sleep depth (Steriade, 2005). Sleep deprivation impairs cognition and performance, as measured on verbal and non-verbal memory tasks (Smith and MacNeill, 1994; Walker et al., 2002a,b), and cognitive and attentional abilities (Linde and Bergstrom, 1992; Harrison and Horne, 1999; Doran et al., 2001; Belenky et al., 2003; Drummond et al., 2006; Kendall et al., 2006), and primarily affects frontal executive functions. In clinical practice, sleep deprivation is an established method to provoke EEG epileptiform abnormalities (Bennett, 1963; Pratt et al., 1968; Jovanovic, 1991; King et al., 1998) and seizures in most types of epilepsy (Dinner, 2002). Neurophysiologically, sleep deprivation modulates the frequency power of EEG rhythms, enhancing the frontal predominance of delta (Kattler et al., 1994; Achermann et al., 2001), with a main effect over the left hemisphere, increasing theta rhythms (Cajochen et al., 1995; Dumont et al., 1999) predominantly over the frontal (Cajochen et al., 1995) and temporal sites (Forest and Godbout, 2000), and increasing alpha in an eyes-open condition (Stampi et al., 1995; Corsi-Cabrera et al., 1996) while decreasing it in an eyes-closed state (Drapeau and Carrier, 2004).

A brain stimulation paradigm has rarely been applied to investigate sleep deprivation. A recent study by Del Felice et al. (2011) looked into its effects on TEPs in a group of healthy volunteers and patients with generalized epilepsy (juvenile myoclonic epilepsy, JME). The authors found that sleep deprivation enhanced cortical excitability, as measured by TEP amplitude, more markedly over the frontal areas in the epileptics, possibly due to involvement of the frontal cortex in the pathogenesis of JME. EEG-TMS was also used to monitor cortical excitability in healthy individuals as a function of time awake (Huber et al., 2013). The authors observed that the immediate cortical response to direct stimulation progressively increases with time awake.

Our data detected a possible theta synchronizing effect of sleep deprivation over the posterior cortical areas, whereas a not significant phenomenon was observed over the frontal electrodes. The almost negligible effect that sleep deprivation exerts on late-response brain oscillation contrasts with the strong effect it demonstrates on TEP. Although we do not have an explanation for this observation, we could suppose a different susceptibility to sleep deprivation effects of the superficial TEPs generators that rely on short interconnections in contrast to the long-loop, deep structures that reverberate in the long-term aftermath of the TMS.

Nonetheless, the reaction we were able to demonstrate seems to bear a physiological meaning. Since theta rhythm is the signature of sleepiness – the so called theta of drowsiness – the response to an external perturbation of a sleepy brain appears to reflect its physiological state: a disturbed brain increments these oscillations in the frequency range more abundant in the stage it is in and over the areas where it is usually represented – i.e., theta over the temporal and parietal. An experimental paradigm aiming at simulating a higher sleep pressure proved an analogous brain reaction: Kirov et al. (2009) applied transcranial slow oscillation stimulation at a frequency of 0.75 Hz during the wake state observing a diffuse theta increase. Although in their experiment a rhythmic entraining effect might have artificially boosted slow brain oscillations, in our view a physiological state of increased slowed rhythms, such as sleep deprivation, has the intrinsic capacity to reverberate at the frequency that is more consistent with its state – theta rhythm in the specific case.

SLEEP AND OSCILLATORY RHYTHMS

No general consensus exists on the generation of ongoing EEG rhythms in wake and in sleep. The prevailing model according to Steriade sees corticofugal slow oscillations (<1 Hz) that group thalamic-generated delta rhythms (1–4 Hz) and spindling activity (7–14 Hz), with delta dominating the EEG and low amplitude alpha (8–12 Hz; Steriade, 2003). When arousing stimuli, either exogenous or endogenous, are delivered, spindling, slow and ultra-slow oscillations are blocked by inhibition of the reticulothalamic (7–14 Hz), thalamocortical (1–4 Hz) and intracortical (<1 Hz) generators. They are replaced by beta (12–18 Hz) and gamma (up to 40 Hz) rhythms paced by the basal forebrain (Steriade, 2003). Instead, during the wake state, alpha is the dominant rhythm, with a low amplitude delta (Steriade and Llinás, 1988; Pfurtscheller and Lopes da Silva, 1999), suggesting a reciprocal inhibition between their generators.

Our data seem to provide the experimental setting to replicate the aforementioned rhythms alternation: during sleep, the brain response to TMS consisted of an early alpha desynchronization over the stimulation site, with a minimal effect over the contralateral omologous areas (possibly due to the transcallosal spread) coupled with an early delta synchronization over the anterior areas and over the stimulation site. Of interest is the main anterior effect on the slow rhythm: the frontal cortex is the main source of the so-called slow traveling wave of sleep (Massimini et al., 2004; Ferri et al., 2005; Murphy et al., 2009) over which there is a higher chance of eliciting, through TMS pulses, waves resembling the physiological oscillation of SWS (Massimini et al., 2004). This mechanism, associated with a recently demonstrated entrainment phenomenon, could contribute to the observed higher delta power over the frontal brain area. As demonstrated by Veniero et al. (2011), stimulating at the frequency of the underlying brain rhythms (alpha in that case) leads to a progressively enhanced oscillatory response in the same frequency band. In our experiment, this seems to hold true over the anterior areas, where the slow wave is physiologically generated, and over the stimulated hemisphere, which is thus the more solicited.

To sum up, our results hint to the change of tagging the brain physiological state by its reaction to external perturbations: the coupled desynchronization of faster, wake-like rhythms, and the rise of slow ones induced by an external perturbation during sleep could indicate that the brain reacts accordingly to its actual state.

CONCLUSION

Our results show a reciprocal synchronizing/desynchronizing effect on slow and fast oscillatory activity in response to focal, standardized TMS after sleep deprivation and sleep, as detected by time-frequency analysis. Nevertheless, this preliminary study has some limitations. Well-designed studies with larger sample size and more detailed data are needed to confirm these conclusions. However, these findings highlight the pronounced interference that external brain stimulation can exert on the cortex modulated by the vigilance state and open up new perspectives regarding automated detection systems of brain state modifications, as well as giving a more detailed insight in the functional modification in pathological conditions. This holds true, for example, in the evaluation of hyperexcitable states, as epilepsy, or states of disturbed consciousness, as in minimal consciousness: the detection of rhythmicity patterns modification could point to a forthcoming clinical manifestation – either a seizure developing or the consciousness level modification, with a potential clinical application.

REFERENCES

Achermann, P., Finelli, L. A., and Borbély, A. A. (2001). Unihemispheric enhancement of delta power in human frontal sleep EEG by prolonged wakefulness. Brain Res. 913, 220–223. doi: 10.1016/S0006-8993(01)02796-2

Avesani, M., Formaggio, E., Fuggetta, G., Fiaschi, A., and Manganotti, P. (2008). Cor- ticospinal excitability in human subjects during nonrapid eye movement sleep: single and paired-pulse transcranial magnetic stimulation study. Exp. Brain Res. 187, 17–23. doi: 10.1007/s00221-008-1274-3

Belenky, G., Wesensten, N. J., Thorne, D. R., Thomas, M. L., Sing, H. C., Redmond, D. P., et al. (2003). Patterns of performance degradation and restoration during sleep restriction and subsequent recovery: a sleep dose–response study. J. Sleep Res. 12, 1–12. doi: 10.1046/j.1365-2869.2003.00337.x

Bennett, D. R. (1963). Sleep deprivation and major motor convulsions. Neurology 13, 953–958. doi: 10.1212/WNL.13.11.953

Bonato, C., Miniussi, C., and Rossini, P. M. (2006). Transcranial magnetic stim- ulation and cortical evoked potentials: a TMS/EEG co-registration study. Clin. Neurophysiol. 117, 1699–1707. doi: 10.1016/j.clinph.2006.05.006

Borbély, A. A., and Achermann, P. (1999). Sleep homeostasis and models of sleep regulation. J. Biol. Rhythms 14, 557–568.

Brignani, D., Manganotti, P., Rossini, P. M., and Miniussi, C. (2008). Modulation of cortical oscillatory activity during transcranial magnetic stimulation. Hum. Brain. Mapp. 29, 603–612. doi: 10.1002/hbm.20423

Cajochen, C., Brunner, D. P., Kräuchi, K., Graw, P., and Wirz-Justice, A. (1995). Power density in theta/alpha frequencies of the waking EEG progressively increases during sustained wakefulness. Sleep 18, 890–894.

Civardi, C., Boccagni, C., Vicentini, R., Bolamperti, L., Tarletti, R., Varrasi, C., et al. (2001). Cortical excitability and sleep deprivation: a transcranial magnetic stimulation study. J. Neurol. Neurosurg. Psychiatry 71, 809–812. doi: 10.1136/jnnp.71.6.809

Corsi-Cabrera, M., Arce, C., Ramos, J., Lorenzo, I., and Guevara, M. A. (1996). Time course of reaction time and EEG while performing a vigilance task during total sleep deprivation. Sleep 19, 563–569.

Davies, C. H., Davies, S. N., and Collingridge, G. L. (1990). Paired-pulse depression of monosynaptic GABA-mediated inhibitory postsynaptic responses in rat hippocampus. J. Physiol. 424, 513–531.

Del Felice, A., Fiaschi, A., Bongiovanni, G. L., Savazzi, S., and Manganotti, P. (2011). The sleep-deprived brain in normals and patients with juvenile myoclonic epilepsy: a perturbational approach to measuring cortical reactivity. Epilepsy Res. 96, 123–131. doi: 10.1016/j.eplepsyres.2011.05.015

Dinner, D. S. (2002). Effect of sleep on epilepsy. J. Clin. Neurophysiol. 19, 504–513. doi: 10.1097/00004691-200212000-00003

Doran, S. M., Van Dongen, H. P., and Dinges, D. F. (2001). Sustained attention performance during sleep deprivation: evidence of state instability. Arch. Ital. Biol. 139, 253–267.

Drapeau, C., and Carrier, J. (2004). Fluctuation of waking electroencephalogram and subjective alertness during a 25-hour sleep-deprivation episode in young and middle-aged subjects. Sleep 27, 55–60.

Drummond, S. P., Paulus, M. P., and Tapert, S. F. (2006). Effects of two nights sleep deprivation and two nights recovery sleep on response inhibition. J. Sleep Res. 15, 261–265. doi: 10.1111/j.1365-2869.2006.00535.x

Dugué, L., Marque, P., and VanRullen, R. (2011). The phase of ongoing oscillations mediates the causal relation between brain excitation and visual perception. J. Neurosci. 31, 11889–11893. doi: 10.1523/JNEUROSCI.1161-11.2011

Dumont, M., Macchi, M. M., Carrier, J., Lafrance, C., and Hébert, M. (1999). Time course of narrow frequency bands in the waking EEG during sleep deprivation. Neuroreport 10, 403–407. doi: 10.1097/00001756-199902050-00035

Ferrarelli, F., Massimini, M., Sarasso, S., Casali, A., Riedner, B. A., Angelini, G., et al. (2010). Breakdown in cortical effective connectivity during midazolam-induced loss of consciousness. Proc. Natl. Acad. Sci. U.S.A. 107, 2681–2686. doi: 10.1073/pnas.0913008107

Ferri, R., Rundo, F., Bruni, O., Terzano, M. G., and Stam, C. J. (2005). Dynamics of the EEG slow-wave synchronization during sleep. Clin. Neurophysiol. 116, 2783–2795. doi: 10.1016/j.clinph.2005.08.013

Forest, G., and Godbout, R. (2000). Effects of sleep deprivation on performance and EEG spectral analysis in young adults. Brain Cogn. 43, 195–200.

Fries, P. (2005). A mechanism for cognitive dynamics: neuronal communi- cation through neuronal coherence. Trends Cogn. Sci. 9, 474–480. doi: 10.1016/j.tics.2005.08.011

Fuggetta, G., Fiaschi, A., and Manganotti, P. (2005). Modulation of cortical oscilla- tory activities induced by varying single-pulse transcranial magnetic stimulation intensity over the left primary motor area: a combined EEG and TMS study. Neuroimage 27, 896–908. doi: 10.1016/j.neuroimage.2005.05.013

Fuggetta, G., Pavone, E. F., Fiaschi, A., and Manganotti, P. (2008). Acute modulation of cortical oscillatory activities during short trains of high-frequency repetitive transcranial magnetic stimulation of the human motor cortex: a combined EEG and TMS study. Hum. Brain. Mapp. 29, 1–13. doi: 10.1002/hbm.20371

Grosse, P., Khatami, R., Salih, F., Kühn, A., and Meyer, B. U. (2002). Corticospinal excitability in human sleep as assessed by transcranial magnetic stimulation. Neurology 59, 1988–1991. doi: 10.1212/01.WNL.0000038762.11894.DA

Harrison, Y., and Horne, J. A. (1999). One night of sleep loss impairs innovative thinking and flexible decision making. Organ. Behav. Hum. Decis. Process. 78, 128–145. doi: 10.1006/obhd.1999.2827

Huber, R., Mäki, H., Rosanova, M., Casarotto, S., Canali, P., Casali, A. G., et al. (2013). Human cortical excitability increases with time awake. Cereb. Cortex 23, 332–338. doi: 10.1093/cercor/bhs014

Ilmoniemi, R. J., Virtanen, J., Ruohonen, J., Karhu, J., Aronen, H. J., Naatanen, R., et al. (1997). Neuronal responses to magnetic stimulation reveal cortical reactivity and connectivity. Neuroreport 8, 3537–3540. doi: 10.1097/00001756-199711100-00024

Izumi, S., Takase, M., Arita, M., Masakado, Y., Kimura, A., and Chino, N. (1997). Transcranial magnetic stimulation-induced changes in EEG and responses recorded from the scalp of healthy humans. Electroen- cephalogr. Clin. Neurophysiol. 103, 319–322. doi: 10.1016/S0013-4694(97) 00007-2

Johnson, K. A., Baylis, G. C., Powell, D. A., Kozel, F. A., Miller, S. W., and George, M. S. (2010). Conditioning of transcranial magnetic stimulation: evidence of sensory-induced responding and prepulse inhibition. Brain Stimul. 3, 78–86. doi: 10.1016/j.brs.2009.08.003

Jovanovic, U. J. (1991). General consideration of sleep and sleep deprivation. Epilepsy Res. Suppl. 2, 205–215.

Kattler, H., Dijk, D. J., and Borbély, A. A. (1994). Effect of unilateral somatosensory stimulation prior to sleep on the sleep EEG in humans. J. Sleep Res. 3, 159–164. doi: 10.1111/j.1365-2869.1994.tb00123.x

Kendall, A. P., Kautz, M. A., Russo, M. B., and Killgore, W. D. (2006). Effects of sleep deprivation on lateral visual attention. Int. J. Neurosci. 116, 1125–1138. doi: 10.1080/00207450500513922

King, M. A., Newton, M. R., Jackson, G. D., Fitt, G. J., Mitchell, L. A., Sil- vapulle, M. J., et al. (1998). Epileptology of the first seizure presentation: a clinical electroencephalographic and magnetic resonance imaging study of 300 consecutive patients. Lancet 352, 1007–1011. doi: 10.1016/S0140-6736(98) 03543-0

Kirov, R., Weiss, C., Siebner, H. R., Born, J., and Marshall, L. (2009). Slow oscil- lation electrical brain stimulation during waking promotes EEG theta activity and memory encoding. Proc. Natl. Acad. Sci. U.S.A. 106, 15460–15465. doi: 10.1073/pnas.0904438106

Komssi, S., Aronen, H. J., Huttunen, J., Kesaniemi, M., Soinne, L., Nikouline, V. V., et al. (2002). Ipsi- and contralateral EEG reactions to transcranial magnetic stim- ulation. Clin. Neurophysiol. 113, 175–184. doi: 10.1016/S1388-2457(01)00721-0

Komssi, S., Kahkonen, S., and Ilmoniemi, R. J. (2004). The effect of stimulus intensity on brain responses evoked by transcranial magnetic stimulation. Hum. Brain Mapp. 21, 154–164. doi: 10.1002/hbm.10159

Linde, L., and Bergstrom, M. (1992). The effect of one night without sleep on problem-solving and immediate recall. Psychol. Res. 54, 127–136. doi: 10.1007/BF00937141

Manganotti, P., Bongiovanni, L. G., Fuggetta, G., Zanette, G., and Fiaschi, A. (2006). Effects of sleep deprivation on cortical excitability in patients affected by juvenile myoclonic epilepsy: a combined transcranial magnetic stimulation and EEG study. J. Neurol. Neurosurg. Psychiatry 77, 56–60. doi: 10.1136/jnnp.2004.041137

Manganotti, P., Formaggio, E., Storti, S. F., De Massari, D., Zamboni, A., Bertoldo, A., et al. (2012). Time-frequency analysis of short-lasting modulation of EEG induced by intracortical and transcallosal paired TMS over motor areas. J. Neurophysiol. 107, 2475–2484. doi: 10.1152/jn.00543.2011

Manganotti, P., Palermo, A., Patuzzo, S., Zanette, G., and Fiaschi, A. (2001). Decrease in motor cortical excitability in human subjects after sleep deprivation. Neurosci. Lett. 304, 153–156. doi: 10.1016/S0304-3940(01) 01783-9

Massimini, M., Ferrarelli, F., Esser, S. K., Riedner, B. A., Huber, R., Murphy, M., et al. (2007). Triggering sleep slow waves by transcranial magnetic stim- ulation. Proc. Natl. Acad. Sci. U.S.A. 104, 8496–8501. doi: 10.1073/pnas.0702 495104

Massimini, M., Ferrarelli, F., Huber, R., Esser, S. K., Singh, H., and Tononi, G. (2005). Breakdown of cortical effective connectivity during sleep. Science 309, 2228–2232. doi: 10.1126/science.1117256

Massimini, M., Huber, R., Ferrarelli, F., Hill, S., and Tononi, G. (2004). The sleep slow oscillation as a traveling wave. J. Neurosci. 24, 6862–6870. doi: 10.1523/JNEUROSCI.1318-04.2004

Massimini, M., Tononi, G., and Huber, R. (2009). Slow waves, synaptic plastic- ity and information processing: insights from transcranial magnetic stimulation and high-density EEG experiments. Eur. J. Neurosci. 29, 1761–1770. doi: 10.1111/j.1460-9568.2009.06720.x

Murphy, M., Riedner, B. A., Huber, R., Massimini, M., Ferrarelli, F., and Tononi, G. (2009). Source modeling sleep slow waves. Proc. Natl. Acad. Sci. U.S.A. 106, 1608–1613. doi: 10.1073/pnas.0807933106

Niedermeyer, E. (1999). "The normal EEG of the walking adult," in Electroen- cephalography: Basic Principles, Clinical Applications and Related Fields, eds E. Niedermeyer and F. Lopes da Silva (Baltimore: Lippincott Williams and Wilkins), 149–173.

Nikouline, V., Ruohonen, J., and Ilmoniemi, R. J. (1999). The role of the coil click in TMS assessed with simultaneous EEG. Clin. Neurophysiol. 110, 1325–1328. doi: 10.1016/S1388-2457(99)00070-X

Noh, N. A., Fuggetta, G., Manganotti, P., and Fiaschi, A. (2012). Long lasting mod- ulation of cortical oscillations after continuous theta burst transcranial magnetic stimulation. PLoS ONE 7:e35080. doi: 10.1371/journal.pone.0035080

Oldfield, R. C. (1971). The assessment and analysis of handedness: the Edinburgh

inventory. Neuropsychologia 9, 97–113. doi: 10.1016/0028-3932(71)90067-4 Panzeri, S., Brunel, N., Logothetis, N. K., and Kayser, C. (2010). Sensory neural codes using multiplexed temporal scales. Trends Neurosci. 33, 111–120. doi: 10.1016/j.tins.2009.12.001

Paus, T., Jech, R., Thompson, C. J., Comeau, R., Peters, T., and Evans, A. C. (1998). Dose-dependent reduction of cerebral blood flow during rapid-rate transcranial magnetic stimulation of the human sensorimotor cortex. J. Neurophysiol. 79, 1102–1107.

Paus, T., Sipila, P. K., and Strafella, A. P. (2001). Synchronization of neuronal activity in the human primary motor cortex by transcranial magnetic stimulation: an EEG study. J. Neurophysiol. 86, 1983–1990.

Pfurtscheller, G., and Lopes da Silva, F. H. (1999). Event-related EEG/MEG syn- chronization and desynchronization: basic principles. Clin. Neurophysiol. 110, 1842–1857. doi: 10.1016/S1388-2457(99)00141-8

Plewnia, C., Rilk, A. J., Soekadar, S. R., Arfeller, C., Huber, H. S., Sauseng, P., et al. (2008). Enhancement of long-range EEG coherence by synchronous bifo- cal transcranial magnetic stimulation. Eur. J. Neurosci. 27, 1577–1578. doi: 10.1111/j.1460-9568.2008.06124.x

Pratt, K. L., Mattson, R. H., Weikers, N. J., and Williams, R. (1968). EEG activation of epileptics following sleep deprivation: a prospective study of 114 cases. Electroen- cephalogr. Clin. Neurophysiol. 24, 11–15. doi: 10.1016/0013-4694(68)90061-8

Rosanova, M., Casali, A., Bellina, V., Resta, F., Mariotti, M., and Massimini, M. (2009). Natural frequencies of human corticothalamic circuits. J. Neurosci. 29, 7679–7685. doi: 10.1523/JNEUROSCI.0445-09.2009

Rossini, P. M., Barker, A. T., Berardelli, A., Caramia, M. D., Caruso, G., Cracco, R. Q., et al. (1994). Non-invasive electrical and magnetic stimulation of the brain, spinal cord and roots: basic principles and procedures for routine clinical application. Report of an IFCN committee. Electroencephalogr. Clin. Neurophysiol. 91, 79–92. doi: 10.1016/0013-4694(94)90029-9

Siegel, M., Warden, M. R., and Miller, E. K. (2009). Phase-dependent neuronal coding of objects in short-term memory. Proc. Natl. Acad. Sci. U.S.A. 106, 21341– 21346. doi: 10.1073/pnas.0908193106

Silber, M. H., Ancoli-Israel, S., Bonnet, M. H., Chokroverty, S., Grigg-Damberger, M. M., Hirshkowitz, M., et al. (2007). The visual scoring of sleep in adults. J. Clin. Sleep Med. 3, 121–131.

Smith, C., and MacNeill, C. (1994). Impaired motor memory for a pursuit rotor task following stage 2 sleep loss in college students. J. Sleep Res. 3, 206–213. doi: 10.1111/j.1365-2869.1994.tb00133.x

Stampi, C., Stone, P., and Michimori, A. (1995). A new quantitative method for assessing sleepiness: the Alpha Attenuation test. Work Stress 9, 368–376. doi: 10.1080/02678379508256574

Steriade, M., and Llinás, R. R. (1988). The functional states of the thalamus and the associated neuronal interplay. Physiol. Rev. 68, 649–742.

Steriade, M. (2003). The corticothalamic system in sleep. Front. Biosci. 8:878–899. doi: 10.2741/1043

Steriade, M. (2005). Sleep, epilepsy and thalamic reticular inhibitory neurons. Trends Neurosci. 28, 317–324. doi: 10.1016/j.tins.2005.03.007

Thut, G., and Miniussi, C. (2009). New insights into rhythmic brain activity from TMS-EEG studies. Trends Cogn. Sci. 13, 182–189. doi: 10.1016/j.tics.2009.01.004

Thut, G., Northoff, G., Ives, J. R., Kamitani, Y., Pfennig, A., Kampmann, F., et al. (2003). Effects of single-pulse transcranial magnetic stimulation (TMS) on func- tional brain activity: a combined event-related TMS and evoked potential study.

Clin. Neurophysiol. 114, 2071–2080. doi: 10.1016/S1388-2457(03)00205-0

Thut, G., and Pascual-Leone, A. (2010). A review of combined TMS-EEG studies to characterize lasting effects of repetitive TMS and assess their useful- ness in cognitive and clinical neuroscience. Brain. Topogr. 22, 219–232. doi: 10.1007/s10548-009-0115-4

Tiitinen, H., Virtanen, J., Ilmoniemi, R. J., Kamppuri, J., Ollikainen, M., Ruohonen, J., et al. (1999). Separation of contamination caused by coil clicks from responses elicited by transcranial magnetic stimulation. Clin. Neurophysiol. 110, 982–985. doi: 10.1016/S1388-2457(99)00038-3

Van Der Werf, Y. D., Sadikot, A. F., Strafella, A. P., and Paus, T. (2006). The neural response to transcranial magnetic stimulation of the human motor cortex. II Thalamocortical contributions. Exp. Brain Res. 175, 246–255. doi: 10.1007/s00221-006-0548-x

Veniero, D., Brignani, D., Thut, G., and Miniussi, C. (2011). Alpha-generation as basic response-signature to transcranial magnetic stimulation (TMS) tar- geting the human resting motor cortex: a TMS/EEG co-registration study. Psychophysiology 48, 381–389. doi: 10.1111/j.1469-8986.2011.01218.x

Walker, M. P., Brakefield, T., Morgan, A., Hobson, J. A., and Stickgold, R. (2002a).

Practice with sleep makes perfect: sleep-dependent motor skill learning. Neuron 35, 205–211. doi: 10.1016/S0896-6273(02)00746-8

11

Modulation of human corticospinal excitability by paired associative stimulation

***Richard G. Carson*[1,2]* *and Niamh C. Kennedy*[2,3]**

[1] *Trinity College Institute of Neuroscience and School of Psychology, Trinity College Dublin, Dublin, Ireland*
[2] *School of Psychology, Queen's University Belfast, Belfast, UK*
[3] *School of Rehabilitation Sciences University of East Anglia, Norwich, UK*

Correspondence:
Richard G. Carson, Trinity College Institute of Neuroscience and School of Psychology, Lloyd Building, Trinity College Dublin, Dublin 2, Ireland
e-mail: richard.carson@tcd.ie

Paired Associative Stimulation (PAS) has come to prominence as a potential therapeutic intervention for the treatment of brain injury/disease, and as an experimental method with which to investigate Hebbian principles of neural plasticity in humans. Prototypically, a single electrical stimulus is directed to a peripheral nerve in advance of transcranial magnetic stimulation (TMS) delivered to the contralateral primary motor cortex (M1). Repeated pairing of the stimuli (i.e., association) over an extended period may increase or decrease the excitability of corticospinal projections from M1, in manner that depends on the interstimulus interval (ISI). It has been suggested that these effects represent a form of associative long-term potentiation (LTP) and depression (LTD) that bears resemblance to spike-timing dependent plasticity (STDP) as it has been elaborated in animal models. With a large body of empirical evidence having emerged since the cardinal features of PAS were first described, and in light of the variations from the original protocols that have been implemented, it is opportune to consider whether the phenomenology of PAS remains consistent with the characteristic features that were initially disclosed. This assessment necessarily has bearing upon interpretation of the effects of PAS in relation to the specific cellular pathways that are putatively engaged, including those that adhere to the rules of STDP. The balance of evidence suggests that the mechanisms that contribute to the LTP- and LTD-type responses to PAS differ depending on the precise nature of the induction protocol that is used. In addition to emphasizing the requirement for additional explanatory models, in the present analysis we highlight the key features of the PAS phenomenology that require interpretation.

Keywords: long-term potentiation, long-term depression, transcranial magnetic stimulation, peripheral nerve stimulation, human, cortex, spike-timing dependent plasticity, translational neuroscience

BACKGROUND

In recent years there has been an explosion of interest in electrophysiological techniques that promote short-term changes in the excitability of human cerebral cortex, including patterned electrical or mechanical excitation of muscles and peripheral nerves, and methods of indirectly stimulating regions of the brain by means of transient magnetic fields or weak electrical currents. At least two motivations can be discerned. The first derives from the belief that interventions based on these techniques have the capacity to augment traditional neurorehabilitation practice, by promoting the physiological changes upon which recovery of function is based (e.g., Harris-Love and Cohen, 2006). The second is that such techniques provide means of studying brain plasticity at a systems level in humans (e.g., Muller-Dahlhaus et al., 2010).

In this context, Paired Associative Stimulation (PAS) has prominence both as a therapeutic intervention (e.g., Jayaram and Stinear, 2008; Castel-Lacanal et al., 2009), and as an experimental method with which to investigate Hebbian principles of synaptic plasticity. In the prototypical form of PAS (Stefan et al., 2000), a single electrical stimulus is directed to a peripheral nerve in advance of a magnetic stimulus delivered to the contralateral primary motor cortex (M1). The inter-stimulus interval is adjusted with a view to ensuring that inputs to M1 initiated by the afferent volley arising from the nerve stimulation occur simultaneously with the magnetic stimulation. Repeated pairing of the two sources of stimulation (i.e., association) over an extended period increases the excitability of corticospinal projections from M1. In circumstances in which the inter-stimulus interval is adjusted such that a corollary of the afferent volley may reach M1 after the magnetic stimulus, a decrease in corticospinal excitability has been reported (Wolters et al., 2003).

The neuroplastic adaptation revealed by PAS appears to exhibit several of the criteria designated for long-term potentiation (LTP) and long-term depression (LTD). Its effects evolve quickly, are reversible; and persist beyond the period of stimulation (McKay et al., 2002; Stefan et al., 2002). Pharmacological agents that interact with NMDA-receptor activity interfere with the outcomes of PAS, supporting the hypothesis that LTP-like changes are implicated (Stefan et al., 2002). In consideration of these properties, and assumptions that the alterations in excitability brought about by PAS were restricted to the cortical representations of muscles innervated by the peripheral nerve that was stimulated electrically, it has been suggested that PAS induced adaptation represents a form of associative LTP (and LTD) that is synapse-specific (Nitsche et al., 2007) and behaves in accordance with Hebbian principles (Stefan et al., 2000, 2004; Quartarone et al., 2003). More specifically, since the polarity of the induced effects appears contingent upon the order of the stimulus-generated cortical events, and the effective inter-stimulus intervals lie within a restricted (milliseconds) range, it has been proposed that the resemblance is to spike-timing dependent plasticity (STDP) (Muller-Dahlhaus et al., 2010).

Subsequent to the first report of this technique in 2000 by Stefan and colleagues, there have been a wide range of derivative investigations concerning, for example, the inter-stimulus intervals (ISIs) that are efficacious (e.g., Wolters et al., 2005; Kumpulainen et al., 2012), the muscles in which the effects can be elicited (e.g., Stefan et al., 2000; Stinear and Hornby, 2005; Carson et al., 2013), and variations in the extent to which they can be induced in various clinical populations (e.g., Castel-Lacanal et al., 2009; Monte-Silva et al., 2009; Bologna et al., 2012). Consideration has also been accorded to the levels of the neuraxis that are subject to influence by PAS (e.g., Stefan et al., 2000; Meunier et al., 2007; Di Lazzaro et al., 2009a,b; Russmann et al., 2009). As this corpus of work has accumulated, large inter-individual differences in response to PAS have been noted (e.g., Fratello et al., 2006). This has given rise to examination of such potential mediating factors as age (Fathi et al., 2010), cortical anatomy (Conde et al., 2012), and the role of specific genetic polymorphisms (Cheeran et al., 2008), among many others.

In view of the large body of empirical evidence that has accumulated, and particularly in light of the variations upon the original protocols that have been implemented, it is perhaps opportune to consider whether the phenomenology of PAS remains consistent with the cardinal features that were first disclosed. Any such assessment necessarily also has bearing upon interpretation of the effects of PAS in relation to specific cellular mechanisms, such as the expression of STDP.

SCOPE OF THE REVIEW

This is an area of enquiry that is already extensive and burgeoning. In the present paper the focus will be maintained upon prototypical forms of PAS, in which stimulation of peripheral afferents is combined with single pulse transcranial magnetic stimulation (TMS) applied to contralateral M1. We pay particular attention to empirical observations that do not concur with standard assumptions, reasoning that these provide the necessary basis upon which to gauge the adequacy of current explanatory models. Consideration is not extended to studies in which PAS has been combined with other forms of non-invasive brain stimulation, for example in assessing the expression of homeostatic plasticity (e.g., Nitsche et al., 2007), or to the mediation of cognitive factors such as locus of attention (Stefan et al., 2004). In addition, the analysis is restricted to the motor system (cf. Schecklmann et al., 2011), and specifically to adaptations within higher brain centers (cf. Taylor and Martin, 2009; Cortes et al., 2011; Leukel et al., 2012).

Principally we characterize the effects of PAS in terms of changes in the excitability of projections from primary motor cortex—assessed through muscle responses evoked by TMS. These are brought about primarily by the trans-synaptic excitation of corticospinal cells. Although the amplitude of the motor-evoked potential (MEP) thus reflects the excitability of neurons in the motor cortex (Rothwell et al., 1991), it is also influenced by the state of the spinal motoneuron pool. While paired-pulse experiments may illuminate the contributory roles of microcircuits within M1, necessarily TMS-based techniques are unable to resolve changes in synaptic weights in the manner in which these are discriminable in reduced preparations (Verhoog et al., 2013).

TIMING DEPENDENCY IN PAS

In foundational reports (Wolters et al., 2003) it was noted that an increase in corticospinal excitability is achieved if the peripheral nerve stimulation is timed such that the initial phase of input to M1 arising as its corollary occurs synchronously with the delivery of a magnetic pulse over that area of cortex. If the relative timing is adjusted such that TMS is applied prior to the time at which a corollary of the peripheral afferent stimulation is anticipated to reach M1, repeated pairings may lead to a subsequent reduction in corticospinal excitability. Since the conclusion that PAS induced effects represent a distinct form of synapse-specific associative plasticity (i.e., STDP) is buttressed by the presence of timing dependency, the associated empirical findings demand particular attention.

UPPER LIMB MUSCLES: EXCITATORY EFFECTS

When the targets are projections to intrinsic hand muscles, the interval between the peripheral nerve stimulus and the TMS pulse is most commonly fixed (across participants) at 25 ms ("PAS25"). This protocol generates sustained increases in corticospinal excitability (e.g., Stefan et al., 2000; Wolters et al., 2003; Sale et al., 2007). It has also been shown that an ISI of 21.5 ms may have similar effects (Weise et al., 2006, 2011). Such increases can however also be obtained when a fixed inter-stimulus interval (ISI) of 35 ms is employed (Stefan et al., 2000).

On other occasions an individualized approach has been employed, whereby the latency of the N20 component of a somatosensory-evoked potential (SEP), elicited in each participant by stimulating the peripheral nerve, is used as a reference. In some instances the magnetic pulse has been timed to coincide with the N20 component (e.g., Ziemann et al., 2004). In other studies it has been delayed by 2 ms ("N20 + 2 PAS") (e.g., Heidegger et al., 2010; Korchounov and Ziemann, 2011; Voytovych et al., 2012). In a recent investigation by Ilic and colleagues in which individual N20 latencies were used, this gave rise to ISIs ranging from 18.7 to 21 ms in a sample of 14 participants (Ilic et al., 2011). In this context, it is also worth noting that the effects of these protocols can vary markedly across participants, even when the ISI is determined on the basis of an individual's SEP. For example, Muller-Dahlhaus et al. (2008) noted that in a sample of twenty-seven people tested using a N20 plus 2 ms ISI, 14 showed the expected increase in corticospinal excitability, whereas the other thirteen exhibited a decrease (mean ratio post-PAS/pre-PAS = 1.00; range = 0.36–1.68). Kang et al. (2011) also failed to induce reliable changes in corticospinal excitability using a 25 ms ISI protocol (see also Fratello et al., 2006).

While for the most part the nature of the processes engaged by these different versions of the PAS protocol (**Table 1**) have not been subject to discrimination, it has been highlighted that the synaptic relays engaged at the latency of the N20 component may be distinct from those that are excited during intervals thereafter (Hamada et al., 2012). Indeed, excitatory effects induced using an ISI of 25 ms can be attenuated by the concurrent application of direct current stimulation to the cerebellum, whereas those brought about via an ISI of 21.5 ms appear to be unaffected by this manipulation (Hamada et al., 2012). A more general point is thereby illustrated. In seeking to appreciate the mechanistic basis of changes in corticospinal excitability instigated by PAS, consideration must necessarily be given to the presence of multiple neural pathways through which the constituent elements of this protocol are liable to exert their influence. With respect to projections to the muscles of the hand, the range of inter-stimulus (single nerve shock; single magnetic impulse) intervals for which excitatory effects can be obtained (18.7–35 ms) represents asynchronies at M1 well within the window necessary for the induction of LTP by STDP in reduced animal preparations (Bi and Poo, 1998; Dan and Poo, 2004, 2006). Nonetheless, this consistency does not in itself imply that a single mechanism is operative at all latencies within this range, or that the effects induced at any given latency are mediated principally by STDP.

In a small number of cases the "classical" PAS protocols—in which a single peripheral afferent stimulus is delivered in association with a single pulse of TMS to the cortex, have been applied to study projections to muscles in the forearm. In these cases [in which the flexor carpi radialis (FCR) has typically been the focus of investigation] the ISI has either been fixed at 20 ms for all participants (Meunier et al., 2007), or determined through subtraction of the FCR M-wave onset latency from the MEP onset latency (to which 6 ms is added as an estimate of the time for the derivate of the afferent volley to travel from sensory to motor cortex). The resulting effects are however smaller than those observed for the intrinsic hand muscles, and in some cases they become clearly expressed only when there is additional cortical excitation promoted by contractions of homologous muscles of the opposite limb (Kennedy and Carson, 2008). We are not aware of attempts to examine the effect of changing ISIs for projections to the forearm muscles, however the intervals that have proved effective are consistent with those employed for muscles in the hand, given that the afferent volley traverses a shorter path (e.g., from a point of stimulation at the elbow) to higher brain centers.

UPPER LIMB MUSCLES: INHIBITORY EFFECTS

In order to induce LTD-type effects in corticospinal projections to the hand (**Table 2**), it has been customary to employ a fixed ISI of 10 ms ("PAS10"), with a view to ensuring that a corollary of the afferent volley arrives at M1 after the magnetic cortical stimulus (e.g., Wolters et al., 2003; Monte-Silva et al., 2009; Thirugnanasambandam et al., 2011a,b; Weise et al., 2011). In a recent study however, Schabrun et al. (2013) reported that MEP amplitudes were reduced by a PAS protocol in which electrical stimulation of the median nerve was applied at fixed intervals of 250, 350, and 450 ms *following* the delivery of TMS to contralateral M1.

In several other investigations individual ISIs have been calculated by means of the SEP N20 latency (e.g., Ziemann et al., 2004; Muller et al., 2007; Potter-Nerger et al., 2009; Ilic et al., 2011; Voytovych et al., 2012). The ISIs calculated by Ilic et al. (2011) on this basis (i.e., N20 latency minus 5 ms) yielded values longer

Table 1 | Upper limb muscles: excitatory effects.

Muscle	Authors	ISI	Total number of stimuli	Stimulation period (mins)	Rate of delivery (Hz)
APB	Fratello et al., 2006	25 ms	140 pairs	23	0.1
APB	Hamada et al., 2012	25/21.5 ms	180 pairs	15	0.2
APB	Heidegger et al., 2010	N20+2	90 pairs	30	0.05
APB	Ilic et al., 2011	N20	200 pairs	15	0.25
APB	Kang et al., 2011	25 ms	225 pairs	15	0.25
FCR	Kennedy and Carson, 2008	18.7 ms (mean)	84 pairs 42 pairs	28 14	0.05 0.05
APB	Korchounov and Ziemann, 2011	N20+2	90 pairs	30	0.05
FCR	Meunier et al., 2007	20 ms	240 pairs	20	0.2
APB	Muller-Dahlhaus et al., 2008	N20+2	225 pairs	15	0.25
APB	Sale et al., 2007	25 ms	Short duration: 132 pairs Long duration: 90 pairs	Short duration: 11 Long duration: 30	Short duration: 0.02 Long duration: 0.05
APB	Stefan et al., 2000	25 ms	90 pairs	30	0.05
APB	Voytovych et al., 2012	N20+2	225 pairs	15	0.25
APB	Weise et al., 2006	21.5 ms	180 pairs	30	0.1
APB	Weise et al., 2011	21.5 ms	180 pairs	30	0.1
APB	Wolters et al., 2003	25 ms	90 pairs	30	0.05
APB	Wolters et al., 2005	N20	180 pairs	30	0.1
APB	Ziemann et al., 2004	N20	200 pairs	15	0.25

Table 2 | Upper limb muscles: inhibitory effects.

Muscle	Authors	ISI	Total number of stimuli	Stimulation period (mins)	Rate of delivery (Hz)
FDI/APB	Amaya et al., 2010	N1-5 ms	200 pairs	13	0.25
APB	De Beaumont et al., 2012	10 ms	200 pairs	13	0.25
APB	Ilic et al., 2011	N20-5	200 pairs	15	0.25
APB	Kang et al., 2011	10 ms	225 pairs	15	0.25
ADM	Monte-Silva et al., 2009	10 ms	90 pairs	30	0.05
APB	Muller et al., 2007	N20-5	225 pairs	15	0.25
FDI	Potter-Nerger et al., 2009	N20-5	200 pairs	15	0.25
APB	Rajji et al., 2011	10 ms	180 pairs	30	0.1
APB	Schabrun et al., 2013	250, 350,450 ms following TMS	90 pairs	30	0.05
ADM	Thirugnanasambandam et al., 2011a	10 ms	90 pairs	30	0.05
ADM	Thirugnanasambandam et al., 2011b	10 ms	90 pairs	30	0.05
APB	Voytovych et al., 2012	N20-5	225 pairs	15	0.25
APB	Weise et al., 2006	10 ms	180 pairs	30	0.1
APB	Weise et al., 2011	10 ms	180 pairs	30	0.1
APB	Wolters et al., 2003	10 ms	90 pairs	30	0.05
APB	Ziemann et al., 2004	N20-5	200 pairs	15	0.25

than the conventional 10 ms interval used to induce inhibition (13.7–16 ms).

A number of investigators have however failed to obtain consistent reductions of corticospinal excitability following administration of a PAS10 protocol (e.g., Kang et al., 2011; Rajji et al., 2011). Weise et al. (2006), recorded a reliable reduction in APB MEP amplitudes at 45–55 min, but not at five other time points following the intervention.

In the only study of which we are aware that has been conducted in non-human primates, Amaya et al. (2010) applied 13 min of PAS to two awake trained rhesus monkeys. On the basis of an estimate of 12 ms for the latency of the N1 component of the SEP generated by contralateral median nerve stimulation, ISIs of 5 and 15 ms were employed (analogous to the PAS-10 and PAS-25 protocols used in humans). Whereas PAS based on an ISI of 15 ms led to reliable facilitation of MEP amplitude (265% of baseline) during a 2 h period following the intervention, no changes in corticospinal excitability were obtained when an ISI of 5 ms was used.

LOWER LIMB MUSCLES

PAS protocols (**Table 3**) are also capable of inducing changes in the excitability of corticospinal projections to the muscles of the lower limb (Uy et al., 2003; Stinear and Hornby, 2005; Mrachacz-Kersting et al., 2007; Kumpulainen et al., 2012). In a study in which common peroneal nerve (CPN) stimulation and bilateral TMS were paired during treadmill walking, an ISI equivalent to the estimated MEP latency for the tibialis anterior (TA) muscle plus 5 ms was employed with a view to producing LTP-like effects. This ISI was gauged to result in a corollary of the CPN stimulation reaching M1 no more than 10 ms prior to TMS (during late swing around heel strike). In a further condition, the ISI was 10 ms shorter than the estimated MEP latency—judged to have ensured that the TMS was delivered prior to the corollary of the peripheral volley arriving in cortex (Stinear and Hornby, 2005). The excitability of corticospinal projections to TA (obtained during the late swing phase of walking prior to and following the 10 min intervention) was increased by the first protocol, and diminished by the second protocol. It emerges however that an ISI (MEP latency + 5 ms) that induces facilitation when the stimulus pairs are delivered during the late swing phase, leads to inhibition of the projections to TA when the PAS is administered during mid swing. Indeed, facilitation could only be induced using this ISI when the application occurred in a narrow time window against a background of voluntary EMG activity in TA (Prior and Stinear, 2006). Nonetheless, it also appears possible to obtain facilitation (assessed during subsequent walking) when this ISI is used at rest, although there is a dependency upon the intensity of the magnetic stimulus (Jayaram et al., 2007). Corresponding inhibitory effects (assessed during walking) have been obtained when PAS is administered at rest using an ISI 8 ms shorter than the estimated MEP latency (Jayaram and Stinear, 2008).

Mrachacz-Kersting et al. (2007) also demonstrated that the effects of PAS directed at the projections to TA were accentuated markedly when the pairing of electrical stimulation of the CPN (at motor threshold) and bilateral magnetic stimulation of M1 was delivered during dorsi-flexion contractions [~5–10% maximum voluntary contraction (MVC)]. On the basis of SEP recordings (N34 peak), it was estimated that the corollary of the afferent volley reached M1 46–57 ms poststimulation. In this context, ISIs of 45, 50, and 55 ms yielded facilitation. In contrast, an ISI of 40 ms—TMS in advance of the estimated arrival of afferent evoked volley at M1, decreased the amplitude of MEPs elicited in TA. Notably however, facilitation of corticospinal projections to TA can also be obtained using ISIs tailored to achieve arrival of sensory mediated inputs to M1 over a range of 15–90 ms *following* cortical stimulation (Roy et al., 2007).

Table 3 | Lower limb muscles.

Muscle	Authors	ISI	Total number of stimuli	Stimulation period (mins)	Rate of delivery (Hz)
TA	Jayaram and Stinear, 2008	MEP latency −8 ms	120 pairs	4	0.5
TA	Jayaram et al., 2007	MEP latency +5 ms	120 pairs	4	0.5
SOL	Kumpulainen et al., 2012	6, 12, 18, and 24 ms	200 pairs	Variable	0.2
TA	Mrachacz-Kersting et al., 2007	20, 30, 40, 45, 50, 55, 60 ms	360 pairs	30	0.2
TA/SOL	Prior and Stinear, 2006	MEP latency +5 ms	120 pairs	10	0.2
TA	Roy et al., 2007	15–90 ms after TMS	90 pairs	15	0.1
TA/SOL	Stinear and Hornby, 2005	MEP latency +5 MEP latency −10	120 pairs	10	0.2
TA	Uy et al., 2003	35 ms	180 pairs	30	0.1

When projections to the soleus (SOL) muscle is the focus of investigation (Kumpulainen et al., 2012), and the first negative peak (P32) of the lower limb SEP (corresponding to the N20 component of the median nerve SEP) is used as a reference, reliable increases in corticospinal excitability have been obtained using an ISI of the P32 latency plus 18 ms. No such changes were registered for ISIs corresponding to the P32 plus 12 or plus 24 ms. A decrease in MEP amplitude was however reported when an ISI of P32 plus 6 ms was employed.

In summary, although the number of completed studies remains relatively small, it is apparent that the range of ISIs that is effective in inducing the facilitation of corticospinal projections to muscles of the lower limb is wider than that employed customarily in experiments on the upper limb, and beyond the upper boundary of intervals used to examine STDP in reduced preparations (e.g., Table 1 of Dan and Poo, 2006). Critically, in this context potentiation of corticospinal output can be achieved using PAS protocols that are likely to result in a corollary of the peripheral afferent volley reaching M1 after magnetic stimulation applied to the same brain region (Roy et al., 2007). Furthermore, the effects of these interventions are generally accentuated when there is additional cortical excitation associated with background contraction of the target muscle (Prior and Stinear, 2006; Mrachacz-Kersting et al., 2007). It has been noted that the physiological effects of (bilateral) magnetic stimulation applied using large double cone coils may differ from those arising from the impulses applied to cortical representations of hand muscles, particularly with respect to the relative contribution of I1 and later waves (Di Lazzaro et al., 2001). In addition, the excitability of M1 circuits projecting to leg muscles appears to be more readily modified by (electrical) peripheral afferent stimulation than those of the intrinsic hand muscles (Roy et al., 2007). These qualifications serve to highlight the limitations of using phenomenology alone as a basis upon which to infer mechanism. More specifically, there exist variants of PAS for which the associated effects fail to exhibit some of the cardinal features upon which attributions of mechanism have previously been based.

TRAINS OF STIMULATION

While with respect to the upper limb, investigations employing single pulse peripheral nerve stimulation appear to corroborate the assumption that the precise inter stimulus interval is critical in determining the nature of PAS induced effects, somewhat different conclusions may be drawn on the basis of experiments in which trains of afferent stimulation have been utilized. In several studies focusing on the state of corticospinal projections to hand and forearm muscles in healthy adults, trains of 500 ms duration consisting of 1 ms square waves delivered at 10 Hz (i.e., 5 stimuli per train) have been employed (Ridding and Taylor, 2001; McKay et al., 2002; Castel-Lacanal et al., 2007; Carson et al., 2013). In a seminal study in which the peripheral stimulation was applied over the motor point of FDI, Ridding and Taylor administered TMS stimuli 25 ms after the *onset* of each train. Following a 30 min intervention, substantial [200 ± 153% (SD)] increases in the amplitude of MEPs elicited in FDI were reported. Using the same protocol, comparable results were reported by McKay et al. (2002). When the TMS is administered 25 ms following the *last* shock of the train, effects of a similar nature are obtained when either the ECR (Castel-Lacanal et al., 2007) or the FCR (Carson et al., 2013) motor point are in receipt of stimulation. In the two variants of the train protocol therefore, there is a disparity of 50 ms with respect to the relative timing of the magnetic stimulus and the proximate peripheral shock. Yet both variants appear effective in potentiating the excitability of descending projections to the target muscle.

Equivalent outcomes were reported when the method introduced by Castel-Lacanal et al. (2007) was applied in stroke survivors, both early in the recovery phase and at 1-year post injury (Castel-Lacanal et al., 2009). In other circumstances in which both the peripheral nerve stimulation and TMS has been applied at 5 Hz over a 2 min interval, increases in the excitability of projections to the APB muscle were obtained if each TMS pulse was delayed by 25 ms with respect to the preceding peripheral (median) nerve stimulus. Reliable changes in corticospinal excitability were not however expressed if the delay was set at 10 ms (Quartarone et al., 2006). In the two cases of which we are aware, PAS protocols based on trains of electrical stimulation applied to the CPN have given rise to weak effects on the excitability of projections to TA that were not expressed consistently within samples of healthy young adults (Perez et al., 2003) or older stroke survivors (Uy et al., 2003).

A REFLECTION UPON TIMING DEPENDENCY

In PAS protocols in which a single shock is applied to a peripheral nerve in the upper limb in close temporal contiguity (<35 ms) with a magnetic pulse delivered over the contralateral hemisphere, the order in which the physiological sequelae exert their effects upon neural circuits within M1 (when paired repeatedly), determines the polarity of the changes in corticospinal excitability that follow. If the corollary of the ascending afferent volley is in advance of excitation arising from TMS, potentiation tends to occur. If the sequence of these events is reversed, inhibition is more likely.

On the basis of the most common PAS variants alone, it is tempting to conclude not only that the order of the stimulus-generated cortical events is critical, but also that the effective inter-stimulus intervals lie within a very restricted range. If however consideration is extended to other contexts in which PAS has been employed, a somewhat different set of inferences is likely to be drawn. This is due to the fact that with respect to projections to the lower limb, PAS protocols that result in a corollary of the peripheral afferent volley reaching M1 tens of milliseconds after the application of TMS result in sustained increases in excitability. Furthermore, when trains of electrical stimulation are applied to the upper limb, the ISIs that are effective in potentiating the corticospinal response extend over a span of at least 50 ms.

As there is a paucity of studies in which ranges of inter-stimulus intervals have been varied systematically, particularly for target muscles in the upper limb, it is not possible to offer definitive conclusions concerning those that might prove effective in inducing facilitation or inhibition of corticospinal projections. As such, some of these questions remain open. Wolters et al. (2003) assessed ISIs of −10, 0, 5, 10, 15, 20, 25, 35, and 50 ms. Although reliable facilitation was seen only at 25 ms and reliable inhibition only at an ISI of −10 ms, intervals greater than 20 ms tended to produce facilitation, whereas ISIs of 0, 5, and 10 ms tended to produce inhibition. Weise et al. (2013) used ISIs adjusted to the N20 latency (i.e., N20 − ISI) of 5.5, 7.0, 8.5, 10, and 11.5 ms, and observed that inhibition of APB could be obtained at adjusted ISIs of 8.5 and 10 ms. Dileone et al. (2010) reported on the basis of a sample of five participants that no changes in MEP amplitude were induced by an ISI of 100 ms. A similar observation was made by Kang et al. (2011) in the context of an investigation in which ISIs of 10 and 25 ms were similarly ineffective. There is certainly considerable variability across individuals. In some people an ISI of 25 ms can depress MEP amplitude, whereas an ISI of 10 ms has a potentiating effect (Huber et al., 2008). In light of the range of inter-stimulus intervals that have proved to be effective in studies of the lower limb, and when trains of peripheral nerve stimulation are applied to the upper limb, the possibility remains that the upper boundary of that range is beyond that which is characteristic of STDP—as studied in reduced preparations. We will return to this issue in some of the sections that follow.

MUSCLE SPECIFICITY OF PAS INDUCED EFFECTS

It has frequently been proposed that PAS induced adaptation represents a form of neuroplastic modification that is synapse-specific (e.g., Nitsche et al., 2007). In this regard, the term "topographical specificity" (e.g., Morgante et al., 2006; Castel-Lacanal et al., 2007; Quartarone et al., 2008) has been used to imply that alterations in excitability brought about by PAS are restricted to the cortical representations of muscles innervated by the peripheral nerve that was stimulated electrically (Stefan et al., 2000). The empirical origins of these suppositions are however difficult to discern. In this section we assess the degree to which the extant literature supports the notion of topographical (i.e., muscle) specificity.

UPPER LIMB MUSCLES: UNITARY PERIPHERAL STIMULUS

In many studies in which PAS protocols are employed, EMG recordings are obtained only from a single (target) muscle. This is typically either the ulnar nerve innervated abductor digiti minimi (ADM), the median nerve innervated abductor pollicis brevis (APB), or the ulnar nerve innervated first dorsal interosseus (FDI). In some cases however potentials evoked in other muscles are recorded prior to and following the administration of PAS. For example, in the seminal study by Stefan et al. (2000), the median nerve was stimulated electrically (at the level of the wrist), and although APB was the primary focus of interest, MEPs were also recorded from ADM and the musculocutaneous nerve innervated biceps brachii (BB) muscle. PAS induced increases in the amplitude of MEPs recorded in each of these three muscles. Although the magnitude of the effect was larger for APB than for BB, the changes registered for the ulnar nerve innervated ADM were not distinguished from those obtained for APB—which is innervated by the nerve that received the electrical stimulation (p. 577). In at least one instance this protocol has yielded effects that are markedly larger for ADM than for APB (Cheeran et al., 2008).

Using precisely the same intervention, Quartarone et al. (2003) reported that for healthy adults, increases in the amplitudes of MEPs recorded in the ulnar nerve innervated FDI were of comparable effect size to those obtained for the (target) APB (see also Rosenkranz and Rothwell, 2006; cf. Quartarone et al., 2008; Elahi et al., 2012). Notably, Potter-Nerger et al. (2009) demonstrated elevations in the amplitude of MEPs recorded from the ulnar nerve innervated FDI, using a median nerve stimulation PAS protocol, and a similar trend for ADM, in the absence of corresponding changes for the APB muscle (see supplementary figure S1). Employing a variation of the Stefan et al. protocol in which the peripheral electrical stimulation was applied to the ulnar nerve at the wrist, Dileone et al. (2010) reported increases in the excitability of corticospinal projections to the target FDI and the median nerve innervated APB, although the latter were most prominent immediately following the cessation of the intervention. In other cases in which the changes in the excitability of corticospinal projections to non-target muscles have not been statistically reliable, the effects have consistently been in the same direction as those induced in the target muscle (e.g., APB target—ADM comparison: Fratello et al., 2006; Morgante et al., 2006; Weise et al., 2011; Popa et al., 2013; APB target—FDI comparison: Quartarone et al., 2009; ADM target—APB comparison: Weise et al., 2006).

Notably, the limited number of studies in which MEPs have been obtained for multiple muscles prior to and following the administration of 10 ms ISI PAS protocols also reveal changes in the excitability of corticospinal projections to muscles (in the hand) which are innervated by peripheral nerves other than the one that is the target of the electrical stimulation. Specifically, Weise et al. (2006, 2011) reported that when the median nerve was stimulated, 10 ms ISI PAS gave rise to decreases in MEP amplitude for the median nerve innervated APB, and increases for the ulnar nerve innervated ADM (see also Weise et al., 2013). Whereas, using a protocol in which TMS was delivered 5 ms in advance of the individual N20 latency of the median nerve SEP, Potter-Nerger et al. (2009) decreases in MEP amplitude were obtained both for the target APB and for the ulnar nerve innervated FDI (see supplementary figure S1).

UPPER LIMB MUSCLES: TRAINS OF PERIPHERAL STIMULATION

When trains of peripheral stimulation are employed, the distributed nature of the effect does not appear to be contingent upon the specific muscle that is the target of the stimulation. Castel-Lacanal et al. (2007) applied PAS comprising 10 Hz (500 ms) trains of electrical stimulation to the ECR motor point (and single pulse TMS), and obtained increases in the magnitude of MEPs that corresponded to large effect sizes for both ECR (eta-squared = 0.27) and FCR (eta-squared = 0.26). Ridding and Taylor (2001) induced a mean increase of 128 ± 132% (SD) in the excitability of corticospinal projections to the median nerve innervated FCR, by means of PAS applied to FDI. Employing the same stimulation protocol, and recording MEPs in ADM and APB, McKay et al. (2002) noted that the increases in corticospinal excitability obtained for FDI were expressed similarly for ADM. A corresponding trend was also apparent for the APB muscle.

Carson et al. (2013) demonstrated that when trains of electrical stimulation were applied to the musculocutaneous nerve innervated BB, the effects of PAS were also expressed in FCR, and in ECR—which is innervated by the radial nerve. When the FCR was the target, increases in the excitability of corticospinal projections to BB and ECR were obtained—in addition to those present for FCR. No impact of either BB or FCR focused PAS was apparent for projections to the lateral head of triceps brachii, which shares with ECR the property of innervation by the radial nerve. In contrast, Quartarone et al. (2006) reported no distributed effects in FDI and ECR, when TMS was delivered over the APB "motor hot spot" and the median nerve was stimulated at the wrist.

LOWER LIMB MUSCLES

Assessing somatotopy in relation to lower limb muscles is complicated by the use in many instances of background contractions as elements of the induction protocol. These necessarily give rise to patterns of facilitation and (e.g., antagonist) inhibition, the effects of which cannot easily be dissociated from those of the PAS. When applied during treadmill walking for example, cycle-phase-specific facilitation of TA arising from electrical stimulation of the CPN paired with TMS, also results in the suppression of MEPs recorded from semimembranosus (SM)—which is innervated by the tibial nerve (TN; Prior and Stinear, 2006). Using a (treadmill walking) PAS protocol designed to decrease the excitability of projections to TA, Stinear and Hornby (2005) reported increases in the area of MEPs recorded to SOL. Using ES delivered to the CPN, and TMS latencies determined from the N34 peak, Mrachacz-Kersting et al. (2007) reported that increases in the amplitude of TA MEPs arising from PAS delivered during weak (~5–10% MVC) dorsiflexion, were not accompanied by similar changes for SOL.

Employing ISIs designed to achieve arrival of CPN stimulation generated inputs to M1 over a range of 15–90 ms following TMS, Roy et al. (2007) observed that when PAS was delivered with the muscles quiescent, increases in the excitability of corticospinal projections were obtained not only for the target TA muscle, but also for the homologous muscle of the opposite limb. In a related context, Roy and Gorassini (2008) reported that electrical stimulation of the TN at the ankle and the posterior tibial nerve (PTN) at the knee had strong facilitatory effects on MEPs at latencies a few milliseconds after the arrival of afferent inputs at the somatosensory cortex, and that these effects were both non-specific and diffuse. Stimulation of TN at the ankle, for example, had "homotopic" (occurring at the corresponding part of the body) effects on projections to abductor hallucis (AH) and "heterotopic" effects on those to TA (see also Uy et al., 2003). Using a PAS protocol in which stimulation was delivered to the TN at the popliteal fossa, Kumpulainen et al. (2012) obtained increases in the excitability of corticospinal projections to SOL, but did not report ("$P > 0.05$") similar outcomes for TA.

A REFLECTION UPON MUSCLE SPECIFICITY

Contrary to received wisdom the empirical evidence indicates that restriction of the effects of PAS to muscles innervated by the peripheral nerve in receipt of electrical stimulation is the exception rather than the rule. Furthermore, there are several reported instances in which changes in the excitability of corticospinal projections induced by classic PAS protocols have been more pronounced for muscles that are innervated by a different nerve (e.g., Cheeran et al., 2008; Potter-Nerger et al., 2009). Indeed, given effects obtained for the ulnar nerve innervated ADM that could not be distinguished from those obtained for APB (innervated by the median nerve that received the electrical stimulation), Stefan et al. (2000) referred in their formative paper to a "somatotopic gradient." The point that the muscle specificity of the changes in corticospinal excitability brought about by PAS is relative rather than absolute, has also been made by other commentators (e.g., Quartarone et al., 2003). In some of the sections that follow we will give further consideration to mechanisms via which somatotopic gradients might emerge.

NEURAL CIRCUITS THROUGH WHICH THE EFFECTS OF PAS ARE MANIFESTED

CORTICAL

Paired pulse TMS is a tool widely used to investigate inhibitory and facilitatory circuits in the human cerebral cortex (Ortu et al., 2008). The technique involves delivery of a conditioning stimulus (s1) and a test stimulus (s2) through the same coil, with the ISI and the intensities of the two pulse being adjusted in a manner appropriate for investigation of the interneuronal circuits that are the focus of interest (Kujirai et al., 1993; Alle et al., 2009; Wagle-Shukla et al., 2009). In regards to PAS, the phenomena that have been investigated by this means include short interval intracortical inhibition (SICI) and long interval intracortical inhibition (LICI) (Kujirai et al., 1993), and intracortical facilitation (ICF).

SHORT INTERVAL INTRACORTICAL INHIBITION (SICI)

The term SICI reflects the elicitation of a response to the test stimulus that is diminished in size when it is preceded by a conditioning stimulus—at intervals typically ranging between 1 and 5 ms. It is thought that the cellular processes underlying this effect are mediated, at least in part, by GABA[a] receptors (Di Lazzaro et al., 2006; Peurala et al., 2008). While it is an over-simplification to consider changes in SICI simply as an index of GABA[a] activity—since there is little direct evidence for this association in humans, benzodiazapines, which are positive modulators of GABA[a], receptor function enhance SICI (Di Lazzaro et al., 2001). In contrast, GABA reuptake inhibitors decrease levels of SICI (Werhahn et al., 1999; Ziemann, 2004). The potential impact that PAS may have upon intracortical circuits mediating the expression of SICI has been investigated in a large number of studies. By and large these have failed to yield consistent changes in SICI following the administration of PAS25 protocols for which an intrinsic hand muscle is the target (Stefan et al., 2002; Quartarone et al., 2003; Rosenkranz and Rothwell, 2006; Sale et al., 2007, 2008; Cirillo et al., 2009; Russmann et al., 2009; Di Lazzaro et al., 2011; Elahi et al., 2012; Schabrun et al., 2013). To some degree this may reflect the fact that the expression of SICI is highly variable both within and between individuals (Wassermann, 2002). While there is very little evidence to indicate that PAS25 has a reliable effect on the manifestation of SICI (see also Ridding and Taylor, 2001; Castel-Lacanal et al., 2007; Roy et al., 2007), this does not preclude the possibility that the efficacy of the intervention is influenced by the state of the inter-neuronal networks to which the SICI technique is sensitive (Ridding and Flavel, 2006). Consistent with this hypothesis, Elahi et al. (2012) demonstrated that when SICI is evoked simultaneously with the administration of a PAS25 protocol, the usual facilitation of corticospinal excitability is not obtained. With respect to PAS10 protocols, we are aware of only two studies in which SICI has been monitored in conjunction with this variant. Both Russmann et al. (2009) and Di Lazzaro et al. (2011) reported decreases in this measure of intracortical inhibition as a result of the intervention.

LONG INTERVAL INTRA-CORTICAL INHIBITION (LICI)

Long interval intra-cortical inhibition (LICI) is measured at ISIs between 50 and 200 ms. It is putatively mediated by GABA[b] receptors (Werhahn et al., 1999; McDonnell et al., 2006). While the effects of a facilitating PAS protocol (N20+2) are blunted by the prior administration of Baclofen (BAC)—a selective GABA[b] receptor agonist, it does not necessarily follow that the state of cortical circuits sampled by the LICI technique will be altered by its administration. Meunier et al. (2012) did however observe that LICI decreased when afferent stimulation was paired (25 ms ISI) with "low intensity" TMS (evoking a MEP of 0.5 mV), but not when an intensity of TMS sufficient to generate an MEP of 1 mV in the target FPB muscle was used. Similarly, Russmann et al. (2009) reported that LICI was reduced by administration of a PAS25 protocol (evoking a MEP of 0.5 mV in FPB), and increased transiently by a PAS10 variant. De Beaumont et al. (2012) found no significant changes in LICI arising from the application of a PAS10 intervention in which afferent stimuli were paired with TMS at an intensity that produced a MEP of 1 mV in the target APB. Notwithstanding other variations in protocol, on the basis of the small number of studies that have been completed, it appears that when the intensity of the cortical stimulus is moderate (leading to 0.5 mV MEPs in intrinsic hand muscles), PAS25 leads to a decrease in LICI, whereas PAS10 may cause an increase in LICI.

INTRACORTICAL FACILITATION (ICF)

The term ICF refers to the elicitation of a response to the test stimulus that is increased in size when it is preceded by a conditioning stimulus—at intervals typically ranging between 7 and 20 ms, in the context of protocols similar to those used to elicit SICI (Kujirai et al., 1993; Ziemann et al., 1996). While it is believed that the net facilitation arises from a strong potentiating effect and a weaker inhibitory component (Hanajima et al., 1998; Hanajima and Ugawa, 2008), pharmacological studies that the dominant element is mediated by glutamatergic M-methyl-D-asparate (NMDA) receptors (Ziemann et al., 1998; Schwenkreis et al., 1999). As benzodiazepines also increase ICF however, a contribution of GABA[a] receptors—expressed through the inhibitory component cannot be excluded (Ziemann, 2008). No changes in ICF have however been reported when PAS25 protocols have been employed, and hand muscles are the focus of interest (Di Lazzaro et al., 2011—15 ms ISI; Elahi et al., 2012 and Sale et al., 2007—10 ms ISI; Schabrun et al., 2013—13 ms). Similarly, no impact upon ICF has been observed when muscles in the lower limb (Roy et al., 2007) or the forearm (Castel-Lacanal et al., 2007) have been investigated. As Elahi et al. (2012) failed to demonstrate that ICF evoked simultaneously with the administration of a PAS25 protocol, exerted an impact upon the usual facilitation of corticospinal excitability, it can also be surmised that the efficacy of the intervention is insensitive to the state of the inter-neuronal networks sampled by the ICF technique.

SHORT-INTERVAL INTRACORTICAL FACILITATION (SICF)

It is also possible to obtain facilitation of a subthreshold test stimulus when a prior conditioning stimulus of threshold or suprathreshold intensity is delivered at discrete intervals of 1.0–1.5 ms, 2.5–3.0 ms and at ≈4.5 ms (Tokimura et al., 1996; Ilic et al., 2002). As the effect is not obtained when transcranial electrical stimulation (TES) is substituted for the magnetic stimulus, a M1 locus for what is termed short-interval intracortical facilitation (SICF) is presumed. In particular, as the effective ISIs are closely related to I-wave periodicity, an instrumental relationship is suspected (e.g., Hanajima and Ugawa, 2008). Benzodiazepines and barbiturates, which enhance the action of GABA[a] receptors, attenuate SICF (Ziemann et al., 1998; Ilic et al., 2002), whereas the NMDA receptor antagonist memantine does not alter the effect. To the best of our knowledge, the impact of PAS upon SICF has been investigated in only one instance. Ridding and Taylor (2001) reported that SICF increased at short ISIs (0.8–1.7 ms) following administration of a protocol that comprised trains of afferent stimulation.

CORTICAL SILENT PERIOD (CSP)

Following the elicitation of a MEP in a contracting peripheral muscle, there occurs a period of EMG silence. While spinal circuitry may be implicated in the early (~50 ms) part of the silent period, the subsequent portion appears to be due to processes operating at the level of the cerebral cortex (Wilson et al., 1993; Ziemann et al., 1993; Brasil-Neto et al., 1995; Chen et al., 1999b; Tergau et al., 1999). The duration of the cortical silent period (CSP) is influenced to a greater degree by TMS intensity than level of muscle contraction (Kojima et al., 2013). As it shares this property with the degree of SICI induced by TMS (i.e., CS intensity), which is not the case for ICF, it has been proposed that the CSP duration is governed by the state of inhibitory interneurons within M1 that also mediate the expression of SICI (Kojima et al., 2013). On the basis of a review of pharmacological interventions it has been suggested previously (Ziemann, 2004) that, as with LICI, the duration of the late part of the CSP is mediated by $GABA^b$ receptors. An elongation of CSP duration following the administration of PAS25 protocols has been reported on numerous occasions (Stefan et al., 2000, 2004; Quartarone et al., 2003; Sale et al., 2007, 2008; Cirillo et al., 2009; De Beaumont et al., 2012; Elahi et al., 2012; cf. Di Lazzaro et al., 2011). In the single study in which this measure has been used to examine a PAS protocol that utilizes trains of afferent stimulation (Ridding and Taylor, 2001), no such prolongation was obtained. In addition, it appears that duration of the CSP is not influenced by a PAS10 protocol (Di Lazzaro et al., 2011; De Beaumont et al., 2012) or a N20-5 protocol (Potter-Nerger et al., 2009).

SHORT AFFERENT INHIBITION (SAI)

The term short afferent inhibition (SAI) refers to the diminution of MEP amplitude that occurs following administration of a prior conditioning afferent stimulus (typically 0.2–1 ms duration at an intensity 2—3 times perceptual threshold or that which evokes a visible twitch in the target muscle) applied to a peripheral nerve. The latency at which the effect is most prominent is 13–19 ms when forearm muscles (FCR and ECR) are the focus of interest, and the nerve is stimulated at the level of the elbow (Bertolasi et al., 1998), and ~20 ms when hand muscles (i.e., FDI and APB) are under investigation and nerve (i.e., median) stimulation is applied at the wrist (Tokimura et al., 2000). It is thought that the effect is produced by modulation of the I2 and I3 waves of the descending corticospinal volley (Tokimura et al., 2000). As scopolamine (an Ach antagonist) reduces SAI, but does not exert a similar influence on SICI, distinct mediating neural circuits are presumed (Di Lazzaro et al., 2000). In addition, the benzodiazepine lorazepam increases SICI, but decreases SAI (Di Lazzaro et al., 2005). Electrophysiological studies of the interactions between SICI and SAI further suggest that these phenomena are expressed via the influence of distinct, but convergent and reciprocally connected, GABAergic inhibitory interneurons that project onto corticospinal neurons (Alle et al., 2009). When MEPs are recorded during the administration of PAS, they are attenuated initially (with respect to pre-intervention controls), most likely as a consequence of SAI type effects. This effect declines through the time course of the induction period (e.g., Di Lazzaro et al., 2011; Elahi et al., 2012; Hamada et al., 2012), presumably due to the overall increase in the excitability of the corticospinal projections brought about by the intervention. When however the amplitude of the MEP obtained following the conditioning afferent stimulus is normalized with respect to the amplitude of a test stimulus alone, no changes in SAI are seen to occur as a result of conventional PAS25 protocols (Stefan et al., 2002; Di Lazzaro et al., 2011; Elahi et al., 2012; Hamada et al., 2012; Schabrun et al., 2013). In this respect therefore, SAI mirrors SICI. The two measures do however diverge in so much as no change in SAI has been reported following PAS10 (Di Lazzaro et al., 2011), whereas in this context a decrease in SICI is obtained (Russmann et al., 2009; Di Lazzaro et al., 2011).

LONG AFFERENT INHIBITION (LAI)

The attenuation of MEP amplitude that is also obtained when the interval between the peripheral afferent stimulation and the subsequent TMS is in the region of 200 ms is referred to as long-latency afferent inhibition (Sailer et al., 2002, 2003). As the amplitude of the F-wave evoked by supramaximal stimulation of the peripheral nerve is not reduced at a conditioning-test interval of 200 ms, the post-synaptic state of spinal motoneurons is not believed to be a principal determinant (Chen et al., 1999a). A contribution of cortical structures in addition to the primary sensory and motor areas, and of sub-cortical elements, to the expression of LAI cannot however be excluded (Classen et al., 2000; Sailer et al., 2003, 2007). On the basis of observations that LAI interacts with (inhibits) LICI, it has been inferred that there is some degree of shared mediation by $GABA^b$ receptors (Sailer et al., 2002), however the neurotransmitters involved in LAI have not yet been corroborated using pharmacological approaches (Ni et al., 2011). Using a PAS25 protocol based on "low intensity" TMS (evoking a MEP of 0.5 mV), Meunier et al. (2012) reported immediate and sustained decreases in LAI (150 ms ISI) evoked for projections to the target FPB—an effect that was broadly similar to that expressed for LICI. No such changes were obtained when an intensity of TMS sufficient to generate an MEP of 1 mV in the target FPB muscle was used in the delivery of PAS. Consistent with these outcomes, Russmann et al. (2009) demonstrated a reduction in LAI (150 ms ISI) evoked in FPB that followed the time course of decreases in LICI induced by a PAS25 (low intensity TMS) protocol (there was no consistent change attributable to PAS10). In contrast, marked increases in LAI (240 ms ISI) were observed following PAS25, whereas decreases were seen following PAS10 (Russmann et al., 2009).

SPINAL

In the small number of studies that have sought to examine potential changes in excitability at the level of the spinal cord following PAS, F-waves have most commonly been obtained, even though this technique has characteristics that limit its effectiveness as a test of spinal motoneuron excitability, a problem that is particular acute when comparisons are drawn with responses evoked by cortical magnetic stimulation (Carson et al., 2004; Taylor, 2006). Investigations utilizing this approach have generally failed to obtain indications of changes in spinal motoneuron excitability following PAS (Stefan et al., 2000; Wolters et al., 2003; Quartarone et al., 2006; Meunier et al., 2007; Mrachacz-Kersting et al., 2007; Thabit et al., 2010). Converging findings have however been derived using electrical transmastoid (cervicomedullary) stimulation, which activates corticospinal axons below the level of the cortex (Ugawa et al., 1991; Taylor et al., 2002). As this technique is uncomfortable it has been used sparingly in PAS studies, and in each case a very small number of participants has been assessed (Stefan et al., 2000; McKay et al., 2002; Wolters et al., 2003).

Employing FCR as the target muscle, and using a PAS protocol in which median nerve stimulation was paired with TMS, Meunier et al. (2007), reported that changes in the slope of the H reflex recruitment curve occurred in parallel with intervention induced increases in corticospinal excitability. A similar pattern was obtained in the small number of participants from whom H-reflexes could be elicited in APB, when a PAS25 protocol was used with this muscle as the target. In a follow up study, it was demonstrated that the PAS-induced change in the H-reflex is mediated by a decrease of presynaptic Ia inhibition of FCR terminals (Lamy et al., 2010). On the basis of the evidence currently available, it is not possible to resolve whether this effect is contingent upon alteration of descending inputs to presynaptic interneurons acting on the Ia pathway, or changes in presynaptic networks at the spinal level. It has been remarked that presynaptic [primary afferent depolarization (PAD)] interneurons, which receive extensive projections from Ia, Ib, and cutaneous afferents, may play an instrumental role in the latter regard (Lamy et al., 2010). It is also worth noting in this context that conventional PAS protocols (e.g., Stefan et al., 2000) employ a level of peripheral nerve stimulation (i.e., 3 × perceptual threshold) that is sufficient to elicit a contraction of the target muscle (Kennedy and Carson, 2008), and thus generate secondary reafference. The implications of this will be given further consideration in sections that follow. Roy et al. (2007) failed to obtain changes in the amplitude of H-reflexes recorded in TA, arising from a PAS protocol that induced increases in corticospinal excitability.

A REFLECTION ON THE EXPRESSION OF PAS-INDUCED EFFECTS

The most direct source of evidence available in humans—that based on recording corticospinal volleys via electrodes implanted in the cervical epidural space (of 4 individuals), indicates that the PAS25 protocol does not alter the first wave of descending excitation generated by TMS given subsequently, but increases the amplitude of later waves (Di Lazzaro et al., 2009a). The complementary finding (from 2 individuals) is that the PAS10 protocol does not alter the first wave of descending excitation, but decreases the amplitude of later waves (Di Lazzaro et al., 2009b). In light of these results, and given indications that the post-synaptic state of spinal motoneurons is not altered by PAS, it is reasonable to conclude that the observed changes in corticospinal excitability are mediated principally at the level of the cortex. Is it also possible to resolve specific circuits within cortex that are implicated?

The summary conclusions that can be drawn from the studies described above are that (corticospinal) excitability enhancing PAS protocols (e.g., PAS25) do not alter expressions of SICI, ICF, or SAI. They do however elongate the CSP, and may decrease LICI and LAI (when the peripheral stimulation applied during PAS is paired with low intensity TMS). Inhibitory protocols (e.g., PAS10) have been investigated less thoroughly. As a consequence, it is possible to surmise only that they tend to decrease SICI, and have no apparent influence on the CSP.

On the basis of indications that TMS invoked silent periods were shortened by the delivery of (single pulse) high-intensity peripheral nerve stimulation over a range of intervals from 30 ms before to 70 ms after TMS (with the largest effect present at 20 ms before), Hess et al. (1999) concluded that the somatosensory input generated by the peripheral stimulation has privileged access to inhibitory interneuronal circuits within M1. In respect of observations that both the extent of LICI and the duration of the CSP increased with eliciting stimulus intensity, Hammond and Vallence (2007) proposed that the long-latency inhibitory circuits that mediate the LICI effect, are also those through which afferent feedback from the contracting muscle acts to modulate the time course of the silent period (see also Taylor et al., 1997; Thabit et al., 2010; Farzan et al., 2013). Given the equivalent pattern of variation that is obtained for LICI, LAI and the duration of the CSP, it might therefore be surmised that the state of these long latency inhibitory circuits is altered by facilitatory variants of PAS. Is it possible that the changes in late I-waves engendered by excitability enhancing forms of PAS reflect tonic modification of GABA[b]mediated projections operating via these circuits (e.g., Humeau et al., 2003).

With respect to LAI, it is notable that the measure itself does not exhibit muscle specificity. If the conditioning stimulus is applied to the median nerve at the wrist, in a fashion similar to that used in PAS protocols, the inhibition of MEP amplitude that is observed at an ISI of 200 ms is obtained not only for APB (median nerve innervated), but also for the FDI (Chen et al., 1999a; Abbruzzese et al., 2001), FCR (Abbruzzese et al., 2001), and ECR (Chen et al., 1999a) muscles. When an ISI of 100 ms is used, median nerve stimulation evokes equivalent levels of LAI in projections to APB, ADM, and FDI (Kotb et al., 2005). Similarly in relation to SAI, if the median nerve is stimulated at the wrist and an ISI ≈20 ms is employed, inhibition is obtained not only for APB, but also for FDI (Tokimura et al., 2000; Kotb et al., 2005; Devanne et al., 2009), ADM (Kotb et al., 2005), and ECR (Devanne et al., 2009). Median nerve stimulation at the antecubital fossa and radial nerve stimulation in the spiral groove each generate comparable SAI in projections to both FCR and ECR. If the ISI is defined in relation to the N20 component of the SEP, ISIs of N20, N2+2, and N20+4 elicit SAI in both FDI and APB when either the median and ulnar nerve are stimulated. In both cases, the level of inhibition is accentuated by increasing the intensity of afferent stimulation (Fischer and Orth, 2011). As such, with respect to both SAI and LAI there is a parallel with the lack of muscle specificity that characterizes the effects of PAS.

While consideration of the intracortical neural circuits that mediate the expression of phenomena such as SAI and LAI may provide insights in relation to those that are instrumental in relation to the effects of PAS, in any such assessment, it is necessary to maintain a conceptual distinction between circuits that may be necessary for the induction of changes in corticospinal output, but which are not altered functionally by the administration of PAS, and those that are modified acutely by PAS. In some but not necessarily all of these latter cases, the PAS induced changes may impact upon the excitability of descending corticospinal projections as registered through responses to TMS (i.e., at rest), or on voluntary motor output. For example, while it may be the case that a lack of muscle specificity is a characteristic shared by SAI, LAI and the effects of PAS, only the expression of long-latency afferent inhibition (LAI) but not that of SAI is altered by the intervention. Furthermore, although levels of SICI are not altered by PAS25, increases in corticospinal excitability normally induced by this protocol are blocked when SICI is evoked simultaneously with its administration (Elahi et al., 2012; see also Weise et al., 2013). In seeking to understand the roles played by specific circuits within cortex in mediating the effects of PAS, it would be extremely useful to have further interference studies of this type. To date however, pharmacological studies have provided the main source of evidence upon which to derive causal inferences, albeit at a systems level.

PHARMACOLOGY OF PAS-INDUCED EFFECTS

As there are authoritative and comprehensive reviews dealing with the pharmacology of neuroplastic responses to non-invasive brain stimulation (Nitsche et al., 2012), and of cortical excitability measures (Ziemann, 2004, 2008; Paulus et al., 2008), we hereby provide only a summary pertinent to PAS that draws in part upon these previous works. Indeed, we explicitly adopt the structure of presentation of Nitsche et al. (2012)—conceiving of the glutamatergic system, voltage-gated ion channels and the GABAergic system as "drivers" of neuroplastic adaptation, and referring to the dopaminergic, cholinergic, serotonergic, and adrenergic systems as "modulators" of neuroplastic adaptation.

THE GLUTAMATERGIC SYSTEM—A DRIVER OF NEUROPLASTIC ADAPTATION

As the N-methyl-d-aspartate (NMDA) receptor antagonist dextromethorphan (150 mg dose) blocks both the excitability enhancing effects of PAS25 (Stefan et al., 2002) and the excitability reducing effects of PAS10 (Wolters et al., 2003), a generalized dependence upon on NMDA receptor activation has been deduced. This drug is however also thought to act as a non-selective serotonin reuptake inhibitor, and as a sigma-1 receptor agonist with influence upon calcium signaling.

VOLTAGE-GATED ION CHANNELS—A DRIVER OF NEUROPLASTIC ADAPTATION

It has been reported that the voltage-gated sodium channel blocker lamotrigine tends to reduce the facilitating effect of a N20+2 PAS protocol (Heidegger et al., 2010). Nimodipine, which blocks L-type (long-lasting) voltage-gated calcium channels, eliminates the excitability reducing effects of PAS10 when given as a 30 mg dose (Wolters et al., 2003). It is thought that when applied chronically, but not acutely, in experimental systems, Gabapentin inhibits calcium currents through an influence on the trafficking of voltage-gated Ca^{2+} channels (Hendrich et al., 2008; but see also Eroglu et al., 2009). Administration of the drug (1100 mg) does not impact on the usually obtained effects of N20+2 PAS (Heidegger et al., 2010). Although the precise mode of action of the anticonvulsant levetiracetam has not always been clear, it is now believed that it inhibits voltage-gated Ca^{2+} channels (Vogl et al., 2012). A 3000 mg dose of this drug abolishes the increases in MEP amplitude otherwise induced by N20+2 PAS (Heidegger et al., 2010).

THE GABAERGIC SYSTEM—A DRIVER OF NEUROPLASTIC ADAPTATION

The facilitating effects of N20+2 PAS are blunted by 50 mg of the $GABA^b$ receptor agonist baclofen (McDonnell et al., 2007). They are also diminished by administration of diazepam (20 mg)—a positive allosteric (binding to a specific subunit on the $GABA^a$ receptor at a site distinct from the that of the endogenous GABA molecule) modulator of GABA (Heidegger et al., 2010). Tiagabine (25 mg) that is thought to act as a selective GABA reuptake inhibitor, permitting increased GABA availability for postsynaptic receptor binding, exerts a similar action (Heidegger et al., 2010). On the other hand, topiramate—having pharmacological properties that may include augmentation of $GABA^a$ mediated inhibition (blockage of voltage-dependent sodium channels), has no such effects in 100 mg dosage (Heidegger et al., 2010).

THE DOPAMINERGIC SYSTEM—A MODULATOR OF NEUROPLASTIC ADAPTATION

Thirugnanasambandam et al. (2011b) delivered low (25 mg), medium (100 mg), or high (200 mg) doses of levodopa prior to PAS in 12 healthy volunteers. In low dose, levodopa abolished the usual effects of both PAS10 and PAS25 variants. In medium dosage, the induced effects were indistinguishable from those obtained in placebo conditions. At high dosage, the prior delivery of levodopa gave rise to an inhibitory influence of the PAS25 protocol on MEP amplitude, whereas the impact of PAS10 could not be differentiated from the placebo condition. This set of outcomes contrasts with the results of Kuo et al. (2008) who observed that a 100 mg dose of levodopa enhances the magnitude and duration of increases in corticospinal excitability induced by PAS25.

Administration of 400 mg of the selective dopamine D2 and D3 receptor antagonist sulpiride (with the intent of increasing the relative contribution of D1 receptors to dopaminergic activity) eliminates the inhibitory effects of PAS10, but has no impact upon increases in excitability brought about by PAS25. When however sulpiride (400 mg) was given in combination with 100 mg of levodopa, the inhibitory effect of PAS10 was preserved (and a typical profile of response to PAS25 obtained) (Nitsche et al., 2009). A 2 mg dose of the selective dopamine D2 receptor agonist Cabergoline does not appear to influence the excitability enhancing effects of N20+2 PAS (Korchounov and Ziemann, 2011). The D2 receptor agonist ropinirole exhibits an inverted "U"-shaped dose–response curve, whereby both high (1.0 mg) or low (0.125 mg) dosages of the drug impair the effects of a PAS25 protocol, whereas the attenuation exhibited following a medium dose (0.5 mg) is less pronounced. In contrast, ropinirole has no apparent impact upon the impact of PAS10 (Monte-Silva et al., 2009).

Haloperidol exhibits high affinity dopamine D2 receptor antagonism. When a 2.5 mg dose of the drug is given 2 h in advance of a N20+2 protocol, the usual facilitating effects of this intervention are not obtained (Korchounov and Ziemann, 2011). Methylphenidate acts primarily to inhibit the reuptake of dopamine and to a lesser extent norepinephrine, thus increasing the extracellular concentrations of these neurotransmitters. The prior delivery of 40 mg of this agent has no apparent impact upon the efficacy of N20+2 PAS (Korchounov and Ziemann, 2011).

THE CHOLINERGIC SYSTEM—A MODULATOR OF NEUROPLASTIC ADAPTATION

If the activity of the two major acetylcholine receptor subtypes [muscarinergic (mAChR) and nicotinergic (nAChR)] is promoted by administration of the cholinesterase inhibitor rivastigmine (3 mg), the positive impact on corticospinal excitability of PAS25 is enhanced relative to a placebo condition, between 20 and 30 min following the cessation of paired stimulation. The inhibitory effects of PAS10 are also accentuated, and particularly pronounced during a period from 25 min to 2 h post stimulation (Kuo et al., 2007). In contrast however, the cholinesterase inhibitor Tacrine (40 mg) does not appear to alter the effects of a N20+2 protocol (Korchounov and Ziemann, 2011). Using transdermal patches able to deliver 15 mg of nicotine (i.e., a nAChR receptor agonist) over 16 h, Thirugnanasambandam et al. (2011a) reported that when paired stimulation commenced 6 h following application of the patch, the effects of PAS25 were not distinguished from a placebo condition. On the other hand, the usual inhibitory influence of PAS10 was eliminated by the administration of nicotine. Biperiden is a M1 muscarinic receptor (mAChR) antagonist. When an 8 mg dose is delivered 2 h before N20+2 PAS, there is marked attenuation of the increases in corticospinal excitability otherwise obtained in placebo conditions (Korchounov and Ziemann, 2011).

THE SEROTONERGIC SYSTEM—A MODULATOR OF NEUROPLASTIC ADAPTATION

Batsikadze et al. (2013) administered 20 mg of the selective serotonin reuptake inhibitor (SSRI) citalopram 2 h prior to the commencement of PAS. In the presence of the drug there was a failure to obtain the diminution of MEP amplitude otherwise obtained in the 30 min following PAS10. There was however no consistent impact of citalopram on the usual excitability enhancing effects of a PAS25 protocol.

THE ADRENERGIC SYSTEM—A MODULATOR OF NEUROPLASTIC ADAPTATION

The mode of action of methylphenidate is such that it leads to increased extracellular concentrations of both norepinephrine (i.e., noradrenaline) and dopamine. As noted above, it has no apparent influence on the effects of N20+2 PAS (Korchounov and Ziemann, 2011). Prazosin is an alpha-adrenergic antagonist that is specific for the alpha-1 receptors. The prior delivery of 1 mg of the drug eliminates the increases in MEP amplitude otherwise induced by a N20+2 protocol (Korchounov and Ziemann, 2011).

A REFLECTION ON PHARMACOLOGICAL STUDIES OF PAS-INDUCED EFFECTS

Pharmacological studies such as those described above are conceptually powerful in so much as they offer the prospect of causal inference with respect to cellular pathways that are necessary for realizing the effects of non-invasive stimulation protocols such as PAS. In practice there are caveats. These agents—which are typically introduced by oral administration, act at a systems level i.e., not only upon the neural circuits that may be engaged by a particular intervention. In addition, the drugs used most often in human experimentation do not have an exclusive mode of action. It has been highlighted previously (e.g., Paulus et al., 2008) that strong inferences can generally only be drawn in circumstances in which a set of drugs sharing a specific mode of action exhibit consistency in their effect upon the phenomenon that is the focus of interest. Furthermore, effective blinding of participants is often precluded by the side effects of these agents that may include nausea (e.g., Wolters et al., 2003; Monte-Silva et al., 2009; Korchounov and Ziemann, 2011) and sedation (e.g., Korchounov and Ziemann, 2011). There is a paucity of replication studies, and in only a very small number of investigations have dose dependencies been examined. Indeed, ethical considerations necessarily impose limits on the dosages of many drugs that can reasonably be employed with human volunteers.

These matters notwithstanding, is it possible to discern patterns of variation that intimate the cellular mechanisms mediating responses to PAS. With respect to the notional drivers of neuroplastic adaptation, drugs (with the exception of topiramate) that enhance the effects of GABA lead to diminution of the increases in excitability otherwise brought about by N20+2 PAS protocols. Dextromethorphan acts in part as an NMDA receptor antagonist. Its administration blunts the impact of both PAS25 and PAS10 interventions. In relation to drugs that disrupt the action of voltage-gated calcium channels, the effects of N20+2 PAS are diminished by levetiracetam, and those of PAS10 are reduced by nimodipine. Taken at face value, these studies suggest that the effects of both excitatory *and* inhibitory PAS protocols are dependent on both NMDA receptor activation and voltage-dependent Ca^{2+} channels (cf. Muller-Dahlhaus et al., 2010). In addition, they indicate that GABAergic circuits may also play a regulating role in relation to (corticospinal) excitability enhancing forms of PAS. In this regard, there is as yet no information readily available concerning GABAergic mediation of excitability diminishing variants.

Although designated a *modulator* of neuroplastic adaptation, as revealed by the impact of D2/D3 receptor antagonists, the dopaminergic system appears to assume a necessary role in relation to the changes in corticospinal excitability brought about by PAS. It is also notable that the administration of levodopa provides one of the few instances (Kuo et al., 2008) in which a pharmacological agent accentuates the effects of PAS (see also Kuo et al., 2007). Nonetheless, the complex influence of this particular agent and D2 receptor agonists, in particular the presence of non-linear dose-response relationships, precludes a simple interpretation of the part played by dopamine. The role of the cholinergic system is similarly elaborate. At least one cholinesterase inhibitor appears to enhance the effects of both excitatory and inhibitory PAS protocols. In addition, the nAChR receptor agonist nicotine selectively dissipates the inhibitory influence of PAS10, whereas the mAChR receptor antagonist Biperiden has a similar impact on the efficacy of an excitatory N20+2 protocol.

With respect to the serotonergic system, at least one agent that increases the extracellular level of the neurotransmitter impedes the inhibitory influence of PAS10. Concerning the adrenergic system, alpha-adrenergic blockade exerts an attenuating influence on the otherwise excitatory effects of N20+2 PAS.

Taken together, these studies paint a picture of multiple cellular mechanisms acting via a complex web of relationships that together mediate the changes in corticospinal excitability induced by both excitatory and inhibitory variants of PAS. The current state of knowledge concerning the cellular foundations of PAS-induced neuroplastic adaptation is sufficiently impoverished that predictions in relation to the outcome of any particular pharmacological perturbation are often usurped by the experimental data. For example, dopamine, norepinephrine, and acetylcholine receptor agonists fail to further augment PAS-induced effects in a context in which there is unlikely to have been saturation of corticospinal excitability (Korchounov and Ziemann, 2011). In light of the conclusion that multiple cellular pathways are almost certainly involved in giving expression to the effects of PAS (e.g., Muller-Dahlhaus et al., 2010; Hamada et al., 2012), we turn our consideration now to mechanisms through which the constituent elements of PAS (i.e., peripheral and cortical) may exert their influence.

CONSTITUENT ELEMENTS OF PAS—SENSORY STIMULATION

On the basis of information derived using neuroimaging techniques, the conclusion has been drawn that the form of peripheral afferent stimulation applied in PAS protocols, first engages circuits in the primary somatosensory cortex (S1) within the postcentral gyrus, the second somatosensory area (S2) within the parietal operculum, and the posterior parietal cortex (Korvenoja et al., 1999; Boakye et al., 2000). In relation to mediating the effects of PAS, the temporal characteristics of this engagement are particularly salient. Electrical stimulation of peripheral afferents elicits complex cortical responses that are discernible as SEPs in scalp EEG recordings, and as somatosensory-evoked fields when magnetoencephalography (MEG) is used. There is widespread agreement that the earliest N20 SEP response following electrical stimulation of the median nerve, arises from contralateral (S1) Brodmann area 3b. The balance of evidence now also suggests that the P22 SEP component has its origin in Brodmann area 1 (i.e., S1), rather than for example M1 (Baumgartner et al., 2010). Indeed, a S1 source is in general presumed for short-latency potentials occurring within the first 40 ms following the median nerve stimulus (Allison et al., 1991). Nonetheless, the presence of synchronized neuronal population activity in S2 (registered by MEG) at these latencies, while suggesting an influence of cortical afferents from SI, does not preclude a presence of additional parallel thalamocortical projections to S2 (Karhu and Tesche, 1999). Although there is not yet consensus in relation to the medium latency (>40 ms) components, a distributed pattern of activation that includes not only S1, but also S2 bilaterally, and contralateral posterior parietal cortex is indicated (Hari et al., 1984; Allison et al., 1989a,b, 1992; Forss et al., 1994). These sources continue to be active simultaneously during a period 70–140 ms following the onset of stimulation (Mauguiere et al., 1997). In addition, when trains of afferent stimulation are applied, the offset of the train gives rise to a (P100 and N140) SEP signature distinct from that associated with the individual stimuli (Yamashiro et al., 2008, 2009).

With respect to these temporal features, it is must be emphasized that SEPs (or fields) do not afford unambiguous interpretation. It is well-established that in order to create electrical fields large enough to propagate through the brain, dura, skull, and skin, in the order of 10^7 of neurons must be active simultaneously. While it is clearly possible to isolate and measure modulations of averaged SEP waveforms generated by the mass action of many neurons, it can be argued that such features as the latency of the peak are arbitrary are no more representative of the temporal dynamics of the latent neural processes than the beginning or end of the deflection (Luck, 2005). It is also typically the case that the voltage fluctuations of the components of a SEP waveform inherently overlap with each other in time and space (see Woodman, 2010, for a review). A deeper problem arises from the corresponding implication that it is not possible on the basis of EEG or MEG measurements to infer temporally discrete propagation of a response to a unitary stimulus (Luck, 2005). These issues have implications not simply in relation to the interpretation of somatosensory-evoked field and potentials, they are pertinent to assumptions that might be made concerning the time course over which peripheral afferent stimulation exerts its effects in the context of PAS.

Ambiguity in relation to the routes via which, and the time course over which, the afferent component of PAS protocols might exert its influence upon the output circuits of primary motor cortex is compounded by the customary use of levels of stimulation above MT. The majority of PAS studies employing mixed nerve targets have used an intensity defined as three times perceptual threshold (e.g., Stefan et al., 2000; Wolters et al., 2003; Sale et al., 2007; Tecchio et al., 2008), which corresponds to a level at which motor potentials are generated (Litvak et al., 2007; Kennedy and Carson, 2008). In the case of trains delivered to the motor point of the target muscle, the stimulation intensity is defined explicitly in relation to the evocation of a visible muscle contraction (Ridding and Taylor, 2001; Castel-Lacanal et al., 2007; Kennedy and Carson, 2008; Carson et al., 2013). Necessarily therefore, in addition to the initial ascending afferent volley induced directly by electrical stimulation of the nerve, all current PAS protocols are likely to encapsulate secondary reafference arising from muscle contractions (Schabrun et al., 2012). The extent of the neural activity induced in M1 by such reafference can be substantially greater than that brought about by the direct sensory consequences of peripheral stimulation (Shitara et al., 2013).

There is in addition a related body of evidence concerning the effects of manipulating the intensity of (electrical) peripheral afferent stimulation. When registered using fMRI, contralateral S1 activity scales with levels of stimulation (at least up to MT) (see also Nelson et al., 2004). The bilateral response obtained for S2 and in posterior parietal cortex does not vary in this manner, although a BOLD response in S2 is registered at lower levels of stimulation than in S1, and is augmented when the participant's attention is directed explicitly to the stimulus (Backes et al., 2000).

Similarly, Smith et al. (2003) reported a dose-response relationship for the S1 BOLD response when stimulation was delivered over the quadriceps muscle. Furthermore, the representational overlap of adjacent fingers derived from the BOLD signal in different subdivisions of S1 increases as the intensity of single digit electrical stimulation is increased (Krause et al., 2001).

When median nerve stimulation (0.2 ms pulse) is delivered at 2 Hz, in a range between the sensory threshold (ST) and 1.2 times MT, the amplitude of the components N9, N20, and N20-P25 SEP components increases in proportion to stimulation intensity (cf. Lakhani et al., 2012; Gatica Tossi et al., 2013), an effect that remains evident at 2.5 times MT (Urasaki et al., 1998). While components of the S1 SEP appear to saturate at some point below the pain threshold (PT) (Parain and Delapierre, 1991), MEG recordings suggest that the asymptote of the S2 response occurs at lower stimulation intensities than for the S1 response (Lin et al., 2003). In general the relationship between stimulus intensity and the overall magnitude of the SEP can be characterized as a decelerating power function (Hashimoto et al., 1992). This process, whereby small and desynchronized peripheral volleys are manifested as synchronous cortical potentials has been referred to as CNS amplification (Eisen et al., 1982; Urasaki et al., 1998). Since there is no difference in the extent to which this phenomenon is expressed in the P14 potential that originates from the cervicomedullary junction and the cortical N20/P25 component, it has been concluded that the amplification arises at the cuneate nucleus, and is maintained at the level of S1 (Urasaki et al., 1998).

Studies in cat indicate that stimulation of sensory cortex can induce long-lasting potentiation of synaptic potentials evoked in the motor cortex (Sakamoto et al., 1987). Elevated activity registered by fMRI (Spiegel et al., 1999) and by MEG (Kawamura et al., 1996) is evident in both contralateral S1 and M1 when median nerve stimulation at motor threshold intensity is used. It is notable therefore that when the intensity of peripheral nerve stimulation applied in humans is between 30 and 50% of that required to produce a maximum compound muscle action potential (M-max i.e., well in excess of that used in SAI paradigms), MEPs-evoked subsequently by TMS over M1 are facilitated at ISIs from 25 to 60 ms in APB (following median nerve stimulation at the wrist), and at ISIs from 40 to 65 ms in flexor hallucis brevis (following TN stimulation at the ankle) (Deletis et al., 1992). A similar outcome was noted (Komori et al., 1992) for the thenar muscle at ISIs between 50 and 80 ms when the peripheral shock was set to 10% of M-max. Devanne et al. (2009) reported than even when stimulation intensity is set just above motor threshold, median nerve stimulation (at the wrist) gives rise to marked facilitation of MEPs recorded in APB, FDI, and ECR when ISIs ranging from 40 to 80 ms are employed. When corticospinal excitability is assessed prior to and following the delivery of extended (up to 2 h) sequences of (electrical) peripheral afferent stimuli resembling those used in PAS protocols, intensities close to MT tend to induce facilitation (Kaelin-Lang et al., 2002; Charlton et al., 2003). These findings are consistent with other indications that given a sufficient intensity of afferent stimulation—whether this is achieved by increases in the current/voltage of individual shocks, and/or by a higher frequency of delivery increases in the excitability of corticospinal projections from the primary motor cortex can be induced by this means alone (e.g., Ridding et al., 2000; Khaslavskaia et al., 2002; McKay et al., 2002; Knash et al., 2003; Chipchase et al., 2011; Schabrun et al., 2012, see also Luft et al., 2002).

While the magnitude and duration of the increase in corticospinal excitability induced by PAS25 scales with the number of stimulus pairs (Nitsche et al., 2007), we are not aware of any instances in which the intensity of the afferent stimulation has been manipulated systematically in this context. In so much as the impact of an afferent volley on M1 excitability appears to be proportionately greater for stimulation of nerves in the lower limb than for those in the upper limb—at levels that are ostensibly equivalent when defined in relation to perceptual thresholds (Roy et al., 2007), it may however be possible to derive an indirect indication of the impact of this factor on the effectiveness of PAS protocols. For example, a 30 min period of CP nerve stimulation is sufficient to bring about sustained increases in the excitability of corticospinal projections to TA (Khaslavskaia et al., 2002; Knash et al., 2003), whereas periods of more than 1.5 h are required to induce similar changes in the state of projections to intrinsic hand muscles (e.g., Ridding et al., 2000). It has been noted previously by Roy et al. (2007) that this difference in the potency of the sensory element of PAS may account for the observation that the range of ISIs that is effective for lower limb induction protocols (≈80 ms) is larger than that which is efficacious for muscles in the upper limb (≈35 ms). The more general point to be made is that in addition to the relative timing of its delivery in relation to TMS, the intensity of afferent stimulation may play an instrumental role in determining the magnitude of the effects induced by PAS.

CONSTITUENT ELEMENTS OF PAS—CORTICAL STIMULATION

There exist a number of authoritative reviews concerning the impact of TMS upon corticospinal output (e.g., Huerta and Volpe, 2009; Siebner et al., 2009; Di Lazzaro and Ziemann, 2013). For the present purposes we draw selectively upon this existing body of knowledge, highlighting those features that may be particularly relevant in relation to PAS. TMS evokes high-frequency repetitive discharge of corticospinal neurons. When it is delivered at intensities above the threshold necessary to evoke a motor response in a peripheral muscle, epidural recordings reveal a series of four or more descending volleys each separated by ≈1.5 ms (see Ziemann and Rothwell, 2000; Di Lazzaro et al., 2012; Di Lazzaro and Ziemann, 2013; for reviews). The first of these is thought to originate from the direct ("D") activation of corticospinal axons in the subcortical white matter. Those occurring subsequently are believed to require mediation of the cortical gray matter, and to arise from indirect ("I") trans-synaptic activation of corticospinal neurons.

In PAS induction protocols, it is customary (at least for the upper limb) to employ a relatively focal figure-of-eight stimulating coil, and an angle of application such that the current induced in the brain flows in a posterior to anterior (PA) direction. At subthreshold stimulation intensities, this configuration yields a single I1 wave that is believed to arise from the action of monosynaptic corticocortical connections projecting onto corticospinal neurons

(Di Lazzaro et al., 2008). At the higher stimulation intensities utilized in the administration of PAS (e.g., able to generate a MEP of 1 mV in a hand muscle), further volleys denoted "late I waves" are also generated. It is understood that this repetitive discharge is produced by the activation of complex chains of interneurons that project ultimately onto corticospinal cells (Di Lazzaro et al., 2009a,b). The conclusion that the mechanisms generating these late I-waves are at least partially independent of those giving rise to I1 waves is supported by the observation that the former are suppressed by GABAa receptor inhibitors, whereas I1 waves are not (Di Lazzaro et al., 2008). Of particular note in the present context, the inhibition of the compound MEP produced by the SICI protocol is accompanied by suppression of late I-waves, whereas this is not the case for the I1 wave (Di Lazzaro et al., 1998; Hanajima et al., 1998). A similar differentiation is obtained when LICI protocols employing ISIs of 100 and 150 are employed (Di Lazzaro et al., 2002). Furthermore, SAI of the MEP generated by TMS delivered 1–8 ms after stimulation of the median nerve N20 potential is accompanied by depression of the I2 and I3 waves, whereas the I1 component of the descending volley is relatively unaffected (Tokimura et al., 2000). Taken together, these studies indicate that the M1 networks activated by single pulse TMS at the intensities used customarily in PAS protocols generate I1 waves which contribute to the compound MEP—the standard measure of the efficacy of PAS, in a manner that is relatively impervious to experimental manipulation; and a series of later I-waves that are subject to the modulatory influence of inhibitory GABAa receptor mediated interneuronal networks. Although PAS25 does not alter expressions of SICI or SAI, it increases the amplitude of late I-waves (Di Lazzaro et al., 2009a), whereas PAS10 (which may decrease SICI) appears to decrease their size (Di Lazzaro et al., 2009b). Is it sufficient therefore to restrict consideration of the TMS component of the PAS protocol to its effect on these chains of interneurons with fixed temporal characteristics that produce a periodic bombardment of corticospinal neurons (Amassian et al., 1987), or do its (spatially and temporally) distributed effects also have to be taken into consideration?

There is a large and rapidly expanding literature that concerns the use of imaging techniques such as PET (Fox et al., 1997; Paus et al., 1997), fMRI (Bohning et al., 1997), and EEG registered potentials (ERP) (Ilmoniemi et al., 1997), in conjunction with TMS, to determine patterns of functional brain connectivity. If TMS is applied over a discrete cortical site, the instigated neural activity can be registered as it propagates orthodromically through a network of connected regions (Fox et al., 1997). Augmented by analytic techniques such as structural equation modeling (SEM), which are used to make inferences in relation to causal relationships, these means have be used to determine, for example that there are path connections from primary motor cortex to S2 (bilaterally) (Laird et al., 2008). More generally it has been proposed that the efficacy of protocols such as PAS may depend not only on the characteristics of the stimulated regions, but also upon other elements of the brain network to which they are interconnected (e.g., Cardenas-Morales et al., 2013).

With respect to the "local" effects of TMS, it has variously been adjudged that the spatial extent of the cortical surface that is stimulated extends to 1 cm^2 (Cowey and Walsh, 2000; Wagner et al., 2004; Thielscher and Wichmann, 2009), although these estimates are increased somewhat when conductivity along the major fiber tracts is taken into account (De Lucia et al., 2007). In relation to temporal extent, when studied in cat, single magnetic stimuli applied to visual cortex give rise to episodes of enhanced and suppressed single-unit activity in the context of a general facilitation that persist for 500 ms (Moliadze et al., 2003).

In relation to the distributed effects of TMS in humans, it is apparent that the delivery of single pulse TMS to M1 produces a complex spreading pattern of activation that can be registered (e.g., by EEG) over 300 ms as it encompasses ipsilateral motor, premotor, and parietal regions (Ilmoniemi et al., 1997; Komssi et al., 2002). It is composed of a sequence of negative deflections peaking at ~7, 18, 44, 100, and 280 ms, alternating with positive peaks at ~13, 30, 60, and 190 ms post-TMS (Ferreri et al., 2011, 2012). In evidently triggering polysynaptic circuits, variable delays will be introduced with the result that the TMS will have distinct effects at different synapses (Huber et al., 2008). It now also accepted that the state of the cortex at the time of the TMS (i.e., when conditioned by peripheral afferent input) both determines the overall neuronal response of the stimulated cortex (Ferreri et al., 2012, 2013), and shapes the responsiveness of distinct subpopulations of cortical neurons (Siebner et al., 2009). Thus, the spatial propagation of TMS invoked coherence, and the functional consequences of this spread of synchronized activity, is contingent upon prior events, and indeed upon those immediately following.

On the basis of observations that rTMS delivered at intensities below motor threshold failed to elicit a discernable BOLD response in M1, whereas suprathreshold intensities consistently do so (Baudewig et al., 2001; Bestmann et al., 2004), Lang et al. (2006) have argued that regional changes in synaptic activity induced by magnetic cortical stimulation are driven in large measure by re-afferent feedback arising from the associated muscle contractions. Applying single pulse TMS (<0.2 Hz) Hanakawa et al. (2009) arrived at a similar conclusion having noted that in the directly stimulated M1, elevated BOLD activity was registered only when intensities above motor threshold were applied. In this context, a bilateral elevation of activity in S2 [plus ventral SMA, caudal cingulate zone (CCZ), and bilateral PMd] was also observed. The BOLD response in ipsilateral S1 was enhanced by both subthreshold and suprathreshold intensities of M1 stimulation (Hanakawa et al., 2009). Recent investigations suggest that at least 10% of the BOLD signal change registered in M1 following suprathreshold TMS is attributable to inputs from muscle afferents (Shitara et al., 2013). As we argued above in relation to the effects of the peripheral stimulation, since standard PAS protocols deliver TMS at intensities above motor threshold, it may be assumed that the associated muscle contraction will give rise to a subsequent reafferent volley that is delayed by tens of milliseconds relative to the initial cortical stimulation and maintained for an extended period thereafter. Necessarily this will lengthen the interval over which the TMS pulse may exert an influence on processes that mediate neuroplastic adaptation.

A handful of studies have been conducted with an explicit focus upon variations in functional connectivity engendered by PAS. Huber et al. (2008) observed that changes in TMS-evoked cortical EEG responses (induced by PAS25 and PAS10 interventions) were expressed for up to 200 ms following the magnetic probe. The largest effects were obtained for the region in which SEPs induced by median nerve stimulation overlapped with TMS-evoked potentials (TEPs). An analysis of movement related cortical potentials (MRCP) obtained prior to and following a N20+2 PAS protocol (15 min duration) suggests that the effects of the intervention also extend to disruption of movement-related effective connectivity between PMd and M1 (Lu et al., 2009). Employing the Ridding and Taylor (2001) protocol that utilizes trains of afferent stimulation, Tsuji and Rothwell (2002) noted increases in the cortical N20/P25 (recorded 2 cm posterior to C3—parietal) and P25/N33 (recorded 5 cm anterior to C3—frontal) components of the SEP for 10 min post-intervention, providing further evidence that PAS-induced changes are both spatially and temporally distributed.

The precise nature of the relationship between the immediate local effects of TMS and the distributed changes in network reactivity that follow remain to be resolved (Shafi et al., 2012). Nonetheless, when applied in the context of a PAS protocol, it is clear that this mode of brain stimulation gives rise to consequential variations in neural activity that are not localized in either space nor time.

MEDIATION OF INTERACTIONS BETWEEN THE CONSTITUENT ELEMENTS OF PAS

In light of the foregoing analyses of the constituent elements of PAS, an assumption that there is discrete temporal convergence of activity generated by the two associated sources of stimulation cannot necessarily be sustained. Consideration might therefore be given to the various routes through which neuronal activity generated by TMS applied to M1, and by peripheral nerve stimulation, may converge and interact.

CORTICO-CORTICAL CONNECTIONS FROM SOMATOSENSORY CORTEX TO M1

In spite of initial controversy (Gandevia et al., 1984; Halonen et al., 1988) concerning the relative contribution of muscle afferents and cutaneous fibers to SEPs evoked by electrical stimulation of mixed nerves (e.g., median nerve at the wrist), there is now consensus that the initial (i.e., N20) responses are dominated by cutaneous rather than muscle afferent input (Gandevia and Burke, 1990; Kunesch et al., 1995). On the other hand, EEG potentials associated with movement-generated reafference are largely contingent on input from muscle spindles. The origin of the N20 response to cutaneous inputs is taken to be a deep tangential generator in area 3b (e.g., Desmedt and Ozaki, 1991; McLaughlin and Kelly, 1993). This is consistent with the characteristics of area 3b that have been defined on the basis of comparative studies in primates (Kaas, 1983). It is likely that the source generator for cortical potentials invoked by muscle spindle afference is principally area 3a, although additional contributions from area 2 cannot be excluded (Mima et al., 1996; Mackinnon et al., 2000). This is likewise consonant with the interpretation drawn from comparative studies that that the major driving input to area 3a is from muscle spindle afferents (Kaas, 1983). Thus, the form of peripheral nerve stimulation that is applied in PAS—consisting of an electrical shock (or series) of shocks, will give rise to cutaneous afferent mediated activity in area 3b of primary somatosensory cortex (SI), and also to activity in area 3a and area 2 (Wiesendanger and Miles, 1982) by virtue of contraction induced reafference brought about by the use of stimulation intensities above motor threshold.

Studies in primates (e.g., Jones et al., 1978; Pons and Kaas, 1986; Ghosh et al., 1987; Huerta and Pons, 1990) and in cat (Grant et al., 1975; Zarzecki et al., 1978; Waters et al., 1982; Burton and Kopf, 1984; Yumiya and Ghez, 1984; Porter and Sakamoto, 1988; Avendano et al., 1992) reveal an extensive network of cortico-cortical connections between SI and primary motor cortex (M1) (Burton and Fabri, 1995). Only cells in the superficial layers of M1 (II and III) exhibit short-latency EPSPs—indicative of direct input, in response to microstimulation of area 2 (Kosar et al., 1985; Porter et al., 1990). In contrast, neurons that receive short latency input from area 3a are found in all laminae of the motor cortex, with the exception of layer I (Herman et al., 1985; Huerta and Pons, 1990; Porter et al., 1990). Indeed it has variously been suggested that area 3a should be regarded at the very least as a relay to motor cortex (Jones and Porter, 1980), or even as a part of area 4 (Jones et al., 1978). Regardless of classification, this organization provides a means through which muscle spindle input that is relayed through area 3a can exert a direct influence on pyramidal and multipolar neurons in deep (V and VI) layers of M1 (Porter et al., 1990). Since the former are suspected to have a facilitatory, and the latter an inhibitory influence on corticofugal cells, this may account, in part, for the alternating pattern of MEP facilitation and inhibition that is observed in response to peripheral nerve stimulation at ISIs shorter than 80 ms (Sailer et al., 2002). Relays involving corticocortical input from area 2 to pyramidal cells in layers II/III of M1 (Kaneko et al., 1994a,b) and then to layer V/VI pyramidal neurons (Kaneko et al., 2000) may also play a role in this regard.

In marked contrast, while there are reciprocal connections between area 3b and area 1 in particular, and further projections to area 2 (which are seemingly not reciprocated), projections from area 3b to M1 are sparse (Darian-Smith et al., 1993; Burton and Fabri, 1995), if present at all (Jones et al., 1978). This being the case, it worth reflecting upon the use of the N20 response latency—which is presumed to have a generator in area 3b, as a reference in determining ISIs in PAS protocols, since this region has few if any direct projections to M1, and is not engaged to a significant degree by peripheral input from muscle spindle afferents. When the interval between mixed nerve stimulation and TMS delivered over *S1* is adjusted with a view to ensuring that the cortical stimulus occurs around the time that reafference arising from the muscle contraction is maximal (N20 + 100 ms), changes in tactile sensitivity otherwise observed when the cortical and peripheral stimulation both occur within a 20 ms window are no longer obtained (Litvak et al., 2007). Since the former condition also gives rise to a medial shift in the topography of the multi-channel SEP, these authors concluded that the reafference driven effects observed in the N20 + 100 associative protocol were expressed via selective enhancement of a source in area 3a, whereas when shorter ISIs were employed, a source in area 3b was also implicated (Litvak et al., 2007). It might also be remarked that PAS protocols employing digital nerve stimulation—which may excite mechanoreceptor fibers rather than muscle spindle afferents (and TMS to M1), tends to produce smaller effects than mixed nerve stimulation (e.g., Stefan et al., 2000; Kujirai et al., 2006). Thus, to the extent that muscle spindle afferents represent the most efficacious source of peripheral input in PAS protocols, it may surmised that area 3a—which has projections onto neurons in most layers of M1—including laminae II/III which are believed to represent the origin of late I-waves [and receives substantial inputs from S1 (Huffman and Krubitzer, 2001)], may play a critical role in mediating the changes in corticospinal output that are induced.

Although a direct activation of the motor cortex via sensory afferents from the periphery (Padel and Relova, 1991) cannot be dismissed, studies in monkey demonstrate that the ventral posterior complex of the thalamus, the major sensory thalamic relay, only has minor direct projections to the motor cortex (Darian-Smith and Darian-Smith, 1993; Huffman and Krubitzer, 2001) and thus a structural correlate for direct motor cortex activation after peripheral sensory stimulation has not yet been found. In addition, as highlighted above, while it has been proposed that the P22 SEP component may originate from the precentral motor area, the balance of evidence now indicates that the source is in area 1 (i.e., S1) (Baumgartner et al., 2010). It is also worth noting in this context that while S1 areas 1, 2 and are represented across the ventrobasal complex of the thalamus, area 3a has connectional relationships similar to those for area 4 (Jones et al., 1979), further emphasizing the likelihood that muscle afferent input relayed via area 3a will have a more direct influence on the state of the primary motor cortex, than cutaneous input relayed via other regions of S1.

CEREBELLO-THALAMO-CORTICAL AND THALMO-CORTICAL CONNECTIONS

The point has been made previously that functional neuroplastic adaptation is likely to encompass changes in activity distributed across "non-primary" elements of the sensorimotor network, including the supplementary motor area and lateral premotor cortex, cingulum, insula, posterior parietal cortex, cerebellum, deep gray nuclei and thalamus (Duffau, 2006). As a case in point, as the VL nucleus is the primary relay station in the cerebello-thalamo-cortical pathway (Asanuma and Hunsperger, 1975), it has been proposed that, through receipt of convergent inputs from both the sensorimotor cortex and the spinal cord, the interpositus nucleus of the cerebellum exerts a modulating influence upon motor network responses to sensory stimulation via thalamic projections to premotor and motor cortices (Luft et al., 2005). In this vein, hemicerebellectomy blocks the modulation of cortical motor output associated with repetitive electrical stimulation of the sciatic nerve in the rat (Ben Taib et al., 2005). The state of the motor cortex itself—acting via the intermediate cerebellum, may further serve to tune the gain of polysynaptic responses to peripheral stimulation (Manto et al., 2006). Hamada et al. (2012) demonstrated recently that when either anodal or cathodal transcranial direct current stimulation (tDCS) was applied to the cerebellum during a PAS25 protocol, the usually obtained excitability enhancing effect of this intervention was not exhibited. In contrast, anodal tDCS failed to modulate the impact of a PAS21.5 protocol. Popa et al. (2013) reported that 600 prior rTMS stimuli applied over the posterior cerebellar cortex in either a continuous (cTBS) or an intermittent (iTBS) theta burst pattern, has opposing effects on the efficacy of PAS protocol. The iTBS pattern attenuated the increases in corticospinal excitability brought about by PAS, whereas the cTBS pattern enhanced and prolonged increases in MEP amplitude.

Area 3a of the primary somatosensory cortex receives projections from nuclei of the thalamus classically associated with the motor system, including indirect input from the cerebellum and basal ganglia via the ventral lateral (VL) nucleus (Huffman and Krubitzer, 2001). Thalamic processing of somatosensory input appears however to extend beyond the relaying of primary afferent signals to the cortex. For example, at levels of median nerve stimulation above PT, thalamic SEPs can be elicited for longer than 75 ms after the peripheral shock, with this duration extending to 150 ms when the intensity is set to MT (Klostermann et al., 2009).

It has been noted previously that since afferent input is relayed via the cerebellum and VL to area 4, and inputs from the globus pallidus reach M1 after relaying in VL, the motor cortex is capable of influencing both its own thalamic afferents and those directed to the primary somatosensory cortex (Canedo, 1997). Indeed, low frequency electrical stimulation of the sensorimotor cortex evokes short and long-latency excitatory and inhibitory postsynaptic potentials in VL neurons. In this regard, it has been proposed that the thalamocortical cells operate in two different modes : an oscillatory mode and a tonic (transfer) mode. The particular significance of this characteristic in the present context is the facility for corticothalamic fibers to induce thalamic oscillating activity that renders the thalamic neurons unresponsive to synaptic input—functionally deafferenting the cerebral cortex (Canedo, 1997). It remains to be determined whether TMS applied to M1 is capable of blocking afferent transmission via the thalamus in this fashion. If so, it may cast a different light on the means through which such protocols as PAS10—whereby TMS precedes the cortical corollary of the peripheral stimulus, serves through repetition to decrease the excitability of projections from M1 (see also Schabrun et al., 2012). While it is known that TMS can suppress the perception of subsequent peripheral afferent stimuli (McKay et al., 2003; Yoo et al., 2008), it is not yet possible to exclude the possibility that this phenomenon is due to sensory masking rather than to gating of the ascending volley, for example at the level of the thalamus.

It has been conjectured that a disruption of basal ganglia-thalamocortical loops arising from striatal dopamine depletion may account for the reduced response to PAS25 that is exhibited by patients with Parkinson's disease (Ueki et al., 2006), and in the course of normal ageing (Fathi et al., 2010). As yet however, this proposition has not been studied in detail. It can nonetheless be concluded that there are a number of neural circuits extending beyond the S1-M1 axis, encompassing cerebello-thalamo-cortical and thalmo-cortical pathways that have the potential to mediate changes in M1 excitability brought about by PAS.

MECHANISMS OF NEUROPLASTIC ADAPTATION ENGAGED BY PAS

In reflecting upon the characteristics of the data obtained in their seminal study of PAS, Stefan et al. (2000) emphasized that changes in the excitability of human motor cortex brought about by such exogenous stimulation are likely to proceed via a number of different routes. For example, these authors highlighted the possibility that variations in membrane excitability, such as those demonstrated in experiments concerning conditional learning (Woody and Engel, 1972; Aou et al., 1992), may play an instrumental role. Other commentators have also been careful to acknowledge that a range of cellular mechanisms may be engaged (e.g., Muller-Dahlhaus et al., 2010; Nitsche et al., 2012). Why then is it the case that interpretations of PAS framed in terms of STDP are so pervasive? In the present section we will consider whether the empirical evidence presented above, and more general considerations in relation to the complexity of the *in vivo* human motor system, support this narrow emphasis.

SPIKE TIMING DEPENDENT PLASTICITY (STDP)

LTP and LTD can be induced by a wide variety of experimental protocols. It has been suggested (e.g., Wolters et al., 2005) that STDP occupies a unique position in so much as the polarity of the induced change in synaptic efficacy is determined by the sequence of pre- and postsynaptic neuronal activity (for reviews see Dan and Poo, 2004; Markram et al., 2011). In the classical model of STDP (e.g., Song et al., 2000), strengthening (potentiation) arises if the presynaptic neuron fires no more than 50 ms in advance of the postsynaptic neuron (Feldman, 2000), whereas weakening (depression) occurs if postsynaptic spikes precede presynaptic action potentials—(or transpire without activity in the presynaptic neuron) (Levy and Steward, 1983; Bi and Poo, 1998; Cooke and Bliss, 2006). In addition, there is a sharp transition from strengthening (LTP) to weakening (LTD) at time differences in the region (within 5 ms) of zero (Feldman, 2012).

At most glutamatergic synapses in the CNS the NMDA receptor (i.e., post-synaptic) performs the function of coincidence detection. The binding to AMPA receptors of glutamate released by presynaptic activation, and the resulting postsynaptic depolarization which leads to removal of the Mg2+ block, together permit the influx of Ca2+ though the NMDA receptors (Mayer et al., 1984; Nowak et al., 1984). The magnitude and time course of the calcium flux (and Mg2+ kinetics) determines whether LTP or LTD is induced (e.g., Verhoog et al., 2013). Transient, high calcium-fluxes invoke LTP, whereas sustained moderate calcium fluxes generate LTD, and low calcium fluxes do not induce adaptation (Lisman, 1989; Yang et al., 1999).

In itself, this mechanism is not strictly timing-dependent (and thus Hebbian) in nature, as the level of activity at *individual* synapses and the firing of the postsynaptic neuron need not necessarily be correlated (Thickbroom, 2007). Back-propagating action potentials (BAP)—which pass antidromically into the soma and then to the dendritic tree following the initiation of an action potential, appear however to provide the retrograde signal through which a contingent association could be instantiated. In the context of LTP, the arrival of presynaptic input milliseconds before the BAP reaches the dendrite can facilitate removal of the Mg2+ block on NMDA receptors and thus promote Ca2+ influx, although other types of interactions between the EPSP and the BAP cannot be excluded (Caporale and Dan, 2008). Conjectures in relation to the mediating role for the BAP in LTD are based on the assumption that it produces an afterdepolarization, such that the generation of an EPSP leads to only a moderate Ca2+influx through NMDA receptors. Although, as with the induction of LTP, a number of alternative models have also been proposed (Caporale and Dan, 2008). With respect to both LTP and LTD, the primary mechanisms of STDP are putatively postsynaptic, and instantiated via addition or removal of AMPA receptors (AMPARs) and changes in single-channel conductance (Malinow and Malenka, 2002).

STDP IN CONTEXT

Evidently, there exist forms of neuroplastic adaptation that do not depend on BAPs. In addition, it now widely acknowledged that the relative timing of postsynaptic spikes and presynaptic action potentials is only one of several factors, including firing rate and dendritic depolarization that operate in relation to STDP (Feldman, 2012). If facilitatory and inhibitory forms of PAS differ only in respect of the polarity of STDP (cf. Wolters et al., 2005), one might anticipate that their effects would be expressed via the same electrophysiological measures, and that they would be responsive to the same pharmacological manipulations. As highlighted in the preceding sections however, this is not generally the case. At least two possibilities are thus admitted. In the first instance it is possible that the induction of changes in corticospinal excitability by PAS requires the engagement of cellular mechanisms other than, or in addition to, those associated with STDP. An alternative possibility is that factors that influence the expression of STDP exert differential effects depending on the protocol that is applied (and the neural circuits that are targeted). It is for example, well-established the range of effective timing intervals varies across different modes of stimulation and cell types, as well as across species (Bi and Poo, 2001; Caporale and Dan, 2008).

With respect to interceding factors, the backpropagation of action potentials from the site of initiation on the axon to the dendrites provides a critical element of the associative signal for the induction of STDP (Magee and Johnston, 1997). Yet the full expression of STDP—as opposed to LTD only, requires either the enhancement of BAP propagation, for example by inactivation of A-type potassium channels, and/or additional sources of depolarization, which may include recruitment of dendritic sodium channels (Sjostrom et al., 2001; Sjostrom and Hausser, 2006). In addition, the dendritic tree itself is not static. Rather, it is subject to modification by synaptic activity and by neuromodulators (e.g., Sjostrom et al., 2008). The latter, including norepinephrine and acetylcholine, exert an influence on the BAP by altering the activation and deactivation of various active conductances (Caporale and Dan, 2008). Of perhaps greater significance in the context of PAS is the recognition that while LTP occurs at excitatory glutamatergic synapses, inhibitory projections mediated by GABA also play a significant role in its induction in the hippocampus (Davies et al., 1991; Chapman et al., 1998), and that GABAergic influences must be attenuated for LTP to be induced in motor cortex slices *in vitro* (Hess and Donoghue, 1996). It has been shown recently that the interceding role of GABA extends to STDP. Specifically, the polarity of STDP induced experimentally at corticostriatal synapses in rodents can be reversed by blockade of GABAA receptors (Paille et al., 2013).

Aside from consideration of factors that influence its expression *in vitro*, it is likely that neuroplastic adaptation in general (Daoudal and Debanne, 2003; Zhang and Linden, 2003), and synaptic plasticity in particular (Schulz, 2010), is governed by processes that are much more complex than those traditionally ascribed to STDP. Indeed, the argument has been made persuasively that, *in vivo*, backpropagating action potentials are neither necessary nor sufficient for synaptic plasticity (Lisman and Spruston, 2005). More pointedly these authors have argued that textbook accounts of STDP are sufficiently impoverished as a general model of synaptic plasticity in naturally active neural circuits that they constitute "a dangerous oversimplification" (Lisman and Spruston, 2010). With specific regard to the topic at hand, Thickbroom (2007) has noted that, given the likely temporal dispersion of the nominally coincident inputs contrived in PAS protocols, the effects that emerge are more probably a consequence of increased network activity generated by convergent inputs (i.e., an activity dependent mechanism), rather than STDP. Indeed, there are contemporary models which predict that potentiation will occur during periods of high pre- and post-synaptic activity in a manner that is independent of the temporal order of spikes (Pfister and Gerstner, 2006). Thus, the dependence on timing expressed empirically may reflect the means through which network activity is increased, rather than a signature of STDP.

In animals that are awake, neurons throughout the cerebral cortex have high spontaneous firing rates, and at any given moment multiple synaptic inputs to single neurons are active simultaneously. As a consequence of this high conductance state, the integrative properties of cortical neurons *in vivo* are profoundly different from neurons maintained *in vitro* (Destexhe et al., 2003). The natural system is inherently stochastic such the relationship between input and outputs is probabilistic—defined by the response characteristics of a population of neurons that share common input (Shadlen and Newsome, 1998). On the other hand, many neurons, including pyramidal neurons, have extensive dendritic arborizations and receive and process synaptic input from widespread sources. In the prototypical experiments used to define the canonical characteristics of STDP, unitary EPSPs were evoked by stimulation of a single presynaptic cell, and a single BAP was induced by the brief injection of current into the soma of the postsynaptic cell. Recent work conducted under conditions of spontaneous activity *in vivo* suggest that, with respect to layer V pyramidal neurons in M1, synaptic input and dendritic activity are spread uniformly throughout all branches of the dendritic tree, rather than it being the case that NMDA spikes are localized to a single branch (i.e., functioning as the putative unit of plasticity) (Hill et al., 2013). While to the best of our knowledge there have not yet been corresponding studies focusing on the layer II/III pyramidal neurons in M1 that are thought to mediate the effects of PAS, in light of the foregoing considerations it would seem unlikely if the effects of this form of non-invasive brain stimulation were to be "synapse specific," at least in the sense in which this term is understood in relation to STDP.

While in the reduced preparations that have typically been used to deduce the characteristics of STDP there is only one connection between the pre- and post-synaptic neurons, at the more macroscopic scale relevant to electrophysiological manipulations and recordings in humans, there are multiple pathways via which sensory corollaries of peripheral stimulation may reach and influence the cortex (Hamada et al., 2012). Similarly, the complex temporal structure of natural neural activity is not reflected in the intermittent pairing of stimuli used to investigate STDP in reduced preparations (Jackson, 2012). Thus, there appears to be little by way of an a priori basis for the assumption that STDP plays a prominent role in mediating the effects of PAS. Furthermore, as Lisman and Spruston (2010) have cautioned in specific relation to this form of neural plasticity, "a field must not go beyond the data" (p. 3).

THE EXCEPTIONS THAT MAY DISPROVE THE RULE

It has been highlighted previously (Hamada et al., 2012) that there is a general assumption that only the initial element of the input to S1 arising from peripheral afferent stimulation (as reflected in the latency of the N20 component of the SEP) contributes to the changes in corticospinal excitability brought about by PAS. Yet the cardinal phenomenological features also emerge when the stimulation that is associated with TMS cannot be rendered in terms of a discrete series of time locked events (i.e., of fixed latencies).

Thabit et al. (2010) paired TMS (delivered over M1) with each of a series of contralateral thumb abduction movements, initiated in the context of an over-learned visually cued reaction time task (240 pairs at 0.2 Hz over 20 min). When the magnetic stimulus *preceded* the mean individualized RT by 50 ms, the intervention gave rise to increases in the excitability of corticospinal projections to the target muscle that were sustained for up to 15 min. There was a corresponding increase in the duration of the CSP over this period, however no changes in SICI were observed. With respect to these additional features too therefore, the pattern of outcomes resembled that obtained using conventional facilitatory PAS protocols. A decrease in corticospinal excitability was obtained when TMS was applied 100 ms after the mean RT, however no changes were observed when it was followed by 50 or 150 ms, or when the TMS preceded the mean RT by 100 ms. Intracortical recordings in monkey indicate that that pyramidal cell firing increases 150 ms prior to movement initiation (Evarts, 1966, 1968). The time at which TMS was delivered in order to induce sustained facilitation (50 ms prior) therefore falls well within this interval. Although neighboring neurons in M1 with similar output projections may themselves exhibit synchronous firing (Jackson et al., 2003), since the protocol employed by Thabit et al. (2010) provided no control over the temporal relationship between these physiological events and the excitation brought about by the delivery of TMS over M1, an explanation of the associative effects framed in terms of activity dependent mechanism is more parsimonious than one that makes appeal to the rules of STDP.

The requirement for an alternative model is also suggested by a recent study in which the other element of PAS—peripheral afferent stimulation was paired with motor imagery. Mrachacz-Kersting et al. (2012) delivered electrical stimulation (intensity = MT) to the CPN while the participants imagined the kinaesthetics of a ramp and hold dorsiflexion movement, which was cued visually every 10–12 s for a total of 50 pairings. In separate conditions, the timing of the afferent stimulation was delivered 101 ± 110 ms prior to the start of the imagined movement, 134 ± 115 ms after, and 368 ± 196 ms after the start of the imagined movement. Increases in the excitability of corticospinal projections to TA were reported when the peripheral stimulation ~135 ms following the start of the imagined task, but not in the other conditions (see also Niazi et al., 2012). While these exemplars highlight the importance of the timing relationship between the voluntary engagement of motor output networks and TMS delivery and on the one hand, and that between the unfolding of an imagined movement and the administration of peripheral stimulation on the other, in neither instance can the conclusion be drawn that the constituent events are sufficiently discrete (i.e., in terms of timing) to satisfy the requirements of STDP. There are alternative models however that can account for the cumulative impact of temporally proximate events separated by intervals such as those described above (e.g., Ostojic and Fusi, 2013). It remains the case however, that since the prevailing explanatory accounts of the effects of PAS in humans have been framed in terms of STDP, there are as yet few empirical studies that scrutinize the role of other mechanisms in this context.

WHAT ARE THE FEATURES FOR WHICH ANY MODEL SHOULD ACCOUNT?

If accounts based on STDP, at least as it has been characterized *in vitro*, fail to provide a complete explanation of the effects of PAS in humans, what are the key features that must be encapsulated by alternative models? It is evident for example that the specific intervals (e.g., Schabrun et al., 2013) and the range of intervals (Ridding and Taylor, 2001) that are effective in inducing facilitation or inhibition, vary depending on the corticomotor pathway that is engaged (Roy et al., 2007), and the mode of peripheral stimulation that is employed (e.g., Suppa et al., 2013). Ideally therefore a comprehensive model will encompass this diversity.

It is also apparent that restriction of the effects of PAS to muscles innervated by the peripheral nerve that receives stimulation is the exception rather than the rule. An explanation should therefore be sought for a somatotopic gradient that is relative rather than absolute (e.g., Quartarone et al., 2003). The evidence that has been derived from a limited number of direct investigations suggests that the initial I-wave generated by TMS is not affected by PAS, whereas later I-waves are accentuated by facilitatory, and attenuated by inhibitory variants of the intervention (Di Lazzaro et al., 2009a,b). There is however divergence with respect to other neural circuits through which the effects of PAS are manifested. Excitability enhancing PAS protocols (e.g., PAS25) do not alter expressions of SICI, ICF, or SAI, whereas inhibitory protocols (e.g., PAS10) may decrease SICI. Furthermore, while facilitatory variants decrease LICI and LAI, and elongate the CSP, inhibitory protocols do not appear to influence the CSP. Thus, switches in the polarity of the net change in corticospinal excitability brought about by different variants of PAS are not accompanied by corresponding alterations in the reactivity of neural circuits that act ultimately upon the state of corticospinal neurons. Yet, since the data concerning some aspects of the preceding synopsis are sparse, a number of the characterizations remain incomplete.

With respect to the action of pharmacological agents upon the effects of PAS, NMDA receptor antagonists blunt the impact of both facilitatory (Stefan et al., 2002; Suppa et al., 2013) and inhibitory (Wolters et al., 2003) forms of PAS. It should be noted in this context that a dependence upon NMDA receptors is not an exclusive property of STDP, nor is it restricted to post-synaptic mechanisms. Indeed, NMDA receptor activation has the capacity to enhance inhibitory GABAergic transmission via presynaptic mechanisms mediated by retrograde nitric oxide (NO) signaling (Xue et al., 2011, see also Rodríguez-Moreno et al., 2010; Duguid, 2013). More generally in the context of PAS, drugs that enhance the effects of GABA tend to diminish the increases in corticospinal excitability otherwise brought about by facilitatory protocols. It is well-established that GABA assumes multiple inter-related roles in regulating the excitability of brain networks (Olsen and Sieghart, 2009), encompassing both synaptic activity and extra-synaptic tone (Semyanov et al., 2004). As such, the impact (i.e., on any form of non-invasive brain stimulation) of a drug that interferes with GABA function is subject to a number of possible interpretations. Likewise, the dependence of both excitatory and inhibitory PAS protocols on voltage-dependent Ca^{2+} channels is consistent with both STDP and activity-dependent (Lisman, 1989) models of synaptic plasticity.

It is striking that the dopaminergic system appears to assume a necessary role in relation to the changes in corticospinal excitability brought about by PAS. The influence of dopamine is consistent with a number of different models of neuroplastic adaptation, including those that emphasize stimulus-response contingencies (e.g., Samson et al., 2010), although a specific role of dopamine signaling in relation to STDP has also been mooted (Izhikevich, 2007). Nonetheless, it is apparent that the action of dopamine (and indeed that of other classes of neuromodulator) must necessarily be an element of any comprehensive model of PAS.

CONCLUSIONS

A large body of empirical evidence has accumulated in the period since the cardinal features of PAS in humans were first disclosed, and as variations upon the original protocols have proliferated, deviations from these features have become more numerous. While presenting challenges to assimilation, in seeking to determine the mechanisms that mediate the effects of PAS these variations are a blessing in disguise. Specifically they serve to enforce recognition that the cellular pathways that contribute to the LTP- and LTD-type responses to PAS may differ depending on the precise nature of the induction protocol that is used. For example, in circumstances in which trains of afferent stimulation are applied, it seems likely that classical STDP-type mechanisms will play a diminished role, at least relative to those contexts in which the timing relationship between the peripheral and cortical stimulation can be precisely circumscribed. Furthermore, it need not be assumed that—even within the context of a protocol in which a single parameter such as ISI is manipulated, excitability enhancing and excitability diminishing variants represent a change in the polarity of a specific cellular process. They are not necessarily two sides of the same coin. Indeed, even in relation to a single polarity of effect, relatively minor variations of ISI—in the order of a few milliseconds may alter profoundly the pathways that are instrumentally engaged (e.g. Hamada et al., 2012). The challenge now lies in moving beyond accounts predicated only on the rules of STDP, to encompass the additional physiological mechanisms of action that promote neuroplastic adaptation in natural systems, and appreciate the context-sensitive features of their contributions.

ACKNOWLEDGMENTS

Northern Ireland Department for Employment and Learning. Richard G. Carson thanks Atlantic Philanthropies for their generous support of his research through their funding of the NEIL (Neuro-Enhancement for Independent Lives) programme at Trinity College Institute of Neuroscience.

REFERENCES

Abbruzzese, G., Marchese, R., Buccolieri, A., Gasparetto, B., and Trompetto, C. (2001). Abnormalities of sensorimotor integration in focal dystonia— A transcranial magnetic stimulation study. Brain 124, 537–545. doi: 10.1093/brain/124.3.537

Alle, H., Heidegger, T., Krivanekova, L., and Ziemann, U. (2009). Interactions between short-interval intracortical inhibition and short-latency afferent inhibition in human motor cortex. J. Physiol. (Lond.) 587, 5163–5176. doi: 10.1113/jphysiol.2009.179820

Allison, T., Mccarthy, G., and Wood, C. C. (1992). the relationship between human long-latency somatosensory evoked-potentials recorded from the cortical sur- face and from the scalp. Electroencephalogr. Clin. Neurophysiol. 84, 301–314. doi: 10.1016/0168-5597(92)90082-M

Allison, T., Mccarthy, G., Wood, C. C., Darcey, T. M., Spencer, D. D., and Williamson, P. D. (1989a). Human cortical potentials evoked by stimulation of the median nerve. I. Cytoarchitectonic areas generating short-latency activity.

J. Neurophysiol. 62, 694–710.

Allison, T., Mccarthy, G., Wood, C. C., Williamson, P. D., and Spencer, D. D. (1989b). Human cortical potentials evoked by stimulation of the median nerve.

II. Cytoarchitectonic areas generating long-latency activity. J. Neurophysiol. 62, 711–722.

Allison, T., Mccarthy, G., Wood, C. C., and Jones, S. J. (1991). Potentials evoked in human and monkey cerebral cortex by stimulation of the median nerve. A review of scalp and intracranial recordings. Brain 114, 2465–503. doi: 10.1093/brain/114.6.2465

Amassian, V. E., Stewart, M., Quirk, G. J., and Rosenthal, J. L. (1987). physiological- basis of motor effects of a transient stimulus to cerebral-cortex. Neurosurgery 20, 74–93. doi: 10.1097/00006123-198701000-00022

Amaya, F., Paulus, W., Treue, S., and Liebetanz, D. (2010). Transcranial mag- netic stimulation and PAS-induced cortical neuroplasticity in the awake rhesus monkey. Clin. Neurophysiol. 121, 2143–2151. doi: 10.1016/j.clinph.2010.03.058
Aou, S. J., Woody, C. D., and Birt, D. (1992). Increases in excitability of neurons of the motor cortex of cats after rapid acquisition of eye blink conditioning. J. Neurosci. 12, 560–569.

Asanuma, H., and Hunsperger, R. W. (1975). Functional significance of projection from the cerebellar nuclei to the motor cortex in the cat. Brain Res. 98, 73–92. doi: 10.1016/0006-8993(75)90510-7

Avendano, C., Isla, A. J., and Rausell, E. (1992). area-3a in the cat.2. projections to the motor cortex and their relations to other corticocortical connections. J. Comp. Neurol. 321, 373–386. doi: 10.1002/cne.903210306

Backes, W. H., Mess, W. H., Van Kranen-Mastenbroek, V., and Reulen, J. P. (2000).

Somatosensory cortex responses to median nerve stimulation: fMRI effects of current amplitude and selective attention. Clin. Neurophysiol. 111, 1738–44. doi: 10.1016/S1388-2457(00)00420-X

Batsikadze, G., Paulus, W., Kuo, M. F., and Nitsche, M. A. (2013). Effect of serotonin on paired associative stimulation-induced plasticity in the human motor cortex. Neuropsychopharmacology 17, 127. doi: 10.1038/npp.2013.127

Baudewig, J., Siebner, H. R., Bestmann, S., Tergau, F., Tings, T., Paulus, W., and Frahm, J. (2001). Functional MRI of cortical activations induced by transcranial magnetic stimulation (TMS). Neuroreport 12, 3543–3548. doi: 10.1097/00001756-200111160-00034

Baumgartner, U., Vogel, H., Ohara, S., Treede, R. D., and Lenz, F. A. (2010). Dipole source analyses of early median nerve SEP components obtained from subdural grid recordings. J. Neurophysiol. 104, 3029–41. doi: 10.1152/jn.00116.2010

Ben Taib, N. O., Nordeyn, O. B. T., Manto, M., Mario, M., Pandolfo, M., Massimo, P., et al. (2005). Hemicerebellectomy blocks the enhancement of cortical motor output associated with repetitive somatosensory stimulation in the rat. J. Physiol. (Lond.) 567(Pt 1), 293–300. doi: 10.1113/jphysiol.2005.088229

Bertolasi, L., Priori, A., Tinazzi, M., Bertasi, V., and Rothwell, J. C. (1998). Inhibitory action of forearm flexor muscle afferents on corticospinal outputs to antagonist muscles in humans. J. Physiol. (Lond.) 511, 947–956. doi: 10.1111/j.1469-7793.1998.947bg.x

Bestmann, S., Baudewig, J., Siebner, H. R., Rothwell, J. C., and Frahm, J. (2004).

Functional MRI of the immediate impact of transcranial magnetic stimulation on cortical and subcortical motor circuits. Eur. J. Neurosci. 19, 1950–1962. doi: 10.1111/j.1460-9568.2004.03277.x

Bi, G. Q., and Poo, M. M. (1998). Synaptic modifications in cultured hippocampal neurons: Dependence on spike timing, synaptic strength, and postsynaptic cell type. J. Neurosci. 18, 10464–10472.

Bi, G., and Poo, M. (2001). Synaptic modification by correlated activ ity: Hebb's postulate revisited. Annu. Rev. Neurosci. 24, 139–166. doi: 10.1146/annurev.neuro.24.1.139

Boakye, M., Huckins, S. C., Szeverenyi, N. M., Taskey, B. I., and Hodge, C. J. (2000). Functional magnetic resonance imaging of somatosensory cortex activity pro- duced by electrical stimulation of the median nerve or tactile stimulation of the index finger. J. Neurosurg. 93, 774–783. doi: 10.3171/jns.2000.93.5.0774

Bohning, D. E., Pecheny, A. P., Epstein, C. M., Speer, A. M., Vincent, D. J., Dannels, W., and George, M. S. (1997). Mapping transcranial magnetic stimulation (TMS) fields in vivo with MRI. Neuroreport 8, 2535–2538. doi: 10.1097/00001756-199707280-00023

Bologna, M., Conte, A., Suppa, A., and Berardelli, A. (2012). Motor cortex plasticity in Parkinson's disease: advances and controversies. Clin. Neurophysiol. 123, 640–641. doi: 10.1016/j.clinph.2011.08.021

Brasil-Neto, J. P., Cammarota, A., Valls-Solé, J., Pascual-Leone, A., Hallett, M., and Cohen, L. G. (1995). Role of intracortical mechanisms in the late part of the silent period to transcranial stimulation of the human motor cortex. Acta Neurol. Scand. 92, 383–386. doi: 10.1111/j.1600-0404.1995.tb00151.x

Burton, H., and Fabri, M. (1995). ipsilateral intracortical connections of physio- logically defined cutaneous representations in area-3b and area-1 of macaque monkeys - projections in the vicinity of the central sulcus. J. Comp. Neurol. 355, 508–538. doi: 10.1002/cne.903550404

Burton, H., and Kopf, E. M. (1984). ipsilateral cortical connections from the 2nd and 4th somatic sensory areas in the cat. J. Comp. Neurol. 225, 527–553. doi: 10.1002/cne.902250405

Canedo, A. (1997). Primary motor cortex influences on the descending and ascend- ing systems. Prog. Neurobiol. 51, 287–335. doi: 10.1016/S0301-0082(96)00058-5 Caporale, N., and Dan, Y. (2008). Spike timing-dependent plasticity: a Hebbian learning rule. Annu. Rev. Neurosci. 31, 25–40. doi: 10.1146/annurev.neuro.31. 060407.125639

Cardenas-Morales, L., Volz, L. J., Michely, J., Rehme, A. K., Pool, E. M., Nettekoven, C., et al. (2013). Network connectivity and individual responses to brain stimulation in the human motor system. Cereb. Cortex 8, 8. doi: 10.1093/cer- cor/bht023

Carson, R. G., Nelson, B. D., Buick, A. R., Carroll, T. J., Kennedy, N. C., and Cann, R. M. (2013). Characterizing changes in the excitability of corticospinal projec- tions to proximal muscles of the upper limb. Brain Stimul. 24, 760–768. doi: 10.1016/j.brs.2013.01.016

Carson, R. G., Riek, S., Mackey, D. C., Meichenbaum, D. P., Willms, K., Forner, M., et al. (2004). Excitability changes in human forearm corticospinal pro- jections and spinal reflex pathways during rhythmic voluntary movement of the opposite limb. J. Physiol. (Lond.) 560, 929–940. doi: 10.1113/jphysiol.2004. 069088

Castel-Lacanal, E., Gerdelat-Mas, A., Marque, P., Loubinoux, I., and Simonetta- Moreau, M. (2007). Induction of cortical plastic changes in wrist muscles by paired associative stimulation in healthy subjects and post-stroke patients. Exp. Brain Res. 180, 113–122. doi: 10.1007/s00221-006-0844-5

Castel-Lacanal, E., Marque, P., Tardy, J., De Boissezon, X., Guiraud, V., Chollet, F., Loubinoux, I. et al. (2009). Induction of cortical plastic changes in wrist mus- cles by paired associative stimulation in the recovery phase of stroke patients. Neurorehabil. Neural Repair 23, 366–372. doi: 10.1177/1545968308322841

Chapman, C. A., Perez, Y., and Lacaille, J. C. (1998). Effects of GABA(A) inhi- bition on the expression of long-term potentiation in CA1 pyramidal cells are dependent on tetanization parameters. Hippocampus 8, 289–298. doi: 10.1002/(SiCi)1098-1063(1998)8:<289::AID-HIPO10>3.0.CO;2-X

Charlton, C. S., Ridding, M. C., Thompson, P. D., and Miles, T. S. (2003). Prolonged peripheral nerve stimulation induces persistent changes in excitability of human motor cortex. J. Neurol. Sci. 208, 79–85. doi: 10.1016/S0022-510X(02)00443-4

Cheeran, B., Talelli, P., Mori, F., Koch, G., Suppa, A., Edwards, M., et al. (2008). A common polymorphism in the brain-derived neurotrophic factor gene (BDNF) modulates human cortical plasticity and the response to rTMS. J. Physiol. (Lond.) 586, 5717–5725. doi: 10.1113/jphysiol.2008.159905

Chen, R., Corwell, B., and Hallett, M. (1999a). Modulation of motor cortex excitability by median nerve and digit stimulation. Exp. Brain Res. 129, 77–86. doi: 10.1007/s002210050938

Chen, R., Lozano, A. M., and Ashby, P. (1999b). Mechanism of the silent period following transcranial magnetic stimulation—Evidence from epidural recordings. Exp. Brain Res. 128, 539–542. doi: 10.1007/s002210050878

Chipchase, L. S., Schabrun, S. M., and Hodges, P. W. (2011). Peripheral electri- cal stimulation to induce cortical plasticity: a systematic review of stimulus parameters. Clin. Neurophysiol. 122, 456–463. doi: 10.1016/j.clinph.2010.07.025 Cirillo, J., Lavender, A. P., Ridding, M. C., and Semmler, J. G. (2009). Motor cortex plasticity induced by paired associative stimulation is enhanced in phys- ically active individuals. J. Physiol. (Lond.) 587, 5831–5842. doi: 10.1113/jphysiol.2009.181834

Classen, J., Steinfelder, B., Liepert, J., Stefan, K., Celnik, P., Cohen, L. G., et al. (2000). Cutaneomotor integration in humans is somatotopically organized at various levels of the nervous system and is task dependent. Exp. Brain Res. 130, 48–59. doi: 10.1007/s002210050005

Conde, V., Vollmann, H., Sehm, B., Taubert, M., Villringer, A., and Ragert, P. (2012). Cortical thickness in primary sensorimotor cortex influences the effectiveness of paired associative stimulation. Neuroimage 60, 864–870. doi: 10.1016/j.neuroimage.2012.01.052

Cooke, S. F., and Bliss, T. V. P. (2006). Plasticity in the human central nervous system. Brain 129(Pt 7), 1659–1673. doi: 10.1093/brain/awl082

Cortes, M., Thickbroom, G. W., Valls-Sole, J., Pascual-Leone, A., and Edwards, D. J. (2011). Spinal associative stimulation: a non-invasive stimulation paradigm to modulate spinal excitability. Clin. Neurophysiol. 122, 2254–2259. doi: 10.1016/j.clinph.2011.02.038

Cowey, A., and Walsh, V. (2000). Magnetically induced phosphenes in sighted, blind and blindsighted observers. Neuroreport 11, 3269–3273. doi: 10.1097/00001756-200009280-00044

Dan, Y., and Poo, M. M. (2004). Spike timing-dependent plasticity of neural circuits. Neuron 44, 23–30. doi: 10.1016/j.neuron.2004.09.007

Dan, Y., and Poo, M. M. (2006). Spike timing-dependent plasticity: from synapse to perception. Physiol. Rev. 86, 1033–1048. doi: 10.1152/physrev.00030.2005 Daoudal, G., and Debanne, D. (2003). Long-term plasticity of intrinsic excitability: learning rules and mechanisms. Learn. Mem. 10, 456–465. doi: 10.1101/lm.64103

Darian-Smith, C., and Darian-Smith, I. (1993). Thalamic projections to area- 3a, area-3b, and area-4 in the sensorimotor cortex of the mature and infant macaque monkey. J. Comp. Neurol. 335, 173–199. doi: 10.1002/cne.903350204

Darian-Smith, C., Darian-Smith, I., Burman, K., and Ratcliffe, N. (1993). Ipsilateral cortical projections to areas 3a, 3b, and 4 in the macaque monkey. J. Comp. Neurol. 335, 200–213. doi: 10.1002/cne.903350205

Davies, C. H., Starkey, S. J., Pozza, M. F., and Collingridge, G. L. (1991). Gaba- b autoreceptors regulate the induction of ltp. Nature 349, 609–611. doi: 10.1038/349609a0

De Beaumont, L., Tremblay, S., Poirier, J., Lassonde, M., and Theoret, H. (2012). Altered bidirectional plasticity and reduced implicit motor learning in concussed athletes. Cereb. Cortex 22, 112–121. doi: 10.1093/cercor/ bhr096

De Lucia, M., Parker, G. J. M., Embleton, K., Newton, J. M., and Walsh, V. (2007). Diffusion tensor MRI-based estimation of the influence of brain tissue anisotropy on the effects of transcranial magnetic stimulation. Neuroimage 36, 1159–1170. doi: 10.1016/j.neuroimage.2007.03.062

Deletis, V., Schild, J. H., Beric, A., and Dimitrijevic, M. R. (1992). facil- itation of motor evoked-potentials by somatosensory afferent stimula- tion. Electroencephalogr. Clin. Neurophysiol. 85, 302–310. doi: 10.1016/0168- 5597(92)90106-L

Desmedt, J. E., and Ozaki, I. (1991). seps to finger joint input lack the n20-p20 response that is evoked by tactile inputs—contrast between cortical genera- tors in area-3b and area-2 in humans. Electroencephalogr. Clin. Neurophysiol. 80, 513–521. doi: 10.1016/0168-5597(91)90133-I

Destexhe, A., Rudolph, M., and Pare, D. (2003). The high-conductance state of neo- cortical neurons in vivo. Nat. Rev. Neurosci. 4, 739–751. doi: 10.1038/nrn1198

Devanne, H., Degardin, A., Tyvaert, L., Bocquillon, P., Houdayer, E., Manceaux, A., et al. (2009). Afferent-induced facilitation of primary motor cortex excitability in the region controlling hand muscles in humans. Eur. J. Neurosci. 30, 439–448. doi: 10.1111/j.1460-9568.2009.06815.x

Di Lazzaro, V., Dileone, M., Pilato, F., Capone, F., Musumeci, G., Ranieri, F., et al. (2011). Modulation of motor cortex neuronal networks by rTMS: com- parison of local and remote effects of six different protocols of stimulation. J. Neurophysiol. 105, 2150–2156. doi: 10.1152/jn.00781.2010

Di Lazzaro, V., Dileone, M., Pilato, F., Profice, P., Oliviero, A., Mazzone, P., et al.

(2009a). Associative motor cortex plasticity: direct evidence in humans. Cereb. Cortex 19, 2326–2330. doi: 10.1093/cercor/bhn255

Di Lazzaro, V., Dileone, M., Profice, P., Pilato, F., Oliviero, A., Mazzone, P., et al. (2009b). LTD-like plasticity induced by paired associative stimulation: direct evidence in humans. Exp. Brain Res. 194, 661–664. doi: 10.1007/s00221-009- 1774-9

Di Lazzaro, V., Oliviero, A., Mazzone, P., Pilato, F., Saturno, E., Insola, A., et al. (2002). Direct demonstration of long latency cortico-cortical inhibition in nor- mal subjects and in a patient with vascular parkinsonism. Clin. Neurophysiol. 113, 1673–1679. doi: 10.1016/S1388-2457(02)00264-X

Di Lazzaro, V., Oliviero, A., Profice, P., Meglio, M., Cioni, B., Tonali, P., et al. (2001). Descending spinal cord volleys evoked by transcranial magnetic and electrical stimulation of the motor cortex leg area in conscious humans. J. Physiol. (Lond.) 537, 1047–1058. doi: 10.1113/jphysiol.2001.012572

Di Lazzaro, V., Oliviero, A., Profice, P., Pennisi, M. A., Di Giovanni, S., Zito, G., et al.

(2000). Muscarinic receptor blockade has differential effects on the excitabil- ity of intracortical circuits in the human motor cortex. Exp. Brain Res. 135, 455–461. doi: 10.1007/s002210000543

Di Lazzaro, V., Oliviero, A., Saturno, E., Dileone, M., Pilato, F., Nardone, R., et al. (2005). Effects of lorazepam on short latency afferent inhibition and short latency intracortical inhibition in humans. J. Physiol. (Lond.) 564, 661–668. doi: 10.1113/jphysiol.2004.061747

Di Lazzaro, V., Pilato, F., Oliviero, A., Dileone, M., Saturno, E., Mazzone, P., et al. (2006). Origin of facilitation of motor-evoked potentials after paired mag- netic stimulation: direct recording of epidural activity in conscious humans. J. Neurophysiol. 96, 1765–1771. doi: 10.1152/jn.00360.2006

Di Lazzaro, V., Profice, P., Ranieri, F., Capone, F., Dileone, M., Oliviero, A., et al. (2012). I-wave origin and modulation. Brain Stimul. 5, 512–525. doi: 10.1016/j.brs.2011.07.008

Di Lazzaro, V., Restuccia, D., Oliviero, A., Profice, P., Ferrara, L., Insola, A., et al. (1998). Magnetic transcranial stimulation at intensities below active motor threshold activates intracortical inhibitory circuits. Exp. Brain Res. 119, 265–268. doi: 10.1007/s002210050341

Di Lazzaro, V., Ziemann, U., and Lemon, R. N. (2008). State of the art: physiol- ogy of transcranial motor cortex stimulation. Brain Stimul. 1, 345–362. doi: 10.1016/j.brs.2008.07.004

Di Lazzaro, V., and Ziemann, U. (2013). The contribution of transcranial mag- netic stimulation in the functional evaluation of microcircuits in human motor cortex. Front Neural Circuits 7:00018. doi: 10.3389/fncir.2013.00018

Dileone, M., Profice, P., Pilato, F., Alfieri, P., Cesarini, L., Mercuri, E., et al. (2010). Enhanced human brain associative plasticity in Costello syndrome. J. Physiol. (Lond.) 588, 3445–3456. doi: 10.1113/jphysiol.2010.191072

Duffau, H. (2006). Brain plasticity: from pathophysiological mecha- nisms to therapeutic applications. J. Clin. Neurosci. 13, 885–897. doi: 10.1016/j.jocn.2005.11.045

Duguid, I. C. (2013). Presynaptic NMDA receptors: are they dendritic receptors in disguise? Brain Res. Bull. 93, 4–9. doi: 10.1016/j.brainresbull.2012.12.004

Eisen, A., Purves, S., and Hoirch, M. (1982). central nervous-system amplification– its potential in the diagnosis of early multiple-sclerosis. Neurology 32, 359–364. doi: 10.1212/WNL.32.4.359

Elahi, B., Gunraj, C., and Chen, R. (2012). Short-interval intracortical inhibi- tion blocks long-term potentiation induced by paired associative stimulation. J. Neurophysiol. 107, 1935–1941. doi: 10.1152/jn.00202.2011

Eroglu, C., Allen, N. J., Susman, M. W., O'rourke, N. A., Park, C. Y., Ozkan, E., et al. (2009). Gabapentin receptor alpha2delta-1 is a neuronal thrombospondin receptor responsible for excitatory CNS synaptogenesis. Cell 139, 380–92. doi: 10.1016/j.cell.2009.09.025

Evarts, E. V. (1966). Pyramidal tract activity associated with a conditioned hand movement in the monkey. J. Neurophysiol. 29, 1011–1027.

Evarts, E. V. (1968). Relation of pyramidal tract activity to force exerted during voluntary movement. J. Neurophysiol. 31, 14–27.

Farzan, F., Barr, M. S., Hoppenbrouwers, S. S., Fitzgerald, P. B., Chen, R., Pascual-Leone, A., et al. (2013). The EEG correlates of the TMS- induced EMG silent period in humans. Neuroimage 83C, 120–134. doi: 10.1016/j.neuroimage.2013.06.059

Fathi, D., Ueki, Y., Mima, T., Koganemaru, S., Nagamine, T., Tawfik, A., et al. (2010). Effects of aging on the human motor cortical plasticity stud- ied by paired associative stimulation. Clin. Neurophysiol. 121, 90–93. doi: 10.1016/j.clinph.2009.07.048

Feldman, D. E. (2000). Timing-based LTP and LTD at vertical inputs to layer II/III pyramidal cells in rat barrel cortex. Neuron 27, 45–56. doi: 10.1016/S0896-6273(00)00008-8

Feldman, D. E. (2012). The spike-timing dependence of plasticity. Neuron 75, 556–571. doi: 10.1016/j.neuron.2012.08.001

Ferreri, F., Pasqualetti, P., Maatta, S., Ponzo, D., Ferrarelli, F., Tononi, G., et al. (2011). Human brain connectivity during single and paired pulse transcranial magnetic stimulation. Neuroimage 54, 90–102. doi: 10.1016/j.neuroimage.2010.07.056

Ferreri, F., Ponzo, D., Hukkanen, T., Mervaala, E., Kononen, M., Pasqualetti,

P., et al. (2012). Human brain cortical correlates of short-latency afferent inhibition: a combined EEG-TMS study. J. Neurophysiol. 108, 314–323. doi: 10.1152/jn.00796.2011

Ferreri, F., Vecchio, F., Ponzo, D., Pasqualetti, P., and Rossini, P. M. (2013). Time- varying coupling of EEG oscillations predicts excitability fluctuations in the primary motor cortex as reflected by motor evoked potentials amplitude: an EEG–TMS study. Hum. Brain Mapp. doi: 10.1002/hbm.22306. [Epub ahead of print].

Fischer, M., and Orth, M. (2011). Short-latency sensory afferent inhibition: con- ditioning stimulus intensity, recording site, and effects of 1 Hz repetitive TMS. Brain Stimul. 4, 202–209. doi: 10.1016/j.brs.2010.10.005

Forss, N., Hari, R., Salmelin, R., Ahonen, A., Hamalainen, M., Kajola, M., Knuutila, J.,et al. (1994). activation of the human posterior parietal cortex by median nerve-stimulation. Exp. Brain Res. 99, 309–315. doi: 10.1007/BF00239597

Fox, P., Ingham, R., George, M. S., Mayberg, H., Ingham, J., Roby, J., et al. (1997). Imaging human intra-cerebral connectivity by PET during TMS. Neuroreport 8, 2787–2791. doi: 10.1097/00001756-199708180-00027

Fratello, F., Veniero, D., Curcio, G., Ferrara, M., Marzano, C., Moroni, F., et al. (2006). Modulation of corticospinal excitability by paired associative stimula- tion: reproducibility of effects and intraindividual reliability. Clin. Neurophysiol. 117, 2667–2674. doi: 10.1016/j.clinph.2006.07.315

Gandevia, S. C., and Burke, D. (1990). Projection of thenar muscle afferents to frontal and parietal cortex of human-subjects. Electroencephalogr. Clin.

Neurophysiol. 77, 353–361. doi: 10.1016/0168-5597(90)90057-K

Gandevia, S. C., Burke, D., and Mckeon, B. (1984). The projection of mus- cle afferents from the hand to cerebral-cortex in man. Brain 107, 1–13. doi: 10.1093/brain/107.1.1

Gatica Tossi, M. A., Lillemeier, A. S., and Dinse, H. R. (2013). Influence of stimulation intensity on paired-pulse suppression of human median nerve somatosensory evoked potentials. Neuroreport 24, 451–6. doi: 10.1097/WNR.0b013e3283616378

d Porter, R. (1987). A quantitative study of the distribution of neurons projecting to the precentral motor cortex in the monkey (macaca-fascicularis). J. Comp. Neurol. 259, 424–444. doi: 10.1002/cne.902590309

Grant, G., Landgren, S., and Silfvenius, H. (1975). columnar distribution of u-fibers

from postcruciate cerebral projection area of cats group-1 muscle afferents. Exp. Brain Res. 24, 57–74. doi: 10.1007/BF00236017

Halonen, J. P., Jones, S., and Shawkat, F. (1988). contribution of cutaneous and muscle afferent-fibers to cortical seps following median and radial nerve-stimulation in man. Electroencephalogr. Clin. Neurophysiol. 71, 331–335. doi: 10.1016/0168-5597(88)90035-4

Hamada, M., Strigaro, G., Murase, N., Sadnicka, A., Galea, J. M., Edwards, M. J., et al. (2012). Cerebellar modulation of human associative plasticity. J. Physiol. (Lond.) 590, 2365–2374. doi: 10.1113/jphysiol.2012.230540

Hammond, G., and Vallence, A.-M. (2007). Modulation of long-interval intracortical inhibition and the silent period by voluntary contraction. Brain Res. 1158, 63–70. doi: 10.1016/j.brainres.2007.05.014

Hanajima, R., and Ugawa, Y. (2008). "Paired-pulse measures," in The Oxford Handbook of Transcranial Stimulation, eds E. M. Wassermann, C. M. Epstein, U. Ziemann, V. Walsh, T. Paus, and S. H. Lisanby (New York, NY: Oxford University Press), 103–117

Hanajima, R., Ugawa, Y., Terao, Y., Sakai, K., Furubayashi, T., Machii, K., et al. (1998). Paired-pulse magnetic stimulation of the human motor cortex: dif- ferences among I waves. J. Physiol. (Lond.) 509, 607–618. doi: 10.1111/j.1469-7793.1998.607bn.x

Hanakawa, T., Mima, T., Matsumoto, R., Abe, M., Inouchi, M., Urayama, S., et al. (2009). Stimulus-response profile during single-pulse transcranial magnetic stimulation to the primary motor cortex. Cereb. Cortex 19, 2605–2615. doi: 10.1093/cercor/bhp013

Hari, R., Reinikainen, K., Kaukoranta, E., Hamalainen, M., Ilmoniemi, R., Penttinen, A., Salminen, J., et al. (1984). Somatosensory evoked cerebral magnetic-fields from si and sii in man. Electroencephalogr. Clin. Neurophysiol. 57, 254–263. doi: 10.1016/0013-4694(84)90126-3

Harris-Love, M. L., and Cohen, L. G. (2006). Noninvasive cortical stimulation in neurorehabilitation: a review. Arch. Phys. Med. Rehabil. 87, S84–S93. doi: 10.1016/j.apmr.2006.08.330

Hashimoto, I., Gatayama, T., Yoshikawa, K., Sasaki, M., and Nomura, M. (1992) Input-output relation of the somatosensory system for mechanical air-puff stimulation of the index finger in man. Exp. Brain Res. 88, 645–50. doi: 10.1007/BF00228193

Heidegger, T., Krakow, K., and Ziemann, U. (2010). Effects of antiepileptic drugs on associative LTP-like plasticity in human motor cortex. Eur. J. Neurosci. 32, 1215–1222. doi: 10.1111/j.1460-9568.2010.07375.x

Hendrich, J., Van Minh, A. T., Heblich, F., Nieto-Rostro, M., Watschinger, K., Striessnig, J., et al. (2008). Pharmacological disruption of calcium channel traf- ficking by the alpha2delta ligand gabapentin. Proc. Natl. Acad. Sci. U.S.A. 105, 3628–3633. doi: 10.1073/pnas.0708930105

Herman, D., Kang, R., Macgillis, M., and Zarzecki, P. (1985). Responses of cat motor cortex neurons to cortico-cortical and somatosensory inputs. Exp. Brain Res. 57, 598–604. doi: 10.1007/BF00237846

Hess, A., Kunesch, E., Classen, J., Hoeppner, J., Stefan, K., and Benecke, R. (1999). Task-dependent modulation of inhibitory actions within the primary motor cortex. Experimental brain research. Experimentelle Hirnforschung. Exp. cérèb. 124, 321–330.

Hess, G., and Donoghue, J. P. (1996). Long-term depression of horizontal con- nections in rat motor cortex. Eur. J. Neurosci. 8, 658–665. doi: 10.1111/j.1460-9568.1996.tb01251.x

Hill, D. N., Varga, Z., Jia, H., Sakmann, B., and Konnerth, A. (2013). Multibranch activity in basal and tuft dendrites during firing of layer 5 cor- tical neurons in vivo. Proc. Natl. Acad. Sci. U.S.A. 110, 13618–13623. doi: 10.1073/pnas.1312599110

Huber, R., Maatta, S., Esser, S. K., Sarasso, S., Ferrarelli, F., Watson, A., et al. (2008). Measures of cortical plasticity after transcranial paired associative stim- ulation predict changes in electroencephalogram slow-wave activity during subsequent sleep. J. Neurosci. 28, 7911–7918. doi: 10.1523/JNEUROSCI.1636-08.2008

Huerta, M. F., and Pons, T. P. (1990). Primary motor cortex receives input from area 3a in macaques. Brain Res. 537, 367–371. doi: 10.1016/0006-8993(90) 90388-R

Huerta, P. T., and Volpe, B. T. (2009). Transcranial magnetic stimulation, synaptic plasticity and network oscillations. J. Neuroeng. Rehabil. 6:7. doi: 10.1186/1743- 0003-6-7

Huffman, K. J., and Krubitzer, L. (2001). Thalamo-cortical connections of areas 3a and M1 in marmoset monkeys. J. Comp. Neurol. 435, 291–310. doi: 10.1002/cne.1031

Humeau, Y., Shaban, H., Bissière, S., and Lüthi, A. (2003) Presynaptic induction of heterosynaptic associative plasticity in the mammalian brain. Nature 426, 841–845. doi: 10.1038/nature02194

Ilic, N. V., Milanovic, S., Krstic, J., Bajec, D. D., Grajic, M., and Ilic, T. V. (2011). Homeostatic modulation of stimulation-dependent plasticity in human motor cortex. Physiol. Res. 60, S107–S112.

Ilic, T. V., Meintzschel, F., Cleff, U., Ruge, D., Kessler, K. R., and Ziemann, U. (2002). Short-interval paired-pulse inhibition and facilitation of human motor cor- tex: the dimension of stimulus intensity. J. Physiol. (Lond.) 545, 153–167. doi: 10.1113/jphysiol.2002.030122

Ilmoniemi, R. J., Virtanen, J., Ruohonen, J., Karhu, J., Aronen, H. J., Naatanen, R., et al. (1997). Neuronal responses to magnetic stimulation reveal cortical reactivity and connectivity. Neuroreport 8, 3537–3540. doi: 10.1097/00001756- 199711100-00024

Izhikevich, E. M. (2007). Solving the distal reward problem through linkage of STDP and dopamine signaling. Cereb. Cortex 17, 2443–2452. doi: 10.1093/cer- cor/bhl152

Jackson, A. (2012). "Plasticity in motor cortical connectivity," in Cortical Connectivity, eds R. Chen and J. C. Rothwell (Berlin Heidelberg: Springer), 3–22. doi: 10.1007/978-3-642-32767-4_1

Jackson, A., Gee, V. J., Baker, S. N., and Lemon, R. N. (2003). Synchrony between neurons with similar muscle fields in monkey motor cortex. Neuron 38, 115–125. doi: 10.1016/S0896-6273(03)00162-4

Jayaram, G., Santos, L., and Stinear, J. W. (2007). Spike-timing-dependent plasticity induced in resting lower limb cortex persists during subsequent walking. Brain Res. 1153, 92–97. doi: 10.1016/j.brainres.2007.03.062

Jayaram, G., and Stinear, J. W. (2008). Contralesional paired associative stimulation increases paretic lower limb motor excitability post-stroke. Exp. Brain Res. 185, 563–570. doi: 10.1007/s00221-007-1183-x

Jones, E. G., Coulter, J. D., and Hendry, S. H. (1978). Intracortical connectivity of architectonic fields in the somatic sensory, motor and parietal cortex of monkeys. J. Comp. Neurol. 181, 291–347. doi: 10.1002/cne.901810206

Jones, E. G., and Porter, R. (1980). What is area-3a. Brain Res. Rev. 2, 1–43. doi: 10.1016/0165-0173(80)90002-8

Jones, E. G., Wise, S. P., and Coulter, J. D. (1979). Differential thalamic relationships of sensory-motor and parietal cortical fields in monkeys. J. Comp. Neurol. 183, 833–881. doi: 10.1002/cne.901830410

Kaas, J. H. (1983). What, if anything, is SI? Organization of first somatosensory area of cortex. Physiol. Rev. 63, 206–231.

Kaelin-Lang, A., Luft, A. R., Sawaki, L., Burstein, A. H., Sohn, Y. H., and Cohen, L. G. (2002). Modulation of human corticomotor excitability by somatosensory input. J. Physiol. (Lond.) 540, 623–633. doi: 10.1113/jphysiol.2001.012801

Kaneko, T., Caria, M. A., and Asanuma, H. (1994a). Information-processing within the motor cortex.1. responses of morphologically identified motor cortical-cells to stimulation of the somatosensory cortex. J. Comp. Neurol. 345, 161–171. doi: 10.1002/cne.903450202

Kaneko, T., Caria, M. A., and Asanuma, H. (1994b). Information-processing within the motor cortex.2. intracortical connections between neurons receiving somatosensory cortical input and motor output neurons of the cortex. J. Comp. Neurol. 345, 172–184. doi: 10.1002/cne.903450203

Kaneko, T., Cho, R. H., Li, Y. Q., Nomura, S., and Mizuno, N. (2000). Predominant information transfer from layer III pyramidal neurons to corticospinal neurons. J. Comp. Neurol. 423, 52–65. doi: 10.1002/1096-9861(20000717)423:1<52::AID-CNE5>3.0.CO;2-F

Kang, J. S., Terranova, C., Hilker, R., Quartarone, A., and Ziemann, U. (2011).

Deficient homeostatic regulation of practice-dependent plasticity in writer's cramp. Cereb. Cortex 21, 1203–1212. doi: 10.1093/cercor/bhq204

Karhu, J., and Tesche, C. D. (1999). Simultaneous early processing of sensory input in human primary (SI) and secondary (SII) somatosensory cortices.

J. Neurophysiol. 81, 2017–2025.

Kawamura, T., Nakasato, N., Seki, K., Kanno, A., Fujita, S., Fujiwara, S., and Yoshimoto, T. (1996). Neuromagnetic evidence of pre- and post-central cor- tical sources of somatosensory evoked responses. Electroencephalogr. Clin. Neurophysiol. 100, 44–50. doi: 10.1016/0168-5597(95)00217-0

Kennedy, N. C., and Carson, R. G. (2008). The effect of simultaneous contrac- tions of ipsilateral muscles on changes in corticospinal excitability induced by paired associative stimulation (PAS). Neurosci. Lett. 445, 7–11. doi: 10.1016/j.neulet.2008.08.064

Khaslavskaia, S., Ladouceur, M., and Sinkjaer, T. (2002). Increase in tibialis anterior motor cortex excitability following repetitive electrical stimulation of the com- mon peroneal nerve. Exp. Brain Res. 145, 309–315. doi: 10.1007/s00221-002- 1094-9

Klostermann, F., Wahl, M., Schomann, J., Kupsch, A., Curio, G., and Marzinzik, F. (2009). Thalamo-cortical processing of near-threshold somatosensory stimuli in humans. Eur. J. Neurosci. 30, 1815–1822. doi: 10.1111/j.1460-9568.2009.06970.x

Knash, M. E., Kido, A., Gorassini, M., Chan, K. M., and Stein, R. B. (2003). Electrical stimulation of the human common peroneal nerve elicits lasting facil- itation of cortical motor-evoked potentials. Exp. Brain Res. 153, 366–377. doi: 10.1007/s00221-003-1628-9

Kojima, S., Onishi, H., Sugawara, K., Kirimoto, H., Suzuki, M., and Tamaki, H. (2013). Modulation of the cortical silent period elicited by single- and paired-pulse transcranial magnetic stimulation. BMC Neurosci. 14:43. doi: 10.1186/1471-2202-14-43

Komori, T., Watson, B. V., and Brown, W. F. (1992). Influence of peripheral affer- ents on cortical and spinal motoneuron excitability. Muscle Nerve 15, 48–51. doi: 10.1002/mus.880150109

Komssi, S., Aronen, H. J., Huttunen, J., Kesaniemi, M., Soinne, L., Nikouline, V. V., et al. (2002). Ipsi- and contralateral EEG reactions to transcranial magnetic stimulation. Clin. Neurophysiol. 113, 175–184. doi: 10.1016/S1388- 2457(01)00721-0

Korchounov, A., and Ziemann, U. (2011). Neuromodulatory neurotrans- mitters influence LTP-like plasticity in human cortex: a pharmaco-TMS study. Neuropsychopharmacology 36, 1894–1902. doi: 10.1038/npp.

2011.75

Korvenoja, A., Huttunen, J., Salli, E., Pohjonen, H., Martinkauppi, S., Palva, L. M., et al. (1999). Activation of multiple cortical areas in response to somatosen-sory stimulation: combined magnetoencephalographic and functional magnetic resonance imaging. Hum. Brain Mapp. 8, 13–27.

Kosar, E., Waters, R. S., Tsukahara, N., and Asanuma, H. (1985). Anatomical and physiological properties of the projection from the sensory cortex to the motor cortex in normal cats: the difference between corticocortical and tha- lamocortical projections. Brain Res. 345, 68–78. doi: 10.1016/0006-8993(85) 90837-6

Kotb, M. A., Mima, T., Ueki, Y., Begum, T., Khafagi, A. T., Fukuyama, H., and Nagamine, T. (2005). Effect of spatial attention on human sensorimotor inte-gration studied by transcranial magnetic stimulation. Clin. Neurophysiol. 116, 1195–1200. doi: 10.1016/j.clinph.2004.12.006

Krause, T., Kurth, R., Ruben, J., Schwiemann, J., Villringer, K., Deuchert, M., et al. (2001). Representational overlap of adjacent fingers in multiple areas of human primary somatosensory cortex depends on electrical stimulus inten- sity: an fMRI study. Brain Res. 899, 36–46. doi: 10.1016/S0006-8993(01) 02147-3

Kujirai, K., Kujirai, T., Sinkjaer, T., and Rothwell, J. C. (2006). Associative plasticity in human motor cortex during voluntary muscle contraction. J. Neurophysiol. 96, 1337–1346. doi: 10.1152/jn.01140.2005

Kujirai, T., Caramia, M. D., Rothwell, J. C., Day, B. L., Thompson, P. D., Ferbert, A., et al. (1993). Corticocortical inhibition in human motor cortex. J. Physiol. (Lond.) 471, 501–519.

Kumpulainen, S., Mrachacz-Kersting, N., Peltonen, J., Voigt, M., and Avela, J. (2012). The optimal interstimulus interval and repeatability of paired asso-ciative stimulation when the soleus muscle is targeted. Exp. Brain Res. 221, 241–249. doi: 10.1007/s00221-012-3165-x

Kunesch, E., Knecht, S., Schnitzler, A., Tyercha, C., Schmitz, F., and Freund, H. J. (1995). Somatosensory-evoked potentials elicited by intraneural micros-timulation of afferent nerve-fibers. J. Clin. Neurophysiol. 12, 476–487. doi: 10.1097/00004691-199509010-00007

Kuo, M. F., Grosch, J., Fregni, F., Paulus, W., and Nitsche, M. A. (2007). Focusing effect of acetylcholine on neuroplasticity in the human motor cortex. J. Neurosci. 27, 14442–14447. doi: 10.1523/JNEUROSCI.4104-07.2007

Kuo, M. F., Paulus, W., and Nitsche, M. A. (2008). Boosting focally-induced brain plasticity by dopamine. Cereb. Cortex 18, 648–651. doi: 10.1093/cercor/ bhm098

Laird, A. R., Robbins, J. M., Li, K., Price, L. R., Cykowski, M. D., Narayana, S., et al. (2008). Modeling motor connectivity using TMS/PET and structural equation modeling. Neuroimage 41, 424–436. doi: 10.1016/j.neuroimage.2008. 01.065

Lakhani, B., Vette, A. H., Mansfield, A., Miyasike-Dasilva, V., and McIlroy, W. E. (2012). Electrophysiological correlates of changes in reaction time based on stimulus intensity. PLoS ONE 7:e36407. doi: 10.1371/journal.pone. 0036407

Lamy, J. C., Russmann, H., Shamim, E. A., Meunier, S., and Hallett, M. (2010). Paired associative stimulation induces change in presynaptic inhibition of ia terminals in wrist flexors in humans. J. Neurophysiol. 104, 755–764. doi: 10.1152/jn.00761.2009

Lang, N., Harms, J., Weyh, T., Lemon, R. N., Paulus, W., Rothwell, J. C., et al. (2006). Stimulus intensity and coil characteristics influence the efficacy of rTMS to sup-press cortical excitability. Clin. Neurophysiol. 117, 2292–2301. doi: 10.1016/j. clinph.2006.05.030

Leukel, C., Taube, W., Beck, S., and Schubert, M. (2012). Pathway-specific plasticity in the human spinal cord. Eur. J. Neurosci. 35, 1622–1629. doi: 10.1111/j.1460-9568.2012.08067.x

Levy, W. B., and Steward, O. (1983). Temporal contiguity requirements for long- term associative potentiation/depression in the hippocampus. Neuroscience 8, 791–797. doi: 10.1016/0306-4522(83)90010-6

Lin, Y. Y., Shih, Y. H., Chen, J. T., Hsieh, J. C., Yeh, T. C., Liao, K. K., et al. (2003). Differential effects of stimulus intensity on peripheral and neuromag- netic cortical responses to median nerve stimulation. Neuroimage 20, 909–17. doi: 10.1016/S1053-8119(03)00387-2

Lisman, J. (1989). A mechanism for the Hebb and the anti-Hebb processes underlying learning and memory. Proc. Natl. Acad. Sci. U.S.A. 86, 9574–9578. doi: 10.1073/pnas.86.23.9574

Lisman, J., and Spruston, N. (2005). Postsynaptic depolarization requirements for LTP and LTD: a critique of spike timing-dependent plasticity. Nat. Neurosci. 8, 839–841. doi: 10.1038/nn0705-839

Lisman, J., and Spruston, N. (2010). Questions about STDP as a general model of synaptic plasticity. Front. Synaptic Neurosci. 2:140. doi: 10.3389/fnsyn.2010. 00140

Litvak, V., Zeller, D., Oostenveld, R., Maris, E., Cohen, A., Schramm, A., et al. (2007). LTP-like changes induced by paired associative stimulation of the primary somatosensory cortex in humans: source analysis and associated changes in behaviour. Eur. J. Neurosci. 25, 2862–2874. doi: 10.1111/j.1460-9568.2007.05531.x

Lu, M. K., Bliem, B., Jung, P., Arai, N., Tsai, C. H., and Ziemann, U. (2009). Modulation of preparatory volitional motor cortical activity by paired associa- tive transcranial magnetic stimulation. Hum. Brain Mapp. 30, 3645–3656. doi: 10.1002/hbm.20793

Luck, S. J. (2005). "Ten simple rules for designing ERP experiments," in Event- Related Potentials: A Methods Handbook, ed T. C. Handy (Cambridge, MA: MIT Press), 17–32.

Luft, A. R., Manto, M.-U., and Ben Taib, N. O. (2005). Modulation of motor cor- tex excitability by sustained peripheral stimulation: the interaction between the motor cortex and the cerebellum. Cerebellum 4, 90–96. doi: 10.1080/ 14734220410019084

Luft, A. R., Kaelin-Lang, A., Hauser, T. K., Buitrago, M. M., Thakor, N. V., Hanley, D. F., et al. (2002). Modulation of rodent cortical motor excitability by somatosensory input. Exp. Brain Res. 142, 562–569. doi: 10.1007/ s00221-001- 0952-1

Mackinnon, C. D., Verrier, M. C., and Tatton, W. G. (2000). Motor cortical potentials precede long-latency EMG activity evoked by imposed displace- ments of the human wrist. Exp. Brain Res. 131, 477–490. doi: 10.1007/s002219 900317

Magee, J. C., and Johnston, D. (1997). A synaptically controlled, associative signal for Hebbian plasticity in hippocampal neurons. Science 275, 209–213. doi: 10.1126/science.275.5297.209

Malinow, R., and Malenka, R. C. (2002). AMPA receptor trafficking and synaptic plasticity. Annu. Rev. Neurosci. 25, 103–126. doi: 10.1146/annurev.neuro.25. 112701.142758

Manto, M., Nowak, D. A., and Schutter, D. J. (2006). Coupling between cerebel- lar hemispheres and sensory processing. Cerebellum 5, 187–188. doi: 10.1080/ 14734220600925075

Markram, H., Gerstner, W., and Sjöström, P. J. (2011). A history of spike-timing-dependent plasticity. Front. Synaptic Neurosci. 3:4. doi: 10.3389/ fnsyn.2011.00004

Mauguiere, F., Merlet, I., Forss, N., Vanni, S., Jousmaki, V., Adeleine, P., et al. (1997). Activation of a distributed somatosensory cortical network in the human brain. A dipole modelling study of magnetic fields evoked by median nerve stimulation.1. Location and activation timing of SEF sources. Electroencephalogr. Clin. Neurophysiol. 104, 281–289. doi: 10.1016/S0013-4694(97)00006-0

Mayer, M. L., Westbrook, G. L., and Guthrie, P. B. (1984). Voltage-dependent block by Mg2+ of NMDA responses in spinal cord neurones. Nature 309, 261–263. doi: 10.1038/309261a0

McDonnell, M. N., Orekhov, Y., and Ziemann, U. (2006). The role of GABA(B) receptors in intracortical inhibition in the human motor cortex. Exp. Brain Res. 173, 86–93. doi: 10.1007/ s00221-006-0365-2

McDonnell, M. N., Orekhov, Y., and Ziemann, U. (2007). Suppression of LTP-like plasticity in human motor cortex by the GABA(B) receptor agonist baclofen. Exp. Brain Res. 180, 181–186. doi: 10.1007/s00221-006-0849-0

McKay, D. R., Ridding, M. C., and Miles, T. S. (2003). Magnetic stimulation of motor and somatosensory cortices suppresses perception of ulnar nerve stimuli. Int. J. Psychophysiol. 48, 25–33. doi: 10.1016/S0167-8760(02)00159-9

McKay, D. R., Ridding, M. C., Thompson, P. D., and Miles, T. S. (2002). Induction of persistent changes in the organisation of the human motor cortex. Exp. Brain Res. 143, 342–349. doi: 10.1007/ s00221-001-0995-3

McLaughlin, D. F., and Kelly, E. F. (1993). Evoked-potentials as indexes of adaptation in the somatosensory system in humans—a review and prospectus. Brain Res. Rev. 18, 151–206. doi: 10.1016/0165-0173(93)90001-G

Meunier, S., Russmann, H., Shamim, E., Lamy, J.-C., and Hallett, M. (2012).

Plasticity of cortical inhibition in dystonia is impaired after motor learning and paired-associative stimulation. Eur. J. Neurosci. 35, 975–986. doi: 10.1111/j. 1460-9568.2012.08034.x

Meunier, S., Russmann, H., Simonetta-Moreau, M., and Hallett, M. (2007). Changes in spinal excitability after PAS. J. Neurophysiol. 97, 3131–3135. doi: 10.1152/jn.01086.2006

Mima, T., Terada, K., Maekawa, M., Nagamine, T., Ikeda, A., and Shibasaki, H. (1996). Somatosensory evoked potentials following proprioceptive stimulation of finger in man. Exp. Brain Res. 111, 233–245. doi: 10.1007/BF00227300

Moliadze, V., Zhao, Y. Q., Eysel, U., and Funke, K. (2003). Effect of transcranial magnetic stimulation on single-unit activity in the cat primary visual cortex.

J. Physiol. (Lond.) 553, 665–679. doi: 10.1113/jphysiol.2003.050153

Monte-Silva, K., Kuo, M. F., Thirugnanasambandam, N., Liebetanz, D., Paulus, W., and Nitsche, M. A. (2009). Dose-Dependent Inverted U-shaped effect of dopamine (D-2-Like) receptor activation on focal and nonfocal plastic- ity in humans. J. Neurosci. 29, 6124–6131. doi: 10.1523/JNEUROSCI.0728-09.2009

Morgante, F., Espay, A. J., Gunraj, C., Lang, A. E., and Chen, R. (2006). Motor cortex plasticity in Parkinson's disease and levodopa-induced dyskinesias. Brain 129, 1059–1069. doi: 10.1093/brain/ awl031

Mrachacz-Kersting, N., Fong, M., Murphy, B. A., and Sinkjaer, T. (2007). Changes in excitability of the cortical projections to the human tibialis ante- rior after paired associative stimulation. J. Neurophysiol. 97, 1951–1958. doi: 10.1152/jn.01176.2006

Mrachacz-Kersting, N., Kristensen, S. R., Niazi, I. K., and Farina, D. (2012). Precise temporal association between cortical potentials evoked by motor imagination and afference induces cortical plasticity. J. Physiol. (Lond.) 590(Pt 7), 1669–1682. doi: 10.1113/jphysiol.2011.222851

Muller, J. F. M., Orekhov, Y., Liu, Y., and Ziemann, U. (2007). Homeostatic plastic- ity in human motor cortex demonstrated by two consecutive sessions of paired associative stimulation. Eur. J. Neurosci. 26, 1077–1077. doi: 10.1111/j.1460-9568.2007.05790.x

Muller-Dahlhaus, F., Ziemann, U., and Classen, J. (2010). Plasticity resembling spike-timing dependent synaptic plasticity: the evidence in human cortex. Front. Synaptic Neurosci. 2:34. doi: 10.3389/fnsyn.2010.00034

Muller-Dahlhaus, J. F. M., Orekhov, Y., Liu, Y., and Ziemann, U. (2008). Interindividual variability and age-dependency of motor cortical plasticity induced by paired associative stimulation. Exp. Brain Res. 187, 467–475. doi: 10.1007/s00221-008-1319-7

Nelson, A. J., Staines, W. R., Graham, S. J., and McIlroy, W. E. (2004). Activation in SI and SII: the influence of vibrotactile amplitude during pas- sive and task-relevant stimulation. Brain Res. Cogn. Brain Res. 19, 174–84. doi: 10.1016/j.cogbrainres.2003.11.013

Ni, Z., Muller-Dahlhaus, F., Chen, R., and Ziemann, U. (2011). Triple-pulse TMS to study interactions between neural circuits in human cortex. Brain Stimul. 4, 281–293. doi: 10.1016/j.brs.2011.01.002

Niazi, I. K., Mrachacz-Kersting, N., Jiang, N., Dremstrup, K., and Farina, D. (2012).

Peripheral electrical stimulation triggered by self-paced detection of motor intention enhances motor evoked potentials. IEEE Trans. Neural Syst. Rehabil. Eng. 20, 595–604. doi: 10.1109/TNSRE.2012.2194309

Nitsche, M. A., Kuo, M. F., Grosch, J., Bergner, C., Monte-Silva, K., and Paulus, W. (2009). D-1-receptor impact on neuroplasticity in humans. J. Neurosci. 29, 2648–2653. doi: 10.1523/JNEUROSCI.5366-08.2009

Nitsche, M. A., Muller-Dahlhaus, F., Paulus, W., and Ziemann, U. (2012). The pharmacology of neuroplasticity induced by non-invasive brain stimulation: building models for the clinical use of CNS active drugs. J. Physiol. (Lond.) 590, 4641–4662. doi: 10.1113/jphysiol.2012.232975

Nitsche, M. A., Roth, A., Kuo, M. F., Fischer, A. K., Liebetanz, D., Lang, N., Tergau, F., et al. (2007). Timing-dependent modulation of associative plasticity by general network excitability in the human motor cortex. J. Neurosci. 27, 3807–3812. doi: 10.1523/JNEUROSCI.5348-06.2007

Nowak, L., Bregestovski, P., Ascher, P., Herbet, A., and Prochiantz, A. (1984). Magnesium gates glutamate-activated channels in mouse central neurones. Nature 307, 462–465. doi: 10.1038/307462a0

Olsen, R. W., and Sieghart, W. (2009). GABA A receptors: subtypes provide diversity of function and pharmacology. Neuropharmacology 56, 141–148. doi: 10.1016/j.neuropharm.2008.07.045

Ortu, E., Deriu, F., Suppa, A., Tolu, E., and Rothwell, J. C. (2008). Effects of voli- tional contraction on intracortical inhibition and facilitation in the human motor cortex. J. Physiol. (Lond.) 586, 5147–5159. doi: 10.1113/jphysiol.2008. 158956

Ostojic, S., and Fusi, S. (2013). Synaptic encoding of temporal contiguity. Front. Comput. Neurosci. 7:32. doi: 10.3389/fncom.2013.00032

Padel, Y., and Relova, J. L. (1991). Somatosensory responses in the cat motor cortex.1. identification and course of an afferent pathway. J. Neurophysiol. 66, 2041–2058.

Paille, V., Fino, E., Du, K., Morera-Herreras, T., Perez, S., Kotaleski, J. H., et al. (2013). GABAergic circuits control spike-timing-dependent plasticity. J. Neurosci. 33, 9353–9363. doi: 10.1523/JNEUROSCI.5796-12.2013

Parain, D., and Delapierre, G. (1991). Effects of stimulus intensity increase on short-latency somatosensory evoked potentials: application of polynomial curvature coefficients. Brain Topogr. 4, 31–5. doi: 10.1007/BF01129663

Paulus, W., Classen, J., Cohen, L. G., Large, C. H., Di Lazzaro, V., Nitsche, M., et al. (2008). State of the art: pharmacologic effects on cortical excitability mea- sures tested by transcranial magnetic stimulation. Brain Stimul. 1, 151–163. doi: 10.1016/j.brs.2008.06.002

Paus, T., Jech, R., Thompson, C. J., Comeau, R., Peters, T., and Evans, A. C. (1997).

Transcranial magnetic stimulation during positron emission tomography: a new method for studying connectivity of the human cerebral cortex. J. Neurosci. 17, 3178–3184.

Perez, M. A., Field-Fote, E. C., and Floeter, M. K. (2003). Patterned sensory stim- ulation induces plasticity in reciprocal Ia inhibition in humans. J. Neurosci. 23, 2014–2018.

Peurala, S. H., Muller-Dahlhaus, J. F. M., Arai, N., and Ziemann, U. (2008). Interference of short-interval intracortical inhibition (SICI) and short-interval intracortical facilitation (SICF). Clin. Neurophysiol. 119, 2291–2297. doi: 10.1016/j.clinph.2008.05.031

Pfister, J. P., and Gerstner, W. (2006). Triplets of spikes in a model of spike timing-dependent plasticity. J. Neurosci. 26, 9673–9682. doi: 10.1523/JNEUROSCI.1425-06.2006

Pons, T. P., and Kaas, J. H. (1986). Corticocortical connections of area-2 of somatosensory cortex in macaque monkeys—a correlative anatom- ical and electrophysiological study. J. Comp. Neurol. 248, 313–335. doi: 10.1002/cne.902480303

Popa, T., Velayudhan, B., Hubsch, C., Pradeep, S., Roze, E., Vidailhet, M., et al.

(2013). Cerebellar processing of sensory inputs primes motor cortex plasticity. Cereb. Cortex 23, 305–314. doi: 10.1093/cercor/bhs016

Porter, L. L., and Sakamoto, K. (1988). Organization and synaptic rela- tionships of the projection from the primary sensory to the primary motor cortex in the cat. J. Comp. Neurol. 271, 387–396. doi: 10.1002/cne. 902710307

Porter, L. L., Sakamoto, T., and Asanuma, H. (1990). Morphological and physio- logical identification of neurons in the cat motor cortex which receive direct input from the somatic sensory cortex. Exp. Brain Res. 80, 209–212. doi: 10.1007/BF00228864

Potter-Nerger, M., Fischer, S., Mastroeni, C., Groppa, S., Deuschl, G., Volkmann, J., et al. (2009). Inducing homeostatic-like plasticity in human motor cortex

through converging corticocortical inputs. J. Neurophysiol. 102, 3180–3190. doi: 10.1152/jn.91046.2008

Prior, M. M., and Stinear, J. W. (2006). Phasic spike-timing-dependent plastic- ity of human motor cortex during walking. Brain Res. 1110, 150–158. doi: 10.1016/j.brainres.2006.06.057

Quartarone, A., Bagnato, S., Rizzo, V., Siebner, H. R., Dattola, V., Scalfari, A., et al. (2003). Abnormal associative plasticity of the human motor cortex in writer's cramp. Brain 126, 2586–2596. doi: 10.1093/brain/awg273

Quartarone, A., Morgante, F., Sant'angelo, A., Rizzo, V., Bagnato, S., Terranova, C., et al. (2008). Abnormal plasticity of sensorimotor circuits extends beyond the affected body part in focal dystonia. J. Neurol. Neurosurg. Psychiatry 79, 985–990. doi: 10.1136/jnnp.2007.121632

Quartarone, A., Rizzo, V., Bagnato, S., Morgante, F., Sant'angelo, A., Girlanda, P., et al. (2006). Rapid-rate paired associative stimulation of the median nerve and motor cortex can produce long-lasting changes in motor cortical excitability in humans. J. Physiol. (Lond.) 575, 657–670. doi: 10.1113/jphysiol.2006.114025

Quartarone, A., Rizzo, V., Terranova, C., Morgante, F., Schneider, S., Ibrahim, N., et al. (2009). Abnormal sensorimotor plasticity in organic but not in psychogenic dystonia. Brain 132, 2871–2877. doi: 10.1093/brain/awp213

Rajji, T. K., Liu, S. K., Frantseva, M. V., Mulsant, B. H., Thoma, J., Chen, R., et al. (2011). Exploring the effect of inducing long-term potentiation in the human motor cortex on motor learning. Brain Stimul. 4, 137–144. doi: 10.1016/j.brs.2010.09.007

Ridding, M. C., and Flavel, S. C. (2006). Induction of plasticity in the dominant and non-dominant motor cortices of humans. Exp. Brain Res. 171, 551–557. doi: 10.1007/s00221-005-0309-2

Ridding, M. C., and Taylor, J. L. (2001). Mechanisms of motor-evoked potential facilitation following prolonged dual peripheral and central stimulation in humans. J. Physiol. (Lond.) 537, 623–631. doi: 10.1111/j.1469-7793.2001.00623.x

Ridding, M. C., Brouwer, B., Miles, T. S., Pitcher, J. B., and Thompson, P. D. (2000).

Changes in muscle responses to stimulation of the motor cortex induced by peripheral nerve stimulation in human subjects. Exp. Brain Res. 131, 135–143. doi: 10.1007/s002219900269

Rodríguez-Moreno, A., Banerjee, A., and Paulsen, O. (2010). Presynaptic NMDA receptors and spike timing-dependent depression at cortical synapses. Front. Synaptic Neurosci. 2:18. doi: 10.3389/fnsyn.2010.00018

Rosenkranz, K., and Rothwell, J. C. (2006). Differences between the effects of three plasticity inducing protocols on the organization of the human motor cortex. Eur. J. Neurosci. 23, 822–829. doi: 10.1111/j.1460-9568.2006.04605.x

Rothwell, J. C., Thompson, P. D., Day, B. L., Boyd, S., and Marsden, C. D. (1991).

Stimulation of the human motor cortex through the scalp. Exp. Physiol. 76, 159–200.

Roy, F. D., and Gorassini, M. A. (2008). Peripheral sensory activation of cortical circuits in the leg motor cortex of man. J. Physiol. (Lond.) 586(Pt 17), 4091–4105. doi: 10.1113/jphysiol.2008.153726

Roy, F. D., Norton, J. A., and Gorassini, M. A. (2007). Role of sustained excitability of the leg motor cortex after transcranial magnetic stimulation in associative plasticity. J. Neurophysiol. 98, 657–667. doi: 10.1152/jn.00197.2007

Russmann, H., Lamy, J. C., Shamim, E. A., Meunier, S., and Hallett, M. (2009). Associative plasticity in intracortical inhibitory circuits in human motor cortex. Clin. Neurophysiol. 120, 1204–1212. doi: 10.1016/j.clinph.2009. 04.005

Sailer, A., Cunic, D. I., Paradiso, G. O., Gunraj, C. A., Wagle-Shukla,

A., Moro, E., et al. (2007). Subthalamic nucleus stimulation modu- lates afferent inhibition in Parkinson disease. Neurology 68, 356–363. doi: 10.1212/01. wnl.0000252812.95774.aa

Sailer, A., Molnar, G. F., Cunic, D. I., and Chen, R. (2002). Effects of peripheral sensory input on cortical inhibition in humans. J. Physiol. (Lond.) 544, 617–629. doi: 10.1113/jphysiol.2002.028670

Sailer, A., Molnar, G. F., Paradiso, G., Gunraj, C. A., Lang, A. E., and Chen, R. (2003). Short and long latency afferent inhibition in Parkinson's disease. Brain 126, 1883–1894. doi: 10.1093/brain/ awg183

Sakamoto, T., Porter, L. L., and Asanuma, H. (1987). Long-lasting potentiation of synaptic potentials in the motor cortex produced by stimulation of the sen- sory cortex in the cat: a basis of motor learning. Brain Res. 413, 360–364. doi: 10.1016/0006-8993(87)91029-8

Sale, M. V., Ridding, M. C., and Nordstrom, M. A. (2007). Factors influencing the magnitude and reproducibility of corticomotor excitability changes induced by paired associative stimulation. Exp. Brain Res. 181, 615–626. doi: 10.1007/s00221-007-0960-x

12

Multivariate autoregressive models with exogenous inputs for intracerebral responses to direct electrical stimulation of the human brain

Jui-Yang Chang*[1]*, Andrea Pigorini*[2]*, Marcello Massimini*[2]*, Giulio Tononi*[3]*, Lino Nobili*[4] *and Barry D. Van Veen*[1]**

[1] *Department of Electrical and Computer Engineering, University of Wisconsin, Madison, WI, USA*
[2] *Department of Clinical Sciences, University of Milan, Milan, Italy*
[3] *Department of Psychiatry, University of Wisconsin, Madison, WI, USA*
[4] *Centre of Epilepsy Surgery "C. Munari," Niguarda Hospital, Milan, Italy*

Correspondence:
Barry D. Van Veen, Department of Electrical and Computer Engineering, University of Wisconsin, 3611 Engineering Hall, 1415 Engineering Drive, Madison, WI 53706, USA.
e-mail: vanveen@engr.wisc.edu

A multivariate autoregressive (MVAR) model with exogenous inputs (MVARX) is developed for describing the cortical interactions excited by direct electrical current stimulation of the cortex. Current stimulation is challenging to model because it excites neurons in multiple locations both near and distant to the stimulation site. The approach presented here models these effects using an exogenous input that is passed through a bank of filters, one for each channel. The filtered input and a random input excite a MVAR system describing the interactions between cortical activity at the recording sites. The exogenous input filter coefficients, the autoregressive coefficients, and random input characteristics are estimated from the measured activity due to current stimulation. The effectiveness of the approach is demonstrated using intracranial recordings from three surgical epilepsy patients. We evaluate models for wakefulness and NREM sleep in these patients with two stimulation levels in one patient and two stimulation sites in another resulting in a total of 10 datasets. Excellent agreement between measured and model-predicted evoked responses is obtained across all datasets. Furthermore, one-step prediction is used to show that the model also describes dynamics in pre-stimulus and evoked recordings. We also compare integrated information—a measure of intracortical communication thought to reflect the capacity for consciousness—associated with the network model in wakefulness and sleep. As predicted, higher information integration is found in wakefulness than in sleep for all five cases.

Keywords: intracerebal EEG, evoked response, MVARX model, cross-validation, integrated information

1. INTRODUCTION

The remarkable cognitive abilities of the healthy human brain depend on an exquisite balance between functional specialization of local cortical circuits and their functional integration through long-range connections. Hence, there is considerable interest in characterizing long-range cause and effect or directional interactions in the human brain. Multivariate autoregressive (MVAR) models, sometimes referred to as vector autoregressive (VAR) models, have been widely applied to study directional cortical network properties from both intracranial data (e.g., Bernasconi and König, 1999; Brovelli et al., 2004; Winterhalder et al., 2005; Ding et al., 2006; Korzeniewska et al., 2008) and scalp EEG or MEG (e.g., Babiloni et al., 2005; Malekpour et al., 2012). An MVAR model describes each signal as a weighted combination of its own past values and the past values of other signals in the model—an autoregression—plus an error term. The weights relating the present of one signal to the past of another capture the causal or directed influence between signals. A variety of different metrics for summarizing the directed interactions in MVAR models have been proposed, including directed transfer functions (Kamiński and Blinowska, 1991), directed coherence (Baccalá and Sameshima, 2001), conditional Granger causality (Geweke, 1984), and integrated information (Barrett and Seth, 2011).

MVAR models assume the data is stationary and of constant mean. While stationarity and constant mean may be reasonable assumptions for a relatively short duration of spontaneous data, evoked or event-related data appear to violate these assumptions. For example, the mean or average response to a stimulus varies with time. An MVAR model fit to data with a time-varying mean results in spurious interactions because the assumption of stationarity is violated. Adaptive or time-varying methods have been developed to relax stationarity assumptions (Ding et al., 2000; Möller et al., 2001; Astolfi et al., 2008). For example, a time-varying mean response is removed by subtracting the ensemble average (Ding et al., 2000) and the MVAR model parameters are allowed to vary with time. Adaptive models require specification of an adaptation rate parameter that effectively determines how much of the past data is used to estimate the present model parameters, or equivalently, how fast the model is changing. Models that use fast adaptation are able to track faster changes in the underlying data, but employ less data to estimate model parameters and consequently possess more variability in the estimated model parameters (see Astolfi et al., 2008, for assessment of these issues).

During the pre-surgical evaluation of drug-resistant epileptic patients, direct electrical stimulation of the brain is systematically performed for diagnostic purposes to identify the epileptogenic zone (Munari et al., 1994). Electrical stimulation generates a time-varying response at the recording sites. In this paper we propose describing the response of the brain using stationary MVAR models with an exogenous input (MVARX) derived from the stimulus characteristics. MVARX models are commonly used in econometric time series analysis (Lütkepohl, 2006). The advantage of the MVARX model is that it does not require subtraction of the mean and consequent reduction in signal-to-noise ratio (SNR) or the complication of time-varying models to capture the response evoked by direct electrical stimulation. The model captures both the mean evoked response and the background activity present during the recordings. We demonstrate the effectiveness of the MVARX model using intracerebral recordings from epilepsy patients.

Direct electrical stimulation of the brain presents several modeling challenges. Although the timing and location of the stimulus is known precisely, the response of the brain in the near vicinity of the stimulus cannot be measured due to electrical artifacts and the propagation of the stimulus to more distant sites depends on the topology of axons in the vicinity of the stimulation site (Ranck, 1975). Electrical stimulation creates action potentials in neurons whose axons pass near the stimulus site. These neurons synapse both near and distant to the stimulation site, so the stimulus actually activates multiple, *a priori* unknown areas. The MVARX model explicitly accounts for this effect with a bank of finite impulse response (FIR) filters that capture the impact of the exogenous input, i.e., stimulus, on all recording sites. The exogenous input filter coefficients and the MVAR model parameters are simultaneously estimated from the recordings and knowledge of the stimulation times using a least squares procedure. The exogenous input filter coefficients describe the conduction paths from the stimulus site to each recording site, while the MVAR model parameters capture the causal interactions between recording sites.

The MVARX model is applied to 10 datasets collected from three subjects in wakefulness and NREM sleep. Two stimulation levels are studied in one subject, and two stimulation sites in another. The data consists of the intracranial response to 30 current impulses separated by 1 s. A cross-validation (CV) procedure is introduced for choosing the memory in the MVARX model. We demonstrate that a stationary MVARX model accurately describes the activity evoked by direct electrical stimulation. Comparison to a series of univariate autoregressive models with exogenous inputs (ARX) reveals that causal interactions must be modeled to accurately describe the measured activity. The series of ARX models result in much larger modeling error than the MVARX model. One-step prediction performance is used to demonstrate that the MVARX model also captures spontaneous fluctuations in the recorded data. The MVARX model errors pass a whiteness test while the univariate ARX models do not, further supporting the applicability of the MVARX model.

The MVARX models are employed to contrast integrated information in wakefulness and sleep. Integrated information is a measure of the extent to which the information generated by the causal interactions in the model cannot be partitioned into independent subparts of the system. Hence, integrated information measures the balance between functional specialization and integration represented by the model. Theoretical considerations (Tononi, 2004; Laureys, 2005; Dehaene et al., 2006; Seth et al., 2008) indicate that integrated information should be less in sleep than in wakefulness. This prediction is confirmed in all 10 datasets using our MVARX model.

This paper is organized as follows. Section 2 describes the data and preprocessing procedures. Section 3 defines the MVARX model, introduces the method for estimating the model parameters, including our CV approach for selecting model memory, and presents the residual whiteness test. Section 4 demonstrates the effectiveness of the proposed model using the 10 datasets described above and section 5 applies the MVARX models to contrast integrated information in wakefulness and sleep. This paper concludes with a discussion in section 6. For notation, boldface lower and upper case symbols represent vectors and matrices, respectively, while superscript T denotes matrix transpose and superscript -1 denotes matrix inverse. The trace of a matrix $\mathbf{A}$ is $\mathrm{tr}[\mathbf{A}]$ and the determinant is $\det(\mathbf{A})$. $E\{a\}$ denotes the expectation of a random variable a. The Euclidean norm of a vector $\mathbf{x}$ is $||\mathbf{x}||_2 = \sqrt{\mathbf{x}^T\mathbf{x}}$. The number of elements in a set S is $|S|$. $\mathbf{x} \sim \mathcal{N}(\mu, \Sigma)$ means that the vector $\mathbf{x}$ is normally distributed with mean μ and covariance matrix Σ.

2. DATA

2.1. SUBJECTS AND EXPERIMENTAL PROTOCOL

Three subjects with long-standing drug-resistant focal epilepsy participated in this study. All patients were candidates for surgical removal of the epileptic focus. During pre-surgical evaluation the patients underwent individual investigation with stereotactically implanted intracerebral multilead electrodes for precise localization of the epileptogenic areas (Cossu et al., 2005). All patients gave written informed consent before intracerebral electrode implantation as approved by the local Ethical Committee. Confirmation of the hypothesized seizure focus and localization of epileptogenic tissue in relation to essential cortex was achieved by simultaneous scalp and intracerebral electrode recording, as well as intracerebral stimulation during wakefulness and sleep to further investigate connectivity of epileptogenic and healthy tissue (Valentín et al., 2002, 2005). The decision on implantation site, duration of implantation and stimulation site(s) was made entirely on clinical needs. Stereoelectroencephalography (SEEG) activity was recorded from platinumiridium semiflexible multilead intracerebral electrodes, with a diameter of 0.8 mm, a contact length of 2 mm, an intercontact distance of 1.5 mm and a maximal contact number of 18 (Dixi Medical, Besançon, France) (Cossu et al., 2005). The individual placement of electrodes was ascertained by post-implantation tomographic imaging (CT) scans. Scalp EEG activity was recorded from two platinum needle electrodes placed during surgery at "10–20" positions Fz and Cz on the scalp. Electroocular activity was registered at the outer canthi of both eyes, and submental electromyographic activity was acquired with electrodes attached to the chin. EEG and SEEG signals were recorded using a 192-channel recording system (Nihon-Kohden Neurofax-110) with a sampling rate of 1000 Hz. Data was recorded and exported in EEG Nihon-Kohden format (Nobili et al., 2011, 2012). The data for each channel is obtained using bipolar referencing to a neighboring contact located entirely in the white matter. Intracerebral stimulations were started on the third day after electrode implantation. In eight out of ten cases we discuss, stimulation of strength 5 mA were performed, while for the other two cases stimulation of 1 mA were applied. At each stimulation session, the stimulation is applied at a single channel and SEEG recordings were obtained from all other channels. A single stimulation session consisted of a 30 impulse stimulation train at intervals of 1 s. Each impulse is of 0.2-ms duration. The channels that were stimulated were chosen based on clinical requirements. All patients included in this study were stimulated during wakefulness and stage 4 of NREM sleep. Sleep staging was performed using standard criteria (Rechtschaffen and Kales, 1968). Stimulations which elicited muscle twitches, sensations or cognitive symptoms, were excluded from this study, in order to prevent possible awareness of stimulation or alteration of sleep depth.

In our analysis, we consider a subset of 8–12 recording channels of all channels for each subject, as illustrated in **Figure 1**. The 8–12 channels were selected based on approximately maximizing the distance between the subset of channels that are both artifact free and near the surface of the cortex.

2.2. PREPROCESSING

During each stimulation session, a raw trigger signal that indicates the occurrence of current stimulation with 1 and the absence of stimulation with 0 is collected at a sampling rate of 1000 Hz in addition to the SEEG recordings. We use a Tukey-windowed median filter to remove volume conduction artifacts within 39 ms of each stimulus. First, a median filter of order 19 is applied to the raw data channel by channel. Next, the raw data within a 39-ms window centered at each stimulus is replaced with a weighted average of the raw data and the median filtered data to eliminate the artifact. The weights for the median filtered data take the form of a Tukey window (Bloomfield, 2000, p. 69) and are zero for ± 20 ms away from the stimulus, a cosine rising from 0 to 1 beginning at 19 ms prior to the stimulus and ending at 10 ms prior to the stimulus, unity until 10 ms post-stimulus, and then a cosine decreasing from 1 to 0 ending at 19 ms post-stimulus. The weighting applied to the raw data are one minus those applied to the median filtered data. **Figure 2** illustrates the results of this process. The cleaned data is then lowpass filtered by an FIR filter with passband-edge of 48 Hz and stopband-edge of 49.9 Hz to eliminate 50 Hz powerline contamination, and the lowpass filtered data is downsampled by a factor of 10 to a sampling frequency of 100 Hz. The portion of the downsampled data containing responses to stimulation are further segmented into 30 epochs of data $\mathbf{y}_n^{(j)}$, each of which contains 100 samples. Here superscript (j) denotes epoch index while subscript n denotes time index. The start of each epoch is from 12 samples (0.12 s) before the occurrence of a stimulus and the end is 87 samples (0.87 s) post-stimulus. Similarly, the raw trigger signal is lowpass filtered, downsampled by 10, and partitioned into 100-sample epochs $x_n^{(j)}$.

In principle, filtering the signal may have an impact on model estimation and causality inference (Barnett and Seth, 2011). We minimize the potential impact of filtering by specifying the stopband edge of the lowpass filter close to the post-downsampling Nyquist frequency.

2.3. IDENTIFICATION OF OUTLYING EPOCHS

An automated procedure is employed to exclude epochs that markedly deviate from the majority of epochs due to non-stationary brain activity or other factors. Let $\mathbf{y}_n^{(j)} = [y_{1,n}^{(j)}, y_{2,n}^{(j)}, \ldots, y_{d,n}^{(j)}]^T$ represent the d channels of recordings at

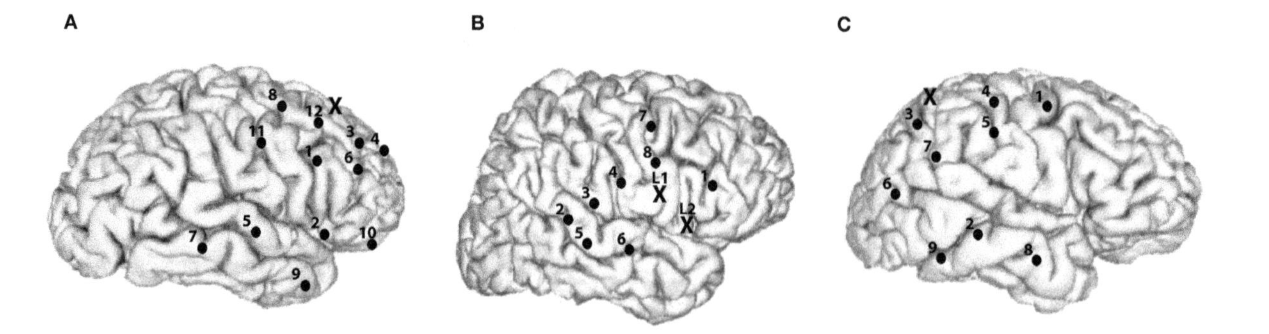

FIGURE 1 | Recording and stimulation electrode placements for the subjects. Black dots represents recording channels while black "X" represents stimulating channel(s). **(A)** Subject A, right hemisphere is shown. 1, Inferior frontal opercular; 2, anterior horizontal lateral fissure; 3, middle frontal gyrus; 4, middle frontal sulcus; 5, superior temporal sulcus; 6, inferior frontal sulcus; 7, middle temporal gyrus; 8, middle frontal gyrus; 9, middle temporal gyrus; 10, orbital gyrus; 11, precentral gyrus; 12, superior frontal sulcus; and X, middle frontal gyrus. **(B)** Subject B, right hemisphere is shown. 1, Inferior frontal gyrus; 2, superior temporal sulcus; 3, posterior lateral fissure; 4, postcentral solcus; 5, superior temporal gyrus; 6, transversal temporal sulcus; 7, superior frontal gyrus; 8, subcentral gyrus; X (L1), precentral gyrus, and X (L2), subcentral sulcus. **(C)** Subject C, right hemisphere is shown. 1, Precentral gyrus; 2, posterior middle temporal gyrus; 3, inferior parietal lobule; 4, postcentral gyrus; 5, postcentral sulcus; 6, angular gyrus; 7, supramarginal gyrus; 8, anterior middle temporal gyrus; 9, inferior temporal gyrus, and X, superior parietal lobule.

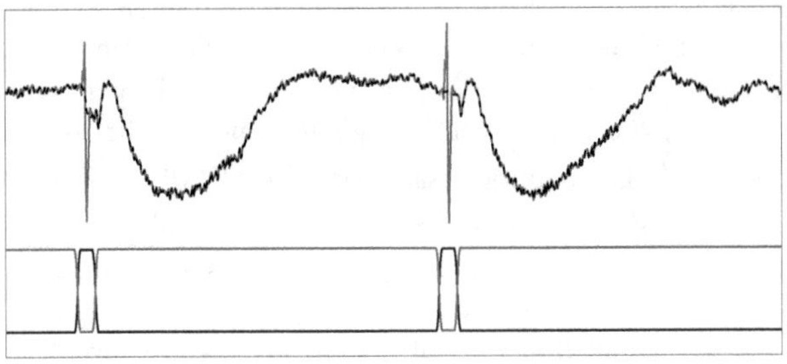

FIGURE 2 | Tukey-windowed median filtering for eliminating volume conduction artifacts. The upper trace depicts an example of raw data (blue solid line) and the Tukey-windowed median filter output (red dashed line). The lower trace depicts the weighting applied to the raw data (blue solid line) and the median filtered data (red solid line) to eliminate the volume conduction artifact.

time $n = 1, 2, \ldots, N_j$ from epochs $j = 1, 2, \ldots, J$. For epoch m, we compute the time-varying mean $\mu_{\mathbf{y}}^{-m}(n)$ and time-varying covariance matrix $\Sigma_{\mathbf{y}}^{-m}(n)$ by excluding the m-th epoch of data. That is,

$$\mu_{\mathbf{y}}^{-m}(n) = \frac{1}{J-1} \sum_{j=1, j\neq m}^{J} \mathbf{y}_n^{(j)} \tag{1}$$

$$\Sigma_{\mathbf{y}}^{-m}(n) = \frac{1}{J-2} \times \sum_{j=1, j\neq m}^{J} \left(\mathbf{y}_n^{(j)} - \mu_{\mathbf{y}}^{-m}(n)\right)\left(\mathbf{y}_n^{(j)} - \mu_{\mathbf{y}}^{-m}(n)\right)^T, \tag{2}$$

for $n = 1, \ldots, 100$. Here $m = 1$ to J and J is 30 for all data sets considered. Then the squared Mahalanobis distance (Penny, 1996) between the epoch m and the other epochs is computed as

$$D^2(m) = \sum_{n=1}^{100} \left(\mathbf{y}_n^{(m)} - \mu_{\mathbf{y}}^{-m}(n)\right)^T \times \left(\Sigma_{\mathbf{y}}^{-m}(n)\right)^{-1} \left(\mathbf{y}_n^{(m)} - \mu_{\mathbf{y}}^{-m}(n)\right). \tag{3}$$

Epochs with $D^2(m)$ exceeding

$$100 \cdot d + 60\sqrt{2 \cdot 100 \cdot d} \tag{4}$$

are declared as outliers and removed from subsequent analysis. Intuitively, if the data is Gaussian, then $D^2(m)$ is Chi-squared distributed with $100 \cdot d$ degrees of freedom. This implies that the threshold rules out an epoch m if $D^2(m)$ exceeds its mean plus 60 standard deviations. Thus this threshold only excludes epochs that have a large deviation from the temporal average of the other epochs. The number of epochs retained for analysis are given in **Table 1**.

Table 1 | Number of non-outlying epochs used in analysis.

Dataset	Wakefulness epochs	Sleep epochs
Subject A, 1 mA	29	25
Subject A, 5 mA	28	22
Subject B, L1	30	24
Subject B, L2	30	29
Subject C	30	29

3. METHODS

3.1. MVARX MODEL

The MVARX model of order (p, ℓ) describes the data as follows (Lütkepohl, 2006):

$$\mathbf{y}_n^{(j)} = \sum_{i=1}^{p} \mathbf{A}_i \mathbf{y}_{n-i}^{(j)} + \sum_{i=0}^{\ell} \mathbf{b}_i x_{n-i}^{(j)} + \mathbf{w}_n^{(j)}, \tag{5}$$

where $x_n^{(j)}$ denotes the input at time n and epoch j. The $d \times d$ matrices $\mathbf{A}_i = \{a_{m,n}(i)\}$ contain autoregressive coefficients describing the influence of channel n on channel m at lag i, and the $d \times 1$ vectors $\mathbf{b}_i = \{b_m(i)\}$ contain filter coefficients from the stimulus to channel m at lag i. The vectors $\mathbf{w}_n^{(j)}$ are $d \times 1$ zero-mean noise vectors with covariance matrix $\mathbf{Q}$ and are assumed to satisfy $E\{\mathbf{w}_n^{(i)}(\mathbf{w}_s^{(j)})^T\} = 0$, for either $i \neq j$ or $n \neq s$. We assume that the epochs are of varying lengths N_j and are possibly disconnected in time to accommodate rejection of outlying epochs. **Figure 3** depicts a schematic diagram of an example MVARX model. The diagram assumes there are three recording electrodes corresponding to the recordings $y_{1,n}$, $y_{2,n}$, and $y_{3,n}$ (the epoch index j is omitted in the figure for simplicity). The intracranial EEG signals recorded at the electrodes contain contributions due to the current stimulus response and background brain activity. The exogenous input x_n represents the current stimulation. If $\mathbf{B} = [\mathbf{b}_0, \ldots, \mathbf{b}_\ell]$ is a $d \times (\ell + 1)$ matrix of exogenous input coefficients, then the i-th row of $\mathbf{B}$, $[\mathbf{B}]_{i,:}$, is the impulse response of the filter representing the unknown transmission characteristics between the current stimulus and the i-th recording channel. The autoregressive coefficients $\mathbf{A} = [\mathbf{A}_1, \ldots, \mathbf{A}_p]$ indicate how past values of the recorded signals affect present values. The autoregressive order p determines the time extent of the past that affect the present values and may be regarded as the memory of the system. The signals $w_{1,n}$, $w_{2,n}$, and $w_{3,n}$ can be interpreted as modeling errors or alternatively as a process that generates spontaneous activity.

Electrodes can be used either as stimulating or recording electrodes but cannot be used simultaneously for recording and stimulation. Moreover, the electrodes closest to the stimulation site are affected by huge electrical artifacts and they cannot be used because of consequent low SNR. Hence the recorded data $\mathbf{y}_n^{(j)}$ contains recordings of the effect of the stimulation at distant sites, not the stimulation itself. Stimulation depolarizes the membranes of neurons passing through the neighborhood of the stimulating electrode, possibly creating action potentials

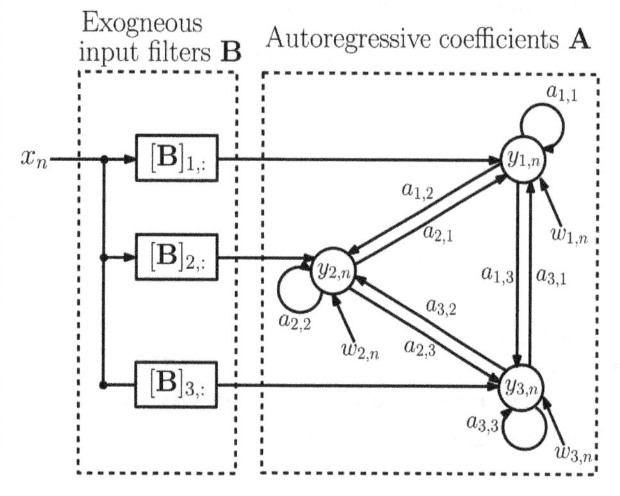

FIGURE 3 | Schematic diagram of the MVARX model. $y_{i,n}$ denotes the recorded signals at the electrodes while x_n represents current stimulation and $w_{i,n}$ is model error, or equivalently, a random input that generates spontaneous activity. $a_{i,j}$ captures the *a priori* unknown connectivity between recording sites while $[\mathbf{B}]_{i,:}$ represents the *a priori* unknown transmission characteristics between the stimulus and recording sites.

in neurons that synapse near the stimulation site and at distant locations (Ranck, 1975), a phenomenon termed fibers of passage. Thus, stimulation generates an "input" that is conveyed to potentially all recording sites in a manner that depends on the axonal topology in the vicinity of the stimulation site. This topology and consequent stimulation effects are usually unknown and described in our MVARX model by the exogenous input filters **B**. In our model we assume the exogenous input is given by the trigger signal associated with delivery of a current pulse, so **B** captures both the shape of the delivered stimulus and the unknown direct propagation of the input to each recording site.

Denote $\mathbf{y}_{n,s}^{(j)}$ and $\mathbf{y}_{n,e}^{(j)}$ as the spontaneous activity and stimulus response to the exogenous input, respectively, at time n from epoch j. Equation (5) can be alternatively expressed as

$$\mathbf{y}_n^{(j)} = \mathbf{y}_{n,s}^{(j)} + \mathbf{y}_{n,e}^{(j)} \tag{6}$$

$$\mathbf{y}_{n,s}^{(j)} = \sum_{i=1}^{p} \mathbf{A}_i \mathbf{y}_{n-i,s}^{(j)} + \mathbf{w}_n^{(j)} \tag{7}$$

$$\mathbf{y}_{n,e}^{(j)} = \sum_{i=1}^{p} \mathbf{A}_i \mathbf{y}_{n-i,e}^{(j)} + \sum_{i=0}^{\ell} \mathbf{b}_i x_{n-i}^{(j)}. \tag{8}$$

Note that in practice $\mathbf{y}_{n,s}^{(j)}$ and $\mathbf{y}_{n,e}^{(j)}$ are not directly observed and cannot be separated from $\mathbf{y}_n^{(j)}$ without knowledge of the MVARX model parameters. The stimulus response component $\mathbf{y}_{n,e}^{(j)}$ is a deterministic term that depends entirely on the stimulus and the model. Given the model parameters $\Theta = [\mathbf{A}, \mathbf{B}]$, we can generate $\mathbf{y}_{n,e}^{(j)}$ by applying the stimulus sequence $\mathbf{x}_n^{(j)}$ to Equation (8) with zero initial conditions. Recall that $\mathbf{w}_n^{(j)}$ is assumed to be zero mean, so $\mathbf{y}_{n,s}^{(j)}$ is a zero mean random process reflecting the spontaneous component of the recordings. It is common in MVAR modeling to subtract the mean prior to estimating MVAR model parameters (Ding et al., 2000). This corresponds to removing the stimulus response $\mathbf{y}_{n,e}^{(j)}$ and is unnecessary with the MVARX model. We shall assume that the stimulus is repeated multiple times such that averaging $\mathbf{y}_{n,e}^{(j)}$ with respect to the stimulus onset times produces the evoked response of the system. This is not required by the model in Equation (5) but is consistent with conventional electrophysiology practice.

The autoregressive parameters **A** model the inherent neural connectivity between sites—how activity at one site propagates to another site. This is evident in Equations (5–8) by the fact that the $\mathbf{A}_i$ are applied to $\mathbf{y}_{n-i}^{(j)}$. If the spontaneous activity $\mathbf{y}_{n,s}^{(j)}$ is very weak relative to $\mathbf{y}_{n,e}^{(j)}$ then the response is described entirely by Equation (8) and the measured data $\mathbf{y}_n^{(j)} \approx \mathbf{y}_{n,e}^{(j)}$. In this case there is a potential modeling ambiguity as there are many different combinations of $\mathbf{A}_i$ and $\mathbf{b}_i$ that could be used to describe $\mathbf{y}_{n,e}^{(j)}$ over a finite duration. For example, $\mathbf{y}_{n,e}^{(j)}$ can be described on $1 \le n \le \ell + 1$ by setting $\mathbf{A}_i = 0$ and only using $\mathbf{b}_i$. We control potential ambiguities associated with relatively weak spontaneous activity by limiting ℓ to a value commensurate with the expected duration of stimulus propagation through fibers of passage. This ensures that **B** is not able to capture long duration interactions associated with feed forward and feedback connectivity between sites. Based on previous experimental evidence (Matsumoto et al., 2004), we set $\ell = 10$ to accommodate a 100 ms duration of propagation through fibers of passage. We will discuss this choice more thoroughly in section 6.

3.2. ESTIMATION OF MVARX MODEL PARAMETERS

Suppose that we have the recordings and inputs $\{(\mathbf{y}_n^{(j)}, x_n^{(j)}) : j = 1, 2, \dots, J, n = 1, 2, \dots, N_j\}$ for J epochs of N_j samples each. Denote $n_0 = \max(p, \ell)$, and suppose that $N_j \ge n_0 + 1$, for all j. Using the first n_0 samples as the initial values, the model in Equation (5) can be rewritten in a simplified form:

$$\mathbf{y}_n^{(j)} = \Theta \mathbf{z}_{n-1}^{(j)} + \mathbf{w}_n^{(j)}, \tag{9}$$

for $j = 1, \dots, J$, $n = n_0 + 1, \dots, N_j$, where the $d \times (dp + \ell + 1)$ matrix $\Theta = [\mathbf{A}, \mathbf{B}]$ and the vector of dimension $dp + \ell + 1$, $\mathbf{z}_{n-1}^{(j)} = [(\mathbf{y}_{n-1}^{(j)})^T, (\mathbf{y}_{n-2}^{(j)})^T, \dots, (\mathbf{y}_{n-p}^{(j)})^T, x_n^{(j)}, x_{n-1}^{(j)}, \dots, x_{n-\ell}^{(j)}]^T$. The vectors $\mathbf{y}_n^{(j)}$, $\mathbf{w}_n^{(j)}$, and $\mathbf{z}_{n-1}^{(j)}$ can be further concatenated as columns of the matrices $\mathbf{Y}_j$, $\mathbf{Z}_j$, and $\mathbf{W}_j$ to write:

$$\mathbf{Y}_j = \Theta \mathbf{Z}_j + \mathbf{W}_j \tag{10}$$

where $\mathbf{Y}_j = [\mathbf{y}_{n_0+1}^{(j)}, \dots, \mathbf{y}_{N_j}^{(j)}]$, $\mathbf{Z}_j = [\mathbf{z}_{n_0}^{(j)}, \dots, \mathbf{z}_{N_j-1}^{(j)}]$, and $\mathbf{W}_j = [\mathbf{w}_{n_0+1}^{(j)}, \dots, \mathbf{w}_{N_j}^{(j)}]$. This expression takes the form of a linear regression model, and we can obtain an ordinary least square (OLS) estimate of $(\Theta, \mathbf{Q})$ as (Lütkepohl, 2006, chap. 10.3):

$$\hat{\Theta} = \left(\sum_{j=1}^{J} \mathbf{Y}_j \mathbf{Z}_j^T\right)\left(\sum_{j=1}^{J} \mathbf{Z}_j \mathbf{Z}_j^T\right)^{-1},$$

$$\hat{\mathbf{Q}} = \frac{1}{N_t}\sum_{j=1}^{J} (\mathbf{Y}_j - \hat{\Theta}\mathbf{Z}_j)(\mathbf{Y}_j - \hat{\Theta}\mathbf{Z}_j)^T, \tag{11}$$

where $N_t = \sum_{j=1}^{J} N_j - n_0 J$. If $\mathbf{w}_n^{(j)}$ is Gaussian, then the OLS estimate $(\hat{\Theta}, \hat{\mathbf{Q}})$ is also the maximum-likelihood estimate of $(\Theta, \mathbf{Q})$ (Lütkepohl, 2006).

3.3. MODEL SELECTION WITH CROSS-VALIDATION

In practice the order p could be chosen using numerous different model selection criteria, including Akaike information criterion and the Bayesian information criterion (McQuarrie and Tsai, 1998; Lütkepohl, 2006). Here we use CV to determine p in a data-driven fashion [see Cheung et al. (2012) for another example of using CV to select model parameters with neurophysiological data]. The data $\mathbf{y}_n^{(j)}$ and input $x_n^{(j)}$ are partitioned into training and test sets. The goal is to choose the value p that produces the best prediction of test data when the model $\Theta = [\mathbf{A}, \mathbf{B}]$ is estimated from the training data. We consider two components in assessing model predictive capability. The first is the one-step prediction error, a measure of the model's ability to track the sample-to-sample and epoch-to-epoch fluctuations in the data. The second is the error between the average evoked response predicted by the model and the measured average response. This measures the quality of the model's response to the stimulus.

Partition the epochs of available data into training sets R_m and test sets S_m and assume there are $m = 1, 2, \ldots, M$ such partitions. Assume the sets S_m are non-overlapping and are of approximately the same size. Let Θ_m be the model estimated from R_m as described in the preceding subsection. The one-step prediction error at time n, $\mathbf{e}_n^{(j)}(\Theta_m)$ is the difference between the recording $\mathbf{y}_n^{(j)}$ and the one-step prediction made by Θ_m using the n_0 samples prior to time n, that is, $\mathbf{z}_{n-1}^{(j)}$:

$$\mathbf{e}_n^{(j)}(\Theta_m) = \mathbf{y}_n^{(j)} - \hat{\mathbf{y}}_n^{(j)}(\Theta_m) \tag{12}$$

where the one-step prediction $\hat{\mathbf{y}}_n^{(j)}(\Theta_m) = \Theta_m \mathbf{z}_{n-1}^{(j)}$. Similarly we define the average response error as

$$\epsilon_n(\Theta_m) = \overline{\mathbf{y}}_n(S_m) - \hat{\overline{\mathbf{y}}}_n(\Theta_m, S_m) \tag{13}$$

where the average evoked response $\overline{\mathbf{y}}_n(S_m) = 1/|S_m| \cdot \sum_{j\in S_m} \mathbf{y}_n^{(j)}$ and the average model response $\hat{\overline{\mathbf{y}}}_n(\Theta_m, S_m)$ over epochs in S_m, $\hat{\overline{\mathbf{y}}}_n(\Theta_m, S_m) = 1/|S_m| \cdot \sum_{j\in S_m} \mathbf{y}_{n,e}^{(j)}(\Theta_m)$. Here $\mathbf{y}_{n,e}^{(j)}(\Theta_m)$ is generated using Θ_m as described following Equation (8). We define a CV score as a weighted combination of the one-step prediction and average response errors averaged over all training/test data partitions

$$\mathrm{CV}(p) = \frac{1}{M}\sum_{m=1}^{M}\left[\frac{\mathrm{CV}_e(p,m)}{w_e} + \frac{\mathrm{CV}_\epsilon(p,m)}{w_\epsilon}\right] \tag{14}$$

where $\mathrm{CV}_e(p, m)$ is the mean square one-step prediction error of a p-th order model $\Theta_m(p)$ in predicting data in S_m:

$$\mathrm{CV}_e(p,m) = \frac{1}{|S_m|}\sum_{j\in S_m}\frac{1}{N_j - n_0}\sum_{n=n_0+1}^{N_j} ||\mathbf{e}_n^{(j)}(\Theta_m(p))||_2^2 \tag{15}$$

and $\mathrm{CV}_\epsilon(p, m)$ is the mean square value of the average response error on S_m:

$$\mathrm{CV}_\epsilon(p,m) = \frac{1}{N}\sum_{n=1}^{N} ||\epsilon_n(\Theta_m(p))||_2^2. \tag{16}$$

Here N is the assumed duration of the average response. The weights w_e and w_ϵ vary the emphasis between the one-step prediction error and average response error. In the analysis below, we set w_e and w_ϵ to the medians of $\mathrm{CV}_e(p, m)$ and $\mathrm{CV}_\epsilon(p, m)$, respectively, for $m = 1, \ldots, M$ and all p considered. This approach places approximately equal emphasis on the two errors. The model order p is chosen as the p that minimizes $\mathrm{CV}(p)$ over the range of p evaluated.

Several practical issues require attention for computing the average response error. First, use of an average evoked response assumes the stimulus is nominally identical for each epoch. Second, care must be taken in computing the average response of the model Θ to the stimulus $x_n^{(j)}$ over epochs in S_m if the effects of preceding stimuli extend into S_m. In such a case the brain is not "at rest" upon the arrival of the new stimulus in S_m, but is still responding to the preceding stimulus. This situation occurs when the response time of the cortex is longer than the inter-stimulus interval. We mimic this aspect of the measured data when computing the average model response by presenting the entire train of stimuli to the model and averaging over the responses corresponding to epochs in S_m.

3.4. MODEL QUALITY ASSESSMENT

A key assumption for the consistency of the OLS estimates is that the residuals $\mathbf{w}_n^{(j)}$ be serially uncorrelated, that is, temporally white. Serial correlation in $\mathbf{w}_n^{(j)}$ may be a sign of mis-specifying the model or incorrect selection of order (p, ℓ) (Hong, 1996; Duchesne and Roy, 2004). We use a consistency test developed in Duchesne and Roy (2004) to validate our models. Denote by $\Gamma_\mathbf{w}(r) = E\{\mathbf{w}_n^{(j)}(\mathbf{w}_{n-r}^{(j)})^T\}$ the covariance at lag r, the hypotheses of interest are:

$$H_0: \; \Gamma_\mathbf{w}(r) = \mathbf{0}, \text{ for all } \mathbf{r} \neq \mathbf{0} \quad \text{vs.}$$

$$H_1: \; \Gamma_\mathbf{w}(r) \neq \mathbf{0}, \text{ for some } \mathbf{r} \neq \mathbf{0}. \tag{17}$$

Let the residual at time n in epoch j be $\hat{\mathbf{w}}_n^{(j)} = \mathbf{y}_n^{(j)} - \hat{\Theta}\mathbf{z}_{n-1}^{(j)}$. Let $q(\cdot)$ be a window function of bounded support L, that is, $q(r) > 0$, for $|r| \leq L$ and $q(r) = 0$ for $|r| > L$. Suppose that the last epoch is of length longer than $(J-1)L$, that is, $N_J > (J-1)L$. The test statistic derived in Duchesne and Roy (2004) for testing H_0 vs. H_1 is

$$T_{N_c} = \frac{N_c \sum_{r=1}^{L} q^2(r)\mathrm{tr}[\mathbf{C}_{\hat{\mathbf{w}}}^T(r)\mathbf{C}_{\hat{\mathbf{w}}}^{-1}(0)\mathbf{C}_{\hat{\mathbf{w}}}(r)\mathbf{C}_{\hat{\mathbf{w}}}^{-1}(0)] - d^2 M_{N_c}(q)}{[2d^2 V_{N_c}(q)]^{1/2}} \tag{18}$$

where $N_c = \sum_{j=1}^{J} N_j - (J-1)L$ and

$$\mathbf{C}_{\hat{\mathbf{w}}}(r) = \frac{1}{N_c}\left[\sum_{j=1}^{J-1}\sum_{n=r+1}^{N_j} \hat{\mathbf{w}}_n^{(j)}(\hat{\mathbf{w}}_{n+r}^{(j)})^T + \sum_{n=r+1+(J-1)(L-r)}^{N_J} \hat{\mathbf{w}}_n^{(J)}(\hat{\mathbf{w}}_{n+r}^{(J)})^T\right], \tag{19}$$

for $r = 0, 1, \ldots, L$, are the estimated residual covariance matrices. The functionals $M_{N_c}(q)$ and $V_{N_c}(q)$ of $q(\cdot)$ and N_c are defined as (Duchesne and Roy, 2004):

$$M_{N_c}(q) = \sum_{i=1}^{L-1}\left(1 - \frac{i}{N_c}\right) q^2(i) \tag{20}$$

$$V_{N_c}(q) = \sum_{i=1}^{L-2}\left(1 - \frac{i}{N_c}\right)\left(1 - \frac{(i+1)}{N_c}\right) q^4(i). \tag{21}$$

We use the Bartlett window defined as $q(j) = 1 - |j/L|, j \leq L$ and $q(j) = 0, j > L$ with a window width $L = \lceil 3N_c^{0.3} \rceil$ as suggested in Duchesne and Roy (2004). For example, in our datasets the longest possible single epoch would have $N_c = 3000$ samples, which leads to the maximum value $L = 34$. Thus the test statistic Equation (18) is based on estimated residual covariance matrices at lags less than or equal to 34. Under the assumption that both $\mathbf{y}_n^{(j)}$ and $x_n^{(j)}$ are stationary, the test statistic is one-sided and asymptotically standard normally distributed (see Duchesne and Roy, 2004, Theorem 1). It declares that the residuals are serially correlated if $T_N > z_{1-\alpha}$ and are white otherwise, where $z_{1-\alpha}$ is the value of the inverse cumulative distribution function of the standard normal distribution at $1 - \alpha$ and α is the significance level of the test.

4. RESULTS

4.1. MODEL PARAMETERS

We have varying definitions and lengths of epochs throughout our data processing procedures. For detection of outlying epochs we choose all epochs to be of length $N_j = 100$ samples based on the time between subsequent current stimuli. In model estimation and assessment of residual whiteness, the epochs are defined as the maximum contiguous segments between the time segments removed by the outlier detection process. This minimizes the impact of the initial conditions $\mathbf{z}_{n_0}^{(j)}$ required at the start of each epoch. Hence, N_j varies across epochs and conditions. In CV, the epoch lengths are set to be equal with $N_j = 100$. This, along with choosing the test sets S_m to contain approximately the same number of epochs, makes the test sets span roughly the same amount of time.

As shown in **Table 1**, the number of outlying epochs is generally larger in sleep than in wakefulness, most likely due to the presence of slow waves during sleep. The number of partitions of the available epochs used in the CV procedure for determining model order p and the corresponding model order is shown in **Table 2**. We did not consider model orders higher than $p = 30$. We also evaluated an unconnected model consisting of d univariate ARX models to assess the importance of the coupling or connectivity between channels. The univariate models were estimated by applying the procedure described above to each channel. With the exception of Subject B, stimulus location 1 (L1), the CV procedure picks a higher model order for the unconnected model and in many cases chooses the maximum order considered.

The whiteness test described in section 3.4 was applied to the residuals from all models using a significance level $\alpha = 0.1$. Note that since exceeding the threshold implies the residuals are not white, use of a relatively large value for α leads to a more stringent test, that is, makes it easier to declare the residuals are not white. The MVARX models passed the whiteness test for every data set, while the unconnected models failed the test for every data set.

4.2. EVOKED RESPONSE MODEL PERFORMANCE

In **Figures 4–6** we compare the average evoked response and average model response for a subset of subjects and conditions. The average responses are generated following the CV approach described in section 3.3. **Figures 4A,B** show the average CV evoked responses $\overline{\mathbf{y}}_n(S) = M^{-1}\sum_{m=1}^{M}\overline{\mathbf{y}}_n(S_m)$ and average CV model responses $\hat{\overline{\mathbf{y}}}_n(\Theta, S) = M^{-1}\sum_{m=1}^{M}\hat{\overline{\mathbf{y}}}_n(\Theta_m, S_m)$ in channels 1, 4, 7, and 11 of Subject A in wakefulness for 1 and 5 mA stimulation, respectively. Here 0 s on the time axis corresponds to the stimulus onset. The averaging is first done within the testing block for each CV partition, then a second phase of averaging is done over the average responses of the test blocks for all CV

Table 2 | Model order parameters for wakefulness and sleep data sets.

	Wakefulness			Sleep		
Dataset	**CV Part.**	**MVARX *p***	**ARX *p***	**CV Part.**	**MVARX *p***	**ARX *p***
Subject A, 1 mA	7	20	30	8	20	30
Subject A, 5 mA	7	26	30	11	26	26
Subject B, L1	10	30	28	8	30	24
Subject B, L2	10	18	22	7	22	30
Subject C	10	16	30	7	12	30

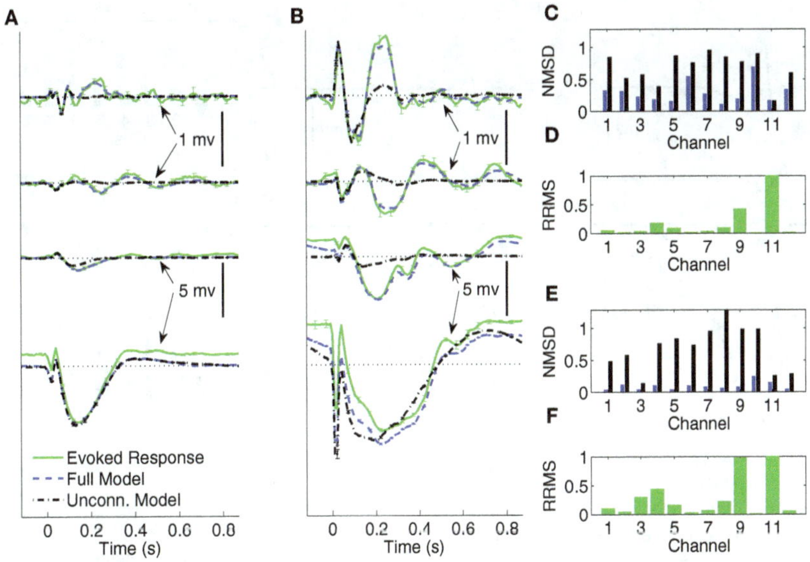

FIGURE 4 | Comparison between average CV evoked and average CV model responses of Subject A to two different stimulation strengths in wakefulness. In panels **(A)** and **(B)** the black dotted lines indicate the origin while the error bars denote the standard error of the mean. **(A)** Average CV evoked and average CV model responses of channels 1, 7, 4, and 11 with 1 mA current stimulation. **(B)** Average CV evoked and average CV model responses of channels 1, 7, 4, and 11 with 5 mA current stimulation. **(C)** Normalized mean-squared difference in each channel for 1 mA stimulation. **(D)** Relative root mean-squared energy in each channel for 1 mA stimulation. **(E)** Normalized mean-squared difference in each channel for 5 mA stimulation. **(F)** Relative root mean-squared energy in each channel for 5 mA stimulation.

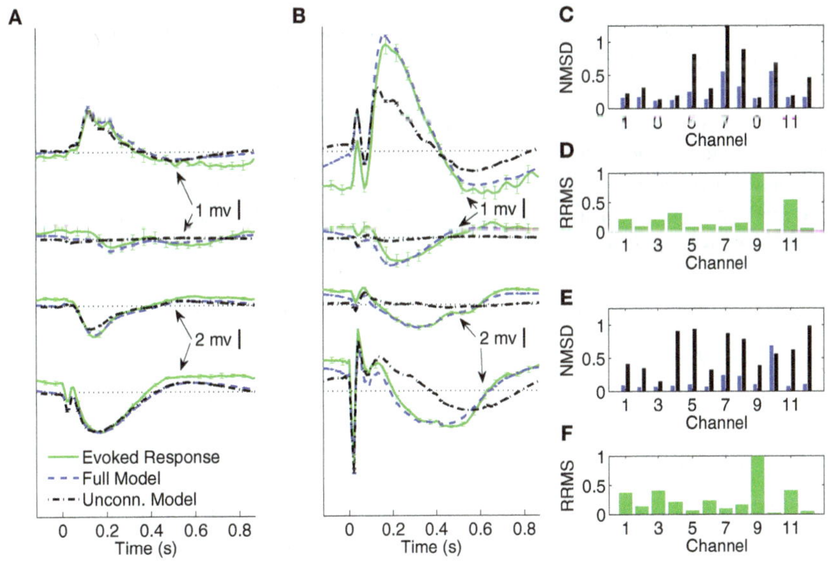

FIGURE 5 | Comparison between average CV evoked and average CV model responses of Subject A to two different stimulation strengths in sleep. In panels **(A)** and **(B)** the black dotted lines indicate the origin while the error bars denote the standard error of the mean. **(A)** Average CV evoked and average CV model responses of channels 1, 7, 4, and 11 with 1 mA current stimulation. **(B)** Average CV evoked and average CV model responses of channels 1, 7, 4, and 11 with 5 mA current stimulation. **(C)** Normalized mean-squared difference in each channel for 1 mA stimulation. **(D)** Relative root mean-squared energy in each channel for 1 mA stimulation. **(E)** Normalized mean-squared difference in each channel for 5 mA stimulation. **(F)** Relative root mean-squared energy in each channel for 5 mA stimulation.

partitions. The average CV model response of the MVARX model (blue dashed line) follows the dynamics of the average CV evoked response (green solid line) in each channel, for both stimulus amplitudes and a range of channel response levels. In contrast, the average CV model response of the unconnected model (red dashed dot line) only tracks the average CV evoked response in channels with the largest amplitudes, even though the univariate model is fit independently to each channel. In the figures,

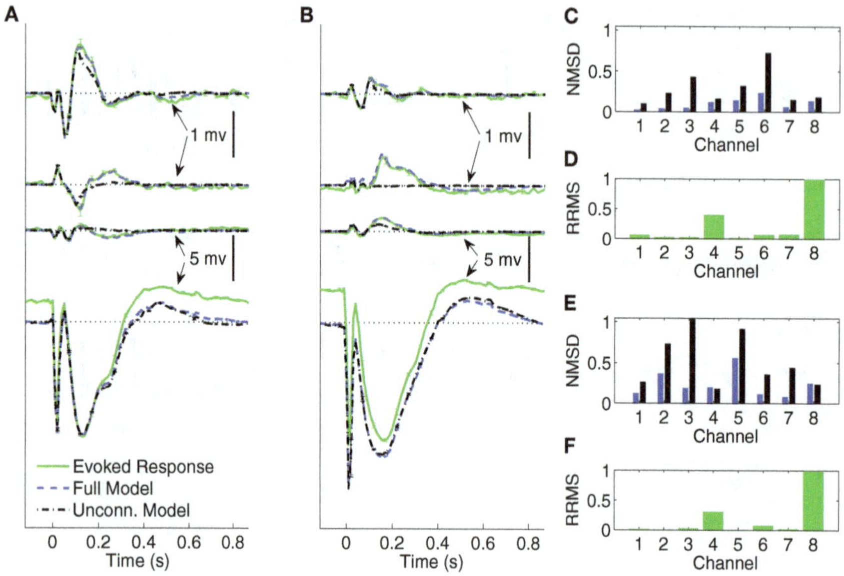

FIGURE 6 | Comparison between average CV evoked responses and average CV model responses of Subject B with two different stimulating locations in wakefulness. In panels **(A)** and **(B)** the black dotted lines indicate the origin while the error bars denote the standard error of the mean. **(A)** Average CV evoked and average CV model responses of channels 1, 3, 6, and 8 when the stimulating channel is L1. **(B)** Average CV evoked and average CV model responses of channels 1, 3, 6, and 8 when the stimulating channel is L2. **(C)** Normalized mean-squared difference in each channel when the stimulating channel is L1. **(D)** Relative root mean-squared energy in each channel when the stimulating channel is L2. **(E)** Normalized mean-squared difference in each channel when the stimulating channel is L1. **(F)** Relative root mean-squared energy in each channel with the stimulating channel is L2.

error bars indicating one standard error are displayed every five samples. **Figures 4C–F** summarize the model performance on a channel-by-channel basis. Let $\bar{y}_{i,n}(S)$ and $\hat{\bar{y}}_{i,n}(\Theta, S)$ be the average CV evoked response and average CV model response at time n in the i-th channel. **Figures 4C,E** depict the normalized mean-squared difference (NMSD) between the average CV evoked and average CV model response for 1 and 5 mA stimulation, respectively, where the NMSD in channel i is defined as

$$\text{NMSD}(i) = \frac{\sum_{n=1}^{N}(\bar{y}_{i,n}(S) - \hat{\bar{y}}_{i,n}(\Theta, S))^2}{\sum_{n=1}^{N}\bar{y}_{i,n}^2(S)}. \tag{22}$$

Figures 4D,F depict the relative root mean-squared (RRMS) energy for 1 and 5 mA stimulations, respectively, for each channel. The RRMS for channel i is defined as the ratio of the root mean-squared energy in channel i to that of the channel with the largest root mean-squared energy. More precisely,

$$\text{RRMS}(i) = \frac{\sqrt{\sum_{n=1}^{N}\bar{y}_{i,n}^2(S)}}{\max\limits_{i'=1,\ldots,d}\sqrt{\sum_{n=1}^{N}\bar{y}_{i',n}^2(S)}}. \tag{23}$$

The unconnected model only gives comparable NMSD to that of full model in channel 11, which has the largest energy. The difference between the MVARX model and the unconnected model in terms of per-channel NMSD is less significant for the 1 mA stimulation, than for the 5 mA stimulation.

Figures 5A,B depict the average CV evoked and average CV model responses for Subject A during NREM sleep with current stimulation of 1 and 5 mA, respectively. The four traces, from top to bottom, show the responses in channels 1, 7, 4, and 11, respectively. Panels (**C**) and (**E**) depict the NMSD, while (**D**) and (**E**) depict RRMS for 1 and 5 mA stimulation, respectively, as a function of channel.

The average CV evoked responses and the average CV model responses in wakefulness for Subject B, with two different stimulating sites L1 and L2, and both with current stimulus of 5 mA, are shown in panels (**A**) and (**B**) of **Figure 6**. The four traces, from top to bottom, depict the responses in channels 1, 3, 6, and 8, respectively. The difference between the two stimulating sites lies mainly in channels with smaller energy, i.e., channels 1, 3, and 6. Panels (**C**) and (**E**) depict NMSD in each channel when the stimulating channel is L1 and L2, respectively. Panels (**D**) and (**F**) show the RRMS in each channel.

Define the normalized mean-squared response difference (NMRD) over all channels as the ratio of the NMRD to the mean-squared average CV evoked response. That is,

$$\text{NMRD} = \frac{\sum_{n=1}^{N}||\bar{\mathbf{y}}_n(S) - \hat{\bar{\mathbf{y}}}_n(\Theta, S)||_2^2}{\sum_{n=1}^{N}||\bar{\mathbf{y}}_n(S)||_2^2}. \tag{24}$$

Figure 7 depicts NMRD of the MVARX models for all five data sets considered. Generally the MVARX models captures the dynamics in average evoked response reasonably well with NMRD no larger than 0.25.

4.3. ONE-STEP PREDICTION MODEL PERFORMANCE

The ability of the model to predict the present recorded value of the data given past recordings reflects a different attribute than

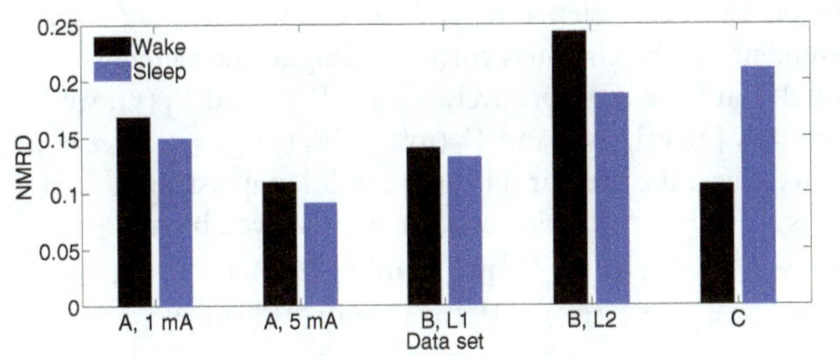

FIGURE 7 | Normalized mean-squared response difference [see Equation (24)] in each dataset.

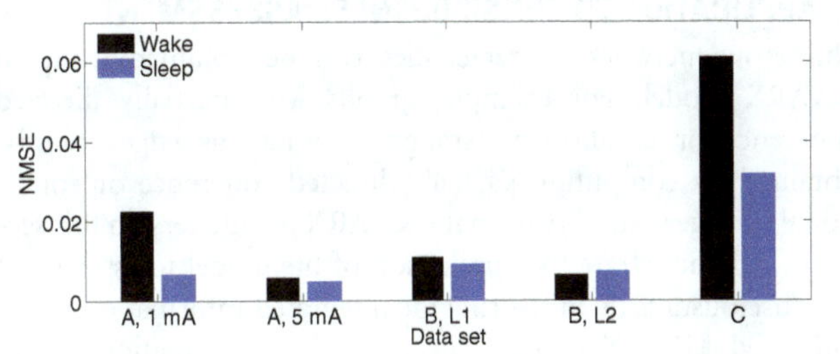

FIGURE 9 | Normalized mean-squared one-step prediction error [see Equation (25)] in each dataset.

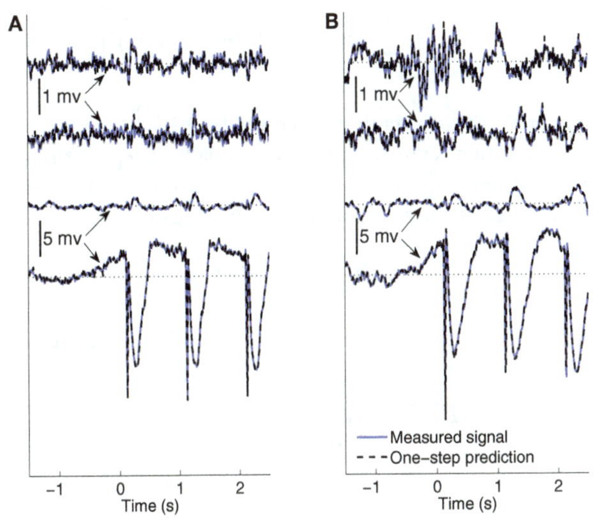

FIGURE 8 | Comparison between recorded signal and one-step prediction of Subject B when the stimulating site is L2. 1.5 s pre-stimulus is shown followed by two-and-a-half epochs of evoked data. The black dotted lines in the panels indicate the origin. The model is estimated from data beginning with the fourth epoch. **(A)** Wake recorded and predicted signals in channels 1, 3, 6, and 8 ordered from top to bottom. **(B)** Non-REM sleep recorded and predicted signals in channels 1, 3, 6, and 8 ordered from top to bottom.

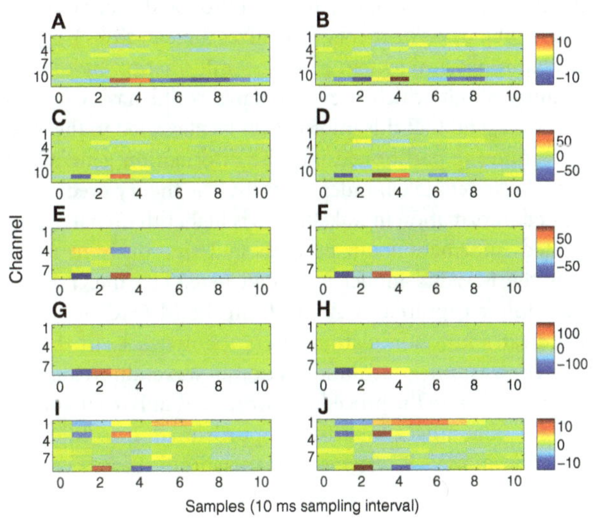

FIGURE 10 | Exogenous input filters B for each channel as a function of time. The identical colormap is used for each row. **(A)** Subject A wake, 1 mA. **(B)** Subject A sleep, 1 mA. **(C)** Subject A wake, 5 mA. **(D)** Subject A sleep, 5 mA. **(E)** Subject B wake, stimulation site L1. **(F)** Subject B sleep, stimulation site L1. **(G)** Subject B wake, stimulation site L2. **(H)** Subject B sleep, stimulation site L2. **(I)** Subject C wake. **(J)** Subject C sleep.

the modeling of the average evoked response. One-step prediction performance indicates the model's ability to follow spontaneous fluctuations in the data. **Figure 8** compares the recording $\mathbf{y}_n^{(j)}$ and one-step prediction $\hat{\mathbf{y}}_n^{(j)}(\Theta)$ of the signals recorded from Subject B for 1.5 s of pre-stimulus data followed by two and a half epochs of evoked data, when the stimulating site is L2. The models used to perform prediction in **Figure 8** are trained from data excluding the data plotted. Panels (**A**) and (**B**) shows the signals in wakefulness and sleep, respectively. Similar results are obtained for the other epochs, subjects, and conditions. The traces show the signals in channels 1, 3, 6, and 8, respectively. These results indicate that the MVARX model performs accurate one-step prediction in wakefulness and sleep and for both pre-stimulus and evoked data segments.

Define the normalized mean-squared one-step (NMSE) prediction error as the ratio of the mean-squared prediction error over the samples to the mean-squared energy. That is,

$$\text{NMSE} = \frac{\frac{1}{J(N-n_0)} \sum_{j=1}^{J} \sum_{n=n_0+1}^{N} ||\mathbf{y}_n^{(j)} - \hat{\mathbf{y}}_n^{(j)}(\Theta)||_2^2}{\frac{1}{JN} \sum_{j=1}^{J} \sum_{n=1}^{N} ||\mathbf{y}_n^{(j)}||_2^2}. \quad (25)$$

As a reference, the NMSE of the model $\Theta = \mathbf{0}$ is approximately 1. The bar diagrams in **Figure 9** show the NMSE of the MVARX models for all five datasets considered. Overall, our models give NMSE less than 0.06 for one-step prediction of the recordings and less than 0.02 in seven of the ten data sets studied.

4.4. B MATRICES

Figure 10 depicts the exogenous input filters **B** matrices estimated for all 10 datasets as color plots. The i-th row of each matrix represents the FIR filter coefficients representing the path from the stimulus site to the i-th channel. Hence, rows with greater extremes of color have the strongest paths from the stimulus site.

5. APPLICATION TO CONSCIOUSNESS ASSESSMENT

Numerous network characteristics can be obtained from an MVARX model. For example, graphs with partially directed coherence or conditional Granger causality as edges can be obtained by computing partially directed coherence or conditional Granger causality from the MVARX parameters. In this section we demonstrate the application of the model to assessment of consciousness by measuring the integrated information of the estimated MVARX model. The integrated information theory (Tononi, 2004, 2008, 2010) starts from two self-evident axioms about consciousness: every experience is one out of many and generates information because it differs in its own way from the large repertoire of alternative experiences; and every experience is one, that is, integrated, because it cannot be decomposed into independent parts. The theory formalizes these notions by postulating that a physical system generates information by reducing uncertainty about which previous states could have caused its present state, and that this information is integrated to the extent that it cannot be partitioned into the information generated by parts of the system taken independently. The theory predicts that integrated information in wakefulness is higher than that in sleep. Integrated information can be measured rigorously in models such as the MVARX model presented here. The integration of information is captured by **A** and **Q** in the MVARX model—**B** only indicates how stimulation enters the network. In this section we contrast integrated information in wakefulness and sleep using a variation on the procedure introduced in Barrett and Seth (2011) for obtaining a bipartition approximation to integrated information in MVAR systems. Our variation is based on use of "effective information" (Kullback–Leibler divergence) (Balduzzi and Tononi, 2008) in place of the difference in mutual information and ensures that integrated information is always positive (Cover and Thomas, 2006).

Suppose $\mathbf{y}_n$ describes a stable MVAR(p) process:

$$\mathbf{y}_n = \sum_{i=1}^{p} \mathbf{A}_i \mathbf{y}_{n-i} + \mathbf{w}_n, \tag{26}$$

where $\mathbf{w}_n$ are i.i.d. zero-mean Gaussian noise vectors with covariance **Q**. Then the MVAR(p) process is wide sense stationary and $\mathbf{y}_n \sim \mathcal{N}(0, \Sigma(\mathbf{y}))$ with $\Sigma(\mathbf{y}) = E\{\mathbf{y}_n \mathbf{y}_n^T\}$. Given that the state at time n, $\mathbf{y}_n = \underline{\mathbf{y}}$, the conditional distribution of the state τ samples prior to sample n, $\mathbf{y}_{n-\tau}$, follows

$$\mathbf{y}_{n-\tau} | (\mathbf{y}_n = \underline{\mathbf{y}}) \sim \mathcal{N}(\Gamma_\tau(\mathbf{y})\Sigma(\mathbf{y})^{-1}\underline{\mathbf{y}}, \Sigma(\mathbf{y}_{n-\tau}|\mathbf{y}_n)) \tag{27}$$

where $\Gamma_\tau(\mathbf{y}) = E\{\mathbf{y}_{n-\tau}\mathbf{y}_n^T\}$ and

$$\Sigma(\mathbf{y}_{n-\tau}|\mathbf{y}_n) = \Sigma(\mathbf{y}) - \Gamma_\tau(\mathbf{y})\Sigma(\mathbf{y})^{-1}\Gamma_\tau(\mathbf{y})^T. \tag{28}$$

Given **A** and **Q**, the matrices $\Sigma(\mathbf{y})$ and $\Gamma_\tau(\mathbf{y})$ for $\tau = 1, \ldots, \rho$, with $\rho \geq p-1$, are computed as described in Barrett and Seth (2011).

Let the set of the channels be $S = \{1, 2, \ldots, d\}$. A bipartiton $\mathcal{B} = \{M^1, M^2\}$, divides the channels into two mutually non-overlapping and non-empty sub-networks, $S = M^1 \bigcup M^2$. Denote two sub-systems $\mathbf{m}_n^1$ and $\mathbf{m}_n^2$ within which are the measurements in the channels corresponding to the elements in M^1 and M^2 at time n, respectively. Given $\Sigma(\mathbf{y})$ and $\Gamma_\tau(\mathbf{y})$, we have $\Sigma(\mathbf{m}^i) = [\Sigma(\mathbf{y})]_{M^i,M^i}$ and $\Gamma_\tau(\mathbf{m}^i) = [\Gamma_\tau(\mathbf{y})]_{M^i,M^i}$, for $i = 1, 2$. Hence, given the present state, the conditional distribution of the sub-system i at τ samples into the past is given by $\mathbf{m}_{n-\tau}^i | (\mathbf{m}_n^i = \underline{\mathbf{m}}^i) \sim \mathcal{N}(\Gamma_\tau(\mathbf{m}^i)\Sigma(\mathbf{m}^i)^{-1}\underline{\mathbf{m}}^i, \Sigma(\mathbf{m}_{n-\tau}^i|\mathbf{m}_n^i))$, for $i = 1, 2$, where $\Sigma(\mathbf{m}_{n-\tau}^i|\mathbf{m}_n^i) = \Sigma(\mathbf{m}^i) - \Gamma_\tau(\mathbf{m}^i)\Sigma(\mathbf{m}^i)^{-1}\Gamma_\tau(\mathbf{m}^i)^T$.

Define the effective information for the system **y** over a lag of τ samples under partition $\mathcal{B}$ as [see Barrett and Seth (2011), (0.32)]

$$\varphi(\mathbf{y}; \tau, \mathcal{B}) = \frac{1}{2}\Big[-\log_2\left(\det(\Sigma(\mathbf{y}_{n-\tau}|\mathbf{y}_n))\right) + \sum_{i=1}^{2} \log_2\left(\det(\Sigma(\mathbf{m}_{n-\tau}^i|\mathbf{m}_n^i))\right)\Big] \text{ bits.} \tag{29}$$

The effective information is the Kullback–Leibler divergence between a system consisting of two mutually independent subsystems $\mathbf{m}_n^1$ and $\mathbf{m}_n^2$ and the system $\mathbf{y}_n$. The integrated information measured at a time difference of τ is defined as

$$\phi(\mathbf{y}; \tau) = \varphi(\mathbf{y}; \tau, \mathcal{B}^{\mathrm{MIB}}) \tag{30}$$

where the minimum information bipartion (MIB) is defined as

$$\mathcal{B}^{\mathrm{MIB}} = \arg\min_{\mathcal{B}} \left(\frac{\varphi(\mathbf{y}; \tau, \mathcal{B})}{K_2(\mathcal{B})} \right) \tag{31}$$

with

$$K_2(\mathcal{B}) = \min(H(\mathbf{m}_n^1), H(\mathbf{m}_n^2)) \tag{32}$$

and the differential entropy of $\mathbf{m}_n^i$, $H(\mathbf{m}_n^i)$ is given by

$$H(\mathbf{m}_n^i) = \frac{1}{2}\log_2\left((2\pi e)^{|M^i|}\det(\Sigma(\mathbf{m}^i))\right). \tag{33}$$

Figure 11 depicts the integrated information of Subject A for stimulus of 5 mA, as the time difference τ varies from 10 to 300 ms. The integrated information in wakefulness is higher than that in sleep. In both wakefulness and sleep, the integrated information increases until the time difference is approximately 100 ms and then remains approximately constant. We further used the CV procedures described in section 3.3 to study the difference between integrated information in wakefulness and sleep. Specifically, we estimated a model from the training set of each CV partition and compute integrated information for each CV partition. This provides M different estimates of integrated information for each data set, where M is the number of CV partitions. We compare the maximum values of the estimates of integrated information for each CV partition in wakefulness and sleep using the Wilcoxon rank sum test, which tests the null (H_0) hypothesis that the measured maximum integrated information values in wakefulness and sleep for all CV partitions are samples from continuous distributions with equal medians, against H_1 that they are not. The p-values of the rank sum test for each conditions are shown in **Table 3**. With the exception of Subject C, all of the cases

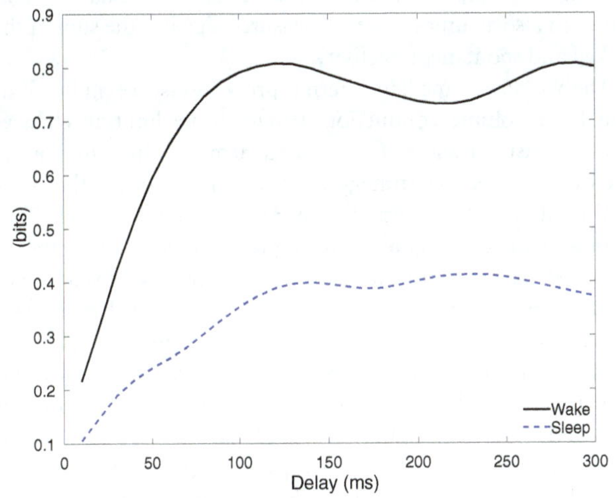

FIGURE 11 | Integrated information of Subject A, when the stimulation current is of 5 mA.

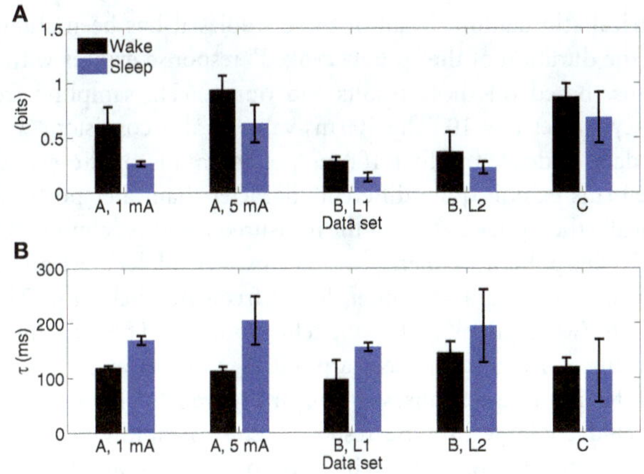

FIGURE 12 | (A) Average maximum values of integrated information with error bars indicating one standard error. **(B)** Average lag at which maximum integrated information is achieved, with error bars indicating one standard error.

have p-values below 0.05, and Subject C is only slightly above 0.05. **Figure 12** depicts the average maximum value of integrated information and average time delay τ at which the maximum value is achieved, where the averaging is done across CV results, and error bars indicates one standard error.

6. DISCUSSION

The results demonstrate the effectiveness of the MVARX model for intracerebral electrical stimulation data. Excellent agreement between measured and modeled evoked responses is found across channels, two stimulus amplitudes, vigilance states, stimulus sites, and subjects (**Figures 4–7**). One-step prediction is used to show that the MVARX model also accurately captures the spontaneous fluctuations in the measured signals (**Figures 8** and **9**). We contrast the MVARX models with a series of univariate ARX models, one for each channel, to illustrate the importance of accounting for the interaction between cortical signals (**Figures 4–6**). In some channels for some subjects/conditions the univariate ARX model describes the evoked response as well as the MVARX model. However, in general modeling interactions between cortical signals is necessary to capture the measured response. For example, in **Figure 4B** the univariate model fails to model the responses in channels 1, 4, and 7 beyond 200 ms after the stimulation.

The MVARX model explicitly represents both evoked and spontaneous (or background) brain activity using a deterministic input term to capture the effect of stimuli and a random input term to generate spontaneous activity. Stimuli generally give rise to a non-zero mean component in the response that varies with time, i.e., is non-stationary. Conventional approaches to MVAR modeling of cortical event-related potentials (e.g., Ding et al., 2000), subtract the ensemble mean of the data before processing to avoid the negative effects of the non-stationary mean on the MVAR model. However, subtraction of the ensemble mean significantly reduces the SNR of the data and is not necessary if the exogenous input is properly accounted for in the modeling procedure.

The effect of the stimulus on each recording channel is addressed by applying a separate filter in each channel to the stimulus signal. The filter coefficients are estimated jointly with the autoregressive model parameters from the measured evoked data. This approach accounts for the generally unknown and different characteristics of the transmission paths from the stimulation to each measurement site. The length of the filters [ℓ samples in Equation (5)] should be limited based on physiological expectations for the stimulus paradigm. Indeed, the autoregressive coefficients $\mathbf{A}_i$ and filters $\mathbf{b}_i$ are estimated simultaneously and the evoked response ($\mathbf{y}_{n,e}^{(j)}$ in Equation (8)) is often much larger than the spontaneous component [$\mathbf{y}_{n,s}^{(j)}$ in Equation (7)]. If ℓ is set equal to the duration of one epoch of $\mathbf{y}_{n,e}^{(j)}$, then it is possible to perfectly model $\mathbf{y}_{n,e}^{(j)}$ using only the $\mathbf{b}_i$ while setting the $\mathbf{A}_i = 0$. We have shown that the MVARX models are capable of characterizing $\mathbf{y}_{n,s}$ by one-step prediction of data not used to estimate the model (see **Figure 8**). Moreover, the model describes the dynamics in $\mathbf{y}_{n,e}$, as was shown in **Figures 4–6**.

In order to define a practical value for ℓ we refer to previous electrophysiological studies on intracerebral evoked potentials (Matsumoto et al., 2004, 2007, 2012). In these studies Matsumoto and colleagues thoroughly discussed the possible

Table 3 | p-values of the Wilcoxon rank sum test of whether integrated information in wakefulness and sleep are different.

	Subject A, 1 mA	Subject A, 5 mA	Subject B, L1	Subject B, L2	Subject C
p-value	3.18e-4	0.0012	2.06e-4	0.0068	0.0553

generator mechanisms of intracerebral potentials evoked by direct electrical stimulation. In all of these studies it has been shown that the duration of the "purely evoked" response expires within 100 ms. Based on these results and our 100 Hz sampling frequency we set $\ell = 10$. The 100 ms value is also consistent with our data. Indeed, the first 100 ms post-stimulus of the evoked waveforms exhibit quite different character than later portions. Typically the initial 100 ms of the measured response contain relatively sharp, high frequency waveforms, while later portions of the response have a smoother, lower frequency behavior. This suggests two regimes in the modeling process. The exogenous input filters account for the sharp initial response, as evident by the filter impulse responses shown in **Figure 10**. Channels having relatively large impulse response tend to rapidly transition from negative to positive maxima over one or two samples, consistent with the sharp features in the early portions of the evoked response. These sharp inputs to the channels are smoothed by the autoregressive component of the model to obtain the later portions of the response. The filter responses depicted in **Figure 10** decay to relatively small values by the 10-th lag (100 ms) and generally contain most of their energy in the first through sixth lags, that is between 10 and 60 ms. This further supports the choice of $\ell = 10$.

The energy transmission characteristics shown in **Figure 10** are consistent with physiological expectations for modeling stimulation of fibers of passage. There is general consistency between wakefulness and sleep in all subjects (**Figure 10**, left column vs. right column) even though the evoked responses differ markedly (**Figure 4** vs. **Figure 5**); channels with strong and weak responses are the same in wakefulness and sleep, and the shape of the responses in each channel are generally very similar. The subtle differences between wakefulness and sleep may be due to changes in neural excitability. Comparing 1 and 5 mA stimulation in Subject A (**Figures 10A,B** and **C,D**) reveals that channel 11 has the strongest response in both stimulation levels and the strength of the response increases roughly by a factor of 5, consistent with the factor of 5 change in the stimulation level. This is because we used the trigger signal to represent the exogenous input without adjusting its amplitude. However, the shape of the response in channel 11 differs slightly, with the 5 mA case having reduced latency by approximately 10 ms and a higher frequency response reflected by the sharper, shorter duration of the filter. This suggests that the higher stimulus level is associated with a faster response. The two stimulation sites L1 and L2 in Subject B (**Figures 10E,F** and **G,H**) both involve channels 8 and 4 as the strongest response, suggesting similar fibers of passage are excited at the two sites. However, the overall gain differs by a factor of 2 and the shape of the response in channel 8 and 4 differ, especially in wakefulness. Subject C (**Figures 10I,J**) exhibits multiple channels with strong linkage to the stimulus site.

Our MVARX approach assumes the dynamic interactions between evoked and spontaneous cortical signals follow the same model, that is, both evoked and spontaneous activity are described by one set of $\mathbf{A}_i$. The excellent one-step prediction performance in the pre-stimulus interval of **Figure 8** combined with the high quality fitting of the evoked responses suggests this is a reasonable assumption, at least for these particular data sets. This approach also assumes that the measured signal is the sum of the evoked and spontaneous activity.

The windowed median filtering procedure successfully eliminated the volume conduction artifact while limiting changes to the measured signal to within ± 20 ms of the stimulation. The outlier detection strategy only eliminates epochs that have significant deviation from the average evoked response. Both of these strategies significantly improve model fidelity to the measured data. Seven times as many outlier epochs were identified in sleep than in wakefulness, likely due to the presence of occasional slow waves during an epoch. However, in seven of the ten data sets we analyzed 28 or more of the 30 available epochs, which indicates our artifact detection procedure is not overly aggressive. Subject A had the most outlier epochs and in the worst case (5 mA, sleep) our procedure eliminated 8 of the possible 30 epochs. The CV strategy for choosing MVAR model order is effective, as demonstrated by the fidelity of the model evoked responses (**Figures 4–7**) and the ability of the models to accurately perform one-step prediction on pre-stimulus data (**Figure 8**). Outlier rejection helps the data meet the stationarity assumption of the MVARX model. While it is unlikely that the data are truly stationary, the accuracy with which the model describes the data and the whiteness of the residuals suggests that the stationarity assumption is reasonable.

As a proof of concept application, we used the MVARX model to assess changes in the level of information integration between wakefulness and deep sleep in human subjects. Using a simple, bipartition approximation we found that, as predicted by theoretical considerations (Tononi, 2004; Seth et al., 2008), integrated information is higher in wakefulness than sleep for each subject/condition, supporting the notion that integrated information reflects the capacity for consciousness. We note that the integrated information results presented here only apply to the recordings analyzed. Analysis of the dependence of integrated information on recording coverage is beyond the scope of this paper. Our findings indicate that the human cerebral cortex is better suited at information integration—being both functionally specialized and functionally integrated—when awake and conscious. In contrast, when consciousness fades in deep sleep, the parameters of the system change in such a way that information integration is diminished, in line with theoretical predictions (Tononi, 2004) and consistent with qualitative evidence obtained from experiments employing transcranial magnetic stimulation and high density EEG (Massimini et al., 2005). We also found that the lag at which the maximum level of information integration is attained is consistently longer in sleep than wakefulness. Maximum information integration in wakefulness occurred at lags of 30–110 ms, while those in sleep were from 70 to 140 ms longer, consistent with the increased low frequency activity of sleep.

ACKNOWLEDGMENTS

This research was supported in part by the National Institute of Biomedical Imaging and Bioengineering under grant R21EB009749.

REFERENCES

Astolfi, L., Cincotti, F., Mattia, D., De Vico Fallani, F., Tocci, A., Colosimo, A., et al. (2008). Tracking the time-varying cortical connectivity patterns by adaptive multivariate estimators. *IEEE Trans Biomed. Eng.* 55, 902–913.

Babiloni, F., Cincotti, F., Babiloni, C., Carducci, F., Mattia, D., Astolfi, L., et al. (2005). Estimation of the cortical functional connectivity with the multimodal integration of high-resolution EEG and fMRI data by directed transfer function. *Neuroimage* 24, 118–131.

Baccalá, L. A., and Sameshima, K. (2001). Partial directed coherence: a new concept in neural structure determination. *Biol. Cybern.* 84, 463–474.

Balduzzi, D., and Tononi, G. (2008). Integrated information in discrete dynamical systems: motivation and theoretical framework. *PLoS Comput. Biol.* 4:e1000091. doi: 10.1371/journal.pcbi.1000091

Barnett, L., and Seth, A. K. (2011). Behaviour of Granger causality under filtering: theoretical invariance and practical application. *J. Neurosci. Methods* 201, 404–419.

Barrett, A. B., and Seth, A. K. (2011). Practical measures of integrated information for time-series data. *PLoS Comput. Biol.* 7:e1001052. doi: 10.1371/journal.pcbi.1001052

Bernasconi, C., and König, P. (1999). On the directionality of cortical interactions studied by structural analysis of electrophysiological recordings. *Biol. Cybern.* 81, 199–210.

Bloomfield, P. (2000). *Fourier Analysis of Time Series: An Introduction.* Wiley Series in Probability and Statistics, 2nd Edn. New York, NY: Wiley-Interscience.

Brovelli, A., Ding, M., Ledberg, A., Chen, Y., Nakamura, R., and Bressler, S. L. (2004). Beta oscillations in a large-scale sensorimotor cortical network: directional influences revealed by Granger causality. *Proc. Natl. Acad. Sci. U.S.A.* 101, 9849–9854.

Cheung, B. L. P., Nowak, R. D., Lee, H. C., van Drongelen, W., and Van Veen, B. D. (2012). Cross validation for selection of cortical interaction models from scalp EEG or MEG. *IEEE Trans. Biomed. Eng.* 59, 504–514.

Cossu, M., Cardinale, F., Castana, L., Citterio, A., Francione, S., Tassi, L., et al. (2005). Stereoelectroencephalography in the presurgical evaluation of focal epilepsy: a retrospective analysis of 215 procedures. *Neurosurgery* 57, 706–718.

Cover, T. M., and Thomas, J. A. (2006). *Elements of Information Theory.* Wiley Series in Telecommunications and Signal Processing, 2nd Edn. New York, NY: Wiley-Interscience.

Dehaene, S., Changeux, J. P., Naccache, L., Sackur, J., and Sergent, C. (2006). Conscious, preconscious, and subliminal processing: a testable taxonomy. *Trends Cogn. Sci. (Regul. Ed.)* 10, 204–211.

Ding, M., Bressler, S. L., Yang, W., and Liang, H. (2000). Short-window spectral analysis of cortical event-related potentials by adaptive multivariate autoregressive modeling: data preprocessing, model validation, and variability assessment. *Biol. Cybern.* 83, 35–45.

Ding, M., Chen, Y., and Bressler, S. L. (2006). *Granger Causality: Basic Theory and Application to Neuroscience.* Weinheim: Wiley-VCH Verlag GmbH & Co. KGaA.

Duchesne, P., and Roy, R. (2004). On consistent testing for serial correlation of unknown form in vector time series models. *J. Multivar. Anal.* 89, 148–180.

Geweke, J. F. (1984). Measures of conditional linear dependence and feedback between time series. *J. Am. Stat. Assoc.* 79, 907–915.

Hong, Y. (1996). Consistent testing for serial correlation of unknown form. *Econometrica* 64, 837–864.

Kamiński, M. J., and Blinowska, K. J. (1991). A new method of the description of the information flow in the brain structures. *Biol. Cybern.* 65, 203–210.

Korzeniewska, A., Crainiceanu, C. M., Kuś, R., Franaszczuk, P. J., and Crone, N. E. (2008). Dynamics of event-related causality in brain electrical activity. *Hum. Brain Mapp.* 29, 1170–1192.

Laureys, S. (2005). The neural correlate of (un)awareness: lessons from the vegetative state. *Trends Cogn. Sci. (Regul. Ed.)* 9, 556–559.

Lütkepohl, H. (2006). *New Introduction to Multiple Time Series Analysis.* Berlin: Springer.

Malekpour, S., Li, Z., Cheung, B., Castillo, E., Papanicolaou, L., Kramer, A., et al. (2012). Interhemispheric effective and functional cortical connectivity signatures of spina bifida are consistent with callosal anomaly. *Brain Connect.* 2, 142–154.

Massimini, M., Ferrarelli, F., Huber, R., Esser, S. K., Singh, H., and Tononi, G. (2005). Breakdown of cortical effective connectivity during sleep. *Science* 309, 2228–2232.

Matsumoto, R., Nair, D. R., Ikeda, A., Fumuro, T., LaPresto, E., Mikuni, N., et al. (2012). Parieto-frontal network in humans studied by cortico-cortical evoked potential. *Hum. Brain Mapp.* 33, 2856–2872.

Matsumoto, R., Nair, D. R., LaPresto, E., Bingaman, W., Shibasaki, H., and Lüders, H. O. (2007). Functional connectivity in human cortical motor system: a cortico-cortical evoked potential study. *Brain* 130, 181–197.

Matsumoto, R., Nair, D. R., LaPresto, E., Najm, I., Bingaman, W., Shibasaki, H., et al. (2004). Functional connectivity in the human language system: a cortico-cortical evoked potential study. *Brain* 127, 2316–2330.

McQuarrie, A. D. R., and Tsai, C.-L. (1998). *Regression and Time Series Model Selection.* River Edge, NJ: World Scientific Pub Co Inc.

Möller, E., Schack, B., Arnold, M., and Witte, H. (2001). Instantaneous multivariate EEG coherence analysis by means of adaptive high dimensional autoregressive models. *J. Neurosci. Methods* 105, 143–158.

Munari, C., Hoffmann, D., Francione, S., Kahane, P., Tassi, L., Lo Russo, G., et al. (1994). Stereo-electroencephalography methodology: advantages and limits. *Acta Neurol. Scand. Suppl.* 152, 56–67.

Nobili, L., De Gennaro, L., Proserpio, P., Moroni, F., Sarasso, S., Pigorini, A., et al. (2012). Local aspects of sleep: observations from intracerebral recordings in humans. *Prog. Brain Res.* 199, 219–232.

Nobili, L., Ferrara, M., Moroni, F., De Gennaro, L., Russo, G. L., Campus, C., et al. (2011). Dissociated wake-like and sleep-like electro-cortical activity during sleep. *Neuroimage* 58, 612–619.

Penny, K. I. (1996). Appropriate critical values when testing for a single multivariate outlier by using the mahalanobis distance. *J. R. Stat. Soc. Ser. C (Appl. Stat.)* 45, 73–81.

Ranck, J. B. (1975). Which elements are excited in electrical stimulation of mammalian central nervous system: a review. *Brain Res.* 98, 417–440.

Rechtschaffen, A., and Kales, A. (eds.). (1968). *A Manual of Standardized Terminology, Techniques and Scoring System for Sleep Stages of Human Subjects.* NIH Publication No. 204. Washington, DC: US Government Printing Office, National Institute of Health Publication.

Seth, A. K., Dienes, Z., Cleeremans, A., Overgaard, M., and Pessoa, L. (2008). Measuring consciousness: relating behavioural and neurophysiological approaches. *Trends Cogn. Sci. (Regul. Ed.)* 12, 314–321.

Tononi, G. (2004). An information integration theory of consciousness. *BMC Neurosci.* 5:42. doi: 10.1186/1471-2202-5-42

Tononi, G. (2008). Consciousness as integrated information: a provisional manifesto. *Biol. Bull.* 215, 216–242.

Tononi, G. (2010). Information integration: its relevance to brain function and consciousness. *Arch. Ital. Biol.* 148, 299–322.

Valentín, A., Alarcón, G., Honavar, M., Garcia Seoane, J. J., Selway, R. P., Polkey, C. E., et al. (2005). Single pulse electrical stimulation for identification of structural abnormalities and prediction of seizure outcome after epilepsy surgery: a prospective study. *Lancet Neurol.* 4, 718–726.

Valentín, A., Anderson, M., Alarcón, G., Garcia Seoane, J. J., Selway, R., Binnie, C. D., et al. (2002). Responses to single pulse electrical stimulation identify epileptogenesis in the human brain *in vivo*. *Brain* 125, 1709–1718.

Winterhalder, M., Schelter, B., Hesse, W., Schwab, K., Leistritz, L., Klan, D., et al. (2005). Comparison of linear signal processing techniques to infer directed interactions in multivariate neural systems. *Signal Process.* 85, 2137–2160.

13

Je pense donc je fais: transcranial direct current stimulation modulates brain oscillations associated with motor imagery and movement observation

Olivia M. Lapenta[1], Ludovico Minati[2], Felipe Fregni[3] and Paulo S. Boggio[1]*

[1] Social and Cognitive Neuroscience Laboratory, Center for Healthy and Biological Sciences, Mackenzie Presbyterian University, Sao Paulo, Brazil
[2] U.O. Direzione Scientifica, Fondazione IRCCS Istituto Neurologico "Carlo Besta," Milano, Italy
[3] Laboratory of Neuromodulation, Harvard Medical School, Spaulding Rehabilitation Hospital, Massachusetts General Hospital, Boston, MA, USA

***Correspondence:**
Paulo S. Boggio, Social and Cognitive Neuroscience Laboratory and Developmental Disorders Program, Center for Health and Biological Sciences, Mackenzie Presbyterian University, Rua Piaui, 181, 10° andar, Sao Paulo, 01241-001, Brazil
e-mail: boggio@mackenzie.br; psboggio@gmail.com

Motor system neural networks are activated during movement imagery, observation and execution, with a neural signature characterized by suppression of the Mu rhythm. In order to investigate the origin of this neurophysiological marker, we tested whether transcranial direct current stimulation (tDCS) modifies Mu rhythm oscillations during tasks involving observation and imagery of biological and non-biological movements. We applied tDCS (anodal, cathodal, and sham) in 21 male participants (mean age 23.8 ± 3.06), over the left M1 with a current of 2 mA for 20 min. Following this, we recorded the EEG at C3, C4, and Cz and surrounding C3 and C4 electrodes. Analyses of C3 and C4 showed significant effects for biological vs. non-biological movement ($p = 0.005$), and differential hemisphere effects according to the type of stimulation ($p = 0.04$) and type of movement ($p = 0.02$). Analyses of surrounding electrodes revealed significant interaction effects considering type of stimulation and imagery or observation of biological or non-biological movement ($p = 0.03$). The main findings of this study were (1) Mu desynchronization during biological movement of the hand region in the contralateral hemisphere after sham tDCS; (2) polarity-dependent modulation effects of tDCS on the Mu rhythm, i.e., anodal tDCS led to Mu synchronization while cathodal tDCS led to Mu desynchronization during movement observation and imagery (3) specific focal and opposite inter-hemispheric effects, i.e., contrary effects for the surrounding electrodes during imagery condition and also for inter-hemispheric electrodes (C3 vs. C4). These findings provide insights into the cortical oscillations during movement observation and imagery. Furthermore, it shows that tDCS can be highly focal when guided by a behavioral task.

Keywords: tDCS, EEG, mu rhythm, motor imagery, action observation, primary motor cortex

INTRODUCTION

I think, therefore I am. This classic Cartesian statement ("Cogito ergo sum") could be revised to "I think, therefore I do" to underscore the notion that the motor neural network is as engaged during motor imagery (Jeannerod, 2001; Decety and Grezes, 2006) as during action execution or observation. The mirror neuron system (MNS) plays a significant role in imitation-based learning and action comprehension (Rizzolatti et al., 2001; Rizzolatti, 2005) being part of a system capable of modulating the plan for action execution through mental simulation via observation and internalization of others' actions (Gallese and Goldman, 1998).

It is well established that movement observation and imagery activates supplementary motor area, premotor cortex and primary motor cortex (M1) (Jeannerod, 2001). Additionally, several studies using transcranial magnetic stimulation (TMS) show imagery induced neuroplasticity as indexed by increased motor evoked potentials (MEPs) and reduced motor threshold (MT) (Fadiga et al., 1999; Roosink and Zijdewind, 2010) with muscle-specific activation pattern (Facchini et al., 2002; Fourkas et al., 2006) predominant at the contralateral hemisphere (Fadiga et al., 1999) and long-lasting effects (Pascual-Leone et al., 1995).

Motor activation during action imagery and observation can also be measured through synchronization (ERS) and desynchronization (ERD) of the Mu rhythm (Pfurtscheller and Aranibar, 1977). Initially described by Gastaut and Bert (1954) and commonly detected in the frequency range 8–13 Hz over the sensory-motor cortex (Pineda, 2008), the Mu rhythm is desynchronized during movement execution, observation and imagery. Increases in M1 excitability and consequently Mu desynchronization seem associated with premotor MNS inputs (Jarvelainen et al., 2001; Muthukumaraswamy and Johnson, 2004). This specific neurophysiological signature is observed with action observation (Buccino et al., 2001; Muthukumaraswamy and Johnson, 2004), imagery of self and other's movements (Hari, 2006; Francuz and Zapala, 2011) and in response to static images that induce sensation of movement (Giromini et al., 2010; Pineda et al., 2011).

In order to better understand the role of the motor cortex in imagery, the use of tools to modify cortical excitability

(CE)—such as non-invasive brain stimulation—is desirable. For instance, anodal transcranial direct current stimulation (tDCS) of the motor cortex enhances CE while cathodal tDCS decreases it (Nitsche and Paulus, 2000, 2001). Furthermore, previous studies have shown that cathodal tDCS coupled with motor imagery leads to decreased MEP while anodal tDCS induces the opposite results (Quartarone et al., 2004). Conversely, combining anodal tDCS with motor observation leads to long-lasting attenuation of neuropathic pain (Soler et al., 2010); therefore the study of combined approach may also provide initial data for a development of novel therapeutic tools.

Here, we aimed to investigate neurophysiological changes as indexed by Mu rhythm associated with combination of tDCS over M1 with movement observation and imagery tasks. Considering the neuromodulatory effects of tDCS we hypothesized that anodal tDCS might increase Mu ERD and cathodal tDCS would decrease it while sham condition should result in the typical Mu rhythm changes associated with motor observation and imagery. Finally, we hypothesized that tDCS induced Mu rhythm would be similar for both movement observation and imagery.

MATERIALS AND METHODS

PARTICIPANTS

Twenty-one right-handed (as verified by the Edinburgh laterality inventory) males (mean age 23.8 ± 3.1) participated in the study which was approved by the institutional ethics committee of the Mackenzie Presbyterian University, Brazil and by the National Ethics Committee (SISNEP, Brazil; CAAE no 0117.0.272.000-11). All participants gave written informed consent.

PROCEDURE

All participants received on different days with an interval between sessions of at least 48 hours, sham, anodal and cathodal tDCS. Current was ramped-up for 20 s until it reached 2 mA; stimulation was then given for 20 min, and finally the device was turned-off with a ramp-down of 20 s. Electrodes were 35 cm^2, therefore, the current density was 0.057 mA/cm2. Active electrode was positioned over the left M1 (C3 according to the EEG 10–20 system) and reference electrode at the supraorbital area (SO) as shown to be the optimal area for M1 stimulation according to neurophysiological, behavioral and modeling studies (Nitsche and Paulus, 2001; Fregni et al., 2005; Foerster et al., 2012). tDCS sessions were randomized and counterbalanced between participants.

For sham tDCS, current was ramped-up for 20 s until it reached 2 mA, then ramped-down in 20 s and turned off without participant knowledge so that the participants felt the same sensation of active stimulation. This procedure has been extensively used and shown to be effective in sham-controlled studies (Nitsche et al., 2008).

Immediately after tDCS, we positioned the EEG net on the participant (this step took approximately 10 min). The participant sat in a comfortable chair at a 110 cm distance from the computer monitor and received detailed instructions before task performance (the experimental design is illustrated in **Figure 1**).

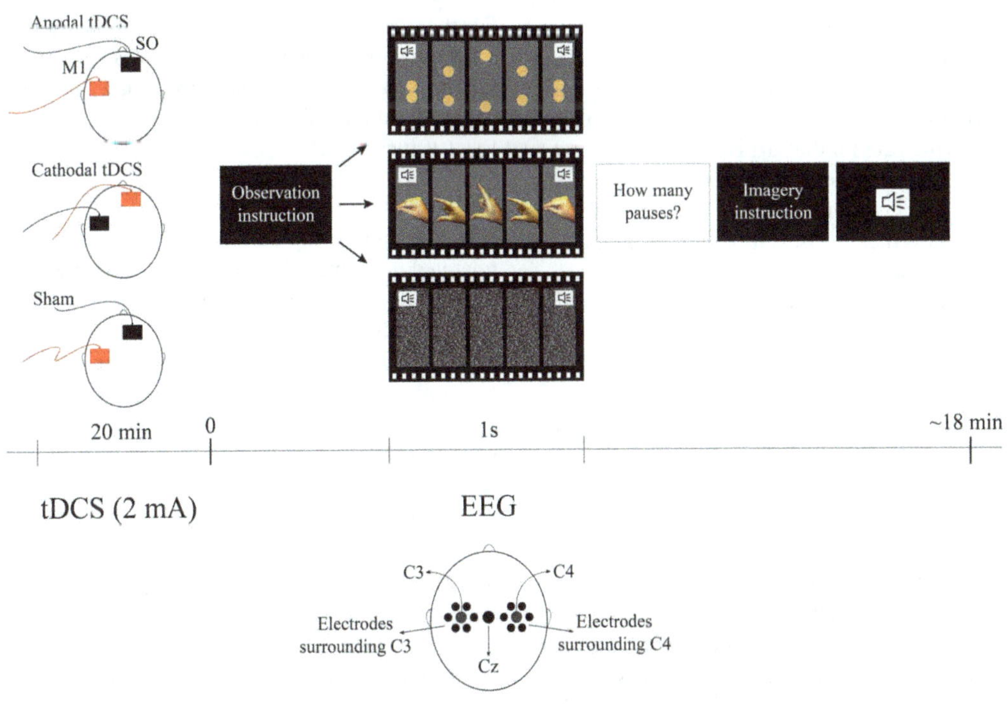

FIGURE 1 | Experimental Design. The order of observation videos was random and always followed by the imagery correspondent condition. The surrounding electrodes are: surround C3 (EGI electrodes: 29, 30, 35, 37, 41, 42), Cz, surround C4 (EGI electrodes: 87, 93, 103, 105, 110, 111). The sound symbols represent the moment when the metronome stimulus occurs pacing each cycle. For tDCS conditions red represents the anode and black represents cathode. SO represents the supraorbital (reference) area.

OBSERVATION AND IMAGERY TASK

The task was comprised of two experimental conditions—observation and imagery—each one having two types of movement—biological and non-biological. The biological observation blocks were videos lasting 80 s, each showing 1 Hz cycles of opening and closing pincer movements of a male right hand. The maximum aperture between the index finger and the thumb was 7.5 cm. For the biological imagery blocks, they were asked to mentally simulate their own right hand in the same movement, pacing at the same rate as it was shown in the observation condition. Similarly, the non-biological observation blocks were videos of 80 s each showing 1 Hz cycles of two spheres moving vertically toward each other and then touching simulating the biological movement. In order to make the non-biological condition closer to the biological one, the maximum distance between the spheres was also 7.5 cm. The diameter of the two spheres was 1.5 cm similarly to the thickness of the distal phalanx as shown in the screen. Finally, the color of the spheres was composed of proportions of Cyan 0%/Magenta 30%/Yellow 70%/Black 0% resulting in a color similar to the presented fingers. For the non-biological imagery blocks, they were asked to mentally simulate the movement of the two spheres paced at the same rate as it was shown in the observation condition. In order to maintain the participant's attention to the task we presented 2–5 pauses of the movement for 1 s in both observation conditions. Participants were asked to mentally count the pauses and report their answers after completing each trial. Both observation and imagery conditions had their own control conditions i.e., for observation control, there was an 80 s video of white noise and for imagery control, participants were asked to imagine the white noise for 80 s. All cycles of 1 Hz for all blocks were accompanied by the sound of a metronome to guide the imagery condition. Each type of block was presented twice in random orders. The observation condition was always presented before their imagery equivalent conditions in order for the participant learn the movement. In summary there was one active condition and two controls for each task (observation and motor imagery)—i.e., (1) the biological motor movement (observation or motor imagery); (2) control 1: non-biological movement and; (3) control 2: no movement control condition. The overall task duration was approximately 18 min.

EEG RECORDING AND DATA REDUCTION

To investigate the effects of tDCS, we recorded the electroencephalogram using a high-density 128 geodesic sensor net (Electrical Geodesic). We processed the original data as follows: (1) Highpass filtering at 1 Hz and Lowpass filtering at 30 Hz; (2) removal of the first and final 10 s of each trial and segmentation of the remaining 120 s (combination of the 60 s from the two equal trials) in 2 s epochs (as in Oberman et al., 2005), (3) artifact detection (difference $>140\,\mu V$ between channels above and below the eyes, a difference $>55\,\mu V$ between channels near the outer canthi, or one or more channels exceeding an amplitude of $200\,\mu V$), (4) re-referencing of scalp potentials to the average reference, (5) baseline correction from 200 ms before each segment. Epochs containing artifacts due to eye blinks, ocular and head movements were automatically rejected. In order to extract the Mu rhythm, we performed a wavelet analyses for the frequency between 8–11 Hz (Francuz and Zapala, 2011) for C3 and C4 and Cz and the electrodes surrounding C3 and C4. Mu ERD was thereafter calculated as a ratio of the power during experimental conditions relative to the respective control condition. This ratio was used to control variability in absolute Mu power as a result of individual differences. Since ratio data are inherently non-normal as a result of lower bounding, a log transform was used for the analysis. This method has been largely used in Mu rhythm analyses (Oberman et al., 2005; Giromini et al., 2010; Pineda et al., 2011).

DATA ANALYSES

Repeated-measures ANOVA were run focusing on specific effects on C3 and C4 or in Cz and the electrodes surrounding C3 and C4. We performed the analysis of the surrounding electrodes taking into consideration previous findings that show a different pattern between C3 and its surrounding area during motor imagery, videlicet ERD and ERS, respectively (e.g., Neuper et al., 2006). For all analyses the dependent variable was the Mu desynchronization index as described earlier. For the main ANOVA we considered the factors condition (observation vs. imagery), movement (biological vs. non-biological), tDCS (anodal vs. cathodal vs. sham), and hemisphere [C3 (EGI number: 36) vs. C4 (EGI number: 104)] and the respective interaction terms. For the secondary ANOVA we considered the factors condition (observation vs. imagery), movement (biological vs. non-biological), tDCS (anodal vs. cathodal vs. sham), and electrodes [surround C3 (EGI number: 29-30-35-37-41-42) vs. surround C4 (EGI number: 87-93-103-105-110-111) vs. Cz] and the respective interaction terms. For the surrounding electrodes ANOVA, we used the mean values of the previously mentioned electrodes (surround C3, surround C4, and Cz values). When appropriate, *post-hoc* comparisons were carried out using Fisher's LSD. Statistical significance refers to a p value < 0.05.

RESULTS

All participants completed the entire experiment. All participants tolerated the stimulation well and no side effects were reported.

With regard to the main ANOVA considering C3 and C4 only, we found significant effects for the factor Movement [$F_{(1, 20)} = 10.2$; $p = 0.005$; $\eta_p^2 = 0.3$] and for the interactions tDCS × Hemisphere [$F_{(2, 40)} = 3.4$; $p = 0.04$; $\eta_p^2 = 0.1$] and tDCS × Movement × Hemisphere [$F_{(2, 40)} = 4.2$; $p = 0.02$; $\eta_p^2 = 0.2$]. Fisher LSD *post-hoc* analyses considering the factors tDCS and hemisphere revealed significant differences between cathodal and anodal tDCS at C3 ($p = 0.016$). As shown in **Figure 2**, cathodal tDCS over C3 resulted in significantly larger Mu desynchronization in this area when compared to anodal tDCS independent of the movement type.

Post-hoc analyses for the three factors (tDCS, type of movement and hemisphere) revealed significant differences between C3 and C4 during biological movement after sham ($p = 0.02$), anodal tDCS ($p = 0.001$), and cathodal tDCS ($p = 0.004$).

Concerning sham tDCS, we found a typical effect of Mu desynchronization during biological movement in the contralateral hemisphere. There was a significant difference for biological and

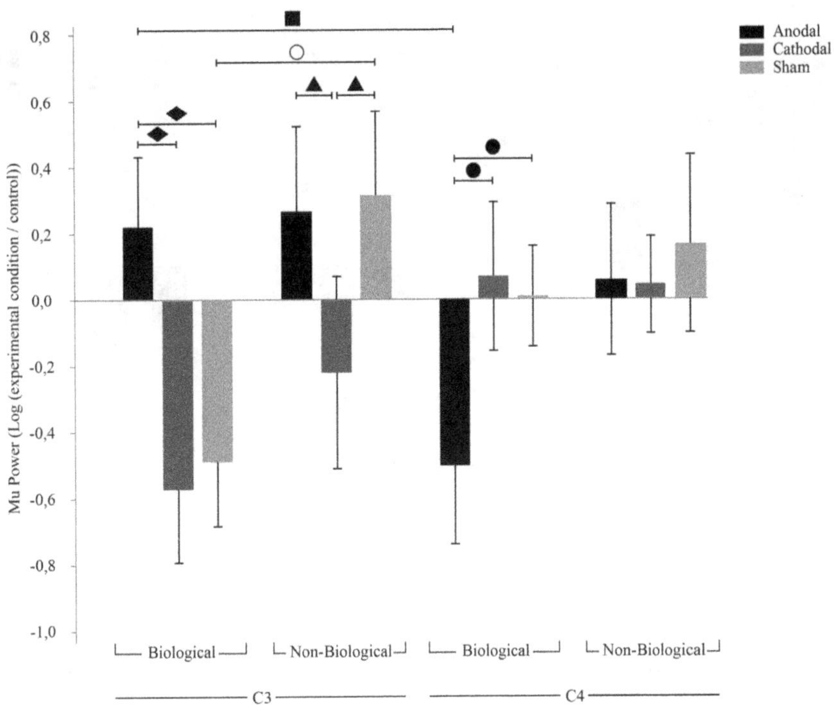

FIGURE 2 | TDCS effects on C3 and C4. Bars mean standard errors. ○, sham tDCS resulted in opposing effects for biological and non-biological conditions at C3 ($p = 0.005$); ■, anodal tDCS resulted in ERS at C3 and ERD at C4 ($p = 0.01$); ▲, cathodal tDCS resulted in Mu ERD compared to anodal ($p = 0.03$) and sham ($p = 0.02$) tDCS at C3 during non-biological movement; ●, anodal tDCS resulted in Mu ERD when compared to cathodal ($p = 0.01$) and sham ($p = 0.02$) tDCS at C4 during biological movement; ◆, anodal tDCS resulted in Mu ERS when compared to cathodal ($p = 0.001$) and sham ($p = 0.002$) tDCS at C3 during biological movement.

non-biological movement at C3 during sham tDCS ($p = 0.005$), i.e., Mu desynchronization at C3 during biological movement and Mu increase during non-biological movement. With regard to anodal tDCS, there was an interesting interhemispheric effect: we observed an absence of Mu desynchronization at C3 (hemisphere contralateral to the movement) and simultaneous Mu desynchronization in C4 (hemisphere ipsilateral to the movement) during biological movement only ($p = 0.01$). Cathodal tDCS resulted also in Mu desynchronization at C3 during non-biological movement compared to sham ($p = 0.02$) and anodal tDCS ($p = 0.03$). In addition, during biological movement observation and imagery there was a smaller desynchronization of Mu in the left hemisphere after anodal tDCS compared to sham ($p = 0.002$) and cathodal tDCS ($p = 0.001$), and a significant Mu desynchronization in the right hemisphere (C4) after anodal tDCS compared to sham ($p = 0.02$) and cathodal tDCS ($p = 0.01$).

Our analysis with C3 and C4 electrodes show that effects are not different for movement observation vs. imagery [$F_{(1, 20)} = 1.05$; $p = 0.32$; $\eta_p^2 = 0.05$].

ANALYSIS OF SURROUNDING ELECTRODES

We then analyzed the electrodes Cz and around C3 and C4 (rather than C3 and C4 themselves), ANOVA revealed a significant effect for the interaction tDCS × Condition × Movement [$F_{(2, 40)} = 3.66$; $p = 0.03$; $\eta_p^2 = 0.15$]. Since there was no effect for the hemisphere of the electrodes, the results of this analysis are referred to as surrounding electrodes data.

Contrary to the effects found in the C3 and C4 electrodes, Fisher LSD *post-hoc* analysis on surrounding electrodes revealed a tendency for sham tDCS to result in synchronization during biological imagery and desynchronization during biological observation ($p = 0.09$). Also, in the surrounding electrodes, after anodal tDCS we found Mu ERD during biological imagery but not during non-biological imagery ($p = 0.028$). On the other hand, after anodal tDCS we observed Mu ERD during non-biological observation while non-biological imagery provoked Mu ERS ($p = 0.048$). Also, biological imagery had different effects in the surrounding electrodes after anodal and cathodal tDCS resulting in Mu ERD and ERS, respectively ($p = 0.011$). Finally, biological observation led to a contrary effect as cathodal tDCS had a higher magnitude effect on Mu ERD compared to anodal ($p = 0.023$) and sham ($p = 0.05$). There was also a tendency for cathodal tDCS to induce Mu ERD in biological observation but not in non-biological observation ($p = 0.06$), and for Mu ERD and ERS during biological imagery after anodal and sham tDCS, respectively ($p = 0.09$). These results are illustrated in **Figure 3**.

DISCUSSION

Motor imagery and observation are extensively correlated with ERD of the Mu rhythm as seen in previous literature. We confirm these findings showing that during biological observation

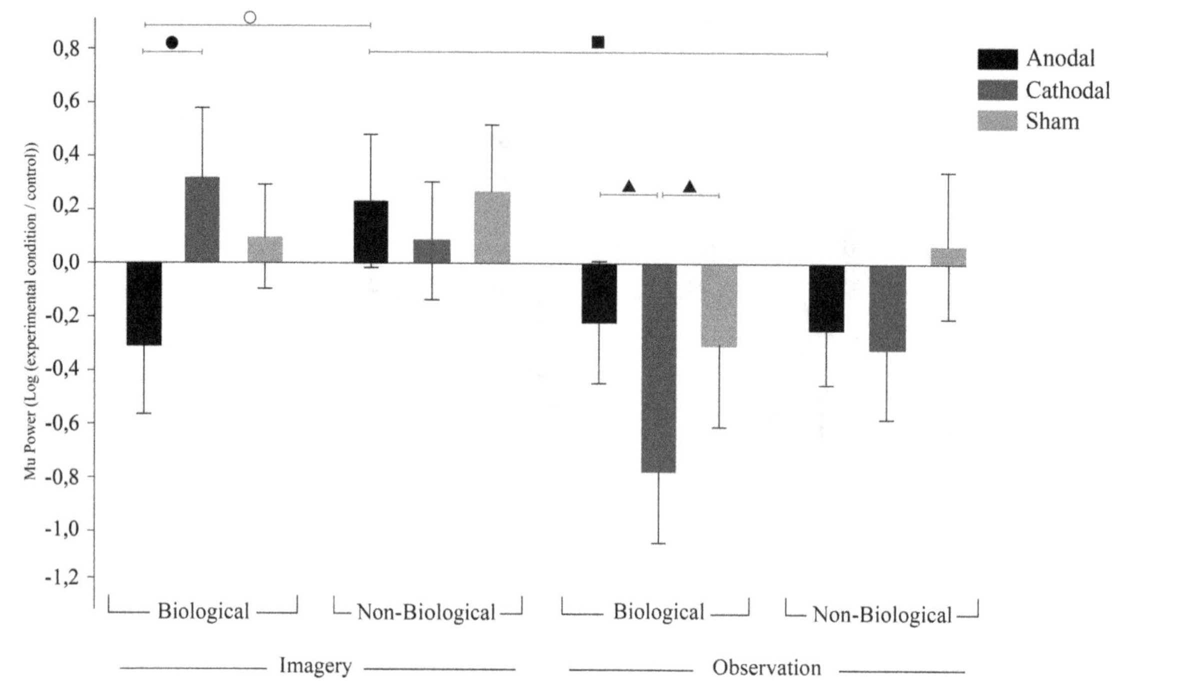

FIGURE 3 | TDCS effects on surrounding electrodes. Bars mean standard errors. ○, after anodal tDCS, biological imagery was significantly different from non-biological imagery ($p = 0.028$); ●, anodal tDCS resulted in Mu ERD when compared to cathodal tDCS in biological imagery ($p = 0.011$); ▲, cathodal tDCS resulted in stronger Mu ERD on biological observation when compared to anodal ($p = 0.023$) and sham ($p = 0.05$) tDCS; and ■, anodal tDCS resulted in Mu ERS on non-biological observation when compared to non-biological imagery ($p = 0.048$).

or imagery primed by sham tDCS, the Mu rhythm is desynchronized at the contralateral hemisphere. Here, we extend previous findings showing that active tDCS induced changes in membrane neuronal threshold is associated with modulation of the Mu rhythm during biological movements.

Our sham findings of Mu desynchronization for biological movement despite of condition (observation vs. imagery) corroborate previous neuroimaging and EEG findings (Ruby and Decety, 2001; Muthukumaraswamy and Johnson, 2004; Michelon et al., 2006; Pfurtscheller et al., 2006) and therefore is in line with the mental simulation theory (Jeannerod, 2001; Rizzolatti, 2005). Furthermore, by showing no differences between movement observation and motor imagery, we extended these findings.

With regard to the active tDCS, both cathodal and anodal stimulation interfered with the Mu rhythm elicited by the tasks. However, contrary to our initial hypothesis, we found that anodal tDCS was related to an increase of Mu power (i.e., synchronization) at C3 while cathodal tDCS resulted in a decrease of Mu power (i.e., desynchronization) at C3. Our hypothesis was based on the notion that anodal would facilitate the neurophysiological processes associated with movement observation and imagery (i.e., Mu desynchronization). However, previous non-invasive stimulation research has reported opposite effects for cathodal and anodal tDCS (Antal et al., 2007; Moliadze et al., 2012; Batsikadze et al., 2013). For instance, Batsikadze et al. (2013) applied cathodal tDCS over M1 for 20 min at 1mA and 2mA intensities and showed decreased and increased CE, respectively. Therefore, the intensity and time of stimulation may result in differential effects and our minor ERD effect might be due to a possible cathodal enhancement on CE as recently demonstrated (Batsikadze et al., 2013).

Still, it is not entirely clear which mechanisms underlie these effects and thus caution is necessary in interpreting these data. However, two main explanations seem possible to comprehend our results. On one hand, our findings might be indicative of the notion that Mu ERD is not generated only in the cortical areas. The fact that anodal tDCS induced Mu ERS is in line with the idea that Mu desynchronization is generated by subcortical systems. Leocani et al. (2005) investigated a sample of patients with multiple sclerosis and showed that ERD during programming of voluntary movement are likely mediated by cortical-subcortical connections as they found delayed ERD onset in patients with more severe subcortical damage. This novel finding might be indicating that simple, learned movements (such as opening and closing of the fingers) are mainly generated by subcortical systems and increased cortical activity may interfere with performance of such movement—here we provide such evidence with neurophysiological data. Similarly Antal et al. (2007) reported decrease of CE when combining hand motor contraction with anodal tDCS, which is aligned with our data considering the similar activation during motor observation, imagery, and execution. On the other hand, these effects might also be due to homeostatic mechanisms. The depolarizing effect of anodal tDCS might have established an enhanced CE at C3 in the baseline which induced a paradoxical effect during the task (a homeostatic effect) resulting in Mu ERS. This mechanism might be useful for neural protection as it avoids a high excitability alteration of the area and possible de-stabilization of neural network properties (Abbott and Nelson, 2000). This hypothesis is strengthened by the reverse effect after cathodal stimulation during biological movement, and furthermore, explains our controversial effect of Mu ERD after cathodal tDCS during non-biological movement. This is particularly underscored by the observation of increased ERS during sham tDCS for the non-biological condition compared to control.

Supporting the homeostatic hypothesis, some previous studies have shown reverse effects of tDCS and TMS resulting from: the combination of both techniques (Siebner et al., 2004), non-invasive brain stimulation with drugs, (Fregni et al., 2006; Kuo et al., 2008) and non-invasive brain stimulation with motor task (Antal et al., 2007). Siebner et al. (2004) found that cathodal tDCS followed by 1 Hz TMS results in a facilitatory effect which is in opposition to commonly reported findings in low frequency TMS studies. In turn, Fregni et al. (2006) found that low-frequency 1 Hz rTMS led to CE enhancement in patients with juvenile myoclonic epilepsy presenting with high plasma valproate level (a drug that reduces CE) and CE decrease for the patient group with low valproate level and control group. In addition, Kuo et al. (2008) showed that combining d-cycloserine with anodal tDCS yielded longer reaction times in a sequential motor learning task. Mainly, Antal et al. (2007) reported decreased CE when combining hand motor contraction with anodal tDCS. This is very aligned with our data considering the similar activation during motor observation, imagery, and execution.

As previously mentioned, caution is necessary when interpreting these data as it is known that tDCS can have effects on subcortical (Polania et al., 2012a) and cortical structures (Polania et al., 2012b) through M1 connections. Further studies testing both our hypotheses are necessary to fully comprehend the generating source of the Mu rhythm, and thus, make possible a more accurate interpretation of these neuromodulatory results.

Contrary to our findings, Matsumoto et al. (2010) reported increased CE and Mu ERD after 10 min of 1 mA anodal tDCS and decreased CE and Mu ERS after cathodal tDCS compared to sham. The differences in the results between our study and Matsumoto's may be explained by methodological differences. In particular, the number of participants has major impact in Mu ERD studies since there is a high variability between participants in Mu oscillatory pattern (Pfurtscheller et al., 2006). Matsumoto and colleagues ran the experiment with six participants whereas we had 21 volunteers. Moreover, we selected the electrodes a priori based on previous literature while Matsumoto et al. (2010) made a posterior selection considering electrodes presenting the higher Mu desynchronization. This method rendered results from Matsumoto's article less specific (as they could not analyze the contrast between C3/C4 and surrounding electrodes—that we showed to be important) and the *post-hoc* selection of electrodes increases the type I error in this study. In addition, another study which demonstrated relative contradictory results is the one from Quartarone et al. (2004) which showed no increase in CE after anodal tDCS companied to motor imagery, arguing that one of the strategies is enough to result in ceiling effect. However, by showing that anodal tDCS does not induce motor imagery increased excitability supports our findings to some extent. Moreover, as it is expected that tDCS alone increases CE, the effect of mental imagery blocking this increase in excitability of anodal tDCS supports our results.

Besides the focal effect under the application area of tDCS, we found interesting hemispheric differences. We analyzed Mu characteristics in C3, C4, and Cz and the electrodes surrounding C3 and C4. One important point here is that, as shown by computational model studies, tDCS has a modulatory effect over a large area application and has also a diffuse widespread action due to the distance between electrodes (Datta et al., 2009). Interestingly, despite of the relative non-focal electrical currents induction by tDCS we could observe specific and opposing effects for C3 and surrounding electrodes during biological imagery. Furthermore, this effect was absent during biological observation (except after anodal tDCS). Finally, we also found opposing effects when comparing the contralateral vs. ipsilateral hemisphere (relative to the movement)—i.e., C3 vs. C4; which is in agreement with inter-hemispheric transcallosal modulation effects as shown behaviorally by other studies (Fregni et al., 2005; Mansur et al., 2005). These results support previous neurophysiological studies showing relatively focal effects of tDCS (Nitsche et al., 2007). Our data extend this finding and demonstrate that tDCS effects can be focalized based on the behavioral task.

The focal ERD/ surrounding ERS theory hypotheses that Mu synchronization occurs to deactivate networks not related to the task (Suffczynski et al., 1999). This hypothesis is supported by our findings as Mu desynchronization over cortical area specifically related to the task followed by an increase of Mu power in motor areas not involved in the task has been previously demonstrated (Pfurtscheller and Neuper, 1994; Neuper et al., 2006; Pfurtscheller et al., 2006).

Interestingly, we found the surrounding ERS effects only during the imagery condition. Similar to our findings, Neuper et al. (2006) have demonstrated surrounding ERS during imagery tasks but not in execution tasks. They registered Mu oscillations over C3 and Cz during cube manipulation and imagery and during foot continuous movement execution and imagery. All tasks showed focal desynchronization, i.e., Mu desynchronization at Cz for foot-related tasks, and at C3 for hand-related tasks. Furthermore, they found Mu synchronization at the area not related to the task during imagery but not execution (e.g., Mu power increase in C3 during imagery of foot movement). Accordingly Pfurtscheller et al. (2006) registered Mu oscillations during 4 types of kinesthetic imagery in the following areas: right hand, left hand, both feet, and thong. They observed Mu ERD in C3 and C4 during both hand motor imagery with evident contralateral dominance and Mu ERD in Cz during feet motor imagery. Also, they report Mu ERS in C3 and C4 (hand area) during motor imagery of feet and tongue. As reported, we found surrounding inhibition for biological imagery but not for biological observation condition. Therefore, it seems plausible that the surrounding inhibition, which reflects an idling or inhibitory state with low cortical neurons excitability (Klimesch et al., 2007), may occur due to removal of motor attention from one modality to another.

The previous studies argued that the execution tasks do not require high directional attention while motor imagery does; thus having a larger focal effect. The high direction of attention seems to be the underlying process of focal Mu ERD associated with Mu surrounding ERS; therefore, our results along with previous literature suggest that motor imagery may have a more focal neuroplastic effect and may be used in rehabilitation approaches. This process seems beneficial to selectively focus and boost the specific recruited area. Considering the aforementioned findings and ours, it is plausible that the imagery tasks demand sustained and focal attention due to their higher complexity as compared to the automaticity of activation during observation. Insofar, observation tasks demand less concentration and can be automated like execution (Neuper et al., 2006).

Our study presents some limitations. Recently, O'Connell et al. (2012) demonstrated that participants receiving 2 mA tDCS judged correctly, more than chance, which stimulation they were receiving (sham vs. active tDCS). We did not directly assess our participants with regard to blinding, therefore possible effects due to correctly guessing which tDCS was being applied might be expected. However, our experiment consisted of three tDCS sessions (two active and one sham) and our results clearly differentiate between the two active conditions—anodal and cathodal effects. Additionally, our methods of ramp up and ramp down of tDCS are similar to previous findings that shows 2 mA as an effective blinding while O'Connell et al. (2012) used 5 s for each ramp up and down. Finally, females composed 75% of O'Connell and colleagues sample; in our experiment, all participants were males. Despite not being directly assessed by previous tDCS experiments, gender effects on tDCS perception may be expected considering previous experiments have shown differential gender effects on pain perception (for a review see Fillingim et al., 2009). A second limitation is that our experiment was performed in a sample of healthy males. Since the effects of tDCS in some tasks appear to differ according to gender (Boggio et al., 2008; Lapenta et al., 2012) further studies should test possible differing effects in females. Furthermore, these results could differ in populations with atypical M1 activation such as psychogenic paresis patients (Liepert et al., 2009, 2011) and autistic patients (Oberman et al., 2005; Théoret et al., 2005; Bernier et al., 2007). Thus, further studies comprising tDCS, EEG, and motor observation and imagery are suggested for better knowledge of possible benefits in populations with atypical brain activation.

In sum, the characteristics of our experiment provide a key differentiation as they allow multiple controls for the effects of the experiment on specific movements and conditions and also on different areas activations in accordance with their involvement in the task. Therefore, our setup allowed evaluation of oscillatory pattern differences relative to the complex task with focal and sustained attention (e.g., imagery) and automated tasks that require less concentration (e.g., observation) extending reports of surrounding effects for movement execution, also considered automatized when compared to imagery. Furthermore, we have shown that tDCS is able to alter Mu rhythm pattern and also that active tDCS priming effects depend on the applied polarity, type of movement, condition, and hemisphere thus introducing a new perspective to the effects of this brain stimulation tool. These novel findings also provide fresh insights regarding possible clinical applications of combined tDCS and motor imagery.

ACKNOWLEDGMENTS

Paulo S. Boggio is supported by a CNPq researcher grant (304164/2012-7). Olivia M. Lapenta was supported by a Master grant (CAPES-PROSUP—IES modality I).

REFERENCES

Abbott, L. F., and Nelson, S. B. (2000). Synaptic plasticity: taming the beast. *Nat. Neurosci. Suppl.* 3, 1178–1183. doi: 10.1038/81453

Antal, A., Terney, D., Poreisz, C., and Paulus, W. (2007). Towards unraveling task-related modulations of neuroplastic changes induced in the human motor cortex. *Eur. J. Neurosci.* 26, 2687–2691. doi: 10.1111/j.1460-9568.2007.05896.x

Batsikadze, G., Moliadze, V., Paulus, W., Kuo, M. F., and Nitsche, M. A. (2013). Partially non-linear stimulation intensity-dependent effects of direct current stimulation on motor cortex excitability in humans. *J. Physiol.* 51, 1987–2000. doi: 10.1113/jphysiol.2012.249730

Bernier, R., Dawson G, Webb, S., and Murias, M., (2007). EEG mu rhythm and imitation impairments in individuals with autism spectrum disorder. *Brain Cogn.* 64, 228–237. doi: 10.1016/j.bandc.2007.03.004

Boggio, P. S., Rocha, R. R., Silva, M. T., and Fregni, F. (2008). Differential modulatory effects of transcranial direct current stimulation on a facial expression go-no-go task in males and females. *Neurosci. Lett.* 447, 101–105. doi: 10.1016/j.neulet.2008.10.009

Buccino, G., Binofski, F., Fink, G., Fadiga, L., Fogassi, L., Gallese, V., et al. (2001). Action observation activates premotor and parietal areas in a somatopic manner: an fMRI study. *Eur. J. Neurosci.* 13, 400–404. doi: 10.1111/j.1460-9568.2001.01385.x

Datta, A., Bansal, V., Diaz, J., Patel, J., Reato, D., and Bikson, M. (2009). Gyri-precise head model of transcranial direct current stimulation: improved spatial focality using a ring electrode versus conventional rectangular pad. *Brain Stimul.* 2, 201–207. doi: 10.1016/j.brs.2009.03.005

Decety, J., and Grezes, J. (2006). The power of simulation: imagining one's own and other's behavior. *Brain Res.* 1079, 4–14. doi: 10.1016/j.brainres.2005.12.115

Facchini, S., Muellbacher, W., Battaglia, F., Boroojerdi, B., and Hallett, M. (2002). Focal enhancement of motor córtex excitability during motor imagery: a transcranial magnetic stimulation study. *Acta Neurol. Scand.* 105, 146–151. doi: 10.1034/j.1600-0404.2002.1o004.x

Fadiga, L., Buccino, G., Craighero, L., Fogassi, L., Gallese, V., and Pavesi, G. (1999). Corticospinal excitability is specifcally modulated by motor imagery: a magnetic stimulation study. *Neuropsychologia* 37, 147–158. doi: 10.1016/S0028-3932(98)00089-X

Fourkas, A. D., Avenanti, A., Urgesi, C., and Aglioti, S. M. (2006). Corticospinal facilitation during first and third person imagery. *Exp. Brain Res.* 168, 143–151. doi: 10.1007/s00221-005-0076-0

Francuz, P., and Zapala, D. (2011). The suppression of the Mu rhythm during the creation of imagery representation of movement. *Neurosci. Lett.* 495, 39–43. doi: 10.1016/j.neulet.2011.03.031

Fregni, F., Boggio, P. S., Mansur, C. G., Wagner, T., Ferreira, M. J. L., Lima, M. C., et al. (2005). Transcranial direct current stimulation of the unaffected hemisphere in stroke patients. *Neuroreport* 16, 1551–1555.

Fregni, F., Boggio, P. S., Valle, A. C., Otachi, P., Thut, G., Rigonatti, S. P., et al. (2006). Homeostatic effects of plasma valproate levels on corticospinal excitability changes induced by 1 Hz rTMS in patients with juvenile myoclonic epilepsy. *Clin. Neurophysiol.* 117, 1217–1227. doi: 10.1016/j.clinph.2006.02.015

Fillingim, R. B., King, C. D., Ribeiro-Dasilva, M. C., Rahim-Williams, B., and Riley, J. L. III. (2009). Sex, gender, and pain: a review of recent clinical and experimental findings. *J. Pain* 10, 447–485. doi: 10.1016/j.jpain.2008.12.001

Foerster, A., Rocha, S., Wiesiolek, C., Chagas, A. P., Machado, G., Silva, E., et al. (2012). Site-specific effects of mental practice combined with transcranial direct current stimulation on motor learning. *Eur. J. Neurosci.* 37, 786–794. doi: 10.1111/ejn.12079

Gallese, V., and Goldman, A. (1998). Mirror neurons and the simulation theory of mind-reading. *Trends Cogn. Sci.* 2, 493–501. doi: 10.1016/S1364-6613(98)01262-5

Gastaut, H., and Bert, J. (1954). EEG changes during cinematographic presentation. *Electroencephalogr. Clin. Neurophysiol.* 6, 433–444. doi: 10.1016/0013-4694(54)90058-9

Giromini, L., Porcelli, P., Viglione, D. J., Parolin, L., and Pineda, J. A. (2010). The feeling of movement: EEG evidence for mirroring activity during the observations of static, ambiguous stimuli in the Rorschach cards. *Biol. Psychol.* 85, 233–241. doi: 10.1016/j.biopsycho.2010.07.008

Hari, R. (2006). Action–perception connection and the cortical mu rhythm. *Prog. Brain Res.* 159, 253–260. doi: 10.1016/S0079-6123(06)59017-X

Jarvelainen, J., Schurmann, M., Avikainen, S., and Hari, R. (2001). Stronger reactivity of the human primary motor cortex during observation of live rather than video motor acts. *Neuroreport* 12, 3493–3495.

Jeannerod, M. (2001). Neural simulation of action: a unifying mechanism for motor cognition. *Neuroimage* 14, 103–109. doi: 10.1006/nimg.2001.0832

Klimesch, W., Sauseng, P., and Hanslmayr, S. (2007). EEG alpha oscillations: the inhibition–timing hypothesis. *Brain Res. Rev.* 53, 63–88. doi: 10.1016/j.brainresrev.2006.06.003

Kuo, M. F., Unger, M., Liebetanz, D., Lang, N., Tergau, F., Paulus, W., et al. (2008). Limited impact of homeostatic plasticity on motor learning in humans. *Neuropsychologia* 46, 2122–2128. doi: 10.1016/j.neuropsychologia.2008.02.023

Lapenta, O. M., Fregni, F., Oberman, L., and Boggio, O. S. (2012). Bilateral temporal cortex transcranial direct current stimulation worsens male performance in a multisensory integration task. *Neurosci. Lett.* 527, 105–109. doi: 10.1016/j.neulet.2012.08.076

Leocani, L., Rovaris, M., Martinelli-Boneschi, F., Annovazzi, P., Filippi, M., Colombo, B., et al. (2005). Movement preparation is affected by tissue damage in multiple sclerosis: evidence from EEG event-related desynchronization. *Clin. Neurophysiol.* 116, 1515–1519. doi: 10.1016/j.clinph.2005.02.026

Liepert, J., Hassa, T., Tüscher, O., and Schmidt, R. (2009). Abnormal motor excitability in patients with psychogenic paresis - a TMS study. *J. Neurol.* 256, 121–126. doi: 10.1007/s00415-009-0090-4

Liepert, J., Hassa, T., Tüscher, O., and Schmidt, R. (2011). Motor excitability during movement imagination and movement observation in psychogenic lower limb paresis. *J. Psychosom. Res.* 70, 59–65. doi: 10.1016/j.jpsychores.2010.06.004

Mansur, C. G., Fregni, F., Boggio, P. S., Ribeiro, M., Gallucci-Neto, J., Santos, C. M., et al. (2005). A sham stimulation-controlled trial of rTMS of the unaffected hemisphere in stroke patients. *Neurology* 64, 1802–1804. doi: 10.1212/01.WNL.0000161839.38079.92

Matsumoto, J., Fujiwara, T., Takahashi, O., Liu, M., Kimura, A., and Ushiba, J. (2010). Modulation of mu rhythm desynchronization during motor imagery by transcranial direct current stimulation. *J. Neuroeng. Rehabil.* 7, 1–5. doi: 10.1186/1743-0003-7-27

Michelon, P., Vettel, J. M., and Zacks, J. M. (2006). Lateral somatotopic organization during imagined and prepared movements. *J. Neurophysiol.* 95, 811–822. doi: 10.1152/jn.00488.2005

Moliadze, V., Atalay, D., Antal, A., and Paulus, W. (2012). Close to threshold transcranial electrical stimulation preferentially activates inhibitory networks before switching to excitation with higher intensities. *Brain Stimul.* 5, 505–511. doi: 10.1016/j.brs.2011.11.004

Muthukumaraswamy, S. D., and Johnson, B. W. (2004). Primary motor cortex activation during action observation revealed by wavelet analysis of the EEG. *Clin. Neurophysiol.* 115, 1760–1766. doi: 10.1016/j.clinph.2004.03.004

Neuper, C., Wortz, M., and Pfurtscheller, G. (2006). ERD/ERS patterns reflecting sensorimotor activation and deactivation. *Prog. Brain Res.* 159, 211–222. doi: 10.1016/S0079-6123(06)59014-4

Nitsche, M. A., Cohen, L. G., Wasserman, E. M., Priori, A., Lang, N., Antal, A., et al. (2008). Transcranial direct current stimulation: state of the art 2008. *Brain Stimul.* 1, 206–223. doi: 10.1016/j.brs.2008.06.004

Nitsche, M. A., Doemkes, S., Karakose, T., Antal, A., Liebetanz, D., Lang, N., et al. (2007). Shaping the effects of transcranial direct current stimulation of the human motor cortex. *J. Neurophysiol.* 97, 3109–3117. doi: 10.1152/jn.01312.2006

Nitsche, M. A., and Paulus, W. (2000). Excitability changes induced in the human motor cortex by weak transcranial direct current stimulation. *J. Physiol.* 527, 633–639. doi: 10.1111/j.1469-7793.2000.t01-1-00633.x

Nitsche, M. A., and Paulus, W. (2001). Sustained excitability elevations induced by transcranial. DC motor cortex stimulation in humans. *Neurology* 57, 1899–1901. doi: 10.1212/WNL.57.10.1899

Oberman, L. M., Hubbard, E. M., McCleery, J. P., Altschuler, E. L., Ramachandran, V. S., and Pineda, J. A. (2005). EEG evidence for mirror neuron dysfunction in autism spectrum disorders. *Cogn. Brain Res.* 24, 190–198. doi: 10.1016/j.cogbrainres.2005.01.014

O'Connell, N. E., Cossar, J., Marston, L., Wand, B. M., Bunce, D., Moseley, G. L., et al. (2012). Rethinking clinical trials of transcranial direct current stimulation: participant and assessor blinding is inadequate at intensities of 2 mA. *PLoS ONE* 7:e47514. doi: 10.1371/journal.pone.0047514

Pascual-Leone, A., Dang, N., Cohen, L. G., Brasil-Neto, J. P., Cammarota, A., and Hallet, M. (1995). Modulation of muscle responses evoked by transcranial magnetic stimulation during the acquisition of new fine motor skills. *J. Neurophysiol.* 74, 1037–1045.

Pfurtscheller, G., and Aranibar, A. (1977). Event-related cortical desynchronization detected by power measurements of scalp EEG. *Electroencephalogr. Clin. Neurophysiol.* 42, 817–826. doi: 10.1016/0013-4694(77)90235-8

Pfurtscheller, G., Brunner, C., Schlogl, A., and Lopes da Silva, F. H. (2006). Mu rhythm (de)synchronization and EEG single-trial classification of different motor imagery tasks. *Neuroimage* 31, 153–159. doi: 10.1016/j.neuroimage.2005.12.003

Pfurtscheller, G., and Neuper, C. (1994). Event-related synchronization of mu rhythm in the EEG over the cortical hand area in man. *Neurosci. Lett.* 174, 93–96. doi: 10.1016/0304-3940(94)90127-9

Pineda, J. A. (2008). Sensorimotor cortex as a critical component of an 'extended' mirror neuron system: does it solve the development, correspondence, and control problems in mirroring? *Behav. Brain Funct.* 47, 1–16. doi: 10.1186/1744-9081-4-47

Pineda, J. A., Giromini, L., Porcelli, P., Parolin, L., and Viglione, D. J. (2011). Mu suppression and human movement responses to the Rorschach test. *Neuroreport* 22, 223–226. doi: 10.1097/WNR.0b013e328344f45c

Polania, R., Paulus, W., and Nitsche, M. (2012a). Modulating cortico-striatal and thalamo-cortical functional connectivity with transcranial direct current stimulation. *Hum. Brain Mapp.* 33, 2499–2508. doi: 10.1002/hbm.21380

Polania, R., Paulus, W., and Nitsche, M. (2012b). Reorganizing the intrinsic functional architecture of the human primary motor cortex during rest with non-invasive cortical stimulation. *PLoS ONE* 7:e30971. doi: 10.1371/journal.pone.0030971

Quartarone, A., Morgante, F., Bagnato, S., Rizzo, V., Sant'Angelo, A., Aiello, E., et al. (2004). Long lasting effects of transcranial direct current stimulation on motor imagery. *Neuroreport* 15, 1287–1291.

Rizzolatti, G. (2005). The mirror neuron system and its function in humans. *Anat. Embryol.* 210, 419–421. doi: 10.1007/s00429-005-0039-z

Rizzolatti, G., Fogassi, L., and Gallese, V. (2001). Neurophysiological mechanisms underlying the understanding and imitation of action. *Nat. Rev.* 2, 661–670. doi: 10.1038/35090060

Roosink, M., and Zijdewind, I. (2010). Corticospinal excitability during observation and imagery of sample and complex hand tasks: implications for motor rehabilitation. *Behav. Brain Res.* 213, 35–41. doi: 10.1016/j.bbr.2010.04.027

Ruby, P., and Decety, J. (2001). Effect of subjective perspective taking during simulation of action: a PET investigation of agency. *Nat. Neurosci.* 4, 546–550. doi: 10.1038/87510

Siebner, H. R., Lang, N., Rizzo, V., Nitsche, M. A., Paulus, W., Lemon, R. N., et al. (2004). Preconditioning of low-frequency repetitive transcranial magnetic stimulation with transcranial direct current stimulation: evidence for homeostatic plasticity in the human motor cortex. *J. Neurosci.* 24, 3379–3385. doi: 10.1523/JNEUROSCI.5316-03.2004

Soler, M. D., Kumru, H., Pelayo, R., Vidal, J., Tornos, J. M., Fregni, F., et al. (2010). Effectiveness of transcranial direct current stimulation and visual illusion on neuropathic pain in spinal cord

injury. *Brain* 133, 2565–2577. doi: 10.1093/brain/awq184
Suffczynski, P., Pijn, J. P., Pfurtscheller, G., and Lopes da Silva, F. H. (1999). "Event-related dynamics of alpha band rhythms: a neuronal network model of focal ERD/surround ERS," in *Event-Related Desynchronization. Handbook of Electroencephalography and Clinical Neurophysiology,* eds
Théoret, H., Halligan, E., Kobayashi, M., Fregni, F., Tager-Flusberg, H., and Pascual-Leone, A. (2005). Impaired motor facilitation during action observation in individuals with autism spectrum disorder. *Curr. Biol.* 15, 84–85. doi: 10.1016/j.cub.2005.01.022

14

tDCS stimulation segregates words in the brain: evidence from aphasia

Valentina Fiori[1], Susanna Cipollari[1], Margherita Di Paola[1,2], Carmelina Razzano[1], Carlo Caltagirone[1,3] and Paola Marangolo[1,4]*

[1] *Istituto Di Ricovero e Cura a Carattere Scientifico Fondazione Santa Lucia, Roma, Italy*
[2] *Dipartimento di Medicina Interna e Sanità Pubblica, Università de L'Aquila, L'Aquila-Coppito, Italy*
[3] *Department of Neurology, University of Tor Vergata, Roma, Italy*
[4] *Department di Medicina, Facoltà di Medicina, Università Politecnica Marche, Ancona, Italy*

Correspondence:
Paola Marangolo, Department of Experimental and Clinical Medicine, Facoltà di Medicina, Università Politecnica delle Marche, Via Tronto 10A, 60020 Ancona, Italia
e-mail: p.marangolo@univpm.it

A number of studies have already shown that modulating cortical activity by means of transcranial direct current stimulation (tDCS) improves noun or verb naming in aphasic patients. However, it is not yet clear whether these effects are equally obtained through stimulation over the frontal or the temporal regions. In the present study, the same group of aphasic subjects participated in two randomized double-blind experiments involving two intensive language treatments for their noun and verb retrieval difficulties. During each training, each subject was treated with tDCS (20 min, 1 mA) over the left hemisphere in three different conditions: anodic tDCS over the temporal areas, anodic tDCS over the frontal areas, and sham stimulation, while they performed a noun and an action naming tasks. Each experimental condition was run in five consecutive daily sessions over three weeks with 6 days of intersession interval. The order of administration of the two language trainings was randomly assigned to all patients. Overall, with respect to the other two conditions, results showed a significant greater improvement in noun naming after stimulation over the temporal region, while verb naming recovered significantly better after stimulation of the frontal region. These improvements persisted at one month after the end of each treatment suggesting a long-term effect on recovery of the patients' noun and verb difficulties. These data clearly suggest that the mechanisms of recovery for naming can be segregated coupling tDCS with an intensive language training.

Keywords: tDCS, brain stimulation, aphasia rehabilitation, lexical deficits, language areas, word recovery

INTRODUCTION

In these last years, a small but growing body of evidence have already indicated that non-invasive brain stimulation techniques, such as transcranial magnetic stimulation (TMS) (Naeser et al., 2005; Martin et al., 2009) and transcranial direct current stimulation (tDCS) (Monti et al., 2008, 2012; Baker et al., 2010; Fiori et al., 2011; Flöel et al., 2011; Fridriksson et al., 2011; Kang et al., 2011; Marangolo et al., 2013), can modulate the language system and, in particular, lexical retrieval. Although, most of these studies suggest that both techniques might be helpful in enhancing noun or verb naming, it is still an open question which stimulated language area might exert the greatest influence.

Some reports, using rTMS or tDCS in the healthy population, have already pointed to a crucial role of the temporal regions, and, in particular of the left Wernicke's area, in noun naming (Töpper et al., 1998; Mottaghy et al., 2006; Sparing et al., 2008). Töpper et al. (1998) have used rTMS to stimulate the left motor cortex, the left Wernicke's area and the right Wernicke's homologous area. A significant shortening of picture naming latencies was present only after stimulation over the left Wernicke's area. The same results were found by Mottaghy et al. (2006). Similarly, in a tDCS study, Sparing et al. (2008) comparing different stimulation conditions (anodic, cathodic, and sham stimulation over the left Wernicke's area and anodic stimulation of the homologous right Wernicke's area) in a group of 15 healthy subjects found faster responses only after anodic tDCS over the left Wernicke's area.

However, other studies have suggested a possible involvement in noun retrieval of the frontal region too. In a group of healthy subjects, Fertonani et al. (2010) found a facilitatory effect for noun naming after anodal tDCS stimulation over the DLPFC. More recently, Holland et al. (2011) targeted left frontal activity using 2 mA-tDCS during an fMRI study of overt spoken picture naming in 10 healthy volunteers. Each of the 107 pictures to be named was presented simultaneously with an auditory cue. Participants were instructed to name the object aloud as quickly and as accurately as possible. Faster naming responses in noun naming correlated with decreased blood oxygen level-dependent signal in Broca's area during the anodic tDCS over this area were found compared to sham stimulation.

To date, contradictory results have been reported also in the brain-damaged populations. Naeser et al. (2005) have shown that the application of slow rTMS suppressing the activation of the anterior portion of the right Broca's homolog (right pars triangularis), for 10 consecutive days, improved noun naming performance in four chronic, non-fluent aphasic subjects. Accordingly, in the same population, Kang et al. (2011) using cathodal tDCS stimulation over the right Broca's homolog area and concomitant noun-retrieval training demonstrated a significantly improved naming accuracy of treated items compared to sham stimulation. Similar results were obtained by Baker et al. (2010) and Monti et al. (2008) during application of anodal (Baker et al., 2010) and cathodal tDCS (Monti et al., 2008) over the left damaged frontal cortex. However, data have been reported where beneficial effects on noun naming during a concomitant language treatment resulted after anodal tDCS over the left temporal cortex (Fiori et al., 2011; Fridriksson et al., 2011; see also Flöel et al., 2011). Fridriksson et al. (2011) found beneficial effects after anodal tDCS over the left temporal cortex on vocal response time during a computerized anomia treatment in eight chronic aphasic participants. Similarly, Fiori et al. (2011) found that anodic tDCS stimulation over the left temporal region (including Wernicke's area) with concomitant language training for five consecutive days led to faster word retrieval in three aphasic patients at the end of treatment and three weeks later [see also Flöel et al. (2011)].

With regard to the recovery of verbs, Cotelli et al. (2006) assessed the effect of TMS applied to the left and right DLPFC on an object and action naming tasks in 15 patients with Alzheimer's disease (AD). In each subject, they found an improvement only for action (see also Cappa et al., 2002; Cotelli et al., 2012).

However, their results were not replicated in a subsequent study (Cotelli et al., 2008) in which rTMS applied to the DLPFC improved both noun and verb naming performance in AD patients not only in early, but also in a more advanced stage of their cognitive decline.

Until recently, only one report has specifically investigated tDCS influence in the improvement of verbs in the aphasic population (Marangolo et al., 2013). In this study, seven chronic subjects participated in an intensive language training for their action naming difficulties. During this training, each subject was treated with tDCS over the left hemisphere in three different conditions: anodic tDCS over the Wernicke's area, anodic tDCS over the Broca's area, and sham stimulation. In all patients, results showed a significantly better response accuracy only after anodic tDCS over the Broca's area.

In summary, the above mentioned studies seem to suggest that both rTMS and tDCS exert a positive influence in word retrieval. Nevertheless, it is still an open question which stimulated area might enhance the greatest effect. In most studies (Naeser et al., 2005; Martin et al., 2009; Baker et al., 2010; Fiori et al., 2011; Flöel et al., 2011; Fridriksson et al., 2011; Kang et al., 2011; see Holland and Crinion, 2012; Monti et al., 2012 for a review), the absence of a control condition through stimulation of another brain region did not allow to univocally attribute the effects to a specific contribution of the targeted region.

One way to resolve this issue is to compare the performance of the same aphasic population both in a noun and action naming task while stimulating different language areas.

This study was designed to investigate whether tDCS, over the frontal and the temporal regions coupled with an intensive language treatment, would differently improve noun and verb recovery in a group of seven participants with chronic aphasia.

MATERIALS AND METHODS

PARTICIPANTS

Seven aphasic subjects (5 men and 2 female) who had suffered a single left hemisphere stroke were included in the study. Inclusion criteria for the study were native Italian proficiency, pre-morbid right handedness, a single left hemispheric stroke at least 6 months prior to the investigation, and no acute or chronic neurological symptoms requiring medication.

The data analyzed in the current study were collected in accordance with the Helsinky Declaration and the Institutional Review Board of the IRCCS Fondazione Santa Lucia, Rome, Italy. Prior to participation, all patients signed informed consent forms.

CLINICAL DATA

In all patients, the MRI revealed an ischemic lesion involving the left hemisphere (see **Figure 1**).

The aphasic disorders were assessed using standardized language tests [the Battery for the analysis of aphasic disorders, BADA test (Miceli et al., 1994); Token test (De Renzi and Vignolo, 1962)]. Subjects were also administered a Neuropsychological Battery (Orsini et al., 1987; Spinnler and Tognoni, 1987; Zimmermann and Fimm, 1994), which excluded the presence of attention and memory deficits that might have confounded the data (see **Table 1**).

The seven subjects were classified as non-fluent aphasics because of their reduced spontaneous speech with short sentences and frequent word-finding difficulties. They had no articulatory deficits with preserved word repetition and reading. In a naming task, all patients had lexical retrieval difficulties [BADA test (Miceli et al., 1994)].

MATERIALS

One hundred and two pictures of concrete nouns [i.e., box ($F = 67$, $L = 7$), pencil ($F = 37$, $L = 6$)] (Snodgrass and Vanderwart, 1980) and 102 videoclip of concrete actions [i.e., to shoot ($F = 63$, $L = 7$), to steal ($F = 36$, $L = 6$)] were used. Nouns and actions were matched for imageability (estimated on the basis of a sample of 21 normal participants along a seven-point scale), number of letters, age of acquisition [estimated on the basis of a sample of 20 normal participants along a nine-point scale; (Lotto et al., 2001)] and surface frequency [taken from De Mauro et al. (1993)]. Both imageability and age-of-acquisition ratings were collected by asking volunteers to judge printed words.

PROCEDURE

Transcranial direct current stimulation (tDCS)

tDCS was applied using a battery driven Eldith (neuroConn GmbH) Programmable Direct Current Stimulator with a pair of surface-soaked sponge electrodes (5 × 7 cm). A constant current of 1 mA intensity was applied on the skin for 20 min. If applied according to safety guidelines, tDCS is considered to be a safe brain stimulation technique with minor adverse effects (Poreisz et al., 2007). To stimulate the left temporal and frontal regions, two different electrode stimulation positions were used: the CP5 of the extended International 10–20 system for EEG electrode placement, which has been found to correspond best to the Wernicke's area (Oliveri et al., 1999; Fiori et al., 2011) and the

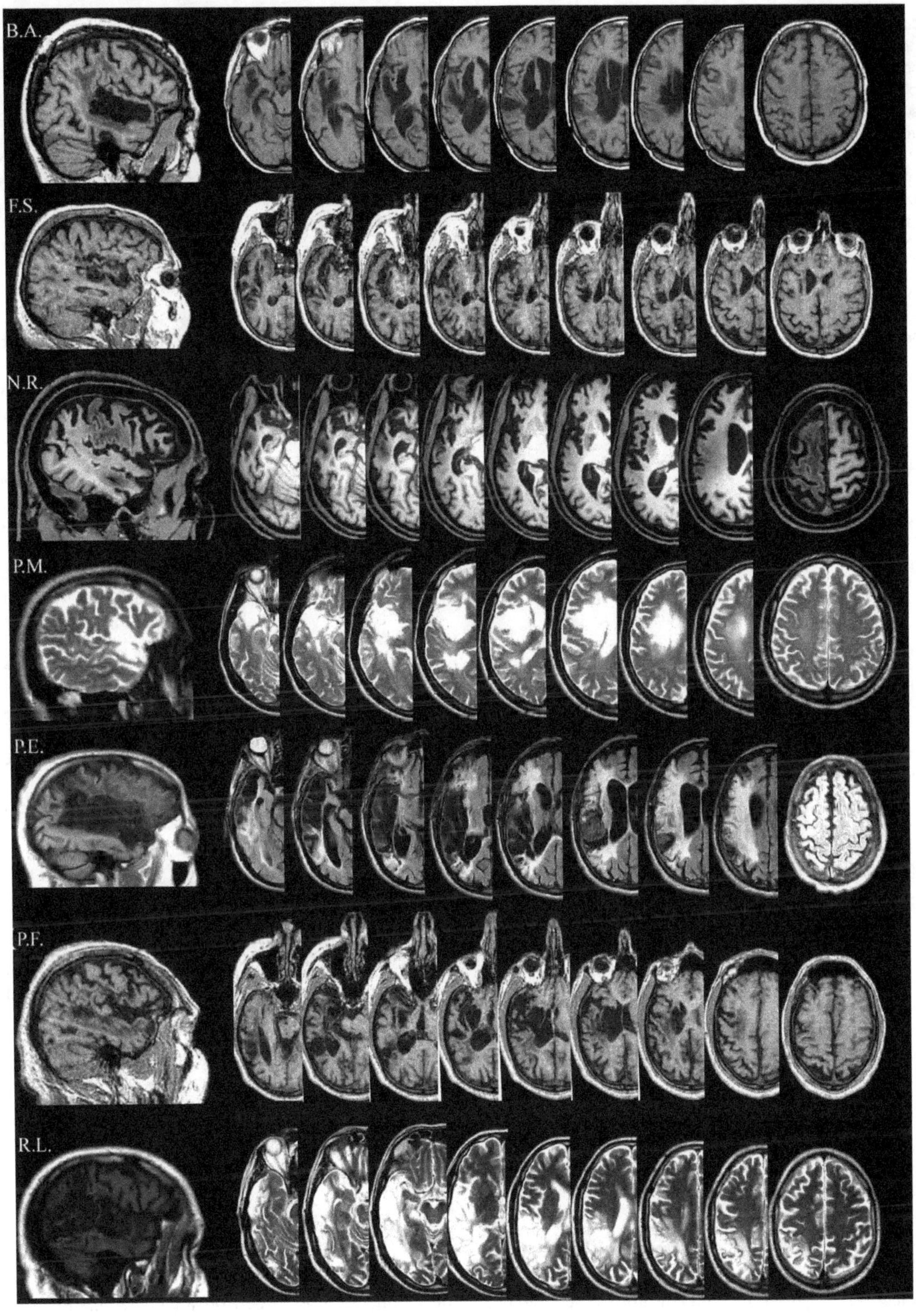

FIGURE 1 | Lesion descriptions for each aphasic patient. B.A.'s lesion is localized in the left temporal cortex involving part of the temporal pole (superior part), the full extension of the superior temporal gyrus (Wernicke's area), and part of the middle temporal gyrus. A sufferance of cerebral white matter running in the angular gyrus and in the post central gyrus, with a relatively sparing of the corresponding parietal cortex is present. The lesion also involves the insula, although part of the insular cortex is spared. **F.S.**'s lesion is mainly localized in the left temporal-insular region. A further damaged area is at the level of the homolateral frontal lobe (mesial portion) involving the white matter running under the middle frontal gyrus. **N.R.**'s lesion is localized in the left fronto-temporo-parietal cortices. At frontal level, the damage laterally involves the inferior frontal gyrus (Broca's area), the middle frontal gyrus, the superior frontal gyrus and the precentral gyrus,

(Continued)

FIGURE 1 | Continued
and medially the medial frontal gyrus and the anterior cingulate gyrus. Posteriorly, the damage involves the temporal pole, the superior and the middle temporal gyrus, the post-central gyrus and the inferior parietal lobule. The lesion also includes the insula. **P.M.**'s lesion is localized in the left fronto-temporo cortices, involving the inferior frontal gyrus (Broca's area), and the temporal pole. The lesion also includes the insula. **P.E.**'s lesion is localized in the left fronto-temporo-parietal cortices, including the inferior frontal gyrus (Broca's area), the inferior part of the pre-central gyrus, the temporal pole, the full extension of the superior temporal gyrus (Wernicke's area), part of the middle temporal lobe, the inferior part of the post-central gyrus, the angular and part of supramarginal gyri. The lesion also includes the insula. **P.F.**'s lesion is mainly localized in the left fronto-temporal cortices, with a minor involvement of the homolateral parietal cortex. The damage includes the temporal pole, part of the superior temporal (Wernicke's area) and of the middle temporal gyri. The lesion also involves the insula. **R.L**'s lesion is localized in the left temporo-parieto-occipital cortices, including the temporal pole, the full extension of the superior temporal gyrus (Wernicke's area), part of the middle temporal lobe, the angular and the supramarginal gyri, the inferior parietal lobule and the superior occipital gyrus.

Table 1 | Sociodemographic and Clinical data of the seven non-fluent aphasic subjects.

Subjects	Sex	Age	Ed. level	Time post-onset	Right Hemip	Right Hemian	Attentional Abilities (scores in percentile > 5 unimpaired)	Memory WM (cut/off 5 ± 2) STM (cut/off 7 ± 2) LTM (cut/off 5.5)
B.A.	F	59	18	3 years and 3 months	+	–	Alertness (tot): 76 Sustained Att (tot): 82 Selective Att (tot): 54	WM: 4 STM: 6 LTM: 10
F.S.	F	71	5	1 year and 6 months	+	–	Alertness (tot): 24 Sustained Att (tot): 21 Selective Att (tot): 31	WM: 5 STM: 6 LTM: 10
N.R.	M	53	13	7 months	+	–	Alertness (tot): 58 Sustained Att (tot): 73 Selective Att (tot): 50	WM: 4 STM: 6 LTM: 10
P.M.	M	52	13	9 months	+	–	Alertness (tot): 88 Sustained Att (tot): 50 Selective Att (tot): 62	WM: 5 STM: 5 LTM: 11
P.E.	M	68	18	1 year and 8 months	+	–	Alertness (tot): 18 Sustained Att (tot): 14 Selective Att (tot): 16	WM: 4 STM: 5 LTM: 6
P.F.	M	44	13	7 years	+	–	Alertness (tot): 99 Sustained Att (tot): 66 Selective Att (tot): 84	WM: 5 STM: 7 LTM: 13
R.L.	M	62	11	4 years and 5 months	–	–	Alertness (tot): 99 Sustained Att (tot): 58 Selective Att (tot): 50	WM: 6 STM: 6 LTM: 13

Results in the Neuropsychological Battery for Attention (Zimmermann and Fimm, 1994) and Memory deficits (Orsini et al., 1987; Spinnler and Tognoni, 1987) are also reported. Ed. Level, Educational Level; Right Hemip, Right Hemiparesis; Right Hemian, Right Hemianopia; WM, Working Memory; STM, Short-Term Memory; LTM, Long-Term Memory.

F5 of the extended International 10-20 system for EEG electrode placement, which correspond best to the Broca's area (Nishitani et al., 2005; Naeser et al., 2010). In both conditions the reference electrode was placed over the contralateral frontopolar cortex (Nitsche and Paulus, 2000; Sparing et al., 2008).

Overall, three different stimulation sessions were carried out: (1) anodic (CP5-A) stimulation of the left Wernicke's area; (2) anodic (F5-A) stimulation of the left Broca's area; and (3) sham stimulation over the Wernicke's area (CP5-S) for four out of seven patients and, for the remaining three, over the Broca's area (F5-S) (**Figure 2**). Sham stimulation was performed exactly like anodic stimulation over the left Wernicke's or Broca's area, but the stimulator was turned off after 30 s (Gandiga et al., 2006). To ensure the double-blind procedure, both the experimenter and the patients were blinded regarding the experimental and the sham conditions and the stimulator was turned on/off by another person.

For each subject, all pictures ($N = 102$) and actions ($N = 102$) were used. Stimuli belonging to each category were subdivided into three groups of 34 items each, matched for frequency,

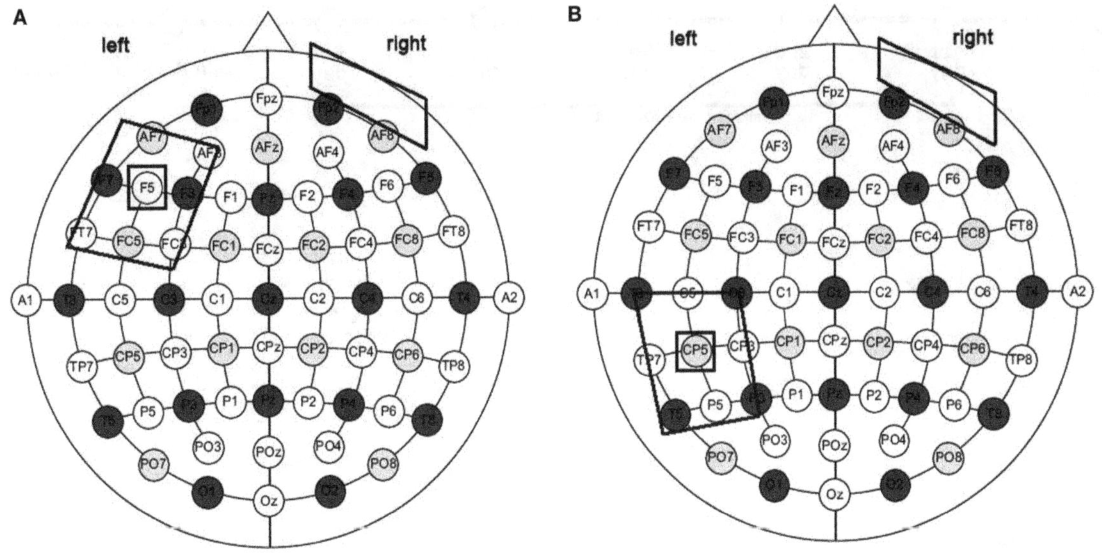

FIGURE 2 | Size and montage parameters of tDCS stimulation. tDCS was applied using a pair of surface-soaked sponge electrodes of 5 × 7 cm. To stimulate the left temporal and frontal regions, two different electrode stimulation positions were used: the CP5 of the extended International 10–20 system for EEG electrode placement **(A)** and the F5 of the extended International 10–20 system for EEG electrode placement **(B)**. In both conditions the reference electrode was placed over the contralateral frontopolar cortex.

length, imaginability, and age of acquisition. For each category, one group of item was used for the left anodic Wernicke's stimulation, one for the left anodic Broca's stimulation and the third one for the sham condition. The assignment of each group of stimuli was randomized across conditions.

TREATMENT

Once the electrodes had been placed on the scalp, the subjects performed the naming tasks while they received 20 min of tDCS. Three out of seven patients began with the noun naming treatment, while the remaining four started with the action naming training. The two treatments were separated by an interval of one month.

For each treatment, subjects were asked to name aloud each picture or videoclip that appeared on the PC screen (screen size 15″, viewing distance 1 m) for 15 s preceded by a fixation point, which lasted 800 ms (see also Raymer et al., 2006, 2007; Conroy and Scowcroft, 2012 for noun and action naming interventions). Only if the subject spontaneously correctly named the picture or the videoclip, the examiner manually recorded the response type on a separate sheet. If the subject failed or did not answer within 15 s, the corresponding written name was presented below the image and the subject was asked to read the word aloud. The subject never listen to the written word spoken aloud by the therapist. The pair of stimuli remained on the screen until the subject read the word or 40 s elapsed (see **Figure 3**). In any cases, subjects were not able to correctly read the word. For both trainings, each stimulation condition was performed in five consecutive daily sessions over three weeks, with six days of intersession interval. The order of items presentation was randomized across sessions. To measure baseline performance, at the beginning of each week and before the training each subject was asked to name the pictures or the videos, one at a time, without help. The order of conditions was randomized across subjects.

FOLLOW-UPS

At 1 and 4 weeks after each treatment, for each stimulation condition, all subjects were again shown the corresponding list of items and asked to name them without help. As before, the examiner manually recorded the answers.

DATA ANALYSIS

Data were analyzed with SPSS 13.0 software. Two different repeated-measures ANOVAs were applied on the mean percentage of response accuracy for nouns and verbs. We have excluded response time as a potential measure because we have found a large variability among patients. Three within-subject factors were included: *Task* [noun naming (NN) vs. verb naming (VN)], *Condition* (anodic Wernicke's area vs. anodic Broca's area vs. Sham) and *Time* [baseline (T1) vs. fifth training day (T5)] which, in the second analysis on the two follow-up sessions, was renamed *End-Post Treatment* factor [end of treatment (T5) vs. first follow-up (F1) vs. second follow-up (F2)]. Interactions were explored using the Scheffè *post-hoc* test.

RESULTS

The analysis showed a significant effect of *Time* [baseline (T1) vs. fifth training day (T5), $F_{(1, 6)} = 160.04$; $p = 0.000$]. Overall, subjects' performance significantly improved on the fifth day of training with respect to baseline [mean = 41%, SEM = 4 (T5) vs. mean = 21%, SEM = 3 (T1) $p = 0.000$]. Neither the *Task* [noun vs. verb naming, $F_{(1, 6)} = 0.05$; $p = 0.831$] nor the *Condition* [Wernicke's vs. Broca's area vs. Sham, $F_{(2, 12)} = 2.37$; $p = 0.673$] effects were significant.

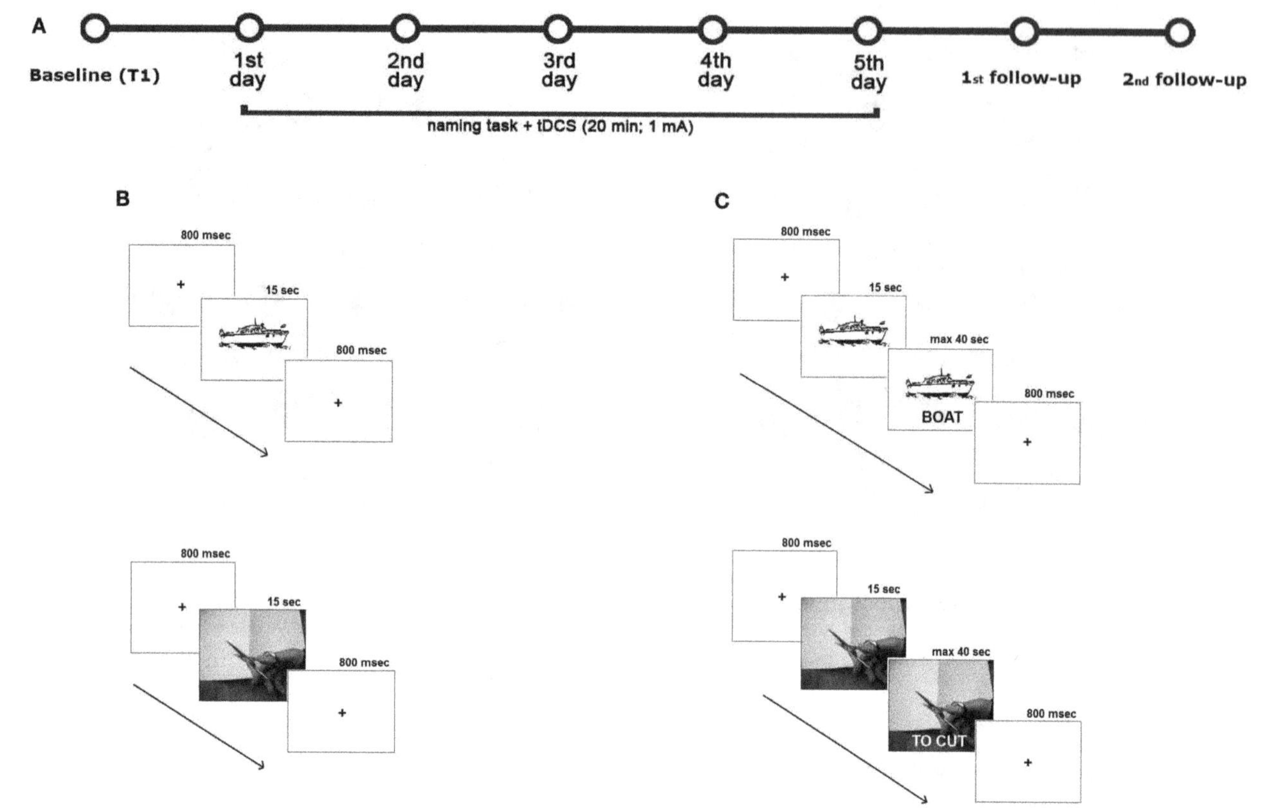

FIGURE 3 | Overview of study design. (A) Subjects underwent two intensive language treatments for their noun and verb difficulties with 30 days of interval between the two trainings. During the two treatments, subjects received 20 min of tDCS. Each stimulation condition was performed in five consecutive daily sessions over three weeks, with six days of intersession interval. To measure baseline performance, at the beginning of each week and before the training each subject was asked to name the picture or the action videoclip, one at a time, without help. To measure the potential, long-term beneficial effects of tDCS two follow-up sessions were also carried 1 and 4 weeks after the end of each treatment condition. Subjects were asked to name aloud each picture or videoclip presented on the PC screen for 15 s and preceded by a fixation point, which lasted 800 ms. If the subject correctly named the item, the examiner manually recorded the response type on a separate sheet **(B)**. If the subject failed or did not answer within 15 s, the corresponding written name of the picture or of the action was presented below the image and the subject was asked to read the word aloud. The pair of stimuli remained on the screen until the subject read the word or 40 s elapsed **(C)**.

The triple interaction *Time* × *Task* × *Condition* was also significant [$F_{(2, 12)} = 60.36$; $p = 0.000$]. The Scheffè *post-hoc* test revealed that the mean percentage of response accuracy for nouns and verbs significantly improved at the end of training in each condition with respect to baseline (differences between T5 vs. T1 for Wernicke's condition: 31%, $p = 0.000$, Broca's condition: 12%, $p = 0.040$, and Sham: 10%, $p = 0.043$ for nouns; differences between T5 vs. T1 for Broca's condition: 42%, $p = 0.000$, Wernicke's condition: 15%, $p = 0.012$, and Sham: 13%, $p = 0.019$ for verbs). However, although for both categories no significant differences emerged between the three conditions at baseline (differences between Wernicke vs. Broca = −2%, $p = 1$; differences between Wernicke vs. Sham = 3%, $p = 0.999$; differences between Broca vs. Sham = 5%, $p = 0.918$ for nouns; differences between Broca vs. Wernicke = −3%, $p = 0.998$; differences between Broca vs. Sham = −7%, $p = 0.684$; differences between Wernicke vs. Sham = −4%, $p = 0.992$ for verbs), at the end of training, there was a clear dissociation on the amount of improvement exerted by the temporal and the frontal stimulation in noun and verb recovery, respectively.

While the mean percentage of correct nouns was significantly greater in the Wernicke's condition with respect to the other two conditions (differences between Wernicke vs. Broca = 17%; $p = 0.002$; differences between Wernicke vs. Sham = 24%; $p = 0.000$; no significant differences between Sham vs. Broca = −7%; $p = 0.571$), the anodic Broca's condition determines the greatest improvement for verb naming with respect to the other two conditions (differences between Broca vs. Wernicke = 24%; $p = 0.000$; differences between Broca vs. Sham = 22%; $p = 0.000$; no significant differences between Sham vs. Wernicke = 2%; $p = 0.999$) (see **Figure 4**).

FOLLOW-UPS

The analysis showed a significant effect of *Condition* [Wernicke's vs. Broca's area vs. Sham, $F_{(2, 12)} = 6.86$; $p = 0.010$] indicating a greater response accuracy for the Wernicke's and Broca's conditions with respect to sham [Wernicke's (mean = 40%, SEM = 3) vs. Broca's (mean = 41%, SEM = 4) vs. Sham condition (mean = 31%, SEM = 3) $p = 0.010$]. Neither the *Task* [$F_{(1, 6)} = 0.00$; $p = 0.978$] nor the *Time* effects [$F_{(2, 12)} = 3.68$; $p = 0.057$] were significant. The interaction *Task* × *Condition* was also significant [$F_{(2, 12)} = 31.85$; $p = 0.000$]. In agreement with previous data, the mean percentage of correct nouns was significantly greater in the Wernicke's condition than in the other two conditions [Wernicke's (mean = 51%, SEM = 5) vs. Broca's (mean = 32%, SEM = 6) vs. Sham conditions (mean = 30%, SEM = 5) $p = 0.000$; no significant differences between Broca's vs. Sham conditions, $p = 0.997$]. On the contrary, the Broca's stimulation exerted again the greatest influence in verbs' accuracy which was significantly higher in this condition than in the other two [Broca's (mean = 50%, SEM = 5) vs. Wernicke's (mean = 29%, SEM = 3) vs. Sham conditions (mean = 32%, SEM = 4) $p = 0.000$; no significant differences between Wernicke's vs. Sham conditions, $p = 0.979$].

Moreover, although no other interactions were significant, *post-hoc* analysis revealed that the greater amount in the mean percentage of correct nouns and verbs found for the Wernicke's and Broca's conditions, respectively, persisted both at the first and the second follow-ups (see **Figure 5**).

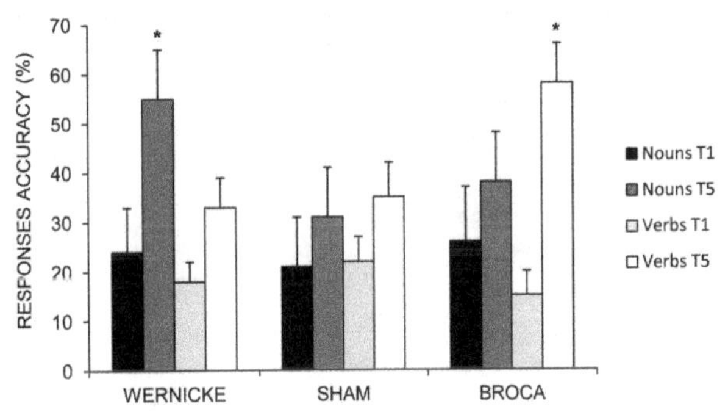

FIGURE 4 | Mean percentage of correct nouns and verbs at baseline (T1) and at the end of treatment (T5) for the left Wernicke's, Broca's and the sham conditions (*0.000). Error bars represent standard error of the mean.

DISCUSSION

Our data suggest that the stimulation of different brain language regions differently affects the amount of improvement in noun and verb naming in a group of seven chronic aphasic patients.

Since previous studies have indicated that the best recovery is observed coupling tDCS with an intensive language treatment (Baker et al., 2010; Fridriksson et al., 2011; Marangolo et al., 2013), we chose to stimulate the patient during a picture naming task comparing the effects during anodic tDCS over the left frontal and temporal areas with a sham condition. In particular, when we analyzed the aphasic subjects' results, we found that all patients significantly recovered in each condition for both categories. This was due to the intensive language training that was performed daily during tDCS application (Bhogal et al., 2003). However, patients were much more accurate in nouns naming after the left temporal stimulation and in verb naming after the left frontal stimulation compared to the other two conditions which did not differ from each other in terms of response accuracy. These results allow us to affirm that the recovery in the two word categories was related to the stimulation of distinct brain regions. A further confirmation on the differential role played by the two regions comes from the follow-up testing which showed that the stimulation of the two language areas still exerted a different influence on the recovery of the two categories at one and four weeks after the end of each treatment.

As stated in the introduction, previous rTMS and tDCS reports with healthy and brain-damaged populations have already indicated a possible involvement of the temporal region in noun's naming (Töpper et al., 1998; Mottaghy et al., 2006; Sparing et al., 2008; Fiori et al., 2011; Flöel et al., 2011; Fridriksson et al., 2011)

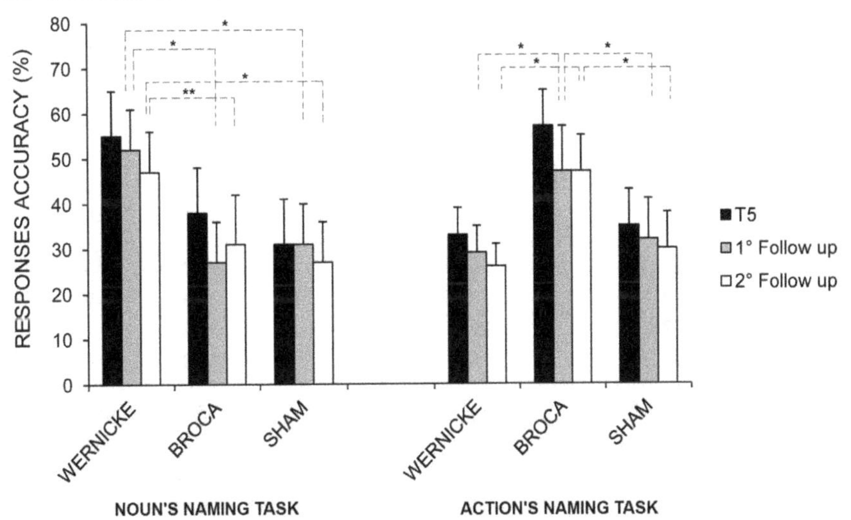

FIGURE 5 | Mean percentage of correct nouns and verbs at the end of treatment (T5), at the first and second follow-ups for the left Wernicke's, Broca's, and sham conditions, respectively (*$p = 0.00$; **$p = 0.03$). Error bars represent standard error of the mean.

and the presence of a close relationship between the stimulation of the frontal region and the recovery of verbs (Cappa et al., 2002; Cotelli et al., 2006, 2008, 2012; Marangolo et al., 2013). However, while more consistent results were reported for verb retrieval, the data were less conclusive for nouns suggesting a possible interest of the frontal regions too (Monti et al., 2008; Baker et al., 2010; Fertonani et al., 2010; Holland et al., 2011; Kang et al., 2011). It might be argued that the facilitatory effect found by Holland et al. (2011) in noun naming after frontal stimulation was not specific to the process of word retrieval *per se* but was related to the activation of a concomitant automatic rehearsal process of the phonological word form exerted by target's spoken name (the auditory cue). In the same vein, it might be the case that in Naeser and Kang et al.'s studies (Naeser et al., 2005; Kang et al., 2011), the beneficial inhibitory influence exerted over the frontal right hemisphere has disengaged a more distributed left hemispheric network which did not necessarily restrict the recovery from nouns to a contribution of the left frontal cortex.

In our opinion, one way to disentangle the above contradictions is to compare within the same population, the performance of the patients in the two naming tasks while stimulating different language regions, as we did in the present study. We believe that our data clearly pointed to the presence of a close relationship between the stimulated region and the amount of recovery found for nouns and verbs. Results from transfer of treatment

Table 2 | Number of correct responses at baseline, post-Broca, post-sham, and post-Wernicke administration of the standardized language tasks (BADA and Token test).

Subj	Conditions	Oral noun naming	Written noun naming	Noun comp	Oral verb naming	Written verb naming	Verb comp	Word reading	Word writing under dictation	Word repetition	Token test
B.A.	Baseline	15/30	0/22	40/40	16/28	0/22	20/20	10/92	0/46	45/45	16/36
	post -Broca (1)	16/30	0/22		17/28	0/22		34/92*	0/46		17/36
	post-Sham (2)	15/30	0/22		18/28	0/22		10/92	0/46		17/36
	post -Wernicke (3)	26/30*	0/22		18/28	0/22		15/92	0/46		25/36
F.S	Baseline	12/30	10/22	40/40	14/28	5/22	20/20	92/92	37/46	45/45	22/36
	post-Broca (2)	14/30	12/22		21/28**	10/22			46/46**		22/36
	post-Sham (1)	12/30	10/22		12/28	5/22			39/46		20/36
	post-Wernicke (3)	27/30*	13/22		20/28	7/22			32/46		26/36
N.R.	Baseline	0/30	0/22	40/40	0/28	0/22	20/20	10/92	0/46	25/45	9/36
	post-Broca (3)	9/30	0/22		10/28**	0/22		10/92	0/46	36/45**	8/36
	post-Sham (2)	9/30	0/22		2/28	0/22		15/92	0/46	30/45	9/36
	post-Wernicke (1)	12/30*	0/22		3/28	0/22		9/92	0/46	36/45	15/36
P.M.	Baseline	0/30	0/22	40/40	0/28	0/22	20/20	10/92	0/46	45/45	11/36
	post-Broca (2)	8/30	2/22		6/28**	0/22		25/92*	5/46		12/36
	post-Sham (3)	10/30	0/22		5/28	0/22		13/92	3/46		13/36
	post-Wernicke (1)	14/30*	1/22		0/28	0/22		15/92	5/46		13/36
P.E.	Baseline	0/30	0/22	40/40	0/28	0/22	20/20	10/92	0/46	13/45	4/36
	post-Broca (2)	5/30	0/22		15/28**	0/22		14/92	0/46	26/45**	6/36
	post-Sham (1)	0/30	0/22		5/28	0/22		15/92	0/46	13/45	4/36
	post-Wernicke (3)	13/30**	0/22		14/28	0/22		10/92	0/46	23/45	10/36
P.F.	Baseline	13/30	0/22	40/40	15/28	0/22	20/20	10/92	0/46	45/45	14/36
	post-Broca (1)	21/30	0/22		15/28	0/22		11/92	0/46		17/36
	post-Sham (3)	17/30	0/22		15/28	0/22		12/92	0/46		15/36
	post-Wernicke (2)	17/30	0/22		21/28	0/22		10/92	0/46		17/36
R.L.	Baseline	11/30	0/22	40/40	14/28	0/22	20/20	55/92	0/46	2/45	10/36
	post-Broca (3)	19/30	0/22		25/28*	0/22		74/92**	0/46	12/45**	10/36
	post-Sham (1)	11/30	0/22		11/28	0/22		55/92	0/46	1/45	9/36
	post-Wernicke (2)	20/30**	0/22		11/28	0/22		60/92	0/46	2/45	11/36

The order of conditions (indicated by the number in brackets) was randomized across subjects. For five out of seven subjects, χ^2(*) test indicated a significant difference before and after the Broca's condition in verb naming and, for six out of seven subjects, before and after the Wernicke's condition in noun naming (< 0.0001; ** < 0.05). Subj, Subjects; Comp, Comprehension.*

effects confirmed this hypothesis. Indeed, at the language tests, in six out of seven patients, there was a significant improvement in noun naming only after stimulation of the temporal region, while the ability to produce verbs significantly increased in five patients only after stimulation of the frontal region. Moreover, after frontal stimulation, some patients showed a significant improvement also in word repetition (N.R., P.E., R.L.) and reading (B.A., P.M., R.L.) while one patient (F.S.) had a significant recovery in writing under dictation task (see **Table 2**). It is widely known that the premotor region, including Broca's area, supports the rehearsal process necessary for refreshing the word memory trace during word repetition (Romero et al., 2006; Trost and Gruber, 2012). It has also been suggested that the premotor cortices play some role in implementing the activity patterns involved in reading and writing (Anderson et al., 1990; Lubrano et al., 2004). In our patients, the hypothesis that could be advanced is that the stimulation of the frontal region co-activated the surrounding premotor areas which lead to an improvement in other language tasks.

Although the neural mechanisms responsible for tDCS stimulation are still not known, some authors have affirmed that anodic stimulation elicits an extended increase in cortical excitability probably due to depolarization of neuronal membrane and to changes in the synaptic connections of the *N*-methyl-D-aspartate (NMDA) receptors involved in long-term potentiation (Nitsche and Paulus, 2000). This happens when the stimulated area is supposed to be directly involved in the investigated language task. However, others (Naeser et al., 2005; Kang et al., 2011) found an improvement also after stimulating through rTMS (Naeser et al., 2005) or tDCS (Kang et al., 2011) the right language homologous areas.

To date, the role played by the right hemisphere in language recovery is more controversial than that of the left regions. Some evidence has suggested that the right activity may support recovery only if homotopic areas take over the function of the lesioned left language areas (Saur et al., 2006, 2008; Turkeltaub et al., 2011) even if they are computationally less efficient. Alternatively, the right hemisphere may limit recovery if its processing is dysfunctional, or if transcallosal projections from the right inhibit the left language areas (Naeser et al., 2005; Martin et al., 2009; Kang et al., 2011). Most of the studies have affirmed that the quality of improvement is dependent on the amount of spared neural tissue in the left hemisphere and, to a lesser extent, on the homologous areas in the right-hemisphere (Heiss and Thiel, 2006). It seems likely that the reactivation of undamaged network areas of the left hemisphere usually leads to a better outcome than the involvement of homotopic contra-lateral regions (Heiss and Thiel, 2006). For this reason, in our study, we choose to stimulate the left hemisphere regions as also suggested by previous tDCS studies which indicated that the stimulation of perilesional spared language areas close to the stimulation site in chronic aphasic patients enhances functional improvement (Baker et al., 2010; Fiori et al., 2011; Fridriksson et al., 2011; Marangolo et al., 2013).

Although some studies have shown that it is difficult to predict the distribution of the current (Baker et al., 2010), others have suggested that during naming the current is distributed around the stimulated region (Holland et al., 2011). The same results were found in an fMRI studies to measure tDCS effects during the stimulation of the motor cortex (Antal et al., 2011, 2012). Since our patients had very different left hemispheric lesions we reasoned that in this way we have targeted the two regions. Considering that all of our patients had left-hemisphere damage, it might be argued that the better recovery observed after the left temporal and frontal stimulation, respectively, for nouns and verbs, was not related to the stimulated areas but to a greater sparing of one of the two region.

However, as shown in **Figure 1**, all of our patients had very different left cerebral stroke which in some cases predominantly involved the posterior (B.A., P.F., and R.L.) or the anterior areas (P.M.) and in others either completely damaged the Wernicke's and Broca's area (N.R., and P.E.) or totally spared the two stimulated regions (F.S.).

We believe that independently of the amount of left spared cerebral tissue, the different improvement found for the two word categories clearly indicate at least a partial segregation of the beneficial effects into a specific brain region. It might be the case that, in our patients, tDCS has enhanced the capacity of the left-hemisphere spared areas close to the stimulated region to make compensatory plastic changes resulting in improved performance.

We are aware that the present approach, due to the small sample used and to the lack of functional magnetic resonance imaging data, does not allows to draw firm conclusions about the underlying neural mechanisms by which tDCS affected subjects' performance.

However, overall, it consents to define some important points about language rehabilitation in persons with aphasia. Indeed, it confirms several previous reports that highlight the importance of coupling tDCS with the naming treatment. Moreover, it clearly suggests the importance to apply different stimulation protocols to the aphasic populations to enhance the best recovery.

REFERENCES

Anderson, S. W., Damasio, A. R., and Damasio, H. (1990). Troubled letters but not numbers domain specific cognitive impairments following focal damage in frontal cortex. *Brain* 113, 749–766. doi: 10.1093/brain/113.3.749

Antal, A., Kovacs, G., Chaieb, L., Paulus, W., and Greenlee, M. W. (2012). Cathodal stimulation of human MT$^+$ leads to elevated fMRI signal: a tDCS-fMRI study. *Restor. Neurol. Neurosci.* 30, 255–263. doi: 10.3233/RNN-2012-110208

Antal, A., Polania, R., Schmidt-Samoa, C., Dechent, P., and Paulus, W. (2011). Transcranial direct current stimulation over the primary motor cortex during fMRI. *Neuroimage* 15, 590–606. doi: 10.1016/j.neuroimage.2010.11.085

Baker, J. M., Rorden, C., and Fridriksson, J. (2010). Using transcranial direct-current stimulation to treat stroke patients with aphasia. *Stroke* 41, 1229–1236. doi: 10.1161/strokeaha.109.576785

Bhogal, S. K., Teasell, R., and Speechley, M. (2003). Intensity of aphasia therapy, impact on recovery. *Stroke* 34, 987–993. doi: 10.1161/01.STR.0000062343.64383.D0

Cappa, S., Sandrini, M., Rossini, P. M., Sosta, K., and Miniussi, C. (2002). The role of the left frontal lobe in action naming: rTMS evidence. *Neurology* 59, 720–723. doi: 10.1212/WNL.59.5.720

Conroy, P., and Scowcroft, J. (2012). Decreasing cues for a dynamic list of noun and verb naming targets: a case-series aphasia therapy study. *Neuropsychol. Rehabil.* 22, 295–318. doi: 10.1080/09602011.2011.641434

Cotelli, M., Manenti, R., Alberici, A., Brambilla, M., Cosseddu, M., Zanetti, O., et al. (2012). Prefrontal cortex rTMS enhances action naming in progressive non-fluent aphasia. *Eur. J. Neurol.* 19, 1404–1412. doi: 10.1111/j.1468-1331.2012.03699.x

Cotelli, M., Manenti, R., Cappa, M. D., Geroldi, C., Zanetti, O., Rossini, P. M., et al. (2006). Effect of transcranial magnetic stimulation on action naming in patients with Alzheimer disease. *Arch. Neurol.* 63, 1602–1604. doi: 10.1001/archneur.63.11.1602

Cotelli, M., Manenti, R., Cappa, S. F., Zanetti, O., and Miniussi, C. (2008). Transcranial magnetic stimulation improves naming in Alzheimer disease patients at different stages of cognitive decline. *Eur. J. Neurol.* 15, 1286–1292. doi: 10.1111/j.1468-1331.2008.02202.x

De Mauro, T., Mancini, F., Vedovelli, M., and Voghera, M. (1993). *Lessico di Frequenza dell'italiano Parlato.* Milano: Etaslibri.

De Renzi, E., and Vignolo, L. A. (1962). The Token Test: a sensitive test to detect receptive disturbances in aphasia. *Brain* 85, 665–678. doi: 10.1093/brain/85.4.665

Fertonani, A., Rosini, S., Cotelli, M., Rossini, P. M., and Miniussi, C. (2010). Naming facilitation induced by transcranial direct current stimulation. *Behav. Brain. Res.* 208, 311–318. doi: 10.1016/j.bbr.2009.10.030

Fiori, V., Coccia, M., Marinelli, C. V., Vecchi, V., Bonifazi, S., Ceravolo, M. G., et al. (2011). Transcranial direct current stimulation improves word retrieval in healthy and nonfluent aphasic subjects. *J. Cogn. Neurosci.* 23, 2309–2323. doi: 10.1162/jocn.2010.21579

Flöel, A., Meinzer, M., Kirstein, R., Nijhof, S., Deppe, M., Knecht, S., et al. (2011). Short-term anomia training and electrical brain stimulation. *Stroke* 42, 2065–2067. doi: 10.1161/STROKEAHA.110.609032

Fridriksson, J., Richardson, J. D., Baker, J. M., and Rorden, C. (2011). Transcranial direct current stimulation improves naming reaction time in fluent aphasia: a double-blind, sham-controlled study. *Stroke* 42, 819–821. doi: 10.1161/STROKEAHA.110.600288

Gandiga, P. C., Hummel, F. C., and Cohen, L. G. (2006). Transcranial DC stimulation (tDCS): a tool for double-blind sham-controlled clinical studies in brain stimulation. *Clin. Neurophysiol.* 117, 845–850. doi: 10.1016/j.clinph.2005.12.003

Heiss, W. D., and Thiel, A. (2006). A proposed regional hierarchy in recovery of post-stroke aphasia. *Brain Lang.* 98, 118–123. doi: 10.1016/j.bandl.2006.02.002

Holland, R., and Crinion, J. (2012). Can tDCS enhance treatment of aphasia after stroke? *Aphasiology* 26, 1169–1191. doi: 10.1080/02687038.2011.616925

Holland, R., Leff, A. P., Josephs, O., Galea, J. M., Desikan, M., Price, C. J., et al. (2011). Speech facilitation by left inferior frontal cortex stimulation. *Curr. Biol.* 21, 1403–1407. doi: 10.1016/j.cub.2011.07.021

Kang, E. K., Kim, Y. K., Sohn, H. M., Cohen, L. G., and Paik, N. J. (2011). Improved picture naming in aphasia patients treated with cathodal tDCS to inhibit the right Broca's homologue area. *Restor. Neurol. Neurosci.* 29, 141–152. doi: 10.3233/RNN-2011-0587

Lotto, L., Dell'Acqua, R., and Job, R. (2001). Le figure PD/DPSS. Misure di accordo sul nome, tipicità, familiarità, età di acquisizione e tempi di denominazione per 266 figure. *G. Ital. Psicol.* 1, 193–210.

Lubrano, V., Roux, F. E., and Démonet, J. F. (2004). Writing-specific sites in frontal areas: a cortical stimulation study. *J. Neurosurg.* 101, 787–798. doi: 10.3171/jns.2004.101.5.0787

Marangolo, P., Fiori, V., Di Paola, M., Cipollari, S., Razzano, C., Oliveri, M., et al. (2013). Differential involvement of the left frontal and temporal regions in verb naming: a tDCS treatment study. *Restor. Neurol. Neurosci.* 31, 63–72. doi: 10.3233/RNN-120268

Martin, P. I., Naeser, M. A., Ho, M., Doron, K. W., Kurland, J., Kaplan, J., et al. (2009). Overt naming fMRI pre- and post- TMS: two nonfluent aphasia patients, with and without improved naming post-TMS. *Brain Lang.* 111, 20–35. doi: 10.1016/j.bandl.2009.07.007

Miceli, G., Laudanna, A., Burani, C., and Capasso, R. (1994). *Batteria per l'analisi dei deficit afasici BADA*. Roma: CEPSAG, Policlinico Gemelli, Università Cattolica del Sacro Cuore.

Monti, A., Cogiamanian, F., Marceglia, S., Ferrucci, F., Mameli, F., Mrakic-Sposta, S., et al. (2008). Improved naming after transcranial direct current stimulation in aphasia. *J. Neurol. Neurosurg. Psichiatry* 79, 451–453. doi: 10.1136/jnnp.2007.135277

Monti, A., Ferrucci, R., Fumagalli, M., Mameli, F., Cogiamanian, F., Ardolino, G., et al. (2012). Transcranial direct current stimulation (tDCS) and language. *J. Neurol. Neurosurg. Psychiatry* 8, 451–453. doi: 10.1136/jnnp-2012-302825

Mottaghy, F. M., Sparing, R., and Töpper, R. (2006). Enhancing picture naming with transcranial magnetic stimulation. *Behav. Neurol.* 17, 177–186.

Naeser, M. A., Martin, P. I., Nicholas, M., Baker, E. H., Seekins, H., Kobayashi, M., et al. (2005). Improved picture naming in chronic aphasia after TMS to part of right Broca's area: an open-protocol study. *Brain Lang.* 93, 95–105. doi: 10.1016/j.bandl.2004.08.004

Naeser, M. A., Martin, P. I., Treglia, E., Ho, M., Kaplan, E., Bashir, S., et al. (2010). Research with rTMS in the treatment of aphasia. *Restor. Neurol. Neurosci.* 28, 511–529. doi: 10.3233/RNN-2010-0559

Nishitani, N., Schürmann, M., Amunts, K., and Hari, R. (2005). Broca's region: from action to language. *Physiology* 20, 60–69. doi: 10.1152/physiol.00043.2004

Nitsche, M. A., and Paulus, W. (2000). Excitability changes induced in the human motor cortex by weak transcranial direct current stimulation. *J. Physiol.* 527, 633–639. doi: 10.1111/j.1469-7793.2000.t01-1-00633.x

Oliveri, M., Rossini, P. M., Traversa, R., Cicinelli, P., Filippi, M. M., Pasqualetti, P., et al. (1999). Left frontal transcranial magnetic stimulation reduces contralesional extinction in patients with unilateral right brain damage. *Brain* 122, 1731–1739. doi: 10.1093/brain/122.9.1731

Orsini, A., Grossi, D., Capitani, E., Laiacona, M., Papagno, C., and Vallar, G. (1987). Verbal and spatial immediate memory span: normative data from 1355 adults and 1112 children. *Ital. J. Neurol. Sci.* 8, 537–548. doi: 10.1007/BF02333660

Poreisz, C., Boros, K., Antal, A., and Paulus, W. (2007). Safety aspects of transcranial direct current stimulation concerning healthy subjects and patients. *Brain Res. Bull.* 72, 208–214. doi: 10.1016/j.brainresbull.2007.01.004

Raymer, A. M., Ciampitti, M., Holliway, B., Singletary, F., Blonder, L. X., Ketterson, T., et al. (2007). Semantic-phonologic treatment for noun and verb retrieval impairments in aphasia. *Neuropsychol. Rehabil.* 17, 244–270. doi: 10.1080/09602010600814661

Raymer, A. M., Singletary, F., Rodriguez, A., Ciampitti, M., Heilman, K. M., and Rothi, L. J. (2006). Effects of gesture+verbal treatment for noun and verb retrieval in aphasia. *J. Int. Neuropsychol. Soc.* 12, 867–882. doi: 10.1017/S1355617706061042

Romero, L., Walsh, V., and Papagno, C. (2006). The neural correlates of phonological short-term memory: a repetitive transcranial magnetic stimulation study. *J. Cogn. Neurosci.* 18, 1147–1155. doi: 10.1162/jocn.2006.18.7.1147

Saur, D., Kreher, B. W., Schnell, S., Kümmerer, D., Kellmeyer, P., Vry, M. S., et al. (2008). Ventral and dorsal pathways for language. *Proc. Natl. Acad. Sci. U.S.A.* 105, 18035–18040. doi: 10.1073/pnas.0805234105

Saur, D., Lange, R., Baumgaertner, A., Schraknepper, V., Willmes, K., Rijntjes, M., et al. (2006). Dynamics of language reorganization after stroke. *Brain* 129, 1371–1384. doi: 10.1093/brain/awl090

Snodgrass, J. G., and Vanderwart, M. (1980). A standardized set of 260 pictures: norms for name agreement, image agreement, familiarity, and visual complexity. *J. Exp. Psychol. Hum. Learn.* 6, 174–215. doi: 10.1037/0278-7393.6.2.174

Sparing, R., Dafotakis, M., Meister, I. G., Thirugnanasambandam, N., and Fink, G. R. (2008). Enhancing language performance with non-invasive brain stimulation-a transcranial direct current stimulation study in healthy humans. *Neuropsychologia* 46, 261–268. doi: 10.1016/j.neuropsychologia.2007.07.009

Spinnler, H., and Tognoni, G. (1987). Standardizzazione e taratura italiana di test neuropsicologici. *Ital. J. Neurol. Sci.* 8(Suppl.), 1–120.

Töpper, R., Mottaghy, F. M., Brugmann, M., Noth, J., and Huber, W. (1998). Facilitation of picture naming by focal transcranial magnetic stimulation of Wernicke's area. *Exp. Brain Res.* 121, 371–378. doi: 10.1007/s002210050471

Trost, S., and Gruber, O. (2012). Evidence for a double dissociation of articulatory rehearsal and non-articulatory maintenance of phonological information in human verbal working memory.

Neuropsychobiology 65, 133–140. doi: 10.1159/000332335

Turkeltaub, P. E., Messing, S., Norise, C., and Hamilton, R. H. (2011). Are networks for residual language function and recovery consistent across aphasic patients? *Neurology* 76, 1726–1734. doi: 10.1212/WNL.0b013e31821a44c1

Zimmermann, P., and Fimm, B. (1994). *Tests d'evaluation de l'attention (TEA)*. St. Lucia; Rome: IRCCS.

15

Concurrent application of TMS and near-infrared optical imaging: methodological considerations and potential artifacts

Nathan A. Parks *

Department of Psychological Science, University of Arkansas, Fayetteville, AR, USA

Correspondence:
Nathan A. Parks, Department of Psychological Science, University of Arkansas, 216 Memorial Hall, Fayetteville, AR 72701, USA
e-mail: naparks@uark.edu

The simultaneous application of transcranial magnetic stimulation (TMS) with non-invasive neuroimaging provides a powerful method for investigating functional connectivity in the human brain and the causal relationships between areas in distributed brain networks. TMS has been combined with numerous neuroimaging techniques including, electroencephalography (EEG), functional magnetic resonance imaging (fMRI), and positron emission tomography (PET). Recent work has also demonstrated the feasibility and utility of combining TMS with non-invasive near-infrared optical imaging techniques, functional near-infrared spectroscopy (fNIRS) and the event-related optical signal (EROS). Simultaneous TMS and optical imaging affords a number of advantages over other neuroimaging methods but also involves a unique set of methodological challenges and considerations. This paper describes the methodology of concurrently performing optical imaging during the administration of TMS, focusing on experimental design, potential artifacts, and approaches to controlling for these artifacts.

Keywords: TMS, near-infrared optical imaging, EROS, fNIRS, connectivity, cortical dynamics

INTRODUCTION

Transcranial magnetic stimulation (TMS) is a brain stimulation technique that uses very strong but very brief magnetic fields to induce electrical currents in the human cerebral cortex (Barker et al., 1985; Hallett, 2007). TMS is a unique and powerful tool for human neuroscience as it is the only method capable of focal and non-invasive stimulation of the healthy human brain. TMS provides a method for assessing the causal role of brain regions in cognitive function with considerable spatial and temporal resolution (Pascual-Leone et al., 2000; Walsh and Cowey, 2000). Since the introduction of TMS in the 1980s (Barker et al., 1985), the technique was swiftly adopted by cognitive neuroscientists and has been used widely to study perceptual, motor, and cognitive processes (Pascual-Leone et al., 2000; Walsh and Cowey, 2000; Hallett, 2007).

Much recent methodological development has focused on combining TMS with other neuroimaging techniques (for reviews see Bestmann et al., 2008; Driver et al., 2009; Siebner et al., 2009; Ilmoniemi and Kičić, 2010; Ziemann, 2011). Combined TMS and neuroimaging approaches offer considerable promise in understanding human brain function as a number of novel research questions can be addressed that were previously unapproachable with TMS or neuroimaging alone. First, TMS-neuroimaging provides a method of causally assessing functional connectivity in cortical networks. Measures of functional connectivity in the human brain have traditionally relied on temporal correlations of activity between brain regions (Biswal et al., 1995; Greicius et al., 2003). Such correlational measures of connectivity are unable to provide causal information, rendering it difficult to determine if coactive regions are truly functionally connected or if they merely coincidentally active at similar points in time. Because activations induced in the cerebral cortex propagate trans-synaptically, the concurrent application of TMS and neuroimaging allows functional connectivity between brain regions to be examined in a causal manner (for review see Bestmann et al., 2008; Driver et al., 2009). This is accomplished by using TMS to activate a targeted cortical region while neuroimaging is employed to measure the consequent inter-regional activations. Second, concurrent TMS and neuroimaging provide direct measures of cortical excitability within a targeted brain region. Traditionally, motor-evoked potentials (MEPs), motor thresholds, and phosphene thresholds have been used to index cortical excitability. Combined TMS and neuroimaging approaches can directly measure levels of cortical excitability by evoking a response with TMS while using neuroimaging to measure the magnitude of the resultant activity. Third, TMS-neuroimaging can be applied to better understand mechanisms of neuroplasticity within the human cerebral cortex. Administration of trains of repetitive TMS (rTMS) or patterned rTMS have been shown to modulate states of cortical neuroplasticity (Pascual-Leone et al., 1994; Chen et al., 1997; Huang et al., 2005). Neuroimaging of TMS-induced plasticity provides important insight into neuroplasticity in human cortex. Last, concurrent TMS and neuroimaging provides invaluable information regarding the action of TMS in the human brain, information that previously inferred primarily from MEPs, phosphenes, and animal studies.

To date, TMS has been combined successfully with a number of neuroimaging methodologies including electroencephalography (EEG; Ilmoniemi et al., 1997; Bonato et al., 2006), functional magnetic resonance imaging (fMRI; Bohning et al., 1998, 1999;

Baudewig et al., 2001; Bestmann et al., 2004), positron emission tomography (PET; Fox et al., 1997, 2006; Paus et al., 1997), functional near-infrared spectroscopy (fNIRS; Hada et al., 2006; Mochizuki et al., 2006; Kozel et al., 2009), and the event-related optical signal (EROS; Parks et al., 2012). With the fervent development of these combined approaches, it is important to document technical considerations, potential pitfalls, artifacts, and confounds introduced by combining TMS with each of these neuroimaging methodologies. Little information is presently available in the literature concerning the concurrent application of TMS and near-infrared optical imaging methods of fNIRS and EROS. This paper bridges this information gap, giving a brief overview of optical imaging methodologies and their concurrent use with TMS. Although the neurophysiological signals that constitute fNIRS and EROS measurements are quite disparate, the methodological challenges and potential sources of TMS-related artifact are common to the two techniques. Associated design considerations, potential artifacts, and approaches to control for artifacts in TMS-fNIRS and TMS-EROS studies are discussed.

NEAR-INFRARED OPTICAL IMAGING

Non-invasive near-infrared optical imaging refers to a category of neuroimaging techniques that measure activity from the human cerebral cortex through changes in the absorption or scattering of near-infrared light that occur as a consequence of events associated with neural activity. Light in the near-infrared range (650–950 nm) largely escapes absorption by water and is primarily scattered in biological tissue. This scattering permits near-infrared wavelengths to penetrate relatively deep into living tissue. When emitted into the human head, near-infrared light will scatter deeply enough to pass through cortical tissue (Villringer et al., 1993) and a proportion of this light will scatter back to the surface of the scalp where it can be measured by a detector. When the distance between emitter and detector (optodes collectively) is known, the path traveled by light is well-defined, giving near-infrared imaging techniques relatively good spatial resolution. The distance separating a near-infrared emitter and detector determines the depth of penetration into the head (Villringer et al., 1993; Gratton et al., 1995; Gratton and Fabiani, 2010). Consequently, non-invasive near-infrared optical imaging is only capable of measuring the most superficial regions of the cerebral cortex as light intensity becomes insufficient across distances of more than 5.5–6.0 cm. Deep cortical regions, subcortical, midbrain, and hindbrain structures are inaccessible to optical imaging. Thus, near-infrared optical imaging approaches can be used only in the study of cortical function in humans. Methods of near-infrared optical imaging place an array (montage) of fiber optic near-infrared emitters and detectors across the scalp. These emitters and detectors are configured so as to measure activity from cortical regions of interest (ROIs) that lie between an emitter and a detector.

Modulations of certain properties of near-infrared light by the cerebral cortex can be used to infer changes in underlying neural activity. Two classes of signals can be measured using near-infrared optical imaging, a slow hemodynamic response which affects the relative absorption of near-infrared wavelengths and a fast optical signal which affects the scattering properties of near-infrared light. These distinct optical signatures of neural activity form the basis of two non-invasive optical imaging techniques—fNIRS and EROS, respectively.

FUNCTIONAL NEAR-INFRARED SPECTROSCOPY (fNIRS)

fNIRS is a near-infrared optical neuroimaging method that provides a measure of the hemodynamic response, an increase in blood oxygenation of the cerebral vasculature that peaks 6–10 s following neural activity (Ogawa et al., 1990; Miezin et al., 2000). The hemodynamic response can be measured with near-infrared light because hemoglobin is a primary absorber of near-infrared wavelengths in biological tissue. Short and long near-infrared wavelengths are absorbed differentially by oxygenated hemoglobin (oxy-Hb) and deoxygenated hemoglobin (deoxy-Hb), oxy-Hb absorbing more at longer wavelengths and deoxy-Hb absorbing more at shorter wavelengths (Jobsis, 1977). The changes in oxy-Hb and deoxy-Hb concentrations associated with the hemodynamic response are measureable as modulations in the intensity of light at different near-infrared wavelengths. By obtaining a sparse near-infrared absorption spectrum using two or more wavelengths, it is possible to measure relative concentrations of oxy-Hb and deoxy-Hb within the cerebral vasculature, yielding an index of neuronal activity via the hemodynamic response (Villringer et al., 1993). The spatial resolution of fNIRS (between 1 and 3 cm) is not as good as that of fMRI, the most comparable measure of the hemodynamic response. However, fNIRS has the advantage of acquiring separable measures of oxy-Hb and deoxy-Hb, which are measured only as a composite in the blood-oxygenation level-dependent (BOLD) response. The temporal resolution of fNIRS is limited by the sluggishness of the hemodynamic response, on the order of several seconds. However, the instrumentation of fNIRS generally permits higher temporal sampling of the which allows the hemodynamic response function to be measured with great precision.

EVENT-RELATED OPTICAL SIGNAL (EROS)

In addition to the slow modulations of near-infrared absorption that occur with changes in blood oxygenation, certain optical properties of neural tissue modulate directly in accordance with neural electrical activity. Numerous *in vivo* and *in vitro* studies have demonstrated that near-infrared light scatters less in active neural tissue as compared to tissue at rest, a phenomenon known as the *fast optical signal* (Frostig et al., 1990; MacVicar and Hochman, 1991; Andrew and MacVicar, 1994; Rector et al., 1997, 2005). These changes in scattering occur simultaneously with neural electrical activity and appear to be the result of neurite swelling caused by the migration of water across ion channels (Foust and Rector, 2007; Lee and Kim, 2010). The fast optical signal can be measured non-invasively from the human brain as a reduction in the intensity of light transmission or as an increase in the time-of-flight (delay) of near-infrared light from a source to a detector (Gratton et al., 1995; Wolf et al., 2002; for review see Wolf et al., 2008; Gratton and Fabiani, 2010). Intensity measures can be used to index the fast optical signal because reduced scattering causes less light to scatter back to the surface thus leading to a transient reduction in measured intensity (Gratton et al., 1995). Delay measures can also index the fast optical signal because reduced scattering causes light, on average, to penetrate deeper into the cortex, travelling a slightly longer path, measurable as an increase in phase delay (Gratton and Fabiani, 2003, 2010). These non-invasive signatures of the fast optical signal form the basis of the EROS neuroimaging technique (also fast optical imaging).

The spatial resolution of EROS is approximately equivalent to that of fNIRS though this resolution can be improved significantly with very high density optode arrangements (Gratton and Fabiani, 2003). The advantage of EROS lies in its measurement of the fast optical signal which gives the technique a temporal resolution on the order of milliseconds. The increased temporal resolution of EROS comes at the cost of signal-to-noise ratio, which is quite low compared to other neuroimaging techniques (Gratton and Fabiani, 2003, 2010).

CONCURRENT APPLICATION OF TMS AND OPTICAL IMAGING: ADVANTAGES AND LIMITATIONS

The simultaneous application of TMS with near-infrared optical imaging is an appealing marriage of techniques, offering several advantages over other concurrent TMS-neuroimaging approaches. First, near-infrared optical signals are not susceptible to electromagnetic interference from TMS pulses as they are based on measures of light intensity or timing. In contrast, TMS-EEG and TMS-fMRI measure electrical and magnetic fields, respectively, requiring considerable technological innovations to overcome TMS-induced electromagnetic artifact (Siebner et al., 2009). Second, optical imaging methods permit TMS stimulation to any target scalp location and are not constrained by the pragmatics of TMS coil positioning in an MRI scanner. Third, optical methods provide unique measures and insights into cortical functions that are distinct from other neuroimaging technologies. fNIRS provides a measure of both oxy-Hb and deoxy-Hb concentrations, allowing for a more detailed study of the human hemodynamic response evoked by TMS. EROS provides a spatially and temporally resolved measure, allowing the inter-regional dynamics of TMS-evoked cortical activity to be examined. Last, optical imaging equipment has become affordable and commercially available, allowing studies of cortical connectivity, excitability, and dynamics to be readily studied in a laboratory setting.

The feasibility and utility of concurrent TMS-fNIRS has been demonstrated in numerous studies conducted in the motor system (Noguchi et al., 2003; Hada et al., 2006; Mochizuki et al., 2006, 2007; Chiang et al., 2007; Kozel et al., 2009; Groiss et al., 2013) and prefrontal cortex (Kozel et al., 2009; Thomson et al., 2011a,b, 2013). These studies have demonstrated clear modulations in blood oxygenation directly beneath the coil (proximal activations; Noguchi et al., 2003; Hada et al., 2006; Mochizuki et al., 2006; Kozel et al., 2009; Groiss et al., 2013) as well as interregionally in cortical areas not directly activated by TMS (distal activations; Mochizuki et al., 2007; Kozel et al., 2009; Groiss et al., 2013). Optical measurement of TMS-evoked hemodynamic responses has been further validated with *in vivo* studies in cats (Allen et al., 2007).

A single study has demonstrated the feasibility of concurrent TMS-EROS and found TMS-evoked activity in the primary motor cortex directly beneath the TMS coil peaking within 16 ms post-pulse and a later activation of contralateral motor cortex occurring within 40 ms of the TMS pulse (Parks et al., 2012). To date, no animal studies have been conducted to examine effects of TMS on the fast optical signal.

There are several limitations associated with combining TMS with non-invasive optical imaging, as compared to other neuroimaging approaches. The primary disadvantage of TMS-optical imaging is the restricted depth of recordings. Both fNIRS and EROS are capable of obtaining functional data from only the most superficial regions of the brain. As such, TMS-induced neural activity can only be examined within the cerebral cortex. TMS-evoked activations within subcortical structures (e.g., basal ganglia) or deep cortical structures (e.g., cingulate) cannot be measured with either fNIRS or EROS. When such ROIs are of interest, optical imaging cannot be used. TMS-fMRI and TMS-PET are currently the only approaches capable of measuring TMS-induced functional activation within such structures.

In addition to the issue of depth, the major limitation of fNIRS is primarily its reliance on the slow hemodynamic response, a problem shared with TMS-fMRI. TMS-fNIRS has relatively good spatial resolution but very poor temporal resolution. This makes TMS-fNIRS well-suited for applications in need of only spatial localization of TMS-evoked responses but prohibits the method from being applied to study neural dynamics. At present, only TMS-EEG and TMS-EROS can yield such temporally precise data in human subjects.

TMS-EROS is also associated with its own set of limitations. The signal-to-noise ratio of EROS is quite low (Gratton et al., 1995; Gratton and Fabiani, 2003, 2010). TMS-EROS requires averaging of between 100 and 300 trials, approximately ten times that of a typical event-related fNIRS study. Given the suggested safety guidelines for the allowable number and frequency of TMS pulses in human subjects, the number of trials required for TMS-EROS averaging can impose significant restrictions on the design of experiments. A further issue of TMS-EROS relates to the supporting literature and prevalence of the technique. Though there is a growing literature applying EROS in the study of human perception and cognition, this literature remains small compared to other neuroimaging techniques. Consequently, there is simply less extant literature from which to draw when designing and interpreting TMS-EROS studies.

Together, TMS-fNIRS and TMS-EROS studies suggest that the concurrent use of TMS and optical imaging can provide useful tools in the study of human cortical connectivity and cerebral dynamics. However, there are several methodological approaches and TMS-related artifacts that should be considered when conducting such studies.

DESIGN CONSIDERATIONS FOR TMS-fNIRS AND TMS-EROS

SINGLE-PULSE vs. REPETITIVE TMS

Single-pulse TMS refers to the intermittent administration of a single magnetic pulse (<1 Hz) to a target region whereas repetitive TMS (≥ 1 Hz) refers to a train of TMS pulses occurring at a set frequency. In the cognitive neurosciences, single-pulse TMS is often employed to examine the chronometry of a cortical ROI whereas rTMS is used to continuously disrupt a brain area or to induce a lasting change in cortical excitability (Pascual-Leone et al., 2000). The choice to use single-pulse TMS vs. rTMS is driven primarily by the research question being asked. Either single-pulse or rTMS may be an appropriate design choice when using TMS as a method of causally assessing cortico-cortical connectivity but certain considerations should be taken when choosing between single-pulse and rTMS with near-infrared optical imaging.

Single-pulse TMS can be easily integrated into both fNIRS and EROS experiments. The use of single-pulse in a TMS-fNIRS experiment generally requires an event-related design. Such event-related designs often require long inter-trial intervals (20–30 s) in order to allow the hemodynamic response to return to baseline before the start of each trial. These long periods can impose major constraints on the type of questions that may be addressed in a single-pulse TMS-fNIRS study. Single-pulse designs are ideal for TMS-EROS as EROS recordings require precise time-locking and averaging of several hundred trials to increase signal-to-noise ratio. RTMS is most appropriate for use in a block design, measuring changes in cortical activity during trains of rTMS as compared to periods of rest (or sham rTMS). The measurement of the hemodynamic response using fNIRS lends itself well to such designs. Blocked rTMS-fNIRS designs can be successfully implemented to perform studies of cortical connectivity and neuroplasticity during rTMS administration or by performing pre-rTMS and post-rTMS fNIRS measurements. EROS is not easily adapted for use in a typical block design as the fast optical signal is a transient response. However, the temporal resolution of EROS may allow time-locking to the individual pulses within a given rTMS train. Such an approach may be used to study the cumulative effects of TMS pulses or variations in cortical response to individual pulses delivered in a high-frequency rTMS train.

The cumulative effects of rTMS should also be considered when designing a TMS-fNIRS or TMS-EROS. There are well-known modulations of cortical excitability associated with administration of rTMS. For example, low-frequency rTMS (1-Hz) to motor cortex has been shown to induce a lasting reduction in cortical excitability that persists for 15 min or more (Chen et al., 1997). Conversely, high-frequency trains of rTMS can induce a lasting increase in the excitability of motor cortex (Pascual-Leone et al., 1994; Huang et al., 2005). Such modulations of cortical excitability may have undesirable interactions as cortical excitability may vary with the number of TMS pulses administered. Depending on the research question being investigated, such temporal variation may or may not be problematic or confounding. The modulatory effects of rTMS should be carefully considered and weighed against the objectives of the experiment.

PROXIMAL vs. DISTAL REGIONS OF INTEREST

TMS-neuroimaging investigations seek to measure TMS-evoked responses from either *proximal* regions of interest (ROIs), those directly beneath the coil, or inter-regional activations that are induced trans-synaptically (*distal* ROIs; **Figure 1**). Performing near-infrared optical imaging on local vs. distal ROIs is a major

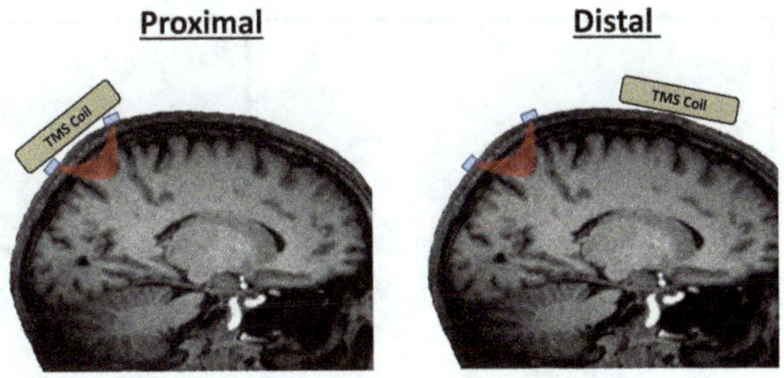

FIGURE 1 | Proximal vs. distal ROIs in TMS-fNIRS and TMS-EROS experiments. Proximal ROIs are those directly activated by a TMS coil. Distal ROIs are those activated trans-synaptically by TMS. Optodes are depicted in blue and the path of near-infrared light between an emitter and detector is depicted in red.

determinant of the technical difficulty of an experiment and the TMS-related artifacts that may come into play. Measuring fNIRS or EROS from a proximal ROI directly beneath the coil presents the greatest challenge as optical emitter and detector fibers (optodes collectively) must be designed to accommodate recordings in the presence of a TMS coil. Furthermore, because of coil proximity, proximal ROI recordings are more susceptible to TMS-related artifacts. Further precautions must be taken to control for TMS-related artifacts when recording from proximal ROIs. Distal ROIs may be recorded much more simply in most scenarios without requiring any special modifications to the optical apparatus and with fewer concerns of TMS-related artifacts.

OPTICAL MONTAGE DESIGN

An optical montage refers to the location and arrangement of emitters and detectors across the scalp to record from the desired cortical ROIs. In a standard TMS-fNIRS or TMS-EROS experiment, optodes are typically secured in place against the scalp with rubber "patches" mounted to the head. For experiments concentrating on distal ROIs, any patch montage can be used so long as the optical mounting apparatus does not limit access of the TMS coil to a targeted scalp location. Performing optical recordings from proximal ROIs presents the greatest technical challenge for TMS-fNIRS and TMS-EROS experiments as the optodes must be mounted against the scalp while still permitting a TMS coil to be positioned close enough to the scalp to activate underlying cortical tissue. The magnetic field generated by a TMS coil falls off rapidly with distance and the introduction of more than a few millimeters of distance can significantly attenuate the efficacy of TMS in underlying cortex (Kozel et al., 2000; McConnell et al., 2001). There are several approaches that may be taken to minimize distance introduced by the placement of an optical patch to measure activity from a proximal ROI. First, a *coil-bounding* optical montage may be incorporated with some TMS coils (Hada et al., 2006). A coil-bounding montage refers to the placement of optodes around the edges or openings of a TMS coil (**Figure 2A**). Coil-bounding montages are ideal as no additional distance is introduced between the TMS coil and the scalp. The drawback of this approach is that the

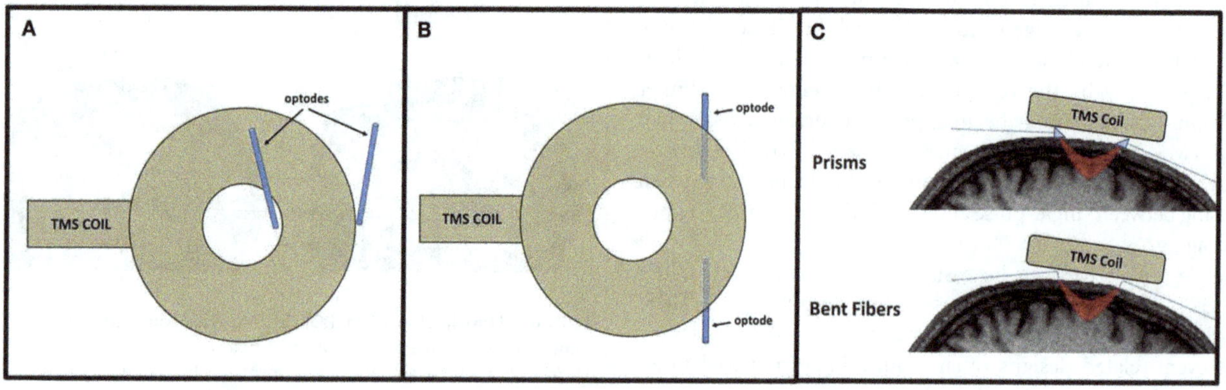

FIGURE 2 | Approaches to TMS-fNIRS and TMS-EROS montages illustrated with a circular coil. In a coil-bounding montage **(A)**, optodes are arranges around inner and outer edges of a TMS coil. A low-profile approach **(B)** positions optodes directly beneath the coil by redirecting light with prisms or bending the tips of fiber optics **(C)**.

placement of optodes becomes constrained by the shape of the TMS coil and does not facilitate optimization of a montage for recording a desired ROI. Furthermore, coil-bounding montages are incompatible with many standard TMS coils because distances introduced by the coil are too great to allow light transmission of adequate intensity between emitters and detectors. A second approach for designing a concurrent TMS-optical montage is to reorient optodes so that they may be mounted in a *low-profile* optical patch directly beneath a TMS coil (**Figure 2B**). Creating a low-profile optical montage can be accomplished either by bending optodes, reorienting their tips at a perpendicular angle (**Figure 2C**; Noguchi et al., 2003; Mochizuki et al., 2006) or by using prisms to redirect light at a perpendicular angle (**Figure 2C**; Näsi et al., 2011; Parks et al., 2012). The advantage of the low-profile approach is that a montage may be designed with freedom, arranging optodes in any desired configuration. The disadvantage of such a montage is, of course, the introduction of additional distance between the coil and cortex which may require TMS of greater intensity to sufficiently stimulate the targeted ROI. A final approach for optical imaging of proximal ROIs is to use specialty coils, designed for optical applications. These coils minimize distances between the coil's stimulating "hot spot" and access to the scalp, allowing optodes to be readily positioned in appropriate locations (Groiss et al., 2013). Such specialty coils allow coil-bounding montages to be constructed with greater freedom and across shorter distances than permitted by standard TMS coil designs.

SAFETY

To ensure subject safety in TMS-fNIRS and TMS-EROS experiments, optodes and mounting apparatus should be MRI-compatible, free of all ferrous material. Additionally, all components must be thoroughly inspected and tested for materials that may present additionally hazard in the presence of strong alternating magnetic fields, such as metallic materials that may become heated with repeated exposure to TMS pulses. So long as these standards are met, there are no additional safety considerations with TMS-fNIRS or TMS-EROS experiments above those associated with the use of TMS alone (Rossi et al., 2009).

POTENTIAL ARTIFACTS IN TMS-fNIRS AND TMS-EROS

ELECTROMAGNETIC ARTIFACTS

As described previously, one advantage of concurrent TMS and optical imaging is that the measurement of near-infrared light is immune to electromagnetic interference. Though light transmission is not affected by TMS pulses, the instrumentation used to measure near-infrared light may be susceptible to electromagnetic interference, particularly in the sensitive photomultiplier tubes (PMTs) that are used to amplify the detection of near-infrared wavelengths (**Figure 3A**).

MOVEMENT ARTIFACTS

The magnetic discharge of a TMS coil causes mechanical deformation, resulting in small movements and vibrations of the coil. Such vibrations can cause small displacements of optodes or transient changes in the pressure of optodes against the scalp. The presence of either form of mechanical agitation at the optode-scalp interface can introduce brief changes in the measurement of light intensity/scatter that will occur systematically with each TMS pulse (*coil movement artifact;* **Figure 3B**). Direct stimulation of the scalp musculature directly beneath the TMS coil can introduce transient muscle contractions that can also cause small but significant optode displacements (*muscle twitch artifact*; **Figure 3B**). Artifacts may also occur as a result of involuntary movements made by the subject due to startle in response to a TMS pulse or through stimulation of cranial nerves and neck muscles. Such *subject movement artifacts* may also lead to large movements of optodes leading to undesirable modulations in intensity/scatter measures (**Figure 3B**).

SENSORY ARTIFACTS

The mechanical deformation of the TMS coil generates a clicking sound, a strong auditory stimulus. The vibrations and scalp stimulation associated with a TMS pulse also cause somatosensory stimulation of the skin and musculature directly below the coil (**Figure 3D**). As with other TMS-neuroimaging approaches, such sensory artifacts are unavoidable as they are precisely time-locked to a TMS pulse. In many cases, sensory artifact can be ruled out based on the optical ROI recorded. For example, an auditory

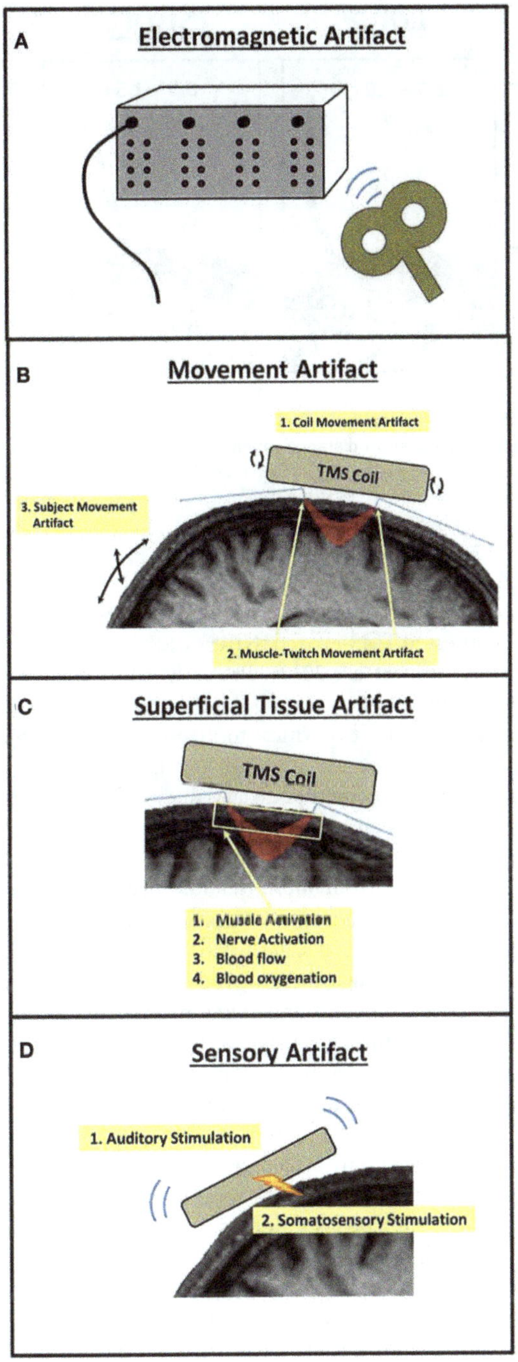

FIGURE 3 | Potential sources of TMS-related artifacts in TMS-fNIRS and TMS-EROS experiments. A TMS pulse may **(A)** introduce interference or noise within the optical imaging instrumentation, **(B)** cause movement of the subject and/or optical fibers, **(C)** induce changes in the absorption and scattering properties of superficial tissue of the scalp and skull, or **(D)** induce neural activations through auditory or somatosensory stimulation.

artifact would not be of major concern when recording fNIRS from primary motor cortex. In other cases, these artifacts must be identified, measured, and ruled out as a source of TMS-evoked cortical activation.

SUPERFICIAL TISSUE ARTIFACTS

Near-infrared light must pass through superficial tissue (e.g., scalp) before penetrating into the cortex then pass through this tissue again as it scatters back to the surface where it is detected. As such, non-invasive optical imaging is sensitive to changes in near-infrared absorption and scattering that occur not only in the cerebral cortex, but also in the superficial tissue of the scalp and skull. During passive optical imaging recordings, physiological activity within superficial tissue presents little problem as this activity is random with respect to the stimuli and tasks presented to the subject. However, TMS induces electrical currents not only in the neural tissue of the cerebral cortex but also in superficial tissue, musculature, and nerves of the scalp and skull. Thus, TMS-induced changes in near-infrared absorption and scattering may also occur in superficial tissue, including changes in superficial blood flow and oxygenation (**Figure 3C**) (Näsi et al., 2011). Such *superficial tissue artifacts*, if present, are not easily disentangled from cortical activations and present the greatest challenge for combined TMS and optical imaging experiments (Näsi et al., 2011).

IDENTIFYING AND CONTROLLING FOR ARTIFACTS IN TMS-fNIRS AND TMS-EROS

PHANTOM TESTS

An optical imaging phantom is a block of material with near-infrared scattering properties approximating that of the human head. Phantoms are typically used to test the integrity of optical fibers and instrumentation but can also provide useful information regarding TMS artifacts. In a phantom test for TMS-related artifacts the phantom is configured with the optical montage and optical data is recorded as TMS pulses are emitted. Phantom TMS tests are useful for identifying two classes of artifact: electromagnetic and coil movement artifact.

A simple test for electromagnetic artifact by positioning the coil several centimeters above a phantom and optical montage and discharging a number of TMS pulses. Because optical signals will always remain constant through a phantom and no physical contact is made between the coil and optodes in this configuration, any TMS-locked changes observed in optical signals are most likely attributable to electromagnetic interference within the optical instrument. Electromagnetic artifacts can be dealt with easily by increasing the distance between the optical imaging instrument and TMS coil (e.g., longer fibers) or by electrically shielding the instrument in a grounded Faraday cage enclosure.

A test of coil movement artifacts can also be performed by positioning the TMS coil in physical contact with the phantom and optode mounting apparatus, approximating the conditions of testing on a human subject's head. Assuming no electromagnetic artifacts were found in the aforementioned test, TMS-related effects in near-infrared signals in this case can be attributed to the displacement of optodes by mechanical contraction of the TMS coil. Coil-movement artifact can be minimized by building additional shock absorption into the optode mounting apparatus (e.g., foam padding) or by introducing a small spatial separation between the coil and optodes so that no physical contact is made during experimental testing.

SHAM AND CONTROL SITE STIMULATION

Sham and control site stimulation are standard control conditions for TMS experiments. These conditions should also be incorporated into the experimental design of a TMS-fNIRS or TMS-EROS study to provide an online control for electromagnetic, movement, and sensory artifacts.

Sham stimulation is commonly performed by positioning the TMS coil over the targeted ROI but orienting the coil perpendicular to the scalp so that magnetic field is emitted into the open air rather than stimulating cortical tissue. Sham stimulation can be used to rule out or identify the presence of electromagnetic artifact, coil movement artifact, subject movement artifact, and sensory artifact. Because sham stimulation does not directly stimulate the scalp or cortex, the occurrence of any significant optical effects under these conditions is artifactual and can be attributed to one or more of the aforementioned sources. Phantom tests may be used to further determine the relative contributions of these artifacts.

Control site stimulation involves positioning the TMS coil over a cortical area deemed to be distant and neutral from the targeted region of interest (e.g., vertex). Control site stimulation provides a method of artifact assessment by approximating the stimulating parameters of an active TMS condition without stimulating the ROI of interest. Like sham stimulation, control site stimulation will also capture electromagnetic artifact, subject movement artifact, and sensory artifact. Control site stimulation will more closely match sensory sensations than sham stimulation, providing a better control of sensory artifact. Control site stimulation may also be used to assess the presence of muscle-twitch artifact as it will directly stimulate the scalp musculature. The complication of control site stimulation is that TMS will actively stimulate cortical tissue and thus could potentially induce true cortical activations via trans-synaptic projections to an ROI. Additionally, control site stimulation could induce a greater degree of movement artifact if coil placement results in greater activation of head and neck musculature. A control site must be carefully selected to avoid the induction of subject movement artifact and cortical activations of ROIs.

SUPERFICIAL CHANNELS

The spatial separation of emitters and detectors determines the depth traveled by near-infrared light. Channels with relatively long source-detector distances penetrate relatively deep into the head, passing through cortical tissue (long channels; ~2.0–5.5 cm; **Figure 4**). Channels with short source-detector distances penetrate superficially, passing only through the scalp and skull (short channels; <1.5 cm; **Figure 4**). Though short channels provide no measure of neural activity, they form a powerful method for identifying TMS-related artifacts. This is accomplished by using short channels to yield a measure of near-infrared absorption and scattering that is confined to superficial tissue of the scalp and skull (Firbank et al., 1998; Medvedev et al., 2008; Näsi et al., 2011; Takahashi et al., 2011; Parks et al., 2012; Fabiani et al., 2013). The presence of electromagnetic, movement, and superficial tissue artifacts will be apparent in these channels. The absence (or presence) of effects in short-distance channels as compared to long-distance channels can be used to eliminate (or confirm) the contribution of artifacts as an explanation of observed TMS-evoked fNIRS or EROS activations (Näsi et al., 2011; Parks et al., 2012). Presently, short channels provide the only means of evaluating the contribution of superficial tissue artifacts. Thus, it is critical to incorporate short channels when designing an optical montage for TMS-fNIRS or TMS-EROS experiments so that superficial tissue artifacts may be ruled out when evaluating and interpreting results.

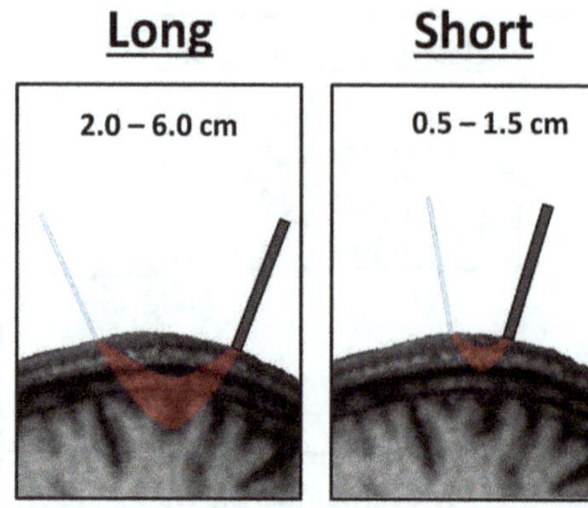

FIGURE 4 | Varying depth of penetration by near-infrared light between long and short distance channels. The path travelled by near-infrared light in a channel with long emitter-detector distances passes through cortical tissue whereas the path of light in a short channel travels only superficially through the scalp and skull.

COREGISTRATION WITH INDIVIDUAL NEUROANATOMY

Cortical ROIs in near-infrared optical imaging are often localized according to standard scalp locations of the 10–20 system (Jasper, 1958). On average, there is good correspondence between a given 10–20 location and underlying neuroanatomy, allowing near-infrared paths through cortex to be modeled relatively accurately based on these positions alone (Okamoto et al., 2004). However, the spatial accuracy of near-infrared optical imaging can be improved significantly by accounting for individual differences in neuroanatomy by coregistering optode locations to a T1-weighted structural MRI obtained for each subject (Whalen et al., 2008). This coregistration is accomplished by digitizing the three-dimensional locations of optodes at the time of experimentation then using fiducial points and statistical fitting procedures to align optode positions to an anatomical MRI collected for each subject (Whalen et al., 2008; Gratton and Fabiani, 2010). The improved spatial localization gleaned from such coregistration procedures can prove indispensable in disentangling true TMS-evoked cortical activations from sensory artifacts.

RECORDING PARAMETERS

Electromagnetic and coil movement artifacts will most likely manifest as transient, short-lived modulations in light transmission. In order to capture the occurrence and pattern of transient TMS-induced artifacts, near-infrared optical imaging data should be acquired with the highest sampling rate possible. Minimal filtering should be applied to optical data when identifying potential artifacts, though digital filtering at a later stage of data preprocessing may be an appropriate method to minimize the contribution of certain artifacts.

SUPPLEMENTARY PSYCHOPHYSIOLOGICAL, PSYCHOPHYSICAL, AND BEHAVIORAL MEASURES

Simultaneously acquired psychophysiological, perceptual, and behavioral measures can be used to increase confidence in the cortical origins of TMS-evoked fNIRS or EROS activations i.e., MEPs, motor/phosphene thresholds, and response times). A corresponding pattern of effects observed between optical activations and supplementary psychophysiological and behavioral measures is unlikely to be the result of a TMS-related artifact. Appropriate supplementary psychophysiological or behavioral measures should be included whenever allowed by the experimental design and logical given the ROIs being investigated.

COIL ORIENTATION

Systematical manipulation of TMS coil orientation may provide a further method of disentangling superficial tissue artifacts from cortical activation. The orientation of a TMS coil is known to vary the cortical response in systematic ways due to differences in underlying cortical geometry interacting with the direction of induced current flow (Sakai et al., 1997; Di Lazzaro et al., 2004). Although the effects of coil orientation have not yet been investigated with either fNIRS or EROS, coil orientation may predict a relative change in activation magnitude for some ROIs (e.g., motor cortex). Superficial tissue artifacts, however, would not be expected to vary systematically with coil orientation. Thus, optical activations of true cortical origin should modulate in a predictable manner with coil orientation whereas superficial tissue artifacts should not. Demonstrating the optical activation pattern predicted by manipulations of coil orientation could potentially be used to infer the cortical origins of observed signals though, to date, such an approach has not been attempted or validated.

ACTIVATION TIMING

In some cases, it may be possible to dismiss artifacts based on the timing of optical activations. For example, the temporal resolution of EROS allows cortical activation to be measured within milliseconds of discharging a TMS pulse. TMS-evoked EROS activations were previously described to peak in cortex beneath the TMS coil within 16 ms (Parks et al., 2012). Because this activation preceded the occurrence of an MEP, somatosensory feedback from the MEP could be excluded as a potential explanation of the effect. The temporally delayed effects of the hemodynamic response in fNIRS may also serve as the basis to logically exclude contributions of certain artifacts to optical activations. Electromagnetic and coil movement artifacts, for example, are likely only to induce transient fluctuations in light transmission, which are unlikely to systematically influence measures of oxy-Hb and deoxy-Hb peaking several seconds later.

STATISTICAL CORRECTION OF TMS ARTIFACTS

Presently, there are no proven methods for filtering or statistical correction of TMS-related artifacts in optical data. However, short-distant channels have been used to understand, measure, and remove superficial signals from fNIRS data (Yamada et al., 2009; Gregg et al., 2010; Takahashi et al., 2011). Independent component analysis has been applied in fNIRS and EROS data to increase signal-to-noise ratio (Kohno et al., 2007; Medvedev et al., 2008). Similar application of such superficial signal regression or blind source separation techniques to concurrent TMS and optical imaging data may provide a future method for the detection and correction of TMS-related artifacts.

CONCLUSIONS

Simultaneous TMS and near-infrared optical imaging provides a flexible and affordable approach to study human cortical dynamics and connectivity. Unique information regarding cortical function, neurovascular coupling, and neuroplasticity can be acquired through measurement of the hemodynamic response (i.e., fNIRS) or fast optical signals (i.e., EROS) concurrently with the administration of TMS. There are a number of technical challenges and TMS-related artifacts associated with TMS-fNIRS and TMS-EROS that must be overcome. In many cases there are straightforward solutions to technical issues and several steps that may be taken to minimize or control for artifactual optical signals.

REFERENCES

Allen, E. A., Pasley, B. N., Duong, T., and Freeman, R. D. (2007). Transcranial magnetic stimulation elicits coupled neural and hemodynamic consequences. *Science* 317, 1918–1921. doi: 10.1126/science.1146426

Andrew, R. D., and MacVicar, B. A. (1994). Imaging cell volume changes and neuronal excitation in the hippocampal slice. *Neuroscience* 62, 371–383. doi: 10.1016/0306-4522(94)90372-7

Barker, A. T., Jalinous, R., and Freeston, I. L. (1985). Non-invasive magnetic stimulation of the human motor cortex. *Lancet* 1, 1106–1107. doi: 10.1016/S0140-6736(85)92413-4

Baudewig, J., Siebner, H. R., Bestmann, S., Tergau, F., Tings, T., Paulus, W., et al. (2001). Functional MRI of cortical activations induced by transcranial magnetic stimulation (TMS). *Neuroreport* 12, 3543–3548. doi: 10.1097/00001756-200111160-00034

Bestmann, S., Baudewig, J., Siebner, H. R., Rothwell, J. C., and Frahm, J. (2004). Functional MRI of the immediate impact of transcranial magnetic stimulation on cortical and subcortical motor circuits. *Eur. J. Neurosci.* 19, 1950–1962. doi: 10.1111/j.1460-9568.2004.03277.x

Bestmann, S., Ruff, C. C., Blankenburg, F., Weiskopf, N., Driver, J., and Rothwell, J. C. (2008). Mapping causal interregional influences with concurrent TMS–fMRI. *Exp. Brain Res.* 191, 383–402. doi: 10.1007/s00221-008-1601-8

Biswal, B., Zerrin Yetkin, F., Haughton, V. M., and Hyde, J. S. (1995). Functional connectivity in the motor cortex of resting human brain using echo−planar mri. *Magn. Reson. Med.* 34, 537–541. doi: 10.1002/mrm.1910340409

Bohning, D., Shastri, A., McConnell, K., Nahas, Z., Lorberbaum, J., Roberts, D., et al. (1999). A combined TMS/fMRI study of intensity-dependent TMS over motor cortex. *Biol. Psychiatry* 45, 385–394. doi: 10.1016/S0006-3223(98)00368-0

Bohning, D. E., Shastri, A., Nahas, Z., Lorberbaum, J. P., Andersen, S. W., Dannels, W. R., et al. (1998). Echoplanar BOLD fMRI of brain activation induced by concurrent transcranial magnetic stimulation. *Invest. Radiol.* 33, 336–340. doi: 10.1097/00004424-199806000-00004

Bonato, C., Miniussi, C., and Rossini, P. M. (2006). Transcranial magnetic stimulation and cortical evoked potentials: a TMS/EEG co-registration study. *Clin. Neurophysiol.* 117, 1699–1707. doi: 10.1016/j.clinph.2006.05.006

Chen, R., Classen, J., Gerloff, C., Celnik, P., Wassermann, E. M., Hallett, M., et al. (1997). Depression of motor cortex excitability by low-frequency transcranial magnetic stimulation. *Neurology* 48, 1398–1403. doi: 10.1212/WNL.48.5.1398

Chiang, T. C., Vaithianathan, T., Leung, T., Lavidor, M., Walsh, V., and Delpy, D. T. (2007). Elevated haemoglobin levels in the motor cortex following 1 Hz transcranial magnetic stimulation: a preliminary study. *Exp. Brain Res.* 181, 555–560. doi: 10.1007/s00221-007-0952-x

Di Lazzaro, V., Oliviero, A., Pilato, F., Saturno, E., Dileone, M., Mazzone, P., et al. (2004). The physiological basis of transcranial motor cortex stimulation in conscious humans. *Clin. Neurophysiol.* 115, 255–266. doi: 10.1016/j.clinph.2003.10.009

Driver, J., Blankenburg, F., Bestmann, S., Vanduffel, W., and Ruff, C. C. (2009). Concurrent brain-stimulation and neuroimaging for studies of cognition. *Trends Cogn. Sci.* 13, 319–327. doi: 10.1016/j.tics.2009.04.007

Fabiani, M., Gordon, B. A., Maclin, E. L., Pearson, M. A., Brumback-Peltz, C. R., Low, K. A., et al. (2013). Neurovascular coupling in normal aging: a combined optical, ERP and fMRI study. *Neuroimage.* doi: 10.1016/j.neuroimage.2013.04.113. [Epub ahead of print].

Firbank, M., Okada, E., and Delpy, D. T. (1998). A theoretical study of the signal contribution of regions of the adult head to near-infrared spectroscopy studies of visual evoked responses. *Neuroimage* 8, 69–78. doi: 10.1006/nimg.1998.0348

Foust, A. J., and Rector, D. M. (2007). Optically teasing apart neural swelling and depolarization. *Neuroscience* 145, 887–899. doi: 10.1016/j.neuroscience.2006.12.068

Fox, P., Ingham, R., George, M. S., Mayberg, H., Ingham, J., Roby, J., et al. (1997). Imaging human intra-cerebral connectivity by PET during TMS. *Neuroreport* 8, 2787–2791. doi: 10.1097/00001756-199708180-00027

Fox, P. T., Narayana, S., Tandon, N., Fox, S. P., Sandoval, H., Kochunov, P., et al. (2006). Intensity modulation of TMS-induced cortical excitation: primary motor cortex. *Hum. Brain Mapp.* 27, 478–487. doi: 10.1002/hbm.20192

Frostig, R. D., Lieke, E. E., Ts'o, D. Y., and Grinvald, A. (1990). Cortical functional architecture and local coupling between neuronal activity and the microcirculation revealed by *in vivo* high-resolution optical imaging of intrinsic signals. *Proc. Natl. Acad. Sci. U.S.A.* 87, 6082–6086. doi: 10.1073/pnas.87.16.6082

Gratton, G., Corballis, P. M., Cho, E., Fabiani, M., and Hood, D. C. (1995). Shades of gray matter: noninvasive optical images of human brain responses during visual stimulation. *Psychophysiology* 32, 505–509. doi: 10.1111/j.1469-8986.1995.tb02102.x

Gratton, G., and Fabiani, M. (2003). The event-related optical signal (EROS) in visual cortex: replicability, consistency, localization, and resolution. *Psychophysiology* 40, 561–571. doi: 10.1111/1469-8986.00058

Gratton, G., and Fabiani, M. (2010). Fast optical imaging of human brain function. *Front. Hum. Neurosci.* 4:52. doi: 10.3389/fnhum.2010.00052

Gregg, N. M., White, B. R., Zeff, B. W., Berger, A. J., and Culver, J. P. (2010). Brain specificity of diffuse optical imaging: improvements from superficial signal regression and tomography. *Front. Neuroenergetics* 2:14. doi: 10.3389/fnene.2010.00014

Greicius, M. D., Krasnow, B., Reiss, A. L., and Menon, V. (2003). Functional connectivity in the resting brain: a network analysis of the default mode hypothesis. *Proc. Natl. Acad. Sci. U.S.A.* 100, 253–258. doi: 10.1073/pnas.0135058100

Groiss, S. J., Mochizuki, H., Furubayashi, T., Kobayashi, S., Nakatani-Enomoto, S., Nakamura, K., et al. (2013). Quadri-pulse stimulation induces stimulation frequency dependent cortical hemoglobin concentration changes within the ipsilateral motor cortical network. *Brain Stimul.* 6, 40–48. doi: 10.1016/j.brs.2011.12.004

Hada, Y., Abo, M., Kaminaga, T., and Mikami, M. (2006). Detection of cerebral blood flow changes during repetitive transcranial magnetic stimulation by recording hemoglobin in the brain cortex, just beneath the stimulation coil, with near-infrared spectroscopy. *Neuroimage* 32, 1226–1230. doi: 10.1016/j.neuroimage.2006.04.200

Hallett, M. (2007). Transcranial magnetic stimulation: a primer. *Neuron* 55, 187–200. doi: 10.1016/j.neuron.2007.06.026

Huang, Y. Z., Edwards, M. J., Rounis, E., Bhatia, K. P., and Rothwell, J. C. (2005). Theta burst stimulation of the human motor cortex. *Neuron* 45, 201–206. doi: 10.1016/j.neuron.2004.12.033

Ilmoniemi, R. J., and Kičić, D. (2010). Methodology for combined TMS and EEG. *Brain Topogr.* 22, 233–248. doi: 10.1007/s10548-009-0123-4

Ilmoniemi, R. J., Virtanen, J., Ruohonen, J., Karhu, J., Aronen, H. J., and Katila, T. (1997). Neuronal responses to magnetic stimulation reveal cortical reactivity and connectivity. *Neuroreport* 8, 3537–3540. doi: 10.1097/00001756-199711100-00024

Jasper, H. H. (1958). The ten-twenty electrode system of the International Federation. *Electroencephalogr. Clin. Neurophysiol.* 10, 371–375.

Jobsis, F. F. (1977). Noninvasive, infrared monitoring of cerebral and myocardial oxygen sufficiency and circulatory parameters. *Science* 198, 1264–1267. doi: 10.1126/science.929199

Kohno, S., Miyai, I., Seiyama, A., Oda, I., Ishikawa, A., Tsuneishi, S., et al. (2007). Removal of the skin blood flow artifact in functional near-infrared spectroscopic imaging data through independent component analysis. *J. Biomed. Opt.* 12, 062111. doi: 10.1117/1.2814249

Kozel, F. A., Nahas, Z., Molloy, M., Lorberbaum, J. P., Bohning, D., Risch, S. C., et al. (2000). How coil–cortex distance relates to age, motor threshold, and antidepressant response to repetitive transcranial magnetic stimulation. *J. Neuropsychiatry Clin. Neurosci.* 12, 376–384. doi: 10.1176/appi.neuropsych.12.3.376

Kozel, F. A., Tian, F., Dhamne, S., Croarkin, P. E., McClintock, S. M., Elliott, A., et al. (2009). Using simultaneous repetitive transcranial magnetic stimulation/functional near infrared spectroscopy (rTMS/fNIRS) to measure brain activation and connectivity. *Neuroimage* 47, 1177–1184. doi: 10.1016/j.neuroimage.2009.05.016

Lee, J., and Kim, S. J. (2010). Spectrum measurement of fast optical signal of neural activity in brain tissue and its theoretical origin. *Neuroimage* 51, 713–722. doi: 10.1016/j.neuroimage.2010.02.076

MacVicar, B. A., and Hochman, D. (1991). Imaging of synaptically evoked intrinsic optical signals in hippocampal slices. *J. Neurosci.* 11, 1458–1469.

McConnell, K. A., Nahas, Z., Shastri, A., Lorberbaum, J. P., Kozel, F. A., Bohning, D. E., et al. (2001). The transcranial magnetic stimulation motor threshold depends on the distance from coil to underlying cortex: a replication in healthy adults comparing two methods of assessing the distance to cortex. *Biol. Psychiatry* 49, 454–459. doi: 10.1016/S0006-3223(00)01039-8

Medvedev, A. V., Kainerstorfer, J., Borisov, S. V., Barbour, R. L., and VanMeter, J. (2008). Event-related fast optical signal in a rapid object recognition task: improving detection by the independent component analysis. *Brain Res.* 1236, 145–158. doi: 10.1016/j.brainres.2008.07.122

Miezin, F. M., Maccotta, L., Ollinger, J. M., Petersen, S. E., and Buckner, R. L. (2000). Characterizing the hemodynamic response: effects of presentation rate, sampling procedure, and the possibility of ordering brain activity based on relative timing. *Neuroimage* 11, 735–759. doi: 10.1006/nimg.2000.0568

Mochizuki, H., Furubayashi, T., Hanajima, R., Terao, Y., Mizuno, Y., Okabe, S., et al. (2007). Hemoglobin concentration changes in the contralateral hemisphere during and after theta burst stimulation of the human sensorimotor cortices. *Exp. Brain Res.* 180, 667–675. doi: 10.1007/s00221-007-0884-5

Mochizuki, H., Ugawa, Y., Terao, Y., and Sakai, K. L. (2006). Cortical hemoglobin-concentration changes under the coil induced by single-pulse TMS in humans: a simultaneous recording with near-infrared spectroscopy. *Exp. Brain Res.* 169, 302–310. doi: 10.1007/s00221-005-0149-0

Näsi, T., Mäki, H., Kotilahti, K., Nissilä, I., Haapalahti, P., and Ilmoniemi, R. J. (2011). Magnetic stimulation-related physiological artifacts in hemodynamic near-infrared spectroscopy signals. *PLoS ONE* 6:e24002. doi: 10.1371/journal.pone.0024002

Noguchi, Y., Watanabe, E., and Sakai, K. L. (2003). An event-related optical topography study of cortical activation induced by single-pulse transcranial magnetic stimulation.*Neuroimage* 19, 156–162. doi: 10.1016/S1053-8119(03)00054-5

Ogawa, S., Lee, T. M., Kay, A. R., and Tank, D. W. (1990). Brain magnetic resonance imaging with contrast dependent on blood oxygenation. *Proc. Natl. Acad. Sci. U.S.A.* 87, 9868–9872. doi: 10.1073/pnas.87.24.9868

Okamoto, M., Dan, H., Sakamoto, K., Takeo, K., Shimizu, K., Kohno, S., et al. (2004). Three-dimensional probabilistic anatomical cranio-cerebral correlation via the international 10–20 system oriented for transcranial functional brain mapping. *Neuroimage* 21, 99–111. doi: 10.1016/j.neuroimage.2003.08.026

Parks, N. A., Maclin, E. L., Low, K. A., Beck, D. M., Fabiani, M., and Gratton, G. (2012). Examining cortical dynamics and connectivity with simultaneous single-pulse transcranial magnetic stimulation and fast optical imaging. *Neuroimage* 59, 2504–2510. doi: 10.1016/j.neuroimage.2011.08.097

Pascual-Leone, A., Valls-Solé, J., Wassermann, E. M., and Hallett, M. (1994). Responses to rapid rate transcranial magnetic stimulation of the human motor cortex. *Brain* 117, 847–858. doi: 10.1093/brain/117.4.847

Pascual-Leone, A., Walsh, V., and Rothwell, J. (2000). Transcranial magnetic stimulation in cognitive neuroscience–virtual lesion, chronometry, and functional connectivity. *Curr. Opin. Neurobiol.* 10, 232–237. doi: 10.1016/S0959-4388(00)00081-7

Paus, T., Jech, R., Thompson, C. J., Comeau, R., Peters, T., and Evans, A. C. (1997). Transcranial magnetic stimulation during positron emission tomography: a new method for studying connectivity of the human cerebral cortex. *J. Neurosci.* 17, 3178–3184.

Rector, D. M., Carter, K. M., Volegov, P. L., and George, J. S. (2005). Spatio-temporal mapping of rat whisker barrels with fast scattered light signals. *Neuroimage* 26, 619–627. doi: 10.1016/j.neuroimage.2005.02.030

Rector, D. M., Poe, G. R., Kristensen, M. P., and Harper, R. M. (1997). Light scattering changes follow evoked potentials from hippocampal Schaeffer collateral stimulation. *J. Neurophysiol.* 78, 1707–1713.

Rossi, S., Hallett, M., Rossini, P. M., and Pascual-Leone, A. (2009). Safety, ethical considerations, and application guidelines for the use of transcranial magnetic stimulation in clinical practice and research. *Clin. Neurophysiol.* 120, 2008–2039. doi: 10.1016/j.clinph.2009.08.016

Sakai, K., Ugawa, Y., Terao, Y., Hanajima, R., Furubayashi, T., and Kanazawa, I. (1997). Preferential activation of different I waves by transcranial magnetic stimulation with a ?gure-of 8-shaped coil. *Exp. Brain Res.* 113, 24–32. doi: 10.1007/BF02454139

Siebner, H. R., Bergmann, T. O., Bestmann, S., Massimini, M., Johansen-Berg, H., Mochizuki, H., et al. (2009). Consensus paper: combining transcranial stimulation with neuroimaging. *Brain Stimul.* 2, 58–80. doi: 10.1016/j.brs.2008.11.002

Takahashi, T., Takikawa, Y., Kawagoe, R., Shibuya, S., Iwano, T., and Kitazawa, S. (2011). Influence of skin blood flow on near-infrared spectroscopy signals measured on the forehead during a verbal fluency task. *Neuroimage* 57, 991–1002. doi: 10.1016/j.neuroimage.2011.05.012

Thomson, R. H., Cleve, T. J., Bailey, N. W., Rogasch, N. C., Maller, J. J., Daskalakis, Z. J., et al. (2013). Blood oxygenation changes modulated by coil orientation during prefrontal transcranial magnetic stimulation. *Brain Stimul.* 6, 576–581. doi: 10.1016/j.brs.2012.12.001

Thomson, R. H., Daskalakis, Z. J., and Fitzgerald, P. B. (2011a). A near infra-red spectroscopy study of the effects of pre-frontal single and paired pulse transcranial magnetic stimulation. *Clin. Neurophysiol.* 122, 378–382. doi: 10.1016/j.clinph.2010.08.003

Thomson, R. H., Maller, J. J., Daskalakis, Z. J., and Fitzgerald, P. B. (2011b). Blood oxygenation changes resulting from suprathreshold transcranial magnetic stimulation. *Brain Stimul.* 4, 165–168. doi: 10.1016/j.brs.2010.10.003

Villringer, A., Planck, J., Hock, C., Schleinkofer, L., and Dirnagl, U. (1993). Near infrared spectroscopy (NIRS): a new tool to study hemodynamic changes during activation of brain function in human adults. *Neurosci. Lett.* 154, 101–104. doi: 10.1016/0304-3940(93)90181-J

Walsh, V., and Cowey, A. (2000). Transcranial magnetic stimulation and cognitive neuroscience. *Nat. Rev. Neurosci.* 1, 73–80. doi: 10.1038/35036239

Whalen, C., Maclin, E. L., Fabiani, M., and Gratton, G. (2008). Validation of a method for coregistering scalp recording locations with 3D structural MR images. *Hum. Brain Mapp.* 29, 1288–1301. doi: 10.1002/hbm.20465

Wolf, M., Morren, G., Haensse, D., Karen, T., Wolf, U., Fauchere, J. C., et al. (2008). Near infrared spectroscopy to study the brain: an overview. *Opto-Electron. Rev.* 16, 413–419. doi: 10.2478/s11772-008-0042-z

Wolf, M., Wolf, U., Choi, J. H., Gupta, R., Safonova, L. P., Paunescu, L. A., et al. (2002). Functional frequency-domain near-infrared spectroscopy detects fast neuronal signal in the motor cortex. *Neuroimage* 17, 1868–1875. doi: 10.1006/nimg.2002.1261

Yamada, T., Umeyama, S., and Matsuda, K. (2009). Multidistance probe arrangement to eliminate artifacts in functional near-infrared spectroscopy. *J. Biomed. Opt.* 14, 064034. doi: 10.1117/1.3275469

Ziemann, U. (2011). Transcranial magnetic stimulation at the interface with other techniques a powerful tool for studying the human cortex. *Neuroscientist* 17, 368–381. doi: 10.1177/1073858410390225

16

Combining functional magnetic resonance imaging with transcranial electrical stimulation

Catarina Saiote, Zsolt Turi, Walter Paulus and Andrea Antal*

Clinic for Clinical Neurophysiology, Universitätsmedizin, Georg-August-Universität, Göttingen, Germany

Correspondence:
Andrea Antal, Clinic for Clinical Neurophysiology, Universitätsmedizin, Georg-August-Universität Göttingen, Robert-Koch-Str. 40, 37075 Göttingen, Germany
e-mail: aantal@gwdg.de

Transcranial electrical stimulation (tES) is a neuromodulatory method with promising potential for basic research and as a therapeutic tool. The most explored type of tES is transcranial direct current stimulation (tDCS), but also transcranial alternating current stimulation (tACS) and transcranial random noise stimulation (tRNS) have been shown to affect cortical excitability, behavioral performance and brain activity. Although providing indirect measure of brain activity, functional magnetic resonance imaging (fMRI) can tell us more about the global effects of stimulation in the whole brain and what is more, on how it modulates functional interactions between brain regions, complementing what is known from electrophysiological methods such as measurement of motor evoked potentials. With this review, we aim to present the studies that have combined these techniques, the current approaches and discuss the results obtained so far.

Keywords: non-invasive brain stimulation, transcranial direct current stimulation (tDCS), transcranial random noise stimulation (tRNS), fMRI, transcranial electrical stimulation (tES), neuromodulation

INTRODUCTION

Non-invasive brain stimulation (NiBS) techniques use externally applied stimulation for inducing neuroplastic changes in the human brain. Sub-threshold transcranial electrical stimulation (tES) is a specific subgroup of NiBS using low-intensity electrical current (usually between 0.4 and 2.0 mA) via two conductive electrodes placed on the scalp (Nitsche et al., 2008). Despite a considerable shunting effect (Miranda et al., 2006), a certain proportion of the weak electrical current penetrates the scalp and causes prolonged but reversible changes in the cortical excitability by modifying spontaneous neural activity of the neurons (Bindman et al., 1964). One of the most studied tES techniques is transcranial direct current stimulation (tDCS),which is based on the application of a constant current (Nitsche and Paulus, 2000), whereas other tES techniques utilize oscillating currents in a various frequency range [(e.g., from 0.1 to 5000 Hz) (for a review see Paulus, 2011)]. Regarding the application of oscillating current we currently have two approaches: In the case of transcranial random noise stimulation (tRNS), several frequencies are applied within a normally distributed frequency spectrum (between 0.1 and 100 Hz for low-frequency tRNS and 101 and 640 Hz for high-frequency tRNS) (Terney et al., 2008), whereas in transcranial alternating current stimulation (tACS) a single sinusoidal - the most common—waveform at a specific frequency (e.g., at 20 Hz) is given (see **Figure 1**) (Antal et al., 2008).

The after-effects of tES dominantly depend on the stimulation parameters, including the stimulation duration, the current intensity, the electrode size, the current density (current intensity/electrode size) (Faria et al., 2011), the type of current (direct, oscillating current, or their combination), additional factors related to the current type (e.g., stimulation frequency in the case of oscillating current) (Antal et al., 2008), the timing of the stimulation (e.g., before, during, or after task performance) (Pirulli et al., 2013), and the electrode montage (i.e., position of the electrodes) (Bikson et al., 2012). It is important to notice however, that other tES-independent factors could also potentially influence the outcome of stimulation, such as the wakefulness of the participants (Huber et al., 2013), the state of participants receiving the stimulation (e.g., during rest or during behavioral/cognitive performance) (Silvanto et al., 2008), the individual differences in the neuroanatomy of the brain, genetic polimorphismus (e.g., Brain derived neurothrophic factor; BDNF) (Antal et al., 2010), handedness (Schade et al., 2012), and the experimental paradigm (e.g., motor, visual, cognitive). The relative contribution of each factor is less clear due to the fact that most of the studies apply remarkably different stimulation parameters and the lack of the studies systematically manipulating each factor while controlling the other parameters.

tES TECHNIQUES AND fMRI

The after-effects induced by sub-threshold tES have been first demonstrated on physiological and behavioral studies (for a review see Stagg and Nitsche, 2011). Transcranial magnetic stimulation (TMS) has been the most commonly used method for evaluating the after-effects of tES on the motor cortex. It is able to detect changes in cortical excitability and depending on the TMS protocol, it can provide information about the influence of tES on aspects of cortico-cortical and cortico-spinal excitability, intracortical inhibition, and facilitation as well as inter-hemispheric interactions (Nitsche et al., 2005). However, this method does not provide information about multifocal brain activation or neural network properties that essentially influence the outcome of stimulation. Functional magnetic resonance imaging (fMRI) has the advantage of providing whole brain data with high spatial precision and with a relatively

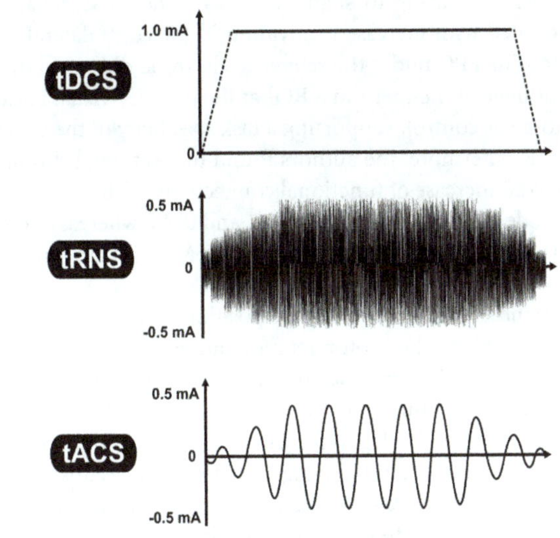

FIGURE 1 | Transcranial electrical stimulation is a specific subgroup of non-invasive brain stimulation techniques, which is based on the application of low-intensity electrical current. While tDCS uses constant current intensity, tRNS and tACS use oscillating current. The vertical axis represents the current intensity in milliamp (mA), while the horizontal axis illustrates the time-course. Abbreviations: tDCS, transcranial direct current stimulation; tRNS, transcranial random noise stimulation; tACS, transcranial alternating current stimulation.

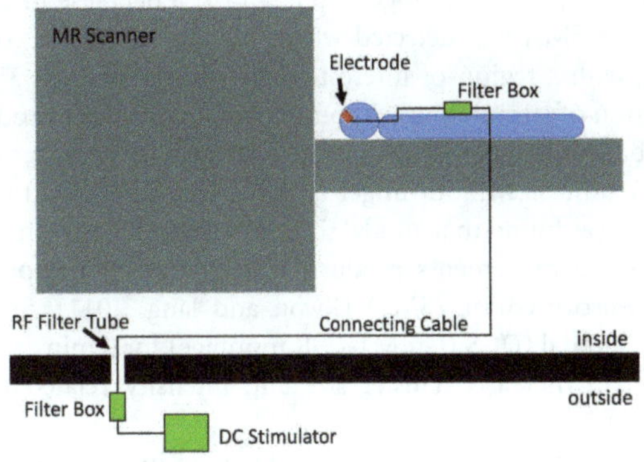

FIGURE 2 | Experimental setup which allows stimulation inside the scanner and also concurrently with fMRI. The electrodes on the subjects' head are connected to a filter box, itself connect by a cable going through the wall of the scanner room. This cable is connected to another filter box, to which the stimulator is connected. Reprinted from Antal et al. (2011), with permission from Elsevier.

high temporal resolution in a safe and non-invasive way. Offers a wide range of possibilities for analyzing brain activity and can, therefore, contribute to further elucidate the effects of tES. Previous studies have demonstrated that transcranial application of electrical currents over the motor cortex with supra-threshold intensity induces local and distant BOLD responses in motor related areas (Brandt et al., 1996; Brocke et al., 2008). Nevertheless, these studies were performed using significantly higher current intensities, and we will focus on sub-threshold tES.

The joint application of tES and fMRI was initially prevented by the technical difficulties regarding both safety of the procedure and quality of the acquired data (see **Figure 2** for a typical setup). The main safety concern is the possibility of heating under the electrodes due to the radio-frequency pulses of the scanner (Lemieux et al., 1997). To prevent this, electrodes wires have been equipped with resistors close to the electrodes. When stimulation is not performed during image acquisition, one has to consider the effect of the stimulation equipment in image quality. This has been shown to cause only a small (3 and 8%) reduction in signal-to-noise ratio (SNR) (Antal et al., 2011) and no distortion in the structural or functional images when electrode cables were unplugged from the stimulator (Polanía et al., 2011). Even though the changes in SNR remain minimal for simultaneous imaging and stimulation (Antal et al., 2011), it is possible to detect artifacts caused by the stimulation. Mild susceptibility artifacts not reaching brain tissue were detected under a frontal electrode (Antal et al., 2011), and B0 field distortions were as well restricted to the scalp (Holland et al., 2011). In a recent study, the artifacts induced by tDCS on functional images were investigated in 2 post-mortem subjects (Antal et al., 2012a,b) In accordance with previous observations, highest artifacts were found in the scalp and in the cerebrospinal fluid (CSF) at the surface and in the ventricles. However, it is relevant to note that the magnitude of the tDCS induced effect was found to be comparable (approximately ½) to that of a physiological BOLD response during finger-tapping using the same imaging sequence. This must be taken into account when interpreting results from concurrent tDCS and fMRI studies. Nevertheless, the technical advances that overcame these difficulties in the last years, have led to an increase in the number of studies combining these tES and fMRI.

The aim of the present article is to review these recent findings about the effect of low-intensity tES on the motor and cognitive functions accompanied by the related brain activity.

MODULATION OF ACTIVATION ELICITED BY MOTOR TASKS

The large majority of early tDCS studies targeted the motor cortex. Likewise, the first attempts to characterize the effects of the stimulation using fMRI focused on motor related brain areas. Baudewig et al. (2001) compared the activation maps elicited by sequential right hand finger movements before and after 5 min of stimulation. Stimulation was delivered during rest, with one electrode place over the hand area of the left primary motor cortex (M1) and the other over the contralateral supraorbital region(CSR) (left M1-CSR montage), at the intensity of 1 mA. The only significant finding was that cathodal tDCS over the M1 reduced the extent of activation in the supplementary motor area (SMA)—an effect still noticeable 15 min after the end of stimulation—suggesting that a reduction in excitability associated with tDCS was accompanied by a reduction in brain activity. In this study, no changes in activation were found in the M1 as an after-effect of stimulation, and the same was described when analyzing how motor-related activation was modulated during tDCS (**Figure 2**) (Antal et al., 2011). In this study, using a block design alternating periods of 20 s rest and tDCS during a finger tapping task, a decrease in activation in the SMA was detected when the anode was placed over the M1, with a region-of-interest (ROI) analysis (**Figure 3**). The application of stimulation without motor task did not produce a detectable effect and neither did the inverse polarity (cathode over the M1) with or without finger tapping. Contrasting with these results, it was found that anodal tDCS simultaneously with grasp-release hand movements modulated activation at the primary somatosensory cortex (SM1) (Kwon and Jang, 2011). Subjects received anodal tDCS (left M1-CSR montage) for 2 min at 1 mA, resulting in increased cluster size and intensity related to the motor task.

A more complex pattern of tDCS induced changes in motor-related activation was described in the study by Stagg et al. (2009). As in the study previously described, tDCS was applied with a left M1-CSR montage with 1 mA intensity, but for a period of 10 min. The participants performed a serial reaction time task before and after stimulation. Whole-brain analysis showed task-related activity increased in the left M1, left PMd, and bilateral SMA when the anode was over the M1. With reversed polarity, bilateral M1, PMd, and posterior parietal cortex (PPC) changes were observed after. For a ROI analysis, the M1 and dorsal premotor cortex (PMd) of both hemispheres as well as the right frontopolar cortex (FPC) were selected and it was found that anodal stimulation was related with an increase in activation in the left M1 comparing to sham, whereas cathodal stimulation was associated with increased activation in the contralateral M1 and PMd. The FPC under the reference electrode did not show a stimulation effect, neither did a ROI at the primary visual cortex (V1) chosen as control, supporting a task specificity of the effects of tDCS. Furthermore, the authors found that cathodal stimulation led to an increase of functional connectivity of the M1 under the electrode with the contralateral M1 and PMd, whereas anodal stimulation did not alter connectivity of left M1 with other motor regions.

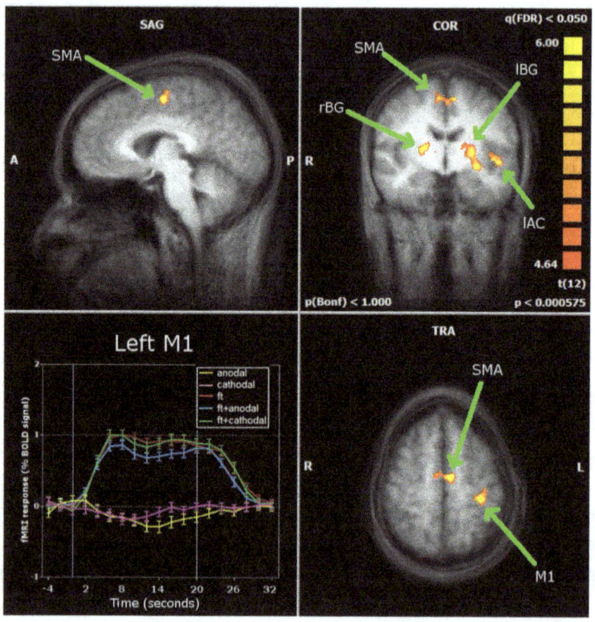

FIGURE 3 | Antal et al. (2011) carried out a ROI analysis on the regions identified by whole brain analysis during finger movements: primary motor cortex (M1), supplementary motor area (SMA), left and right basal ganglia (IBG and rBG) and left auditory cortex (IAC). Neither stimulation alone nor combined with finger movements induced significant changes in the BOLD response of the M1. Only in the SMA was a significant decrease found during anodal stimulation simultaneously with finger movements. Reprinted from Antal et al. (2011), with permission from Elsevier.

In the studies described so far, the position of the M1 electrode was determined by the motor representation of the hand area, detected using TMS, and the motor-task accordingly involved hand movements. Kim et al., 2012 applied anodal tDCS (cathode at CSR) over the leg representation on the right hemisphere for 15 min at 2 mA during rest, for 4 consecutive days. Whole-brain analysis revealed that after the fourth day activation elicited by toe flexion increased in the ipsilateral SMA and decreased in the contralateral M1, bilateral anterior cingulate gyri and right temporal and frontal region, in comparison with sham stimulation. Taken together, these results suggest a complex effect of tDCS, highly dependent on the stimulation paradigm and on the task being performed. This is not surprising, as physiological and behavioral studies have shown: timing between repetition of stimulation sessions as well as duration can be determinant (Monte-Silva et al., 2012), and the changes in the intensity of stimulation can even reverse effects of stimulation on cortical excitability (Batsikadze et al., 2013).

The after-effects of tRNS were also investigated using a finger-tapping task. After 4 min of stimulation (C3-CSR) at 1mA the extent of activation of the left sensorimotor cortex was decreased but no other significant changes were found (Chaieb et al., 2009). When tRNS was applied for 10 min during a visuomotor learning task (left M1-CSR montage), high-frequency tRNS caused a decrease in left frontal cortex activation, comparing with sham stimulation and a further decrease in bilateral frontal cortex and precuneous comparing with low-frequency tRNS (Saiote et al., 2013). This suggests a moderate effect of tRNS on BOLD response, however, it must be said that in this study, no changes due to tDCS were found. These are the only two studies combining tRNS and fMRI, and more are needed to understand how this technique is able to cause excitability (Terney et al., 2008) and behavioral (Fertonani et al., 2011) changes that have already been observed.

VISUAL FUNCTIONS

To our knowledge, only one study investigated the effect of tDCS on visual perception. Combining cathodal tDCS of the right MT+ with a motion perception paradigm, (Antal et al., 2012a,b) observed increased activation of the MT+ after the stimulation (10 min). This effect was site specific, as no effect on the contralateral MT+ or V1 was found and the whole brain analysis did not detect significant changes. However, the results may not be task-specific as they did not depend on the difficulty level and there was not effect of stimulation at a behavioral level, in contrast with previous studies (Antal et al., 2004a,b). However, studies have shown that tDCS is also able to modulate cortical excitability of the visual cortex (Antal et al., 2003), contrast perception (Antal et al., 2001; Kraft et al., 2010) and visual evoked potentials (Antal et al., 2004c; Accornero et al., 2007). Therefore, it would be of interest to conduct more studies to characterize the tES modulation of visual function from primary to higher order level.

tDCS AND THE RESTING BRAIN

Intrinsic brain activity has been measured with BOLD-fMRI during rest to reveal a set of distinct groups of brain regions (networks) showing coherent activity at low-frequencies (0.01—0.1 Hz), which are functionally relevant, and comply with the underlying anatomy (Biswal et al., 1995; De Luca et al., 2006). This prompted the development of several techniques for analyzing resting-state fMRI data without the need to define an expected model of activation and instead based on functional connectivity measures (Van den Heuvel and Hulshoff Pol, 2010). Recent studies have used diverse approaches to analyze the wide-spread effects of tDCS on resting-state brain activity.

Polanía et al. (2011) investigated the effects of 10 min anodal tDCS at 1 mA over the M1 (left M1-CSR montage). They used an approach based on graph theory, which provides a theoretical framework for characterizing local and global properties of networks quantitatively (Stam and Reijneveld, 2007; Bullmore and Sporns, 2009). The simplest measure is the connectivity degree (K), which quantifies the number of connections of a voxel and was found to have increased in the left posterior cingulate cortex (PCC) and right dorsolateral prefrontal cortex (DLPFC). The characteristic path length (L) can provide information about the global character of connections, as it quantifies the minimum number of connections between two voxels, between nodes, thus measuring whether they are directly or indirectly connected. L was found to be increased in the left SM1, pointing toward a decrease of the direct distant connections with the rest of the brain (Polanía et al., 2011). To further characterize the observed changes in the PCC, right DLPFC, and left SM1, these regions were taken as seeds in a correlation analysis and it was found that the left PCC had increased connectivity with other regions from the default mode network (DMN). The DLPFC showed increased connectivity with the right anterior insula (part of executive control network). As for the left SM1, it showed increased connectivity with the left premotor and M1 as well as with the left SM1 and superior parietal cortex. Using other measure derived from graph theory, it was found that after 20 min of anodal stimulation of the right SM1 (C4-CSR montage), eigenvector centrality increased in the right prefrontal cortex, left middle temporal lobe, right fusiform, and middle temporal gyrus and bilateral cerebellum. Eigenvector centrality is a measure of the importance of a node within a network (Lohmann et al., 2010), according to which a high value indicates that a voxel is connected to other important nodes. Thus, this result provides further evidence of tDCS induced functional network reorganization (Sehm et al., 2012). This was compared to bilateral stimulation (anode C4—cathode C3) in which case eigenvector centrality increased in motor areas as the right M1, PMd and bilateral SMA as well bilateral prefrontal cortex. In this study, the dynamics of eigenvector centrality changes during the 20 min stimulation period were also investigated. Bilateral stimulation led to increases within the right M1/PMd (under the anode) but not by unilateral stimulation. Also in secondary motor areas, bilateral stimulation caused eigenvector centrality changes. Both montages caused changes in prefrontal cortex which may reflect an effect of the stimulation on the resting-state network and not specifically related to changes in excitability in the M1. In fact, bilateral vs. unilateral stimulation of the SM1 had previously been studied, although with opposite polarity. Voxel-count and signal intensity were found to be significantly higher after bilateral stimulation on the SM1 (anode left and cathode right SM1) comparing with unilateral stimulation (left SM1-CSR montage), for the short 1 min stimulation duration (Kwon and Jang, 2012).

Besides modulating the network between the M1 and other brain regions, it was found that tDCS interferes with the connections within the M1 itself (Polanía et al., 2012b). Cathodal tDCS over the M1 caused an increase of the clustering coefficient and anodal tDCS a decrease of the minimum path length in the hand/arm area. These changes were not due to alterations of the number of connections, since no significant changes were found regarding the connectivity degree caused by anodal or cathodal stimulation. Therefore, these results suggest that cathodal tDCS reinforces the local functional connections of the arm/hand area and anodal with the connection in other M1 areas. Interestingly, it was also found that the magnitude of changes depended on the baseline efficiency level.

Two studies have focused on the connectivity changes during rest observed after stimulation of the DLPFC. Keeser et al. (2011) applied anodal stimulation to the left DLPFC at 2 mA for 20 min and used independent component analysis (ICA) to identify 4 resting state networks: the DMN, the left and right fronto-parietal network (FPN) and the self-reference network (SRN) and found that, comparing with sham stimulation, there was an increase in connectivity within the DMN, left, and right FPN, which could be interpreted as an enhancement of the level of alertness. In the study by Peña-Gómez et al. (2012) used a right/left DLPFC—CSR montage and applied for 20 min at 2 mA intensity. Resting-state fMRI was measured for 10 min before and after stimulation and analyzed using ICA. The authors compared functional connectivity within the DMN, visual, and motor networks and found decreased functional connectivity when comparing the anterior and posterior regions of the DMN, accompanied by the detection of a new independent component (IC) similar to the anterior part of the DMN. Increased functional connectivity was found between prefrontal and parietal regions within a network showing negative correlation to the DMN (the anti-correlated network) together with the disappearance of parietal ICs, suggesting the merging of components. This effect was observed for both stimulation of the right and left DLPFC, but it was still considered as a specific effect, since no changes in functional connectivity of the motor and visual networks were found.

Evidence has also been provided regarding the influence of tDCS on cortico-subcortical functional connectivity using a seed-based approach (Polanía et al., 2012a). The nucleus accumbens, caudate, putamen, and thalamus were taken as seeds in a multiple regression analysis during resting state, comparing before and after 10 min of anodal or cathodal stimulation over the M1. After anodal tDCS, connectivity between the left thalamus and M1 increased, as well as between the left caudate and superior parietal lobule. Also, connectivity decreased between the left caudate and the PCC. Polarity reversal led to decreased connectivity between the right putamen and left M1 and between the right thalamus and left superior frontal gyrus.

THE SIMULTANEOUS EFFECT OF tDCS ON HIGHER COGNITIVE FUNCTIONS AND ON BRAIN ACTIVITY

The tES-induced after-effects are not only limited to the motor and visual functions or on resting state activity but considerable evidence emerged for a reliable behavioral effect of tES on the cognitive functions (for a recent review see Kuo and Nitsche, 2012). The investigation of the effect of tDCS on cognition combined with fMRI is a particularly interesting approach, since it provides unique information about the tES-induced behavioral changes accompanied by the neural alternations.

Only two studies have directly investigated the effect of stimulation on cognitive functions with the combination of neuroimaging, and both studies used the concurrent application of tDCS and fMRI. Holland et al. (2011) targeted the left inferior frontal cortex (IFC) with anodal tDCS (cathodal electrode over the CSR) and measured neural and behavioral changes in a picture-naming paradigm. The stimulation was 20 min long with an intensity of 2.0 mA resulting in a current density of 0.057 mA/cm^2. They found a significant facilitation in picture naming performance in the active tDCS condition, compared to the sham tDCS condition (using a cross-over design). These behavioral findings were accompanied by a significant reduction of the BOLD response in the left IFC, including the Broca's area. In a more recent study, (Meinzer et al., 2012) investigated the effect of anodal tDCS on a semantic word generation task by stimulating again the left IFC (cathodal over the CSR). Ten minutes long anodal tDCS over the Broca's area at 1.0 mA (with a current density of 0.029 mA/cm^2 under the anodal electrode) improved semantic word generation performance, by increasing the number of the correct answers during active vs. sham tDCS. Interestingly, similar to the findings of Holland and colleagues, this behavioral enhancement was also associated with a selective reduction of the BOLD-response in the left ventral inferior frontal gyrus (vIFG) and with an increased language network connectivity evidenced by a graph-based eigenvector centrality mapping data analysis approach, this latter result suggesting an enhanced efficacy in information processing at the neural network level.

At the present, it is difficult to draw a conclusion from these two studies. The experimental evidence so far suggests that in both cases the tDCS-induced changes in higher cognitive functions were associated with reduced BOLD activity in highly-specific task-related brain regions. These findings are converging despite the strikingly different stimulation protocols concerning the stimulation duration and the intensity. A remaining issue for future studies would be providing further evidences for the relationship between altered cognition and the associated neural changes in the functionally relevant brain regions.

SUMMARY

The aim of this review was to summarize results so far obtained by combining tES and fMRI. Taken together, the studies presented here provide valuable insight to the potential of tES, as a tool to modulate brain activity. Modeling studies estimate a spatially wide distribution of the electric field induced during tDCS (e.g., Bikson et al., 2012), which seems to be confirmed by the whole brain effects of the stimulation on brain activity. However, it is especially interesting that the findings gathered from tDCS-fMRI up to this point, do not show an unspecific change in the neuronal activity, but are found in rather functionally relevant and task-related brain regions. Therefore, despite tDCS and generally tES techniques being considered as a non-focal NiBS methods (compared to TMS for example), it can be that the effects of stimulation are functionally focal. However, it is not clear how much of the dispersion of tES-induced changes is mediated by the functional state of the brain or by the wide reach of the induced electric field. Efforts have been made to improve focality of tDCS so as to enable controlled targeting of the stimulation and a setup for high-definition tDCS has been developed (Datta et al., 2010). Therefore, it would be interesting to see how the focality of physiological effects that has been achieved (Edwards et al., 2013) translates to whole-brain activity and its interplay with functional brain state.

Other tES modalities, namely tACS and tRNS are not expected to act by the same mechanisms as tDCS, not only regarding local physiological changes, but also at a functional and network level. To our knowledge, no study combined fMRI with tACS and only two studies combined it with tRNS (Chaieb et al., 2009). The possibility of differentially interact with rhythmic brain activity is very enticing and calls for more studies regarding these techniques, as knowledge of their effects is quite limited and can be complemented by fMRI.

What also remains to be further elucidated at a whole-brain level, is the temporal evolution of the tES-induced changes, not only in terms of duration of after-effects, but also regarding the influence of protocols and repeated stimulation sessions. As a clinical tool, tDCS has found application in several neurological conditions (Nitsche et al., 2008), such as stroke, depression and Parkinson's disease with a diversity of stimulation paradigms, stressing the importance of understanding the specific effects and dependence of tES on the parameters chosen for its application. Furthermore, the impact of tES on functional brain networks already altered by disease is yet to be studied and related to current clinical findings, as well as compared with that of healthy subjects.

REFERENCES

Accornero, N., Li Voti, P., La Riccia, M., and Gregori, B. (2007). Visual evoked potentials modulation during direct current cortical polarization. *Exp. Brain Res.* 178, 261–266. doi: 10.1007/s00221-006-0733-y

Antal, A., Bikson, M., Datta, A., Lafon, B., Dechent, P., Parra, L. C., et al. (2012a). Imaging artifacts induced by electrical stimulation during conventional fMRI of the brain. *Neuroimage*. doi: 10.1016/j.neuroimage.2012.10.026. [Epub ahead of print].

Antal, A., Kovács, G., Chaieb, L., Cziraki, C., Paulus, W., and Greenlee, M. W. (2012b). Cathodal stimulation of human MT+ leads to elevated fMRI signal: a tDCS-fMRI study. *Restor. Neurol. Neurosci.* 30, 255–263.

Antal, A., Boros, K., Poreisz, C., Chaieb, L., Terney, D., and Paulus, W. (2008). Comparatively weak after-effects of transcranial alternating current stimulation (tACS) on cortical excitability in humans. *Brain Stimul.* 1, 97–105. doi: 10.1016/j.brs.2007.10.001

Antal, A., Chaieb, L., Moliadze, V., Monte-Silva, K., Poreisz, C., Thirugnanasambandam, N., et al. (2010). Brain-derived neurotrophic factor (BDNF) gene polymorphisms shape cortical plasticity in humans. *Brain Stimul.* 3, 230–237. doi: 10.1016/j.brs.2009.12.003

Antal, A., Kincses, T. Z., Nitsche, M. A., and Paulus, W. (2003). Manipulation of phosphene thresholds by transcranial direct current stimulation in man. *Exp. Brain Res.* 150, 375–378.

Antal, A., Nitsche, M. A., Kincses, T. Z., Kruse, W., Hoffmann, K.-P., and Paulus, W. (2004a). Facilitation of visuo-motor learning by transcranial direct current stimulation of the motor and extrastriate visual areas in humans. *Eur. J. Neurosci.* 19, 2888–2892.

Antal, A., Nitsche, M. A., Kruse, W., Kincses, T. Z., Hoffmann, K.-P., and Paulus, W. (2004b). Direct current stimulation over V5 enhances visuomotor coordination by improving motion perception in humans. *J. Cogn. Neurosci.* 16, 521–527.

Antal, A., Varga, E. T., Kincses, T. Z., Nitsche, M. A., and Paulus, W. (2004c). Oscillatory brain activity and transcranial direct current stimulation in humans. *Neuroreport* 15, 1307–1310.

Antal, A., Nitsche, M. A., and Paulus, W. (2001). External modulation of visual perception in humans. *Neuroreport* 12, 3553–3555. doi: 10.1097/00001756-200111160-00036

Antal, A., Polania, R., Schmidt-Samoa, C., Dechent, P., and Paulus, W. (2011). Transcranial direct current stimulation over the primary motor cortex during fMRI. *Neuroimage* 55, 590–596. doi: 10.1016/j.neuroimage.2010.11.085

Batsikadze, G., Moliadze, V., Paulus, W., Kuo, M.-F., and Nitsche, M. A. (2013). Partially non-linear stimulation intensity-dependent effects of direct current stimulation on motor cortex excitability in humans. *J. Physiol.* 7, 1987–2000. doi: 10.1113/jphysiol.2012.249730

Baudewig, J., Nitsche, M. A., Paulus, W., and Frahm, J. (2001). Regional modulation of BOLD MRI responses to human sensorimotor activation by transcranial direct current stimulation. *Magn. Reson. Med.* 45, 196–201.

Bikson, M., Rahman, A., and Datta, A. (2012). Computational models of transcranial direct current stimulation. *Clin. EEG Neurosci.* 43, 176–183. doi: 10.1177/1550059412445138

Bindman, L. J., Lippold, O., and Redfearn, J. (1964). The action of brief polarizing currents on the cerebral cortey of the rat (1) during current flow and (2) in the production of long-lasting aftereffect. *J. Physiol.* 172, 369–382.

Biswal, B., Yetkin, F. Z., Haughton, V. M., and Hyde, J. S. (1995). Functional connectivity in the motor cortex of resting human brain using echo-planar, M. R. I. *Magn. Reson. Med.* 34, 537–541. doi: 10.1002/mrm.1910340409

Brandt, S. A., Davis, T. L., Obrig, H., Meyer, B.-U., Belliveau, J. W., Rosen, B. R., et al. (1996). Functional magnetic resonance imaging shows localized brain activation during serial transcranial stimulation in man. *Neuroreport* 7, 734–736. doi: 10.1097/00001756-199602290-00013

Brocke, J., Schmidt, S., Irlbacher, K., Cichy, R. M., and Brandt, S. A. (2008). Transcranial cortex stimulation and fMRI: electrophysiological correlates of dual-pulse BOLD signal modulation. *Neuroimage* 40, 631–643. doi: 10.1016/j.neuroimage.2007.11.057

Bullmore, E., and Sporns, O. (2009). Complex brain networks: graph theoretical analysis of structural and functional systems. *Nat. Rev. Neurosci.* 10, 186–198. doi: 10.1038/nrn2575

Chaieb, L., Kovacs, G., Cziraki, C., Greenlee, M., Paulus, W., and Antal, A. (2009). Short-duration transcranial random noise stimulation induces blood oxygenation level dependent response attenuation in the human motor cortex. *Exp. Brain Res.* 198, 439–444. doi: 10.1007/s00221-009-1938-7

Datta, A., Bansal, V., Diaz, J., Patel, J., Reato, D., and Bikson, M. (2010). Gyri –precise head model of transcranial DC stimulation: Improved spatial focality using a ring electrode versus conventional rectangular pad. *Brain Stimul.* 2, 201–207. doi: 10.1016/j.brs.2009.03.005

De Luca, M., Beckmann, C. F., De Stefano, N., Matthews, P. M., and Smith, S. M. (2006). fMRI resting state networks define distinct modes of long-distance interactions in the human brain. *Neuroimage* 29, 1359–1367. doi: 10.1016/j.neuroimage.2005.08.035

Edwards, D., Cortes, M., Datta, A., Minhas, P., Wassermann, E. M., and Bikson, M. (2013). Physiological and modeling evidence for focal transcranial electrical brain stimulation in humans: a basis for high-definition tDCS. *Neuroimage* 74, 266–275. doi: 10.1016/j.neuroimage.2013.01.042

Faria, P., Hallett, M., and Miranda, P. C. (2011). A finite element analysis of the effect of electrode area and inter-electrode distance on the spatial distribution of the current density in tDCS. *J. Neural Eng.* 8, 066017.

Fertonani, A., Pirulli, C., and Miniussi, C. (2011). Random noise stimulation improves neuroplasticity in perceptual learning. *J. Neurosci.* 31, 15416–15423. doi: 10.1523/JNEUROSCI.2002-11.2011

Holland, R., Leff, A. P., Josephs, O., Galea, J. M., Desikan, M., Price, C. J., et al. (2011). Speech facilitation by left inferior frontal cortex stimulation. *Curr. Biol.* 21, 1403–1407. doi: 10.1016/j.cub.2011.07.021

Huber, R., Mäki, H., Rosanova, M., Casarotto, S., Canali, P., Casali, A. G., et al. (2013). Human cortical excitability increases with time awake. *Cereb. Cortex* 23, 332–338. doi: 10.1093/cercor/bhs014

Keeser, D., Meindl, T., Bor, J., Palm, U., Pogarell, O., Mulert, C., et al. (2011). Prefrontal transcranial direct current stimulation changes connectivity of resting-state networks during fMRI. *J. Neurosci.* 31, 15284–15293. doi: 10.1523/JNEUROSCI.0542-11.2011

Kim, C. R., Kim, D.-Y., Kim, L. S., Chun, M. H., Kim, S. J., and Park, C. H. (2012). Modulation of cortical activity after anodal transcranial direct current stimulation of the lower limb motor cortex: a functional MRI study. *Brain Stimul.* 5, 462–467. doi: 10.1016/j.brs.2011.08.002

Kraft, A., Roehmel, J., Olma, M. C., Schmidt, S., Irlbacher, K., and Brandt, S. A. (2010). Transcranial direct current stimulation affects visual perception measured by threshold perimetry. *Exp. Brain Res.* 207, 283–290. doi: 10.1007/s00221-010-2453-6

Kuo, M.-F., and Nitsche, M. A. (2012). Effects of transcranial electrical stimulation on cognition. *Clin. EEG Neurosci.* 43, 192–199. doi: 10.1177/1550059412444975

Kwon, Y. H., and Jang, S. H. (2011). The enhanced cortical activation induced by transcranial direct current stimulation during hand movements. *Neurosci. Lett.* 492, 105–108. doi: 10.1016/j.neulet.2011.01.066

Kwon, Y., and Jang, S. (2012). Onsite-effects of dual-hemisphere versus conventional single-hemisphere transcranial direct current stimulation. *Neural Regen. Res.* 7, 1889–1894.

Lemieux, L., Allen, P. J., Franconi, F., Symms, M. R., and Fish, D. R. (1997). Recording of EEG during fMRI experiments: patient safety. *Magn. Reson. Med.* 38, 943–952. doi: 10.1002/mrm.1910380614

Lohmann, G., Margulies, D. S., Horstmann, A., Pleger, B., Lepsien, J., Goldhahn, D., et al. (2010). Eigenvector centrality mapping for analyzing connectivity patterns in fMRI data of the human brain. *PLoS ONE* 5:e10232. doi:10.1371/journal.pone.0010232

Meinzer, M., Antonenko, D., Lindenberg, R., Hetzer, S., Ulm, L., Avirame, K., et al. (2012). Electrical brain stimulation improves cognitive performance by modulating functional connectivity and task-specific activation. *J. Neurosci.* 32, 1859–1866. doi: 10.1523/JNEUROSCI.4812-11.2012

Miranda, P. C., Lomarev, M., and Hallett, M. (2006). Modeling the current distribution during transcranial direct current stimulation. *Clin. Neurophysiol.* 117, 1623–1629. doi: 10.1016/j.clinph.2006.04.009

Monte-Silva, K., Kuo, M.-F., Hessenthaler, S., Fresnoza, S., Liebetanz, D., Paulus, W., et al. (2012). Induction of late LTP-like plasticity in the human motor cortex by repeated non-invasive brain stimulation. *Brain Stimul.* 6, 424–432. doi: 10.1016/j.brs.2012.04.011

Nitsche, M. A., Cohen, L. G., Wassermann, E. M., Priori, A., Lang, N., Antal, A., et al. (2008). Transcranial direct current stimulation: State of the art 2008. *Brain Stimul.* 1, 206–223. doi: 10.1016/j.brs.2008.06.004

Nitsche, M. A., and Paulus, W. (2000). Excitability changes induced in the human motor cortex by weak transcranial direct current stimulation. *J. Physiol.* 527, 633–639. doi: 10.1111/j.1469-7793.2000.t01-1-00633.x

Nitsche, M. A., Seeber, A., Frommann, K., Klein, C. C., Rochford, C., Nitsche, M. S., et al. (2005). Modulating parameters of excitability during and after transcranial direct current stimulation of the human motor cortex. *J. Physiol.* 568, 291–303. doi: 10.1113/jphysiol.2005.092429

Paulus, W. (2011). Transcranial electrical stimulation (tES - tDCS; tRNS, tACS) methods. *Neuropsychol. Rehabil.* 21, 602–617. doi: 10.1080/09602011.2011.557292

Peña-Gómez, C., Sala-Lonch, R., Junqué, C., Clemente, I. C., Vidal, D., Bargalló, N., et al. (2012). Modulation of large-scale brain networks by transcranial direct current stimulation evidenced by resting-state functional MRI. *Brain Stimul.* 5, 252–263.

Pirulli, C., Fertonani, A., and Miniussi, C. (2013). The role of timing in the induction of neuromodulation in perceptual learning by transcranial electric stimulation. *Brain Stimul.* 6, 683–689. doi: 10.1016/j.brs.2012.12.005

Polanía, R., Paulus, W., Antal, A., and Nitsche, M. A. (2011). Introducing graph theory to track for neuroplastic alterations in the resting human brain: a transcranial direct current stimulation study. *Neuroimage* 54, 2287–2296. doi: 10.1016/j.neuroimage.2010.09.085

Polanía, R., Paulus, W., and Nitsche, M. A. (2012a). Modulating cortico-striatal and thalamo-cortical functional connectivity with transcranial direct current stimulation. *Hum. Brain Mapp.* 33, 2499–2508.

Polanía, R., Paulus, W., and Nitsche, M. A. (2012b). Reorganizing the intrinsic functional architecture of the human primary motor cortex during rest with non-invasive cortical stimulation. *PLoS ONE* 7:e30971. doi:10.1371/journal.pone.0030971

Saiote, C., Polanía, R., Rosenberger, K., Paulus, W., and Antal, A. (2013). High-Frequency TRNS Reduces BOLD Activity during Visuomotor Learning. *PLoS ONE* 8:e59669. doi: 10.1371/journal.pone.0059669

Schade, S., Moliadze, V., Paulus, W., and Antal, A. (2012). Modulating neuronal excitability in the motor cortex with tDCS shows moderate hemispheric asymmetry due to subjects' handedness: a pilot study. *Restor. Neurol. Neurosci.* 30, 191–198.

Sehm, B., Schäfer, A., Kipping, J., Margulies, D., Conde, V., Taubert, M., et al. (2012). Dynamic modulation of intrinsic functional connectivity by transcranial direct current stimulation. *J. Neurophysiol.* 108, 3253–3263. doi: 10.1152/jn.00606.2012

Silvanto, J., Muggleton, N., and Walsh, V. (2008). State-dependency in brain stimulation studies of perception and cognition. *Trends Cogn. Sci.* 12, 447–454. doi: 10.1016/j.tics.2008.09.004

Stagg, C. J., and Nitsche, M. A. (2011). Physiological basis of transcranial direct current stimulation. *Neuroscientist* 17, 37–53. doi: 10.1177/1073858410386614

Stagg, C. J., O'Shea, J., Kincses, Z. T., Woolrich, M., Matthews, P. M., and Johansen-Berg, H. (2009). Modulation of movement-associated cortical activation by transcranial direct current stimulation. *Eur. J. Neurosci.* 30, 1412–1423.

Stam, C. J., and Reijneveld, J. C. (2007). Graph theoretical analysis of complex networks in the brain. *Nonlinear Biomed. Phys.* 1, 3. doi: 10.1186/1753-4631-1-3

Terney, D., Chaieb, L., Moliadze, V., Antal, A., and Paulus, W. (2008). Increasing human brain excitability by transcranial high-frequency random noise stimulation. *J. Neurosci.* 28, 14147–14155. doi: 10.1523/JNEUROSCI.4248-08.2008

Van den Heuvel, M. P., and Hulshoff Pol, H. E. (2010). Exploring the brain network: a review on resting-state fMRI functional connectivity. *Eur. Neuropsychopharmacol.* 20, 519–534. doi: 10.1016/j.euroneuro.2010.03.008

17

Transcranial alternating current stimulation: a review of the underlying mechanisms and modulation of cognitive processes

Christoph S. Herrmann[1,2]*, Stefan Rach[1,2], Toralf Neuling[1] and Daniel Strüber[1,2]

[1] *Experimental Psychology Lab, Center of excellence Hearing4all, Department for Psychology, Faculty for Medicine and Health Sciences, Carl von Ossietzky Universität, Ammerländer Heerstr, Oldenburg, Germany*
[2] *Research Center Neurosensory Science, Carl von Ossietzky Universität, Oldenburg, Germany*

***Correspondence:**
Christoph S. Herrmann, Department of Experimental Psychology, Carl von Ossietzky Universität, Ammerländer Heerstr. 114-118, D-26129 Oldenburg, Germany
e-mail: christoph.herrmann@uni-oldenburg.de

Brain oscillations of different frequencies have been associated with a variety of cognitive functions. Convincing evidence supporting those associations has been provided by studies using intracranial stimulation, pharmacological interventions and lesion studies. The emergence of novel non-invasive brain stimulation techniques like repetitive transcranial magnetic stimulation (rTMS) and transcranial alternating current stimulation (tACS) now allows to modulate brain oscillations directly. Particularly, tACS offers the unique opportunity to causally link brain oscillations of a specific frequency range to cognitive processes, because it uses sinusoidal currents that are bound to one frequency only. Using tACS allows to modulate brain oscillations and in turn to influence cognitive processes, thereby demonstrating the causal link between the two. Here, we review findings about the physiological mechanism of tACS and studies that have used tACS to modulate basic motor and sensory processes as well as higher cognitive processes like momory, ambiguous perception, and decision making.

Keywords: alpha, EEG, electroencephalogram, gamma, oscillations, transcranial direct current stimulation, transcranial alternating current stimulation, transcranial magnetic stimulation

INTRODUCTION

Transcranial electric stimulation (tES) is the superordinate term for a class of non-invasive brain stimulation techniques comprising direct current (DC), alternating current (AC), and random noise (RN) stimulation (Paulus, 2011). The principle of using electric currents to stimulate the human body and brain is not new (see Priori, 2003 for a review). The applied currents can either be constant over time, as is the case with transcranial direct current stimulation (tDCS), or they can alternate at a certain frequency, which is referred to as transcranial alternating current stimulation (tACS). Stimulation with a RN frequency spectrum is known as transcranial random noise stimulation (tRNS). Here, we want to focus on tACS, since this method is particularly well suited to modulate physiologically relevant brain oscillations in a frequency-specific manner. Oscillations and DCs can be combined to more complex waveforms. If DC and AC are combined for transcranial stimulation, this is referred to as oscillatory tDCS (otDCS, Groppa et al., 2010). The AC does not need to be sinusoidal but may as well be rectangular or have even more complex shapes (**Figure 1**).

Numerous elegant studies during the last few decades have demonstrated a close association between brain oscillations and cognitive functions (for reviews, see Başar et al., 2001; Engel et al., 2001; Herrmann et al., 2004). The link has, however, always been established by correlating oscillatory brain activity with specific cognitive processes. Therefore, the issue of whether brain oscillations reflect a fundamental mechanism in cortical information processing or just an epiphenomenon is still unresolved. It has been argued that if oscillations were essential for any cognitive function, then this function should be altered by selectively interfering with these oscillations (Sejnowski and Paulsen, 2006). This has been considered to be a very difficult question to answer empirically in healthy humans until recently (Rees et al., 2002). One possibility to address this important issue is to study abnormal oscillatory activity in patients with neuropsychiatric disorders (Herrmann and Demiralp, 2005; Schnitzler and Gross, 2005; Uhlhaas and Singer, 2006). For example, it has been shown that the degree of cognitive deficits in patients with attention deficit hyperactivity disorder (ADHD) is correlated with an amplitude reduction of gamma-band oscillations in a memory paradigm (Lenz et al., 2008). However, complex diseases are usually not the result of one single symptom like disturbed gamma oscillations. Therefore, such studies provide evidence for an association between clinical symptoms and deviances in brain oscillations but do not provide causal links. Probing a causal role of oscillations for cognition has been promoted by recent developments of non-invasive human brain stimulation techniques that allow for driving brain oscillations within the range of observable, physiologically relevant frequencies. For one such technique—repetitive transcranial magnetic stimulation (rTMS)—the capability to entrain brain oscillations has been demonstrated recently (Thut et al., 2011). Compared to otDCS and tACS, rTMS is spatially more precise and neurons are excited directly by each TMS pulse (Thut et al., 2011). On the one hand, rTMS delivers

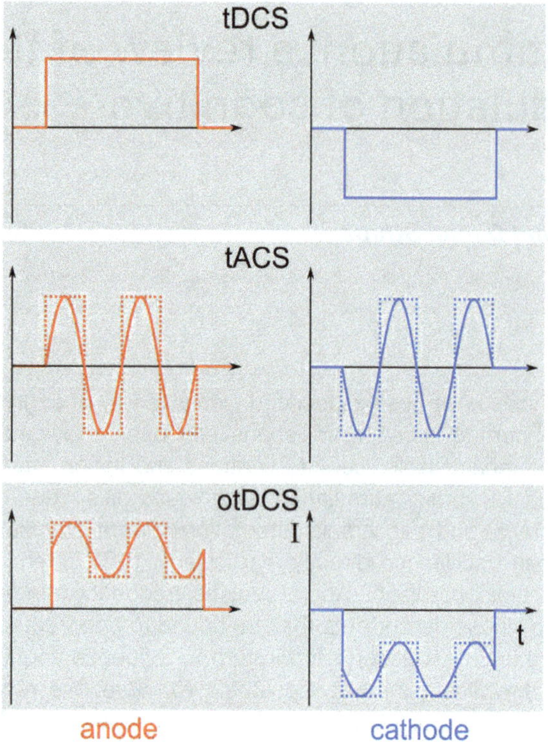

FIGURE 1 | Different stimulation paradigms. Top: During tDCS, a direct current will be switched on for a duration of typically a few minutes. **Middle:** In contrast, tACS uses alternating currents for stimulation that can either be sinusoidal (solid line) or rectangular (dotted line). **Bottom:** Combining tDCS and tACS results in oscillatory tDCS (otDCS), where the alternating current is superimposed onto a direct current. The alternating current can again be sinusoidal or rectangular.

brief bursts of about 100 μs duration that can be repeated at the frequency that is believed to be responsible for a certain cognitive effect. On the other hand, as depicted in **Figure 2**, repetitive bursts span a wide range of frequencies. Thus, care must be taken when ascribing rTMS-induced effects to the repetition frequency of rTMS. A recent article nicely mentions the criteria required to consider an effect to be based upon rhythmic entrainment of brain oscillations (Thut et al., 2011). In the case of tACS it is less likely to entrain brain oscillations other than the stimulation frequency, since the sinusoidal currents are strictly bound to only one frequency. Nevertheless, the finding of frequency specific rTMS effects on behavior (e.g., Romei et al., 2011) demonstrates that rTMS mainly entrains oscillations at the stimulation frequency and not at the broad-band responses of the single pulses.

In addition, tACS does not generate sounds that could interfere with the experimental paradigm and can be applied in the absence of somatosensory sensations—thus allowing for easy control conditions.

PHYSIOLOGICAL MECHANISM OF tACS

Recently, the physiological mechanisms that underlie the observed tACS effects have been revealed via intracranial recordings in animals (Fröhlich and McCormick, 2010). The authors stimulated ferrets intracranially and simultaneously recorded local field potentials (LFPs) and multiunit activity (MUA). Before stimulating the animals, *in vivo* recordings demonstrated that neuronal spikes in MUAs were synchronized to the oscillatory LFPs (**Figure 3**, left). Subsequently, cortical slices were stimulated *in vitro* and MUA was recorded simultaneously revealing that weak sinusoidal voltages ($\leq$0.5 V/m) were able to elicit spiking activity (**Figure 3**, right). Intriguingly, the spiking activity synchronized to different driving frequencies, suggesting that neuronal firing can be entrained to the electrically applied field (not shown here). Furthermore, Fröhlich and McCormick (2010) were able to demonstrate that steep transient voltage changes lead to stronger neural firing than slow transients albeit reaching the same voltage maximum [see supplemental information of Fröhlich and McCormick (2010)]. This indicates that not only absolute voltage levels determine neural firing but the temporal dynamics of voltage changes are important.

From that study, however, it was not clear whether weak currents can also penetrate the skull and still have similar effects upon neural activity. Ozen et al. (2010) have addressed this question by stimulating rats with electrodes on the surface of the skull while recording neural activity intracranially. These authors were able to show that an intracranial electric field as low as $\sim$1 V/m was sufficient to synchronize neural firing to a specific phase of the extracranially applied sinusoidal current. The current that has to be applied extracranially to achieve this electric field depends upon multiple parameters, such as skull thickness, electrode placement, and the like. This issue will be addressed in Section Modeling current flow.

A recent experiment in humans revealed that changes of cortical excitation depend non-linearly upon the intensity of tACS (Moliadze et al., 2012). Primary motor cortex was stimulated with tACS at 140 Hz while motor evoked potentials (MEPs) were simultaneously recorded in response to single TMS pulses. Low stimulation intensities of 0.2 mA resulted in cortical inhibition as indexed by increased motor thresholds. High intensities of 1 mA resulted in decreased thresholds, i.e., excitation. Intermediate intensities of 0.6 and 0.8 mA had no effect on motor threshold. This seems to indicate that inhibitory neurons are more susceptible to electric stimulation and are stimulated already at lower intensities. Excitatory neurons are less susceptible and require stronger stimulation but dominate the inhibitory neurons leading to a net effect of excitation. At intermediate intensities, inhibitory and excitatory effects cancel each other out.

An important step for tACS was to show its effectiveness in modulating oscillatory brain activity in humans. In this context, Zaehle et al. (2010) demonstrated that tACS applied at participants' individual EEG alpha frequency resulted in an enhancement of the EEG alpha amplitude after 10 min of stimulation. EEG was recorded offline, i.e., three minutes before and after applying tACS. After tACS, spectral power was significantly increased specifically in the range of the individual alpha frequency (IAF $\sim 10 \pm 2$ Hz) as compared to before tACS, indicating that this stimulation method can interfere with ongoing brain oscillations in a frequency-specific way despite its low amplitude and its transcranial application. A recent study

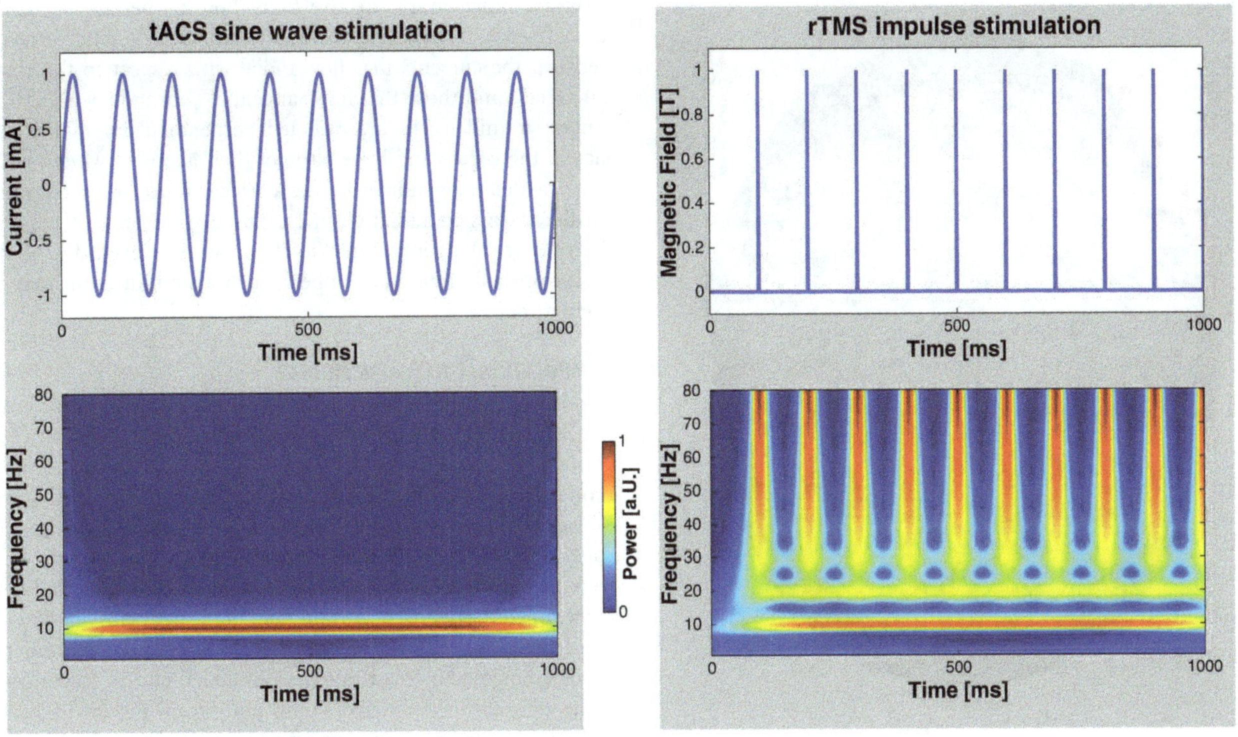

FIGURE 2 | Comparison of rTMS and tACS. Left: tACS uses sinusoidal currents which are restricted to one frequency as shown by a time-frequency wavelet transform. **Right:** rTMS, however, spans a wide range of frequencies in addition to the frequency of repetition. Note, that these diagrams depict only the stimulation currents/fields—not possible artifacts that may be elicited in the human brain.

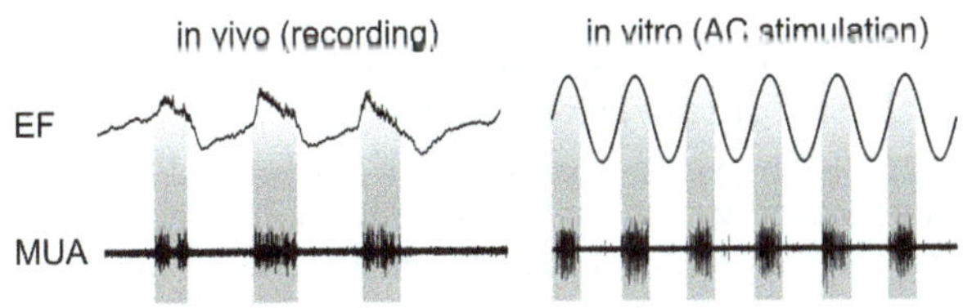

FIGURE 3 | Physiological mechanisms of tACS. Left: *In vivo* recordings in ferrets show that spontaneous neuronal activity seen in MUA synchronizes to certain phases of LFPs. **Right:** Stimulating slices of cortex electrically with sinusoidal currents results in a similar synchronization. Interestingly, the inter-burst frequency of the spontaneously occurring activity can be speeded up and slowed down resulting in neural entrainment [adapted from Fröhlich and McCormick (2010)].

by Neuling et al. (2013) replicated and extended the findings of Zaehle et al. (2010) by showing that the tACS-induced alpha amplitude enhancement remains present for at least 30 min after stimulation offset. Interestingly, alpha amplitude was only enhanced when the effective intracranial alpha tACS amplitude exceeded the endogenous alpha amplitude (eyes-open condition), but not when the former was weaker than the latter (eyes-closed condition).

Further insights into the effect of tACS can be expected from simultaneously recording hemodynamic responses with functional magnetic resonance imaging (fMRI), as has been done for brief impulses of TES (Brocke et al., 2008). While this procedure seems challenging for tDCS due to hemodynamic artifacts, it appears feasible for tACS (Antal et al., 2013).

MODELING CURRENT FLOW

A series of modeling studies has investigated how much of the weak extracranially applied current (typically around 1 mA in tACS) arrives intracranially. Early studies have used spherical head models to address this issue (Miranda et al., 2006). Later approaches used more realistically shaped head models that were derived from MRI recordings (Holdefer et al., 2006; Wagner et al., 2007). A large amount of the current is short-circuited by the well-conducting skin. Nevertheless, significant current densities can be modeled intracranially that result from the extracranial stimulation. Miranda et al. (2006) demonstrated that 2 mA of tDCS results in 0.1 A/m^2 of intracranial current density[1] corresponding to an electric field of 0.22 V/m. Neuling et al. (2012b) used a very fine-grained finite element model to show that 1 mA of tDCS/tACS applied to human visual cortex results in an intracranial current density of 0.1 A/m^2 amounting to a cortical electric field of 0.417 V/m when assuming a gray matter conductivity of 0.24 S/m (**Figure 4**). Compared to the thresholds for synchronizing neural spikes to electric fields derived from intracranial recordings in animals

[1] Note, that intracranial current density refers to current flow in cortex and is different from electrode current density as reported elsewhere in this article.

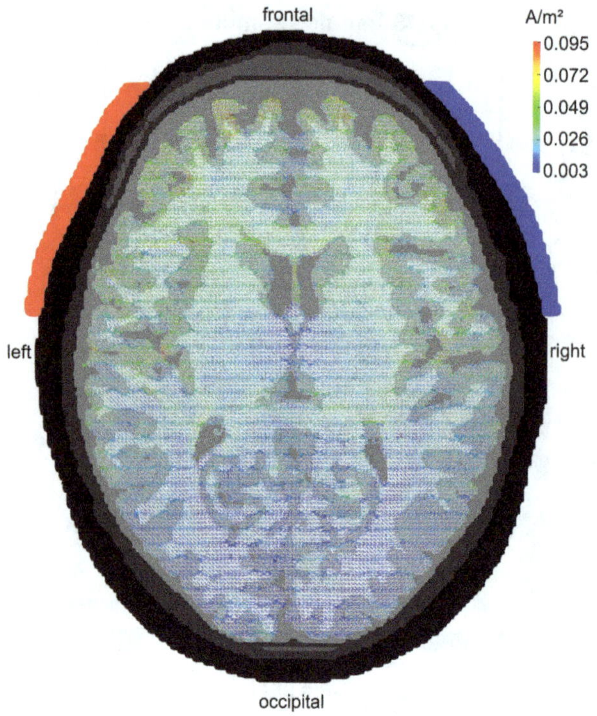

FIGURE 4 | Modeling tACS-induced intracranial current flow. Axial view of a human brain visualizing the current density distribution of tDCS/tACS applied at electrode locations F7 (anode, red) and F8 (cathode, blue). A clear maximum in anterior brain areas can be seen. Current densities are 20 times stronger in frontal as compared to occipital cortex. However, tDCS/tACS with large electrodes is not as focal as TMS. Reprinted from Neuling et al. (2012b) with permission of the authors.

(0.5–1 V/m) this would suggest that 1 mA of tDCS/tACS would be near or below threshold whereas 2 mA would be well above threshold.

Recent modeling studies demonstrate that focality of tDCS/tACS can be significantly enhanced when multiple small electrodes, e.g., EEG electrodes, are used instead of the typical 5 × 7 cm sponge electrodes (Faria et al., 2009; Dmochowski et al., 2011). However, even the usage of small electrodes suffers from the fact that at least two electrodes are required to apply a current to the human head. Therefore, two foci of current density result from the use of equally sized anode and cathode or from a small stimulation electrode and a larger return electrode. This problem can be overcome by using a so-called 4 × 1 ring electrode configuration (Datta et al., 2009). This montage uses four electrodes arranged in a ring for one polarity of stimulation, e.g., cathode, and another single electrode placed in the middle of the ring for the other polarity, e.g., anode. A single region of current density results from this electrode arrangement. The stimulated region can be located in a specific brain area by appropriate electrode placement.

Electric stimulation of brain tissue in animals revealed that the axon–especially the axon hillock–but not the soma is susceptible to electric fields (Nowak and Bullier, 1998). In addition, it has been demonstrated that electric fields along an axon are much more effective than those perpendicular to the axon (Ranck, 1975). This has led to the idea of differentiating between the currents that flow radial with respect to the cortical surface and those that flow tangential (Miranda et al., 2012). Since pyramidal cells are oriented perpendicularly to the surface of the cortex and large parts of their axons in white matter are oriented tangentially to the cortex surface, it is tempting to directly assign radial electric fields to the soma of pyramidal cells and tangential ones to the axon. However, due to the anisotropy of white matter fibers, such a simplification may be premature.

COMPUTATIONAL NETWORK MODELS

Beside their above mentioned physiological work, Fröhlich and McCormick (2010) also set out to simulate neural responses to direct and sinusoidal currents. They used the Hodgkin-Huxley model (Hodgkin and Huxley, 1952) in order to simulate how a network of 400 pyramidal neurons and 64 inhibitory interneurons responds to applied DC and AC fields. Importantly, they were able to demonstrate that the frequency of the applied field determined the degree of entrainment of the neural oscillations. If the driving frequency was close to the intrinsic frequency, membrane voltages showed strong periodic fluctuations. In contrast, if the external field differed significantly from the intrinsic frequency, no such entrainment was observed. These findings are in line with theoretical considerations of entrainment (Pikovsky et al., 2003).

Using the tACS parameters from Zaehle et al. (2010) as a reference, Merlet et al. (2013) simulated scalp EEG activity under tACS compared to no stimulation. Effects of tACS on EEG mean alpha power were modeled for different frequencies from 4 to 16 Hz in steps of 1 Hz. The strongest increase in alpha power was found at 10 Hz tACS, with progressively decreasing effects for the neighboring frequencies (8/9 Hz and 11/12 Hz). Outside the 8–12 Hz band, no significant tACS effects were found. These simulation findings correspond to the experimental results in humans by Zaehle et al. (2010). Furthermore, the modeled results demonstrated that alpha tACS is most efficient at the intrinsic frequency (10 Hz for the model).

Reato et al. (2010) used a simplified version of the Hodgkin Huxley model in which 800 excitatory and 200 inhibitory hippocampal neurons were modeled according to the integrate-and-fire model of Izhikevich (2003). The results demonstrated that:

1. DC stimulation mainly affects the firing rate.
2. AC stimulation up- and down-regulates the firing rate in an oscillatory manner without changing the average firing rate over a longer time interval (**Figure 5**).
3. AC stimulation at the frequency of endogenous oscillations mainly affects spike timing.
4. Even low amplitudes of electrical stimulation corresponding to a cortical electric field of 0.2 V/m result in enhanced coherence between spikes and the driving oscillation.

Interestingly, these simulations demonstrate a neural mechanism which could be responsible for the cross-frequency coupling

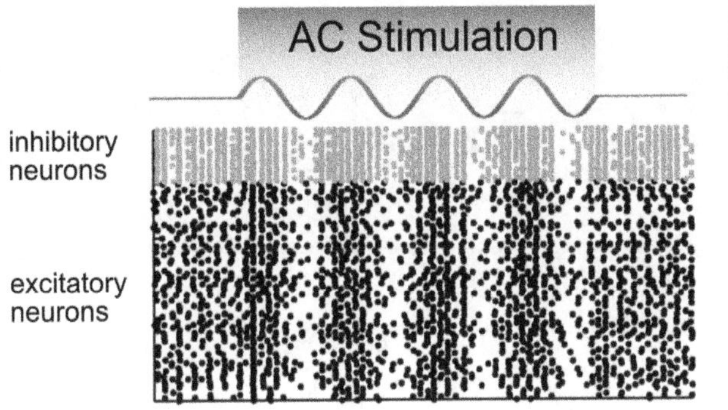

FIGURE 5 | Model predictions of how a network of neurons would behave in response to AC stimulation. The firing rates of inhibitory (gray) and excitatory (black) neurons are up- and down-regulated in phase with the AC current. In these raster plots, each dot represents a neural spike. Adapted from Reato et al. (2010).

that has been found in electrophysiological recordings (Jensen and Colgin, 2007). It has been repeatedly demonstrated that the phase of theta oscillations modulates the amplitude of gamma oscillations (Canolty et al., 2006; Demiralp et al., 2007), i.e., theta oscillations spread out cortically and their phase modulates gamma amplitudes. If the cortex were stimulated electrically at a frequency in the theta range, these artificial theta oscillations could spread out in the same way as physiological fields have been shown to do. The phase of these oscillations could then modulate the amplitude of gamma oscillations.

Due to the strong artifact that tACS produces during the time of stimulation, so far, effects on electrophysiology have only been shown for EEG after stimulation as compared to before stimulation (Marshall et al., 2006; Zaehle et al., 2010). However, the above stimulation experiments in animals and the simulation experiments in "silicon cells" explain only how electric stimulation affects electrophysiology at the time of stimulation. In order to simulate also the after-effects of their EEG experiment, Zaehle et al. (2010) used a neural network composed of Izhikevich neurons. They used a single neuron that was driven by an external current and 2500 neurons that were connected to the driven neuron by axons with variable delay times resulting in 2500 resonance loops with different resonance frequencies (**Figure 6**). During stimulation with a 10 Hz spike train, spike-timing-dependent-plasticity (STDP) modulated those synapses that were incorporated into loops with resonance frequencies close to the frequency of the driving force (100 ms$\sim$10 Hz). This finding suggests that synaptic plasticity was responsible for the observed after-effect of tACS. Along the same lines, neuroplastic changes have also been proposed as the mechanism underlying tACS after-effects by other authors (Antal and Paulus, 2012).

MOTOR AND COGNITIVE FUNCTIONS MODULATED BY tACS

MOTOR PROCESSES

Probing tACS/otDCS effects on the primary motor cortex bears the advantage to objectively measure changes of cortico-spinal excitability with MEPs after TMS. Compared to, e.g., phosphene ratings in the visual domain, MEPs do not rely on subjective experience of the participants. MEPs are used as a dependent variable that is usually compared from a baseline before stimulation to one or more time points during and after stimulation. Encouraging evidence with regard to motor excitability and behavior has been reported by existing studies, whereas conclusive electrophysiological results are largely missing, due to a general lack of concurrent EEG measurements. Exceptions are studies by Antal et al. (2008) and Pogosyan et al. (2009), which combined tACS and EEG. Therefore, effects on behavior, excitability, and electrophysiological effects will be reviewed in separate sections.

Effects on motor cortex excitability

The first study utilizing tACS and anodal/cathodal otDCS to investigate effects on the motor cortex was conducted by Antal et al. (2008). This exploratory study intended to compare oscillatory TES protocols to established constant current TES protocols. The authors analyzed MEP amplitudes before and after tACS/otDCS with different durations and frequencies. No effects on MEPs were found. Subsequent studies indicated that the weak after effects could be attributed to the stimulation parameters, e.g., comparatively short stimulation durations (2–10 min) and weak stimulation intensities (tACS: 0.25 A/m^2; otDCS: 0.16 A/m^2; current density in the electrode[2]). For example, otDCS studies with at least 10 min of stimulation and mean intensities of 0.63 A/m^2 were able to reveal after-effects (Bergmann et al., 2009; Groppa et al., 2010). Depending on the polarity, cortico-spinal excitability could be increased or decreased (Groppa et al., 2010). However, these effects do not differ from control conditions utilizing tDCS, suggesting that the DC portion of the stimulation currents caused the observed effects. Additionally, with a maximal intensity of 0.62 A/m^2, polarity dependent effects have only been demonstrated for tDCS but not for otDCS, indicating that not the maximal intensity but the overall current (mean intensity: tDCS, 0.62 A/m^2; otDCS: 0.31 A/m^2) was relevant for the effects (Groppa et al., 2010). Unfortunately, EEG was not recorded in these studies to differentiate effects of otDCS compared to tDCS.

Studies using tACS revealed bidirectional excitability shifts both during and after stimulation. Short tACS with different frequencies (5, 10, 20, 40 Hz; 90 s; 0.14 A/m^2) revealed that only during 20 Hz tACS motor excitability increased (Feurra et al., 2011a). Likewise, a study by Schutter and Hortensius (2011) yielded no increased excitability after 10 Hz tACS (10 min; 0.298 A/m^2) but after a combined frequency stimulation (5 Hz followed by 20 Hz; 5 min each; 0.298 A/m^2), although the specific contributions of the applied frequencies cannot be differentiated. Vice versa, tACS with 15 Hz (20 min; 0.80 A/m^2) decreased excitability after stimulation (Zaghi et al., 2010). Moliadze et al. (2010) applied tACS at frequencies outside traditional EEG frequency bands in the so called ripple range (80, 140, and 250 Hz; 10 min; 0.63 A/m^2). Only stimulation with 140 Hz resulted in sustained excitability enhancement of the motor cortex for up to 1 h after

[2]Note, that here current density refers to the current density in the electrode and is computed by dividing the total stimulation current (e.g., 1 mA) by the area of the electrode (e.g., 35 cm^2).

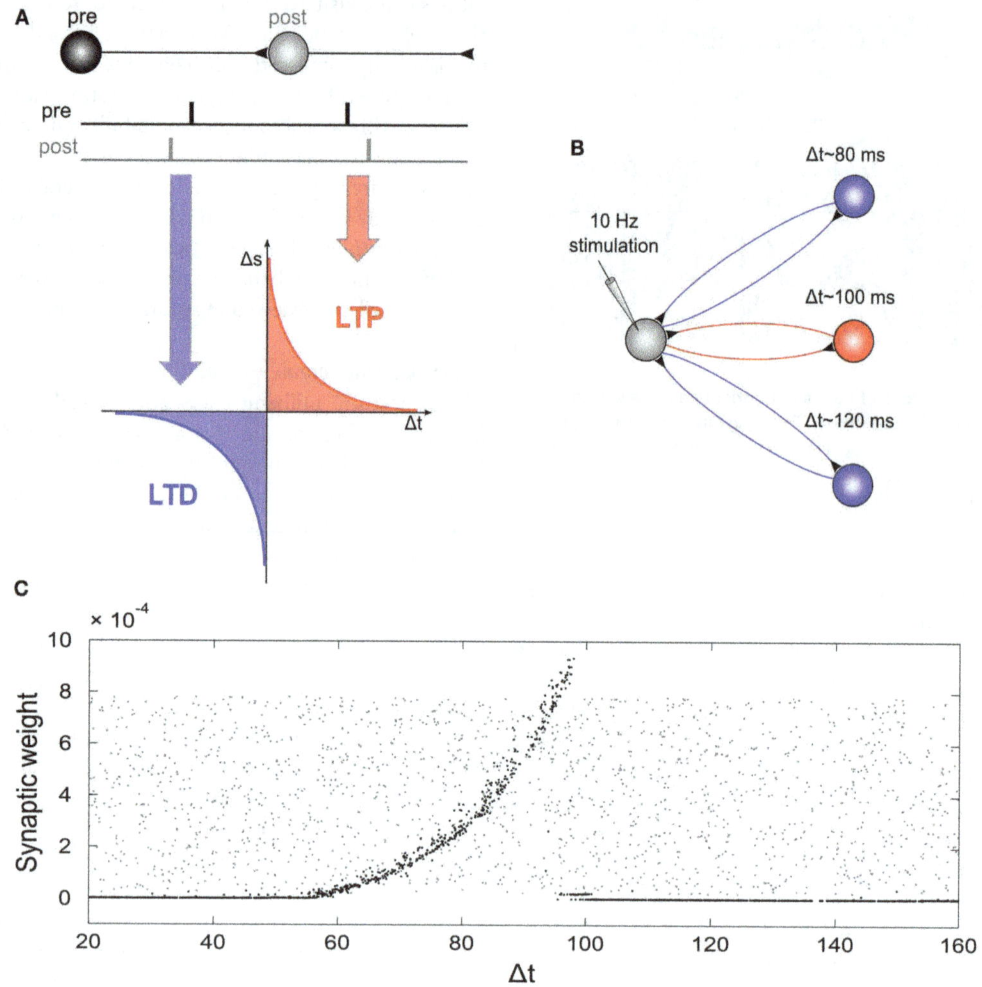

FIGURE 6 | Network simulation of tACS. (A) Spike timing dependent plasticity: synaptic weights are increased if a post-synaptic potential follows a pre-synaptic spike (long-term potentiation, LTP) and decreased if a post-synaptic potential occurs prior to a pre-synaptic spike (long-term depression, LTD). **(B)** Schematic illustration of the network: A driving neuron establishes a recurrent loop with each neuron of a hidden layer. The total synaptic delay, Δt, (i.e., the sum of both delays of the loop) varied between 20 and 160 ms. The driving neuron was stimulated with a spike train of 10 Hz repetition rate. **(C)** Synaptic weights of the back-projection as a function of the total synaptic delay of the recurrent loops: Gray dots display synaptic weights at the start of the simulation, black dots represent synaptic weights after the end of simulation. External stimulation of the driving neuron at 10 Hz resulted in increased weights for recurrent loops with a total delay between 60 and 100 ms, and dramatically reduced synaptic weights for loops with total delays outside this interval. Note, that the highest synaptic weights are observed at 100 ms, i.e., for loops with a resonance frequency near the stimulation frequency. Reprinted from Zaehle et al. (2010) with permission of the authors.

stimulation. Even higher frequencies (1000, 2000, and 5000 Hz; 10 min; 0.20 A/m^2) are also able to modulate cortical excitability (Chaieb et al., 2011). Increased excitability has been reported during and up to 90 min after stimulation. This effect was most pronounced for 5000 Hz and was interpreted as an interference with neuronal membrane excitation but not entrainment of neural oscillations.

Behavioral effects

Diverse behavioral effects after applying different tACS frequencies raise the possibility to causally link specific frequencies to distinct functions. A significant role takes the beta rhythm (15–30 Hz) as the "natural frequency" of motor regions (Rosanova et al., 2009). Beta synchrony correlates with slower voluntary movement (Gilbertson et al., 2005). In the same way, tACS with 20 Hz slowed down voluntary movement, indicating a causal relationship (Pogosyan et al., 2009; Joundi et al., 2012; Wach et al., 2013).

Applying two different tACS frequencies allows to dissociate frequency-behavior relationships. Joundi et al. (2012) found that 20 Hz tACS (5 s; ~0.26 A/m^2) slowed down voluntary movement, but 70 Hz tACS with the same parameters increased the performance, extending correlative studies which found increased gamma band activity (30–70 Hz) during voluntary movement (Muthukumaraswamy, 2010). Besides the 20 Hz slowing effect, Wach et al. (2013) observed an increased behavioral variability after 10 Hz tACS with the same parameters (10 min, 0.29 A/m^2). The authors attributed the 10 Hz effect to a disruption of an internal pacemaker represented by activity in the alpha range. Interestingly, both effects occurred at different time points: the 20 Hz effect was found immediately after stimulation, but not after 30 min, conversely to the 10 Hz effect.

Electrophysiological effects

A major drawback of the present studies on the effects of tACS/otDCS is the lack of electrophysiological evidence. This is rather unfortunate in light of the assumption that tACS and otDCS interact with oscillatory brain activity. Although studies on the effects of tACS/otDCS on motor processes imply the promising advantage to demonstrate changes in the EEG, so far, only few studies reported electrophysiological results. Stimulation with different frequencies (1, 10, 15, 30, 45 Hz) yielded no EEG effects after tACS/otDCS with different frequencies (Antal et al., 2008). But, as mentioned above, weak stimulation intensity could explain absent effects.

Future studies, combining tACS/otDCS and EEG, could be helpful in two different aspects. First, changes in EEG frequency bands, e.g., parameters like power and synchrony, could be related to the previously reported behavioral effects, further strengthening the assumption of a causal oscillation-behavior relationship. Second, by comparing the specific effects after tACS/otDCS and tDCS, contributions of the constant and time varying part of the stimulation could be disentangled. Particular attention should be paid to frequencies that are predominant in the EEG during specific tasks, because tACS/otDCS might only be effective to entrain physiologically relevant rhythms (Thut et al., 2011).

SENSORY PROCESSING

Phosphenes induced by tACS: cortical or retinal origin?

The earliest effect of tACS on the human visual system was reported by Kanai et al. (2008). These authors studied the influence of different tACS frequencies on the detection of phosphenes induced by tACS over visual cortex (stimulation electrode of 3 × 4 cm placed 4 cm above the inion; reference electrode of 9 × 6 cm placed at the vertex). Participants were stimulated at 5 different intensities (125, 250, 500, 750, and 1000 μA) with 12 frequencies ranging from 4 to 40 Hz in randomized order with each frequency being applied 5 s in the light and 5 s in the dark, consecutively. After stimulation, participants had to rate the phosphenes in both conditions with respect to a standard phosphene induced by tACS with 16 Hz at 1000 μA in the light (maximum current density under the stimulation electrode 0.83 A/m^2). The results indicated that the effectiveness of tACS indeed varied with stimulation frequency and that this effect was moderated by the surrounding light conditions. In a dark room, stimulation was most effective in the range of 10–12 Hz, whereas in a light room, phosphene thresholds were lowest for stimulation in a frequency range between 14 and 20 Hz. In a second experiment, these results were replicated by measuring phosphene detection thresholds. The authors explained their results with the change of dominant oscillation frequencies in the natural EEG with respect to different light conditions: in darkness, the most prominent oscillations are found in the alpha range (8–12 Hz), which are, however, suppressed and replaced by higher frequencies in the light.

Although Kanai et al. (2008) assumed that their finding of tACS-induced phosphenes results from an excitatory tACS effect on parts of the visual cortex, this view has been questioned subsequently by Schwiedrzik (2009). This author referred to earlier work demonstrating that AC can reliably excite retinal ganglion cells and that the frequency at which this effect occurs depends upon the dark adaptation of the retina (Schwarz, 1947). Phosphenes are absent when retinal ganglion cells are inhibited due to pressure on the eyeball (Rohracher, 1935). In line with this argumentation favoring a retinal phosphene origin, it has been demonstrated that a more anterior placement of tACS electrodes over fronto-central areas leads to stronger phosphenes than a more posterior placement over occipito-central regions (Schutter and Hortensius, 2010). These findings have been replicated recently by Kar and Krekelberg (2012). However, Paulus (2010) argues that the intracranial electric field induced by typical tACS studies is below published thresholds of retinal sensitivity.

In a further attempt to identify the visual cortex as the site of interaction between tACS and the visual system, Kanai et al. (2010) delivered TMS impulses to the visual cortex while tACS was applied to the posterior part of the brain at different frequencies. The threshold needed to evoke a phosphene via TMS was recorded depending on tACS frequency. The results demonstrated that excitability is modulated by tACS in a frequency-dependent manner with maximal excitation at 20 Hz stimulation frequency as indexed by lowest phosphene thresholds. While this finding does not rule out a retinal origin of phosphenes for the previous study (Kanai et al., 2008), it supports the hypothesis that tACS modulates excitability of the visual cortex.

Visual, auditory, and somatosensory processing

In a visual study on contrast perception, Laczó et al. (2012) applied tACS in the gamma range (40, 60, 80 Hz) with the stimulation electrode (4 × 4 cm) over the central visual cortex and the reference (7 × 4 cm) over the vertex. Using a stimulation current of 1500 μA, the maximum current density in the stimulation electrode was 0.94 A/m^2. Participants had to detect stationary random dot patterns in a four-alternative forced-choice paradigm. Results revealed that contrast sensitivity was not modulated by tACS, whereas contrast discrimination thresholds decreased during 60 Hz tACS relative to sham stimulation, but not during 40 or 80 Hz.

Brignani et al. (2013) presented leftward or rightward tilted low-contrast Gabor patches for 30 ms within the left or right visual hemifield, while participants received either sham stimulation or tACS at 6, 10, or 25 Hz with 1000 μA intensity (maximum current density in the electrode: 0.63 A/m^2). The stimulation electrode (16 cm^2) was placed over the left or right parietal-occipital regions and the reference (35 cm^2) over the vertex. Participants had to report whether a Gabor patch was present or not (detection task) and whether it was tilted to the left or right (discrimination task). It was hypothesized that entraining alpha oscillations via 10 Hz tACS would increase the inhibitory alpha-effects at the target region of the stimulated hemisphere, thereby decreasing the accuracy in perceiving stimuli presented in the contralateral hemifield. Although the results demonstrated the expected accuracy decrease for 10 Hz tACS compared to sham and 25 Hz tACS, this effect was only found for the detection task and it was not hemifield-specific. The lack of hemispheric specificity might be due to the bi-hemispheric reference electrode. Moreover, the accuracy effects obtained with 10 Hz tACS did not differ significantly from those of 6 Hz tACS, leaving the issue of frequency specificity uncertain.

In an auditory detection paradigm, Neuling et al. (2012a) revealed dependencies between auditory detection performance and the phase of alpha oscillations over the temporal cortex. Participants were stimulated with otDCS at 10 Hz (DC of 1000 μA, modulated by a sinusoidal current of 425 μA) while having to detect a 500 Hz tone embedded in white noise at seven different signal-to-noise ratios (ranging from −4 to 8 dB). Electrodes were placed at temporal locations (cathode over left temporal cortex; anode over right temporal cortex). Results indicated that detection thresholds were modulated by the phase of the otDCS stimulation, demonstrating a causal link between oscillatory phase and perception. Furthermore, alpha power in the spontaneous EEG after stimulation was significantly increased relative to pre-stimulation alpha power, replicating the results of Zaehle et al. (2010).

Feurra et al. (2011b) studied the frequency-dependency of tactile sensations induced by tACS. The stimulation electrode (3 × 4 cm) was placed over the right somatosensory cortex, the reference electrode (5 × 7 cm) over the left posterior parietal cortex. The stimulation intensity of 1500 μA resulted in a maximum current density of 0.63 A/m^2 in the stimulation electrode. Participants were stimulated at 35 different frequencies ranging from 2 to 70 Hz in randomized order for 5 s each and had to rate the presence and intensity of tactile sensations in their left hand. Results showed that stimulation in the alpha (10–14 Hz) and high gamma (52–70 Hz) range was significantly more effective in eliciting tactile sensations than stimulation in the delta (2–4 Hz) or the theta (6–8 Hz) range. Furthermore, beta stimulation (16–20 Hz) was more effective than that in the theta range.

Together, most of the studies on sensory processing demonstrate frequency-dependent perceptual consequences of tACS within different modalities and, thereby, the effectiveness of tACS in modulating ongoing rhythmic brain activity. However, the study by Brignani et al. (2013) represents a case of uncertain frequency specificity, i.e., yielding expected null results for one but not for another control frequency. Therefore, these findings are neither evidence against nor in favor of the possibility of tACS to modulate brain oscillations. In addition to frequency, the study by Neuling et al. (2012a) underlines the importance of oscillatory phase in entraining brain oscillations via tACS.

HIGHER COGNITIVE PROCESSES

Memory

Anodal otDCS has been used to study the functional roles of different brain oscillations in the formation of declarative memories during sleep and wakefulness. Marshall et al. (2006) focused on the association between slow oscillatory brain activity (<1 Hz) and sleep-dependent memory consolidation. After a learning period, participants were stimulated bilaterally at frontolateral locations with otDCS at 0.75 Hz (maximum current density in electrode: 5.17 A/m^2) to boost slow oscillations that occur naturally during non-rapid eye movement (non-REM) sleep. Stimulation was applied for five 5-min periods separated by 1 min intervals without stimulation, during which EEG activity was analyzed. The results demonstrated a stimulation-induced increase of slow wave sleep (SWS) during the stimulation-free epochs, as reflected by an EEG power increase in the 0.5–1.0 Hz band. Slow frontal spindle activity (8–12 Hz) was also enhanced. On the behavioral level, the memory improvement after sleep compared with evening performance before sleep was stronger following otDCS than sham stimulation. Furthermore, both the electrophysiological and behavioral effects were frequency specific, since otDCS at 5 Hz (theta-tDCS) did not improve memory and reduced the power of slow oscillations.

Recently, the impact of theta-tDCS on memory consolidation and EEG activity has been investigated in more detail (Marshall et al., 2011). Using the same experimental setup as Marshall et al. (2006), theta-tDCS during non-REM sleep impaired memory consolidation and reduced both slow oscillations and frontal spindle activity. Thus, the theta-tDCS results were opposite to the effects induced by slow oscillatory stimulation, but they replicated the findings of the control condition using otDCS at 5 Hz from Marshall et al. (2006). Whereas these findings support a functional role for these oscillations in sleep-dependent memory consolidation during non-REM sleep, applying theta-tDCS during REM sleep did not affect consolidation, but produced a strong and widespread increase of gamma (25–45 Hz) power. These findings indicate a synchronizing effect of the theta rhythm on gamma oscillations that has no direct impact on memory consolidation during REM sleep (Marshall et al., 2011).

Whereas the study by Marshall et al. (2006) demonstrated a causal role of slow oscillations in declarative memory consolidation during sleep, Kirov et al. (2009) examined the impact of the same otDCS protocol on EEG and memory when applied during wakefulness. In analogy to the Marshall et al. (2006) study, stimulation of the participants started ~20 min after the end of the learning period and EEG was recorded until 1 h after stimulation has ended. Recall performance was tested after a 7 h retention period following learning. Electrophysiologically, otDCS at 0.75 Hz induced an EEG power increase in the slow oscillation frequency band that was restricted to frontal sites, however, the most pronounced and widespread power enhancement was found in the theta band (4–8 Hz). At the behavioral level, stimulation of the waking brain had no effect on memory consolidation after learning. Interestingly, when Kirov et al. (2009) applied stimulation during the learning period, i.e., while the material had to be encoded, learning performance improved as assessed by immediate recall performance.

Together, these studies demonstrate that the effects of otDCS on oscillatory EEG activity and related memory processes depend critically on the prevailing brain-state, i.e., whether stimulation was applied during wakefulness (Kirov et al., 2009), non-REM sleep (Marshall et al., 2006), or REM sleep (Marshall et al., 2011). A similar brain-state dependency of oscillatory brain stimulation has been shown for the visual (Kanai et al., 2008) and motor domain (Bergmann et al., 2009).

Using a working memory task, Polanía et al. (2012) tested the relevance of fronto-parietal theta phase-coupling for cognitive performance. In a first EEG experiment, the authors found an increase of phase synchronization between left frontal and parietal electrode sites at 4–7 Hz during memory matching. Furthermore, reaction times in the matching periods were faster when the phase lag between frontal and parietal oscillations was near to 0°. In a subsequent tACS experiment, Polanía et al. (2012) stimulated this fronto-parietal network with an oscillatory current at 6 Hz with a relative 0 or 180° phase difference or applied sham stimulation. As hypothesized by the authors, reaction times decreased during synchronization of fronto-parietal regions with 0° phase lag and increased during desynchronization with 180° compared to sham stimulation. Applying tACS at a control frequency of 35 Hz had no effect. These tACS results provide causal evidence for the relevance of theta phase-coupling during cognitive performance in a working memory task.

Ambiguous perception

In a recent study with ambiguous visual stimuli, Strüber et al. (2013) applied 40 Hz tACS over occipital-parietal regions of both hemispheres while bistable apparent motion stimuli were presented which can be perceived as moving either horizontally or vertically (**Figure 7A**, top). In this paradigm, the switch between horizontal and vertical apparent motion is likely to involve a change in interhemispheric functional coupling. When 40 Hz tACS was applied with 180° phase difference between hemispheres (**Figure 7A**, bottom), the proportion of horizontal motion perception decreased significantly compared to sham stimulation (**Figure 7B**). Furthermore, EEG was recorded offline, i.e., 3 min before (pre-tACS) and after (post-tACS) applying tACS. After tACS, the interhemispheric gamma-band coherence increased between left and right parietal-occipital electrodes as compared to pre-tACS. This was not the case for sham stimulation (**Figure 7C**). Interestingly, when 40 Hz tACS was applied with 0° phase difference between hemispheres or with a control frequency of 6 Hz no behavioral or EEG-effects were observed (not shown here). These results were interpreted as evidence in favor of a causal role for gamma band oscillations in the perception of bistable apparent motion stimuli. It was further hypothesized that the external desynchronization of gamma oscillations via 40 Hz tACS with 180° interhemispheric phase difference might impair interhemispheric motion integration by a functional decoupling of the hemispheres.

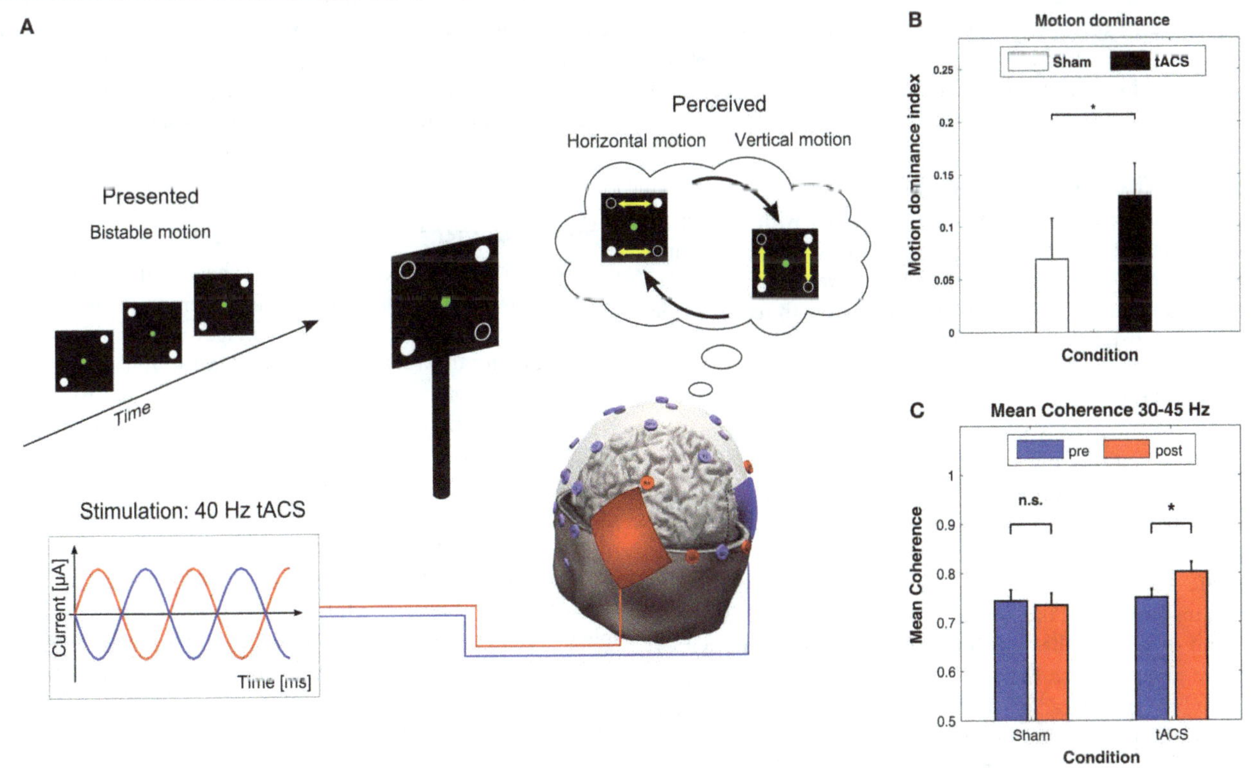

FIGURE 7 | Effects of 40 Hz tACS with 180° phase difference between hemispheres. (A) Configuration of the bistable apparent motion display together with the EEG and tACS electrode montage. EEG electrodes that were used for analyzing interhemispheric coherence are indicated in red. The tACS sponge electrodes were placed bilaterally over the parietal-occipital cortex. This montage leads to 40 Hz stimulation with 180° phase difference between hemispheres. **(B)** The motion dominance index is significantly enhanced during 40 Hz tACS (black bar) as compared to sham stimulation (white bar), indicating that 40 Hz tACS results in a longer total duration of perceived vertical motion (*$P < 0.05$). Error bars display the standard error of the mean. **(C)** Mean coherence within the 30–45 Hz frequency band shows a significant increase from pre-tACS to post-tACS (right), but not from pre-sham to post-sham (left). Error bars correspond to standard errors of the mean; *$P < 0.05$. Adapted from Strüber et al. (2013) with permission of the authors.

This study by Strüber et al. (2013), together with the abovementioned findings of Polanía et al. (2012), demonstrates that tACS can be used to couple or decouple inter-areal oscillatory activity either between or within hemispheres, which strongly supports the role of phase synchronization for large-scale neuronal integration (Engel et al., 2001; Varela et al., 2001; Siegel et al., 2012).

Decision-making

Sela et al. (2012) applied theta tACS to either the left or right dorsolateral prefrontal cortex (DLPFC) while participants performed a task that requires decision-making under risk. The rationale was to examine the laterality effects on risk-taking behavior. Stimulation was delivered during the task for 15 min (starting 5 min before task) using tACS with a frequency of 6.5 Hz and an intensity of 1 mA. One group of participants received tACS over the left hemisphere, one over the right, and another group received sham stimulation. EEG was not recorded. Only left hemispheric stimulation resulted in a significant effect on behavior, in that participants adopted a riskier decision-making strategy compared to right hemispheric stimulation and sham. According to the authors, these findings demonstrate a causal influence of both the DLPFC and theta oscillations on decision-making style. However, Sela et al. (2012) did not apply a control frequency, leaving the issue of frequency-specificity of the reported effects unaddressed. In this context, Feurra et al. (2012) pointed out that the inclusion of other frequencies that have been related to risky decision-making could have changed the pattern of results.

OPEN QUESTIONS/FUTURE PERSPECTIVES

The reviewed studies are rather heterogeneous with respect to the experimental design and subsequent results. In the following sections, we critically discuss experimental parameters, as well as giving suggestions to overcome major concerns with regard to the validity of the results of tACS studies.

STIMULATION FREQUENCY

If the goal of a study is to demonstrate that tACS can modulate brain oscillations, the stimulation frequency should coincide with an existing brain oscillation, i.e., should be applied in a frequency range from delta (~0.5–4 Hz) to high gamma (~200 Hz). If a further goal of the study is to demonstrate that tACS can modulate a cognitive process which is associated with a certain brain oscillation, the stimulation frequency should match the brain oscillation that has been reported to correlate with a cognitive process. Since EEG frequencies vary inter-individually, this may require to adapt the stimulation frequency to the individual frequency that needs to be determined via EEG as in the case of stimulation at participants' IAF (Zaehle et al., 2010).

STIMULATION INTENSITY

In the past, two procedures have been used to address the problem of stimulation intensity. Either all participants were stimulated at the same intensity or intensity was adapted to an individual threshold (e.g., phosphene or somatosensory threshold). Both procedures have certain advantages and disadvantages. If all participants are stimulated at the same intensity, this reduces the effort for determining individual thresholds, but, on the other hand, makes it possible that some participants sense the stimulation (via skin sensation or phosphenes), whereas others do not. This could, in principle, introduce a confound since more sensitive participants would be able to differentiate between stimulation and sham blocks, whereas less sensitive participants would not. To tackle this issue, two procedures have been established that conceal which block is currently performed. The first procedure is to fade-in the stimulation amplitude over a time interval of ~30 s. This reduces the skin sensations and has been applied frequently in tDCS studies where it is referred to as ramping-in. The second procedure consists of a short stimulation period at the beginning of a sham block which is faded out after ~30 s. This procedure mimics a stimulation block, because the stimulation is usually not felt consistently but only during the first seconds following the start of a stimulation block. When stimulation intensities are adapted to individual thresholds, confounds due to phosphenes or skin sensations can be excluded as alternative explanations for any observed effects. An obvious disadvantage of this method is that the intracranial current density can vary considerably across subjects. This problem, however, applies to both procedures as different skull thicknesses may also result in a significant variation of intracranial current densities. An ideal solution would be to acquire individual MR images in order to perform finite element modeling for each participant. Of course, this would require great effort both in terms of measurement time and computation time. Thus, if modeling is not feasible, the pros and cons of the different procedures have to be carefully balanced.

ELECTRODE MONTAGE

As indicated above, modeling studies have demonstrated that current flow is not always maximal underneath the stimulation electrode. In addition, new montages with multiple small electrodes offer the advantage of more focal stimulation as compared to two large electrodes. However, small electrodes also make skin sensations more likely due to increased current density if the intensity is kept constant. Again, the ideal solution would be to acquire individual MR images and to determine where to place electrodes based on the desired target region within the brain. At least two tools are currently freely available that allow this: SIMNIBs (http://simnibs.org) and Bonsai (http://neuralengr.com/bonsai). If this is not feasible, it would be desirable to compare the intended electrode montage with published modeling studies. For example, Neuling et al. (2012b) reported intracranial current density distributions of multiple electrode montages that have previously been used in cognitive experiments and therapeutic applications.

CONTROL CONDITIONS

A hitherto unsolved question is how to design an optimal control condition. Such a control or placebo condition should be identical to the stimulation or verum condition with respect to treatment duration, all possible sensations, time of day, experimenter, etc. but should not achieve the same cognitive or therapeutic effect.

In addition, it would be desirable to carry out the two conditions in a double-blind procedure, i.e., neither experimenter nor participant know whether the verum or placebo stimulation is applied. One approach to achieve this goal would be to adapt stimulation intensities to be below certain thresholds for each participant—thus assuring that neither verum nor placebo stimulation can be sensed. However, as noted above, this results in significant variation of stimulation intensity across participants which is undesirable for comparable effects. Therefore, another approach is to apply identical stimulation intensity in all participants above threshold. In that case, participants will sense the onset of stimulation in both conditions. In the placebo condition, however, the stimulation will be ramped down after a few seconds. If the only goal of a study were to demonstrate that tACS has an effect as compared to no stimulation, the placebo condition could be sham stimulation. If, however, frequency specificity of tACS effects were to be demonstrated, the placebo conditions need to be a tACS stimulation at different frequencies. The study by Brignani et al. (2013) raises the question for appropriate control frequencies, since the use of multiple control frequencies was only partially successful. Ideally, the placebo conditions should apply two frequencies above and below the frequency of the verum condition demonstrating that the cognitive effect is absent or diminished at those control frequencies (Thut et al., 2011). Importantly, the frequency of the placebo condition should not be related to other cognitive effects such as memory which might be involved in the cognitive process at hand. It has to be noted, however, that currently no clear procedure has been established that defines the number of control frequencies or the distance in Hertz from the frequency of the verum condition in order to unequivocally demonstrate frequency specificity.

CONCLUSION

An increasing number of studies on sensory, motor, and even higher cognitive processing demonstrates the effectiveness of tACS in modulating ongoing rhythmic activity in the human brain which, in turn, affects behavior. Interestingly, it has been demonstrated that, in addition to amplitude and frequency, also oscillatory phase plays a crucial role. Our understanding of the electrophysiological mechanisms of tACS has profited enormously from recent animal studies and computer simulations. In addition, realistically shaped models of the human head and brain have been successfully applied to further our knowledge of the intracranial current flow induced by tACS. Until recently, associations between cognitive processes and brain oscillations have been established via correlation. Using tACS offers the unique possibility to demonstrate a causal link between brain oscillations of a specific frequency and a specific cognitive process. If the brain oscillation is manipulated, the associated cognitive function is expected to co-vary. In case such co-variations can be demonstrated, a causal role of the oscillatory process must be assumed for the associated cognitive process. Recordings in animals have demonstrated convincingly that sinusoidal currents can entrain endogenous brain oscillations. However, so far, simultaneous recordings of EEG during tACS were not feasible due to strong artifacts. For future investigations, it would be worthwhile to combine electrophysiological recordings with tACS in order to shed further light on the neural mechanisms of brain entrainment.

ACKNOWLEDGMENTS

The work was supported by the Deutsche Forschungsgemeinschaft (DFG) with grants RA 2357/1-1 (Stefan Rach, Daniel Strüber) and SFB/TRR 31 (Christoph S. Herrmann).

REFERENCES

Antal, A., Bikson, M., Datta, A., Lafon, B., Dechent, P., Parra, L. C., et al. (2013). Imaging artifacts induced by electrical stimulation during conventional fMRI of the brain. *Neuroimage*. doi: 10.1016/j.neuroimage.2012.10.026. [Epub ahead of print].

Antal, A., Boros, K., Poreisz, C., Chaieb, L., Terney, D., and Paulus, W. (2008). Comparatively weak after-effects of transcranial alternating current stimulation (tACS) on cortical excitability in humans. *Brain Stimul.* 1, 97–105. doi: 10.1016/j.brs.2007.10.001

Antal, A., and Paulus, W. (2012). Investigating neuroplastic changes in the human brain induced by transcranial direct (tDCS) and alternating current (tACS) stimulation methods. *Clin. EEG Neurosci.* 43, 175. doi: 10.1177/1550059412448030

Başar, E., Başar-Eroglu, C., Karakaş, S., and Schürmann, M. (2001). Gamma, alpha, delta, and theta oscillations govern cognitive processes. *Int. J. Psychophysiol.* 39, 241–248. doi: 10.1016/S0167-8760(00)00145-8

Bergmann, T. O., Groppa, S., Seeger, M., Mölle, M., Marshall, L., and Siebner, H. R. (2009). Acute changes in motor cortical excitability during slow oscillatory and constant anodal transcranial direct current stimulation. *J. Neurophysiol.* 102, 2303–2311. doi: 10.1152/jn.00437.2009

Brignani, D., Ruzzoli, M., Mauri, P., and Miniussi, C. (2013). Is transcranial alternating current stimulation effective in modulating brain oscillations? *PLoS ONE* 8:e56589. doi: 10.1371/journal.pone.0056589

Brocke, J., Schmidt, S., Irlbacher, K., Cichy, R. M., and Brandt, S. A. (2008). Transcranial cortex stimulation and fMRI: electrophysiological correlates of dual-pulse BOLD signal modulation. *Neuroimage* 40, 631–643. doi: 10.1016/j.neuroimage.2007.11.057

Canolty, R. T., Edwards, E., Dalal, S. S., Soltani, M., Nagarajan, S. S., Kirsch, H. E., et al. (2006). High gamma power is phase-locked to theta oscillations in human neocortex. *Science* 313, 1626–1628. doi: 10.1126/science.1128115

Chaieb, L., Antal, A., and Paulus, W. (2011). Transcranial alternating current stimulation in the low kHz range increases motor cortex excitability. *Restor. Neurol. Neurosci.* 29, 167–175. doi: 10.3233/RNN-2011-0589

Datta, A., Bansal, V., Diaz, J., Patel, J., Reato, D., and Bikson, M. (2009). Gyri-precise head model of transcranial DC stimulation: improved spatial focality using a ring electrode versus conventional rectangular pad. *Brain Stimul.* 2, 201–207. doi: 10.1016/j.brs.2009.03.005

Demiralp, T., Bayraktaroglu, Z., Lenz, D., Junge, S., Busch, N. A., Maess, B., et al. (2007). Gamma amplitudes are coupled to theta phase in human EEG during visual perception. *Int. J. Psychophysiol.* 64, 24–30. doi: 10.1016/j.ijpsycho.2006.07.005

Dmochowski, J. P., Datta, A., Bikson, M., Su, Y., and Parra, L. C. (2011). Optimized multi-electrode stimulation increases focality and intensity at target. *J. Neural Eng.* 8:046011. doi: 10.1088/1741-2560/8/4/046011

Engel, A. K., Fries, P., and Singer, W. (2001). Dynamic predictions: oscillations and synchrony in top-down processing. *Nat. Rev. Neurosci.* 2, 704–716. doi: 10.1038/35094565

Faria, P., Leal, A., and Miranda, P. C. (2009). Comparing different electrode configurations using the 10-10 international system in tDCS: a finite element model analysis. *Annu. Int. Conf. IEEE Eng. Med. Biol. Soc.* 2009, 1596–1599. doi: 10.1109/IEMBS.2009.5334121

Feurra, M., Bianco, G., Santarnecchi, E., Del Testa, M., Rossi, A., and Rossi, S. (2011a). Frequency-dependent tuning of the human motor system induced by transcranial oscillatory potentials. *J. Neurosci.* 31, 12165–12670.

doi: 10.1523/JNEUROSCI.0978-11. 2011

Feurra, M., Paulus, W., Walsh, V., and Kanai, R. (2011b). Frequency specific modulation of human somatosensory cortex. *Front. Psychol.* 2:13. doi: 10.3389/fpsyg.2011.00013

Feurra, M., Galli, G., and Rossi, S. (2012). Transcranial alternating current stimulation affects decision making. *Front. Syst. Neurosci.* 6:39. doi: 10.3389/fnsys.2012.00039

Fröhlich, F., and McCormick, D. A. (2010). Endogenous electric fields may guide neocortical network activity. *Neuron* 67, 129–143. doi: 10.1016/j.neuron.2010.06.005

Gilbertson, T., Lalo, E., Doyle, L., Di Lazzaro, V., Cioni, B., and Brown, P. (2005). Existing motor state is favored at the expense of new movement during 13–35 Hz oscillatory synchrony in the human corticospinal system. *J. Neurosci.* 25, 7771–7779. doi: 10.1523/JNEUROSCI.1762-05. 2005

Groppa, S., Bergmann, T. O., Siems, C., Mölle, M., Marshall, L., and Siebner, H. R. (2010). Slow-oscillatory transcranial direct current stimulation can induce bidirectional shifts in motor cortical excitability in awake humans. *Neuroscience* 166, 1219–1225. doi: 10.1016/j.neuroscience.2010.01.019

Herrmann, C. S., and Demiralp, T. (2005). Human EEG gamma oscillations in neuropsychiatric disorders. *Clin. Neurophysiol.* 116, 2719–2733. doi: 10.1016/j.clinph.2005.07.007

Herrmann, C. S., Munk, M. H. J., and Engel, A. K. (2004). Cognitive functions of gamma-band activity: memory match and utilization. *Trends Cogn. Sci.* 8, 347–355. doi: 10.1016/j.tics.2004.06.006

Hodgkin, A. L., and Huxley, A. F. (1952). A quantitative description of membrane current and its application to conduction and excitation in nerve. *J. Physiol.* 117, 500–544.

Holdefer, R. N., Sadleir, R., and Russell, M. J. (2006). Predicted current densities in the brain during transcranial electrical stimulation. *Clin. Neurophysiol.* 117, 1388–1397. doi: 10.1016/j.clinph.2006.02.020

Izhikevich, E. M. (2003). Simple model of spiking neurons. *IEEE Trans. Neural Netw.* 14, 1569–1572. doi: 10.1109/TNN.2003.820440

Jensen, O., and Colgin, L. L. (2007). Cross-frequency coupling between neuronal oscillations. *Trends Cogn. Sci.* 11, 267–269. doi: 10.1016/j.tics.2007.05.003

Joundi, R. A., Jenkinson, N., Brittain, J.-S., Aziz, T. Z., and Brown, P. (2012). Driving oscillatory activity in the human cortex enhances motor performance. *Curr. Biol.* 22, 403–407. doi: 10.1016/j.cub.2012.01.024

Kanai, R., Chaieb, L., Antal, A., Walsh, V., and Paulus, W. (2008). Frequency-dependent electrical stimulation of the visual cortex. *Curr. Biol.* 18, 1839–1843. doi: 10.1016/j.cub.2008.10.027

Kanai, R., Paulus, W., and Walsh, V. (2010). Transcranial alternating current stimulation (tACS) modulates cortical excitability as assessed by TMS-induced phosphene thresholds. *Clin. Neurophysiol.* 121, 1551–1554. doi: 10.1016/j.clinph.2010.03.022

Kar, K., and Krekelberg, B. (2012). Transcranial electrical stimulation over visual cortex evokes phosphenes with a retinal origin. *J. Neurophysiol.* 108, 2173–2178. doi: 10.1152/jn.00505.2012

Kirov, R., Weiss, C., Siebner, H. R., Born, J., and Marshall, L. (2009). Slow oscillation electrical brain stimulation during waking promotes EEG theta activity and memory encoding. *Proc. Natl. Acad. Sci. U.S.A.* 106, 15460–15465. doi: 10.1073/pnas.0904438106

Lacz6, B., Antal, A., Niebergall, R., Treue, S., and Paulus, W. (2012). Transcranial alternating stimulation in a high gamma frequency range applied over V1 improves contrast perception but does not modulate spatial attention. *Brain Stimul.* 5, 484–491. doi: 10.1016/j.brs.2011.08.008

Lenz, D., Krauel, K., Schadow, J., Baving, L., Duzel, E., and Herrmann, C. S. (2008). Enhanced gamma-band activity in ADHD patients lacks correlation with memory performance found in healthy children. *Brain Res.* 1235, 117–132. doi: 10.1016/j.brainres.2008.06.023

Marshall, L., Helgadóttir, H., Mölle, M., and Born, J. (2006). Boosting slow oscillations during sleep potentiates memory. *Nature* 444, 610–613. doi: 10.1038/nature05278

Marshall, L., Kirov, R., Brade, J., Mölle, M., and Born, J. (2011). Transcranial electrical currents to probe EEG brain rhythms and memory consolidation during sleep in humans. *PLoS ONE* 6:e16905. doi: 10.1371/journal.pone.0016905

Merlet, I., Birot, G., Salvador, R., Molaee-Ardekani, B., Mekonnen, A., Soria-Frish, A., et al. (2013). From oscillatory transcranial current stimulation to scalp EEG changes: a biophysical and physiological modeling study. *PLoS ONE* 8:e57330. doi: 10.1371/journal.pone.0057330

Miranda, P. C., Lomarev, M., and Hallett, M. (2006). Modeling the current distribution during transcranial direct current stimulation. *Clin. Neurophysiol.* 117, 1623–1629. doi: 10.1016/j.clinph.2006.04.009

Miranda, P. C., Mekonnen, A., Salvador, R., and Ruffini, G. (2012). The electric field in the cortex during transcranial current stimulation. *Neuroimage* 70C, 48–58. doi: 10.1016/j.neuroimage. 2012.12.034

Moliadze, V., Antal, A., and Paulus, W. (2010). Boosting brain excitability by transcranial high frequency stimulation in the ripple range. *J. Physiol.* 588, 4891–4904. doi: 10.1113/jphysiol.2010.196998

Moliadze, V., Atalay, D., Antal, A., and Paulus, W. (2012). Close to threshold transcranial electrical stimulation preferentially activates inhibitory networks before switching to excitation with higher intensities. *Brain Stimul.* 5, 505–511. doi: 10.1016/j.brs.2011.11.004

Muthukumaraswamy, S. D. (2010). Functional properties of human primary motor cortex gamma oscillations. *J. Neurophysiol.* 104, 2873–2885. doi: 10.1152/jn.00607.2010

Neuling, T., Rach, S., and Herrmann, C. S. (2013). Orchestrating neuronal networks: sustained after-effects of transcranial alternating current stimulation depend upon brain states. *Front. Hum. Neurosci.* 7:161. doi: 10.3389/fnhum.2013.00161

Neuling, T., Rach, S., Wagner, S., Wolters, C. H., and Herrmann, C. S. (2012a). Good vibrations: oscillatory phase shapes perception. *Neuroimage* 63, 771–778. doi: 10.1016/j.neuroimage.2012.07.024

Neuling, T., Wagner, S., Wolters, C. H., Zaehle, T., and Herrmann, C. S. (2012b). Finite-element model predicts current density distribution for clinical applications of tDCS and tACS. *Front. Psychiatry* 3:83. doi: 10.3389/fpsyt.2012.00083

Nowak, L. G., and Bullier, J. (1998). Axons, but not cell bodies, are activated by electrical stimulation in cortical gray matter. I. Evidence from chronaxie measurements. *Exp. Brain Res.* 118, 477–488. doi: 10.1007/s002210050304

Ozen, S., Sirota, A., Belluscio, M. A., Anastassiou, C. A., Stark, E., Koch, C., et al. (2010). Transcranial electric stimulation entrains cortical neuronal populations in rats. *J. Neurosci.* 30, 11476–11485. doi: 10.1523/JNEUROSCI.5252-09.2010

Paulus, W. (2010). On the difficulties of separating retinal from cortical origins of phosphenes when using transcranial alternating current stimulation (tACS). *Clin. Neurophysiol.* 121, 987–991. doi: 10.1016/j.clinph.2010.01.029

Paulus, W. (2011). Transcranial electrical stimulation (tES - tDCS; tRNS, tACS) methods. *Neuropsychol. Rehabil.* 21, 602–617. doi: 10.1080/09602011.2011.557292

Pikovsky, A., Rosenblum, M., and Kurths, J. (2003). *Synchronization: a Universal Concept in Nonlinear Sciences.* Cambridge: Cambridge University Press.

Pogosyan, A., Gaynor, L. D., Eusebio, A., and Brown, P. (2009). Boosting cortical activity at Beta-band frequencies slows movement in humans. *Curr. Biol.* 19, 1637–1641. doi: 10.1016/j.cub.2009.07.074

Polanía, R., Nitsche, M. A., Korman, C., Batsikadze, G., and Paulus, W. (2012). The importance of timing in segregated theta phase-coupling for cognitive performance. *Curr. Biol.* 22, 1314–1318. doi: 10.1016/j.cub.2012.05.021

Priori, A. (2003). Brain polarization in humans: a reappraisal of an old tool for prolonged non-invasive modulation of brain excitability. *Clin. Neurophysiol.* 114, 589–595. doi: 10.1016/S1388-2457(02)00437-6

Ranck, J. B. (1975). Which elements are excited in electrical stimulation of mammalian central nervous system: a review. *Brain Res.* 98, 417–440. doi: 10.1016/0006-8993(75)90364-9

Reato, D., Rahman, A., Bikson, M., and Parra, L. C. (2010). Low-intensity electrical stimulation affects network dynamics by modulating population rate and spike timing. *J. Neurosci.* 30, 15067–15079. doi: 10.1523/JNEUROSCI.2059-10.2010

Rees, G., Kreiman, G., and Koch, C. (2002). Neural correlates of consciousness in humans. *Nat. Rev. Neurosci.* 3, 261–270. doi: 10.1038/nrn783

Rohracher, H. (1935). Über subjektive Lichterscheinungen bei Reizung mit Wechselströmen. *Zeitschrift für Sinnesphysiologie* 66, 164–181.

Romei, V., Driver, J., Schyns, P. G., and Thut, G. (2011). Rhythmic TMS over parietal cortex links distinct brain frequencies to global versus local visual processing. *Curr. Biol.* 21, 334–337. doi: 10.1016/j.cub.2011.01.035

Rosanova, M., Casali, A., Bellina, V., Resta, F., Mariotti, M., and Massimini, M. (2009). Natural frequencies of human corticothalamic circuits. *J. Neurosci.* 29, 7679–7685. doi: 10.1523/JNEUROSCI.0445-09.2009

Schnitzler, A., and Gross, J. (2005). Normal and pathological oscillatory communication in the brain. *Nat. Rev. Neurosci.* 6, 285–296. doi: 10.1038/nrn1650

Schutter, D. J., and Hortensius, R. (2010). Retinal origin of phosphenes to transcranial alternating current stimulation. *Clin. Neurophysiol.* 121, 1080–1084. doi: 10.1016/j.clinph.2009.10.038

Schutter, D. J., and Hortensius, R. (2011). Brain oscillations and frequency-dependent modulation of cortical excitability. *Brain Stimul.* 4, 97–103. doi: 10.1016/j.brs.2010.07.002

Schwarz, F. (1947). Über die elektrische Reizbarkeit des Auges bei Hell- und Dunkeladaptation. *Pflügers Arch.* 66, 76–86. doi: 10.1007/BF00362672

Schwiedrzik, C. M. (2009). Retina or visual cortex? The site of phosphene induction by transcranial alternating current stimulation. *Front. Integr. Neurosci.* 3:6. doi: 10.3389/neuro.07.006.2009

Sejnowski, T. J., and Paulsen, O. (2006). Network oscillations: emerging computational principles. *J. Neurosci.* 26, 1673–1676. doi: 10.1523/JNEUROSCI.3737-05d.2006

Sela, T., Kilim, A., and Lavidor, M. (2012). Transcranial alternating current stimulation increases risk-taking behavior in the balloon analog risk task. *Front. Neurosci.* 6:22. doi: 10.3389/fnins.2012.00022

Siegel, M., Donner, T. H., and Engel, A. K. (2012). Spectral fingerprints of large-scale neuronal interactions. *Nat. Rev. Neurosci.* 13, 121–134. doi: 10.1038/nrn3137

Strüber, D., Rach, S., Trautmann-Lengsfeld, S., Engel, A. K., and Herrmann, C. S. (2013). Antiphasic 40 Hz oscillatory current stimulation affects bistable motion perception. *Brain Topogr.* doi: 10.1007/s10548-013-0294-x. [Epub ahead of print].

Thut, G., Schyns, P. G., and Gross, J. (2011). Entrainment of perceptually relevant brain oscillations by non-invasive rhythmic stimulation of the human brain. *Front. Psychol.* 2:170. doi: 10.3389/fpsyg.2011.00170

Uhlhaas, P. J., and Singer, W. (2006). Neural synchrony in brain disorders: relevance for cognitive dysfunctions and pathophysiology. *Neuron* 52, 155–168. doi: 10.1016/j.neuron.2006.09.020

Varela, F., Lachaux, J. P., Rodriguez, E., and Martinerie, J. (2001). The brainweb: phase synchronization and large-scale integration. *Nat. Rev. Neurosci.* 2, 229–239. doi: 10.1038/35067550

Wach, C., Krause, V., Moliadze, V., Paulus, W., Schnitzler, A., and Pollok, B. (2013). Effects of 10 Hz and 20 Hz transcranial alternating current stimulation (tACS) on motor functions and motor cortical excitability. *Behav. Brain Res.* 241, 1–6. doi: 10.1016/j.bbr.2012.11.038

Wagner, T., Fregni, F., Fecteau, S., Grodzinsky, A., Zahn, M., and Pascual-Leone, A. (2007). Transcranial direct current stimulation: a computer-based human model study. *Neuroimage* 35, 1113–1124. doi: 10.1016/j.neuroimage.2007.01.027

Zaehle, T., Rach, S., and Herrmann, C. S. (2010). Transcranial alternating current stimulation enhances individual alpha activity in human EEG. *PLoS ONE* 5:e13766. doi: 10.1371/journal.pone.0013766

Zaghi, S., De Freitas Rezende, L., De Oliveira, L. M., El-Nazer, R., Menning, S., Tadini, L., et al. (2010). Inhibition of motor cortex excitability with 15Hz transcranial alternating current stimulation (tACS). *Neurosci. Lett.* 479, 211–214. doi: 10.1016/j.neulet.2010.05.060

18

Orchestrating neuronal networks: sustained after-effects of transcranial alternating current stimulation depend upon brain states

Toralf Neuling[1], Stefan Rach[1,2] and Christoph S. Herrmann[1,2]*

[1] *Experimental Psychology Lab, University of Oldenburg, Oldenburg, Germany*
[2] *Research Center Neurosensory Science, University of Oldenburg, Oldenburg, Germany*

Correspondence:
Christoph S. Herrmann, Experimental Psychology Lab, University of Oldenburg, Ammerländer Heerstraße 114–118, 26111 Oldenburg, Germany.
e-mail: christoph.herrmann@uni-oldenburg.de

The interest in transcranial alternating current stimulation (tACS) has significantly increased in the past decade. It has potential to modulate brain oscillations in a frequency specific manner, offering the possibility to demonstrate a causal nature of oscillation behavior relationships. TACS is a strong candidate as a tool for clinical applications, however, to fulfill this potential, certain parameters have yet to be evaluated. First, little is known about long-lasting after-effects of tACS with respect to the modulations of rhythmic brain activity. Second, the power of endogenous brain oscillations might play a crucial role in the efficacy of tACS. We hypothesize that the after-effects of tACS depend on the endogenous power of oscillations. To this end, we modulated the power of endogenous occipital alpha oscillations via tACS. In two experiments, participants either had their eyes open or closed to keep endogenous alpha power either low or high while they were stimulated for 20 min with their individual alpha frequency (IAF) and simultaneously performing a vigilance task. After-effects on IAF power were evaluated over a course of 30 min with a pre stimulation period serving as baseline. After-effects were strongly dependent on IAF power. Enhanced IAF power was observed for at least 30 min after tACS under conditions of low endogenous IAF power, whereas, IAF power could not be further enhanced by tACS under conditions of high IAF power. The current study demonstrates, for the first time, a long lasting effect after tACS on endogenous EEG power in the range of the stimulation frequency. Additionally, we present conclusive evidence that the power of the endogenous oscillations has a critical impact on tACS efficacy. Long lasting after-effects foster the role of tACS as a tool for non-invasive brain stimulation and demonstrate the potential for therapeutic application to reestablish the balance of altered brain oscillations.

Keywords: EEG, transcranial alternating current stimulation, tACS, alpha, brain state

INTRODUCTION

Brain oscillations play a crucial role in motor, perceptual, and cognitive processes (Başar et al., 2001; Herrmann et al., 2004; Buzsáki, 2006; Schroeder and Lakatos, 2009) and alterations of these oscillations can be linked to psychiatric disorders (Herrmann and Demiralp, 2005; Uhlhaas et al., 2008). Previous experiments demonstrated associations by correlating behavior and brain oscillations. However, non-invasive brain stimulation techniques, combined with electroencephalography (EEG), offer the possibility to demonstrate a *causal* relationship (for recent reviews see: Thut et al., 2011a; Miniussi et al., 2012).

Oscillatory brain activity is evoked by neuronal network activity of different spatial scales (Buzsáki and Draguhn, 2004). These oscillations, which manifest as changes of extracellular electric fields, in turn, can serve as a feedback signal to structure the activity of the neurons that generated it (Fröhlich and McCormick, 2010). Transcranial electrical stimulation (TES) with weak sinusoidally varying currents is a non-invasive brain stimulation technique that can mimick endogenous electric fields and is thought to directly modulate ongoing oscillatory brain activity as suggested by numerous studies (e.g., Marshall et al., 2006; Antal et al., 2008; Kanai et al., 2008; Pogosyan et al., 2009; Zaehle et al., 2010; Feurra et al., 2011; Neuling et al., 2012a; Polania et al., 2012). Oscillating TES includes transcranial alternating current stimulation (tACS) and tACS with a DC-offset as referred to as oscillating transcranial direct current stimulation (otDCS), see Herrmann., et al. (in revision, this issue) for an overview. TACS/otDCS produces periodic changes of cortical excitability over time with a specific frequency. As a consequence, the power of the spontaneous brain activity in the range of the stimulation frequency can be enhanced (Marshall et al., 2006; Zaehle et al., 2010; Neuling et al., 2012a).

Although immediate after-effects on brain activity have been demonstrated via EEG, the duration and contributing parameters of these after-effects remain largely unknown. This knowledge would provide not only a foundation for further neuroscientific studies on the causal relevance of brain oscillations, but also for clinical applications to re-establish a balance in altered brain oscillations (Kuo and Nitsche, 2012). Only by determining the long term after-effects of tACS, it is possible to work toward a successful treatment of dysfunctional brain oscillations.

It has been argued that only physiologically meaningful brain rhythms can be entrained (Thut et al., 2011a). Based on this view, brain rhythms can either be entrained depending on the *state* (ongoing) or *function* (task-related) of the oscillations. With regard to state, this means, for example, that sleep-like slow wave oscillations can be entrained in sleep (Marshall et al., 2006) but not in waking state (Bergmann et al., 2009) and stimulation in the alpha rhythm is more effective in the dark compared to beta stimulation, whereas it is opposite in light (Kanai et al., 2008). Entrainment of functional rhythms includes the modulation of task-related oscillations (Romei et al., 2010; Thut et al., 2011b; Brignani et al., 2013). Although the current study focuses on the state-dependency of physiological tACS after-effects, the results are expected to generalize to task-related oscillations, as we assess general properties of oscillations.

In the context of synchronization the problem is: "Under which conditions the observed [...] frequency of oscillations in an externally periodically driven system will come into coincidence with the frequency of the driving? Usually these conditions are quantified in terms of the power and the mismatch between the frequency of the external force and the natural (internal) frequency of the oscillator" (Osipov et al., 2007, pg. 35). This means that a neuronal network with strong oscillatory power should not be as prone to a certain external periodic force as a network with weaker oscillatory power. *In vitro* experiments revealed that neuronal network activity can be entrained by sinusoidal electric fields with an intensity similar to that of the endogenous electric field of that network (Fröhlich and McCormick, 2010). The same study also found that entrainment works best if the external and internal frequency match. It would be desirable to demonstrate this interaction of the external and internal oscillation with tACS to contribute to the understanding and feasibility of this brain stimulation method.

The goal of this study was to discern for how long endogenous brain oscillations are enhanced post tACS and how the baseline power of the endogenous oscillations modulates this effect. To this end, we conducted two experiments focusing on the occipito-parietal alpha rhythm (8–12 Hz) that was recorded via EEG. Participants either had their eyes closed or open (in a dark room) while they received tACS with their individual alpha frequency (IAF). Without any visual stimulation (closed eyes), the endogenous alpha power is increased compared to visual stimulation (open eyes) as already discovered by Berger (1929). We hypothesize that this experimental modulation of endogenous alpha power results in a weak after-effect of tACS on endogenous alpha power when participants keep their eyes closed and a comparatively strong after-effect if participants keep their eyes open.

METHODS

Two experiments were conducted in which participants had their eyes either closed (Experiment 1) or open (Experiment 2). Except for participants, all materials and methods were the same for both experiments.

PARTICIPANTS

Subjects gave written informed consent before participation. Participants were university students and were paid for participation. All participants were medication-free at the time of the experiments. They reported no hearing deficits, presence or history of epilepsy, neurological or psychiatric disorders, cognitive impairments, intracranial metal or cochlear implants. All participants were right handed, according to the Edinburgh handedness inventory (Oldfield, 1971). In a single blind study design, participants were assigned to either experimental (*stim*) or control group (*sham*). In a debriefing after the experiment, participants were informed about the hypotheses and whether they belonged to the *stim* or *sham* group. The experimental protocol was approved by the ethics committee of the University of Oldenburg and was conducted in accordance with the Declaration of Helsinki.

Experiment 1: eyes closed

Twenty-four healthy, right-handed subjects participated in the study. Four participants were excluded due to technical problems which corrupted the EEG data. One participant was excluded because the sensation threshold of the stimulation was as low as 0.1 mA. Nineteen subjects (12 female) with an age of 22.9 ± 0.8 (mean ± standard error of the mean, SEM) years were used for data analysis. *Stim* and *sham* groups did not differ significantly in age (stim: 23.5 ± 1.4 years; sham: 22.3 ± 1.1 years; independent t-test: $t_{17} = 0.68, P = 0.51$), gender (stim: 7 female; sham: 5 female, $\chi^2_1 = 0.43$ ($n = 19$), $P = 0.52$), individual alpha frequency (IAF) (stim: 9.9 ± 0.3 Hz; sham: 10.3 ± 0.3 Hz, independent t-test: $t_{17} = 1.01$, $P = 0.33$), or threshold (see below) (stim: 905 ± 122 μA; sham: 844 ± 35 μA, independent t-test: $t_{17} = 0.58, P = 0.57$).

Experiment 2: eyes open

Thirty healthy, right-handed subjects participated in the study. One participant reported in the post experiment interview that he kept his eyes closed for most of the time. To take account of other participants who might not have reported that they left their eyes closed, we z-transformed the participant's mean IAF power in the post stimulation period. A high z-score indicates that this value deviates from the distribution of the other values. All participants with a z-score higher than 1.65 ($\alpha < 0.05$, one-tailed) were rejected from further analyses. Twenty-two subjects (12 female) with a mean age of 25.1 ± 0.6 years remained for data analysis. *Stim* and *sham* group did not significantly differ in age (stim: 24.2 ± 0.6 years; sham: 26.1 ± 1.1 years; independent t-test: $t_{20} = 1.53, P = 0.14$), gender (stim: 5 female; sham: 7 female, $\chi^2_1 = 0.73$ ($n = 22$), $P = 0.39$), IAF (stim: 10.3 ± 0.2 Hz; sham: 10.3 ± 0.5 Hz, independent t-test: $t_{20} = 0$, $P = 1.00$), and threshold (see below) (stim: 877 ± 48 μA; sham: 1200 ± 154 μA, independent t-test: $t_{20} = 1.996, P = 0.06$).

EEG

The experiments were performed in a dark room with the participants seated in a recliner. The EEG was measured from 25 sintered Ag-AgCl electrodes mounted in an elastic cap (Easycap, Falk Minow, Munich, Germany) with a standard 10–20 system layout, and vertical EOG, referenced to the nose. The ground electrode was positioned on the forehead at Fpz. Electrode impedance was kept below 10 kΩ. Signals were recorded using Brain Vision Recorder (Brain Products GmbH, Gilching, Germany) with an online low pass filter (250 Hz). When an electrode reached 70% saturation, a DC reset was applied. Sampling rate was 500 Hz and amplified in the range of ±3.2768 mV at a resolution of 0.1 μV. Stimulus markers and EEG data were digitally stored on hard disk for further offline analysis. No offline filters were applied.

ELECTRICAL STIMULATION

The tACS was applied via two surface conductive-rubber electrodes (5 × 7 cm) enclosed in saline-soaked sponges (Neuroconn, Ilmenau, Germany) centered at Cz and Oz underneath the EEG recording cap (see **Figure 2A**). Stimulation electrode positions were chosen in order to affect the occipital cortex (**Figure 1**). The impedance was kept below 10 kΩ. An alternating, sinusoidal current at the IAF of each participant was applied using a battery-operated stimulator system (Eldith, Neuroconn, Ilmenau, Germany). The intensity of the sinusoidal current was adjusted individually to the highest intensity at which the stimulation was not noticed by the participants. To obtain this threshold, we started with an intensity level of 1500 μA (peak-to-peak). If the subject indicated no skin sensation or phosphene perception, we increased the intensity in steps of 100 μA. As soon as the participant either indicated skin sensation or phosphene perception, we decreased the intensity in steps of 100 μA. Each intensity step was applied for approximately 20 s, without fade-in/out. The obtained threshold level was used as stimulation intensity. The experimental group received 20 min of stimulation. In the beginning, and at the end, the stimulation was faded-in and faded-out for 10 s. In the control group, sham stimulation was applied. While all other stimulation parameters were the same as in the experimental group, the control group received only 30 s of stimulation, a procedure that has been used in previous studies (e.g., Polania et al., 2012).

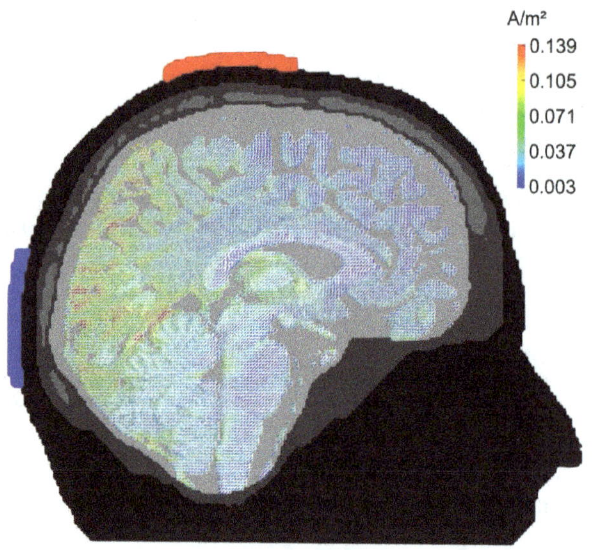

FIGURE 1 | Current density distribution. Results of a finite-element model simulation of tACS (Neuling et al., 2012a). Simulation electrodes are centered at electrode positions Cz and Oz of the 10/20 system. Current densities are highest in the posterior cortex.

DESIGN

The experimental procedure is illustrated in **Figure 2B**. After the EEG and TES electrodes were attached, the participant's IAF was estimated. Participants were asked to keep their eyes closed while the spontaneous EEG was recorded for 90 s. Afterwards, raw EEG data of electrode Pz was split into one-second segments. Segments containing artefacts were rejected. A fast Fourier transformation (FFT) was performed on the first 50 artifact-free segments and the resulting spectra were averaged. The power peak in the alpha range (8–12 Hz) was considered as IAF and used as stimulation frequency. Subsequently, the stimulation intensity was determined. Now, the EEG was recorded for 5 min which served as a baseline (*pre*-EEG), before tACS or sham stimulation was applied for 20 min. Afterwards, the EEG was recorded for 30 min (*post*-EEG).

During EEG recording, the subjects performed a simple auditory detection task and were instructed to either close their eyes (Experiment 1) or leave their eyes open (Experiment 2). In Experiment 2, participants were asked to fixate on a cross that was presented in the center of a computer screen. The auditory detection task was introduced to ensure vigilance during the course of the experiment (**Figure 2C**). With an inter stimulus interval of 10 to 12 s a tone was presented for 500 ms via loudspeakers. In 80% of the presentations this was a 500 Hz tone and in 20% of the presentations this was a 1000 Hz tone. Subjects were instructed to press a button when the 1000 Hz tone was presented.

After the experiment, participants were at first asked to guess if they were stimulated at all or perceived phosphenes during the stimulation and were subsequently debriefed. Additionally, a questionnaire assessed possible adverse effects.

QUESTIONNAIRE ON ADVERSE EFFECTS

To obtain possible adverse effects for tACS a translated version of a questionnaire introduced by Brunoni et al. (2011) was used. The following side-effects were inquired: headache, neck pain, scalp pain, tingling, itching, burning sensation, skin redness, sleepiness, trouble concentrating and acute mood change. Specifically, participants were asked to indicate the intensity of the side-effect (1, absent; 2, mild; 3, moderate; 4, severe) and if they attributed the side-effect to the tACS (1, none; 2, remote; 3, possible; 4, probable; 5, definite).

DATA ANALYSIS

Data analysis was performed using MATLAB R2012a (The MathWorks Inc, Natick, MA, USA) and EEGLAB 11.0.4.3 (Delorme and Makeig, 2004). For statistical analysis, SPSS 20.0 (IBM Corp, Armonk, NY, USA) was used.

EEG data

Data analysis was conducted in accordance with the approach introduced by Zaehle et al. (2010). The *post*-EEG was divided into 10 epochs of 3 min each. Each of the data epochs (*pre*-EEG,

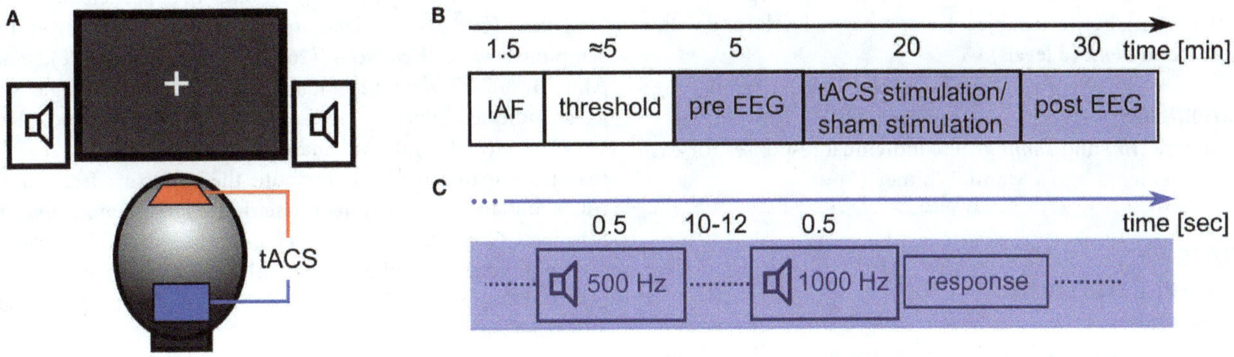

FIGURE 2 | Experimental details. (A) Experimental setup: tACS electrodes were centered at electrode positions Cz and Oz of the 10/20 system. Subjects were seated in front of a computer screen with a gray fixation cross on a black background (Experiment 2). Auditory stimuli were delivered through stereo speakers. **(B)** Sequence of the experiment: at first, the participant's IAF was obtained with their eyes closed, before the thresholds for skin sensation and phosphene perception were acquired. In the following 55 min, participants had to perform a detection task with either closed (Experiment 1) or open eyes (Experiment 2). In the first 5 min of this period, the EEG was recorded (*pre* EEG) and served as a baseline. Subsequently, 20 min of stimulation (tACS or sham) were applied. Afterwards, the EEG was recorded for 30 min (*post* EEG). **(C)** Detection task: every 10–12 s, a tone was presented for 500 ms. 80% of those were standards (500 Hz) and 20% were targets (1000 Hz). Subjects had to respond with a button press to each presentation of the target stimulus.

10× *post*-EEG) from each participant was split into 180 one-second segments. Segments containing artefacts (eye movements, muscle activity), acoustical stimulation or a motor response were rejected from further analysis. The first 120 segments of each data set without artefacts were used for further analysis. After subtracting the mean value of each segment to avoid DC distortion of the spectra at 0 Hz, an FFT was applied on each segment and the resulting 120 spectra for each data set were averaged. The parieto-occipital electrode Pz was chosen for power analysis. To evaluate power changes in the range of the IAF ± 2 Hz, the individual mean spectral powers were calculated. In order to account for individual differences, the power data were normalized to the alpha-power of the pre-EEG measurement. To discern the specificity of the power changes, we additionally analyzed frequency bands below (*lower band*, IAF −5 to −3 Hz) and above (*upper band*, IAF +3 to +5 Hz) the IAF.

A recent study conducted by our group aimed to reveal differences in coherence before and after tACS (Strüber et al., under revision). Therefore, we calculated changes of coherence in the alpha-range (7.8–11.7 Hz). We computed the mean magnitude squared coherence (Equation 1) between EEG electrodes P3 and P4 in the *pre*-EEG, which served as a baseline.

$$C_{xy}(f) = \frac{|P_{xy}(f)|^2}{P_{xx}(f)P_{yy}(f)} \qquad (1)$$

The magnitude squared coherence (C) for a specific frequency (f) is a function of the power spectral densities of two signals x (P3) and y (P4) and the cross power spectral density of the two signals (P_{xy}(f)). The coherence ranges between 0 (no coherence) and 1 (perfect coherence). In order to account for individual differences, the average coherence for each *post*-EEG epoch was normalized to the individual coherence baseline.

For statistical analysis of the tACS after-effect, normalized spectral power/ coherence was entered into a Two-Way analysis of variance (ANOVA) with repeated measurements with between subject factor *group* (2 levels) and within subject factor *time* (10 levels). In case Mauchly's test detected violation of sphericity, Greenhouse-Geisser corrected values are reported. This applies for all ANOVAs conducted. To further elaborate on the duration of the power after-effect, we examined when the alpha-power returned to baseline. Therefore, one sample *t*-tests against 1, which represents the baseline alpha power, were conducted. This means, if the mean of the relative alpha-power is 1 after stimulation, the power does not differ from the baseline power and the *t*-test against 1 is not significant. Bonferroni correction was applied to account for multiple comparisons.

To discern whether or not alpha topographies after tACS differed between tACS and sham groups, we calculated Spearman's rank correlation coefficients between the relative IAF power between tACS and sham groups for each electrode, whereby a high correlation would indicate a similar topography. To assess, whether or not an increase in IAF power from pre to post stimulation was locally specific, we chose a subset of electrodes (frontal: Fz, temporal: FT9/FT10, parietal: Pz) based on their position relative to the stimulation electrodes and entered the normalized IAF power into a Two-Way ANOVA with repeated measurements with between subject factor *group* (2 levels) and within subject factor *electrode* (4 levels). For *post-hoc* analyses, Bonferroni corrected 2-sample *t*-tests (one-tailed) were applied.

Behavioral data

We analyzed the behavioral performance of the auditory detection task for the *pre*-block, the *stimulation*-block and the *post*-block. Reaction times exceeding 1500 ms were considered as misses and excluded from further analysis. Furthermore, we calculated the sensitivity index *d'* (Wickens, 2001), the difference between the *z*-transformed hit rate and the false alarms rate. In the stimulation and post block, the same number of targets and standards as presented in the pre block were randomly chosen. We entered the behavioral data into Two-Way ANOVAs with repeated measurements with between subject factor *group* (2 levels) and within subject factor *block* (3 levels).

QUESTIONNAIRE

To compare *stim* and *sham* group, individual responses for each item were entered into a Mann–Whitney *U* test.

RESULTS

EXPERIMENT 1: EYES CLOSED

Debriefing

None of the participants indicated phosphenes during stimulation. Twenty-six percent of the participants indicated that they assumed to be stimulated. The judgments did not differ between the *stim* and the *sham* group (stim: 20%, sham: 33%, $\chi^2_1 = 0.15$ ($n = 19$), $P = 0.70$). None of the responses on the items of the questionnaire differed between *stim* and *sham* group (Mann–Whitney *U* test: for all responses, $p > 0.05$).

Most common symptoms among the participants were *Sleepiness* (89%) and *Concentration* (63%). Other common symptoms were *Headache* (26%), *Neck pain* (26%), *Scalp pain* (37%), *Tingling* (26%), and *Itching* (16%). Single subjects indicated *Burning sensation, Skin redness,* and *Acute mood change.* Qualitative analysis of the responses revealed that participants did not attribute the adverse effects to the tACS, but to the experimental setting (*dark room; Headache, Sleepiness, Concentration*), design ("monotonous task": *Sleepiness, Concentration*) and the fluids below the electrodes ("EEG gel" and "saline solution"; *Tingling, Itching, Burning sensation, Skin redness*).

Behavioral data

As depicted in **Figure 3AI**, reaction times did not differ between groups or across blocks. Behavioral effects were tested with a Two-Way ANOVA with repeated measurements with the between subject factor *group* (2 levels) and the within subject factor *time* (3 levels: *pre, stim, post*). The ANOVA revealed no

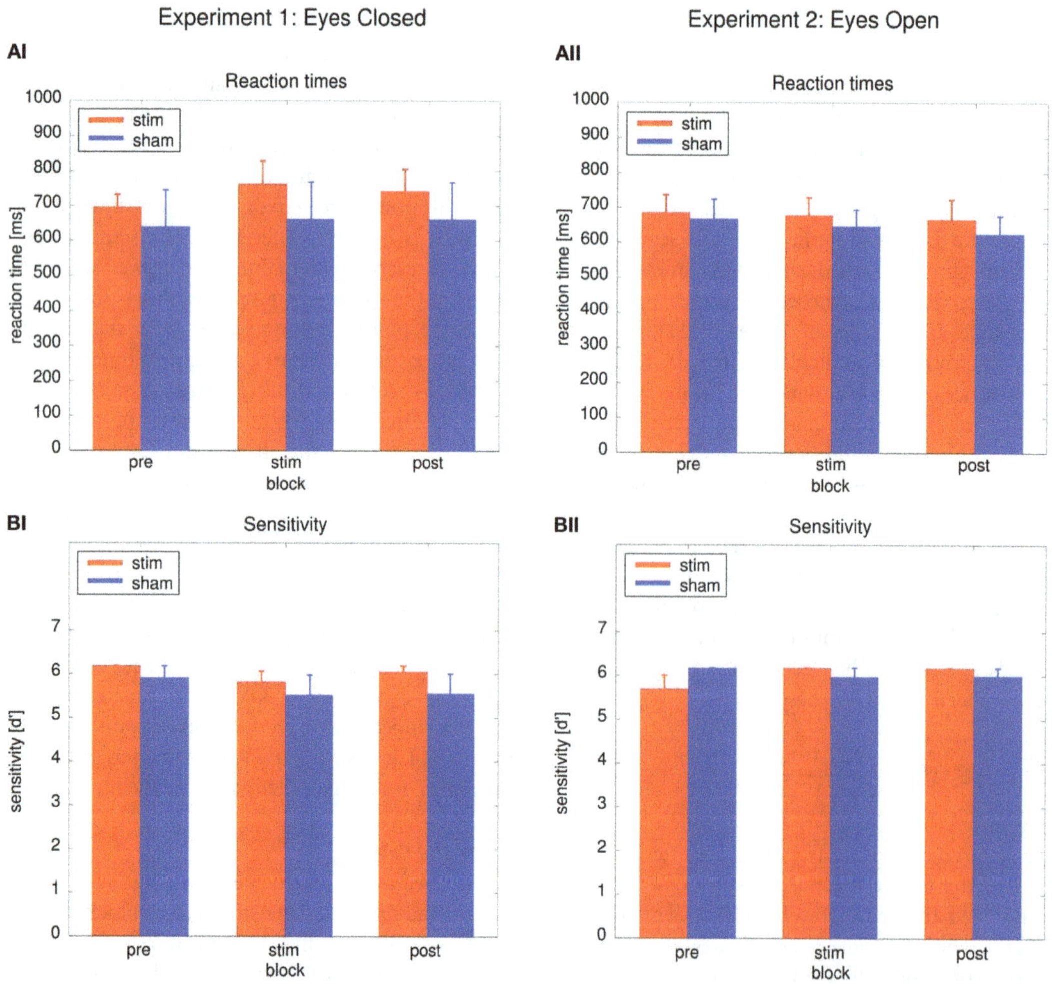

FIGURE 3 | Behavioral results. Left: Experiment 1, right: Experiment 2; red: tACS stimulation group, blue: sham stimulation group. **(AI,AII)** Reaction times: average reaction times for the *stim* and the *sham* group for the three blocks of the detection task. Bars indicate the mean ± SEM. **(BI,BII)** Sensitivity *d'*: average *d'* for the *stim* and the *sham* group for the three blocks of the detection task. Bars indicate the mean ± SEM.

significant effects (*group*: $F_1 = 0.31, P = 0.59$; *time*: $F_{1.39} = 0.12$, $P = 0.81$; *group* × *time*: $F_{1.39} = 1.104$, $P = 0.33$). Sensitivity analysis demonstrated that both groups were able to perform the detection task. Sensitivity was not significantly different between both groups (**Figure 3BI**). An ANOVA yielded no significant results (*group*: $F_1 = 0.99, P = 0.33$; *time*: $F_2 = 2.17, P = 0.13$; *time* × *group*: $F_2 = 0.23, P = 0.799$). The absence of significant behavioral differences between the groups confirm that sham stimulation was successful.

Electrophysiological data

The mean FFT power spectra of the *pre* and *post* EEG reveal no difference between *stim* and *sham* group in any frequency band (**Figure 4AI**). The timecourse of the IAF power (**Figure 4BI**) and the corresponding topographies (**Figure 5A**) do not differ between groups ($r = 0.98, P < 0.001$). A Two-Way ANOVA with repeated measurements on the normalized IAF power with the between subject factor *group* (2 levels) and the within subject factor post EEG *time* (10 levels) was conducted. The ANOVA revealed no significant main effects or interactions (*group*: $F_1 = 1.75, P = 0.20$; *time*: $F_{2.58} = 1.09, P = 0.36$; *group* × *time*: $F_{2.58} = 1.01, P = 0.39$). Likewise, no *group* effects were found for the *lower* ($F_1 = 2.273, P = 0.15$) or *upper* frequency band ($F_1 = 0.002, P = 0.97$).

Subsequently, one sample *t*-tests against 1 (corresponding to baseline IAF power) were performed to test for a power increase after tACS and sham stimulation (**Figure 4CI**) compared to baseline IAF power, which revealed no significant power increase after tACS (*stim*: $t_9 = 0.61, P = 0.55$) or sham stimulation (*sham*: $t_8 = 0.16, P = 0.28$). Similar results were found for the *lower* (*stim*: $t_9 = 0.89, P = 0.40$; *sham*: $t_8 = 1.10, P = 0.30$) and *upper* frequency band (*stim*: $t_9 = 1.72, P = 0.12$; *sham*: $t_8 = 0.55, P = 0.59$).

Alpha coherence was increased in the *stim* group compared to the *sham* group (**Figures 6A** upper/**B** left). This was confirmed by a Two-Way ANOVA with repeated measurements on the normalized alpha coherence with the between subject factor *group* (2 levels) and the within subject factor post EEG *time* (10 levels). The ANOVA revealed a significant main effect of *group* ($F_1 = 5.41, P = 0.03, \eta^2 = 0.24$). Neither a main effect of *time* ($F_{3.63} = 1.76, P = 0.15$) nor a significant interaction *group* × *time* ($F_{3.63} = 1.59, P = 0.19$) were observed.

EXPERIMENT 2: EYES OPEN

Debriefing

As in the eyes closed condition, no participant indicated phosphene perception during stimulation. Overall, 50% of the participants indicated that they assumed to be stimulated. The responses did not differ between the *stim* and the *sham* group (stim: 45%, sham: 54%, $\chi^2_1 = 0.67$ ($n = 22$), $P = 0.67$). None of the responses on the items of the questionnaire differed between *stim* and *sham* group (Mann–Whitney *U* test: for all responses, $p > 0.05$).

Most common symptoms among the participants were *Sleepiness* (45%) and *Concentration* (36%). Single subjects indicated *Headache, Tingling, Burning sensation* and *Skin redness*. Qualitative analysis of the responses revealed that participants did not attribute the adverse effects to the tACS, but to the experimental setting (*dark room; Headache, Sleepiness, Concentration*), design ("monotonous task": *Sleepiness, Concentration*) and the fluids below the electrodes ("EEG gel" and "saline solution"; *Tingling, Itching, Burning sensation, Skin redness*).

Behavioral data

Performance between the *stim* and *sham* group did not differ throughout the experiment, as illustrated in **Figures 3AII, BII**. To confirm this result, Two-Way ANOVAs with repeated measurements with the between subject factor *group* (2 levels) and the within subject factor *block* (3 levels) were performed. The ANOVAs revealed no significant effects neither for reaction times (*group*: $F_1 = 0.19, P = 0.67$; *time*: $F_2 = 0.95, P = 0.395$; *group* × *time*: $F_2 = 0.167, P = 0.80$) nor sensitivity *d'* (*group*: $F_1 = 0.04, P = 0.84$; *time*: $F_2 = 1.141, P = 0.65$; *group* × *time*: $F_2 = 2.47, P = 0.097$).

Sensitivity analysis confirmed that both groups were able to perform the detection task. The absence of significant *group* effects on the behavior confirm that sham stimulation was successful.

Electrophysiological data

Endogenous power in the alpha range was enhanced after tACS, but not after sham stimulation (**Figure 4AII**). However, tACS and sham group did not differ with regard to alpha topography ($r = 0.97, P < 0.001$) as illustrated in **Figure 5B**. The difference between *stim* and *sham* group with regard to the increase in IAF alpha power after stimulation is also visible over time, as illustrated in **Figure 4BII**. This was confirmed by a Two-Way ANOVA with repeated measurements on the normalized IAF power with the between subject factor *group* (2 levels) and the within subject factor post EEG *time* (10 levels). Significant main effects of *group* ($F_1 = 5.84, P = 0.025, \eta^2 = 0.23$) and *time* ($F_{4.71} = 6.86, P < 0.001, \eta^2 = 0.26$) were observed, but the interaction *group* × *time* was not significant ($F_{4.71} = 1.52, P = 0.19$). No *group* effects were found for the *lower* ($F_1 = 0.21, P = 0.96$) and *upper* frequency band ($F_1 = 1.67, P = 0.21$). Additionally, no difference in the topographies of IAF power between groups could be demonstrated.

Subsequent one-sample *t*-tests against 1 (corresponding to baseline IAF power) revealed that IAF power is enhanced compared to base line after tACS ($t_{10} = 4.28, P = 0.002, d = 1.27$) but not after sham stimulation ($t_{10} = 2.13, P = 0.06$) as illustrated in **Figure 4CII**. On average, the normalized IAF power after tACS is 148 ± 37%. The effect is not found for the *lower* (*stim*: $t_{10} = 1.38, P = 0.19$; *sham*: $t_{10} = 1.82, P = 0.10$) and *upper* frequency band (*stim*: $t_{10} = 1.97, P = 0.08$; *sham*: $t_{10} = 0.55, P = 0.59$).

The significant main effect of *group* demonstrated that *stim* and *sham* groups significantly differed with regard to their IAF power increase. Additionally, compared to baseline, only the group that received tACS had increased IAF power. To get detailed information on how long the IAF power was increased in the *stim* group, we performed one-sample *t*-tests (Bonferroni corrected) against 1 (corresponding to baseline IAF power) for each timepont of the *post* stimulation block. This procedure revealed that

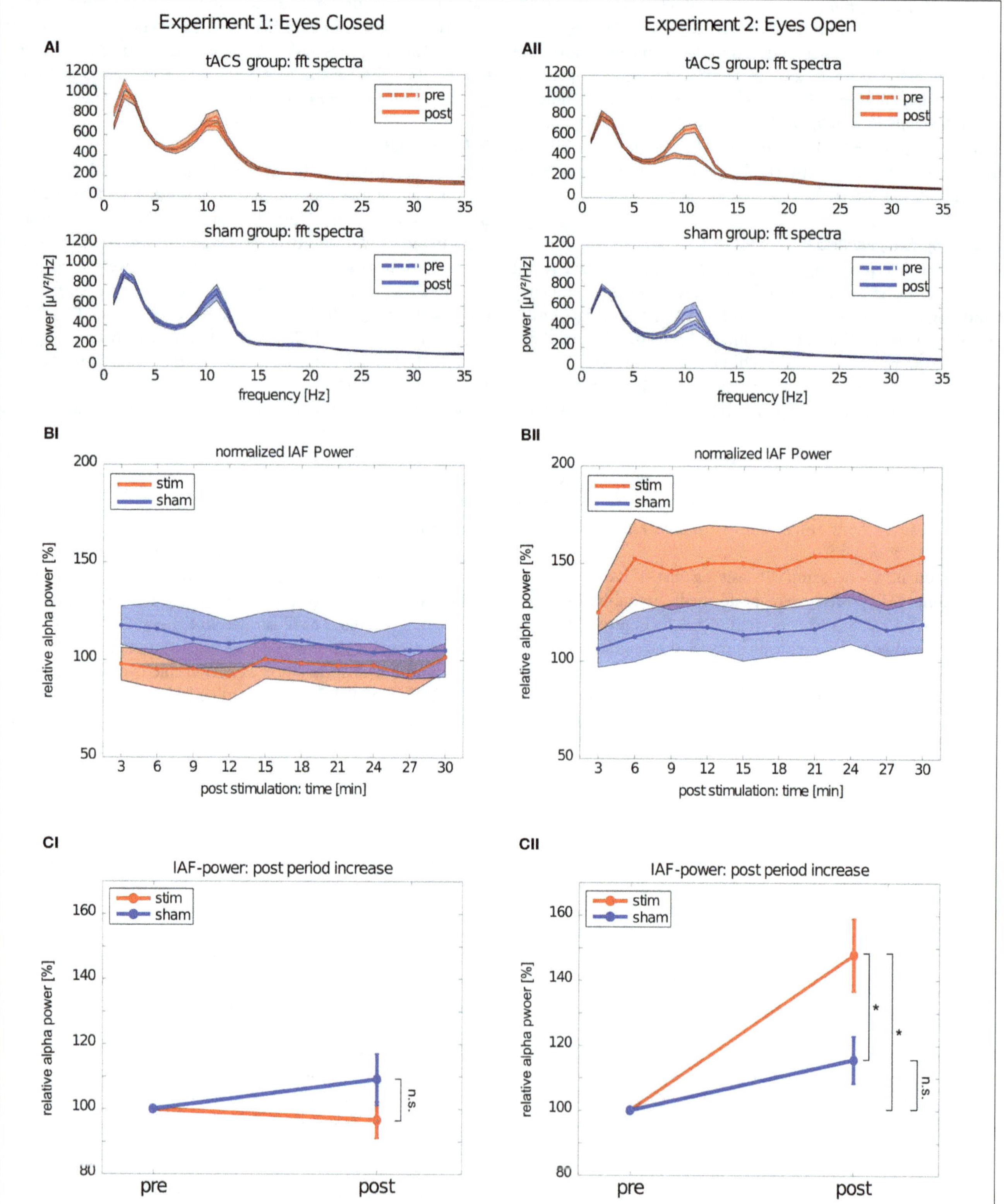

FIGURE 4 | Changes in power. Left: Experiment 1, right: Experiment 2; red: tACS stimulation group, blue: sham stimulation group. **(AI,AII)** Average power spectra: average FFT power spectra for the *pre* EEG and the *post* EEG. Solid lines depict the mean, shaded areas depict the SEM. **(BI,BII)** Timecourse of IAF power after stimulation: change of the IAF power over the whole *post* EEG block. Solid lines depict the mean, shaded areas depict the standard deviation. **(CI,CII)** Average IAF power before and after stimulation: change of the average normalized IAF power from *pre* EEG to *post* EEG (mean ± SEM). Asterisks depict significant differences.

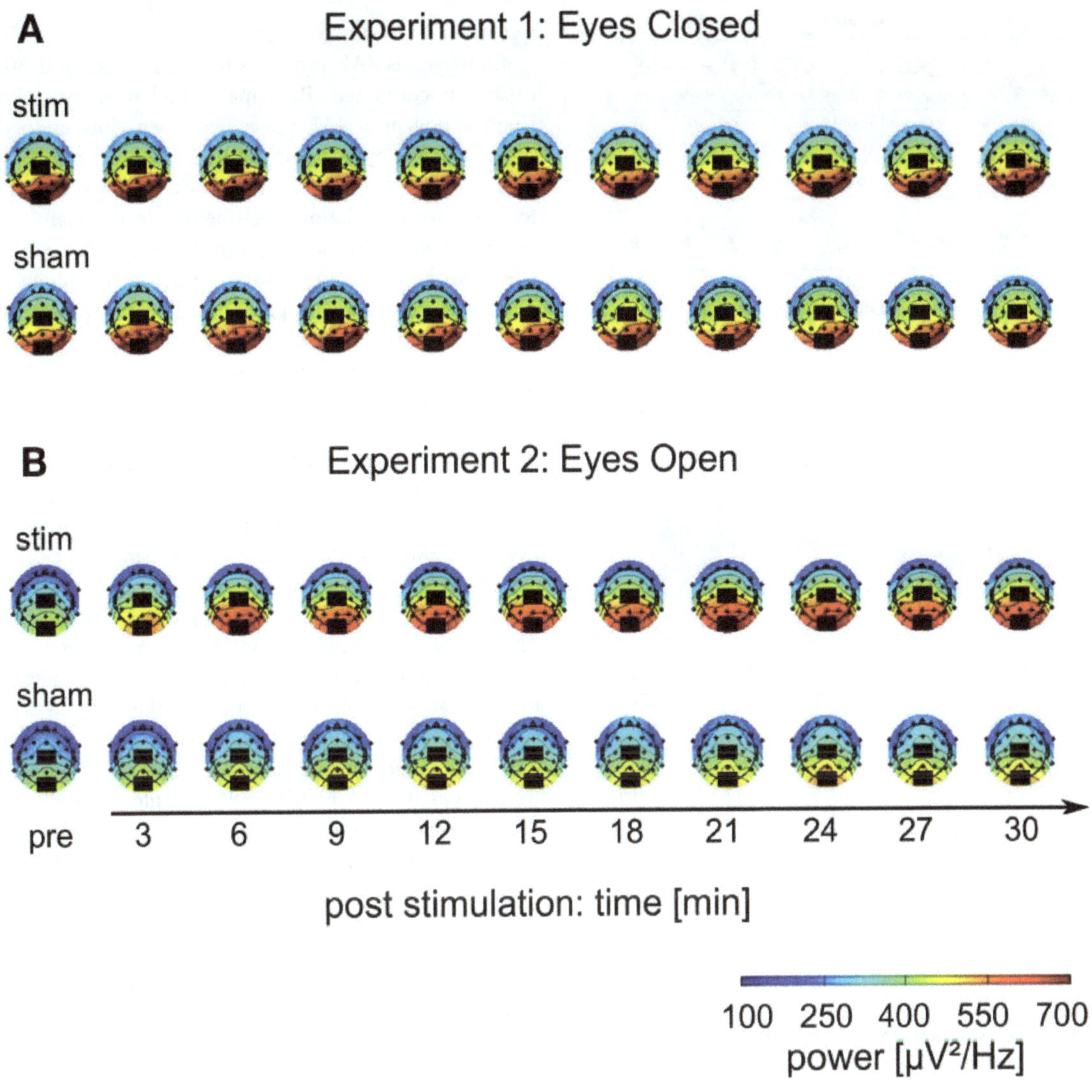

FIGURE 5 | Topographies of IAF power. (A) Experiment 1, **(B)** Experiment 2; colors depict power. Black rectangles illustrate the placement of the stimulation electrodes.

the IAF power of the *stim* group did not return to baseline during the whole timecourse of the *post* stimulation block (all $P < 0.05$, $d > 1.15$).

A Two-Way ANOVA with repeated measurements with between subject factor *group* (2 levels) and within subject factor *electrode* (4 levels) revealed a significant main effect of *electrode* ($F_3 = 2.98$, $P = 0.038$, $\eta^2 = 0.13$). The main effect of *group* ($F_1 = 3.14$, $P = 0.08$) did not reach significance, but the interaction *groups* × *electrode* ($F_3 = 2.588$, $P = 0.06$) showed a trend. The interaction fails to meet the 5% level of significance only by a small margin, indicating that the alpha power increase was indeed locally specific. *Post-hoc t*-tests revealed that IAF power differed significantly only at electrode Pz between groups ($P < 0.05$, $d = 1.08$), differences at the other electrodes were not significant (Fz: $P = 0.38$, FT9: $P = 0.52$, FT10: $P = 0.38$).

Alpha coherence did not differ between groups (**Figures 6A** lower/**B** right). This was confirmed by a Two-Way ANOVA with repeated measurements on the normalized alpha coherence with the between subject factor *group* (2 levels) and the within subject factor post EEG *time* (10 levels). Neither significant main effects of *group* ($F_1 = 1.35$, $P = 0.26$) and *time* ($F_{3.95} = 1.04$, $P = 0.39$) nor a significant interaction *group* × *time* ($F_{3.95} = 0.72$, $P = 0.58$) was observed.

In order to further elaborate on the coherence effect in the tACS stimulation groups, we correlated the *pre* stimulation coherence for all subjects of both eyes open and eyes closed tACS stimulation groups with their average *post* stimulation change in coherence (**Figure 6C**). The correlation was $r = -0.33$, which means that the lower *pre* stimulation coherence the higher the increase in the *post* stimulation period. However, the correlation was not significant ($P = 0.145$).

For a demonstration that the physiological after-effect of tACS differed for the eyes closed experiment compared to the eyes open experiment, additional Three-Way ANOVAs were conducted with

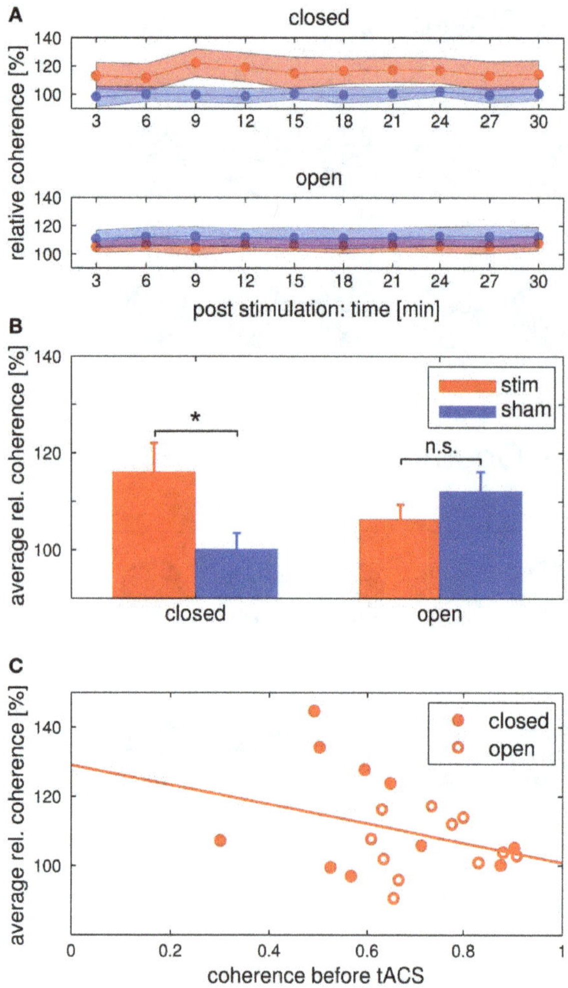

FIGURE 6 | Changes in alpha coherence. Red: tACS stimulation group, blue: sham stimulation group. **(A)** Timecourse of coherence after stimulation: change of the alpha coherence over the whole *post* EEG block. Solid lines depict the mean, shaded areas depict the standard deviation. Upper: closed eyes, lower: open eyes. **(B)** Relative difference in coherence after stimulation: average alpha coherence of the whole *post* EEG block. Solid lines depict the mean, shaded areas depict the standard deviation. Bars indicate the mean ± SEM, asterisks indicate significant differences. In the closed eyes condition, alpha coherence was increased in the tACS stimulation group compared to the sham stimulation group. **(C)** Correlation of *pre* alpha coherence and coherence chance *post* stimulation: lower pre stimulation coherence yields higher coherence increases after tACS. Red discs: participants of the eyes closed experiment, red circles: participants of the eyes open experiment. The solid red line depicts the regression curve.

between subject factors *condition* (2 levels; eyes closed/open) and *group* (2 levels; stim/sham) and the within subject factor *time* (10 levels). The interaction *condition* × *group* was significant for both ANOVAs (*power*: $F_1 = 5.104, P = 0.012, \eta^2 = 0.16$; *coherence*: $F_1 = 6.841, P = 0.013, \eta^2 = 0.16$).

DISCUSSION

We have reported novel findings regarding the duration of frequency-specific after-effects of tACS stimulation in endogenous EEG power. In addition, evidence is provided that the endogenous oscillatory power of the entrained frequency has a crucial impact on the efficacy of tACS.

Endogenous IAF power before (baseline) and 30 min after tACS was compared. Participants had their eyes either closed (high endogenous IAF power) or open (low endogenous IAF power). In the eyes closed experiment, no effects on oscillatory power were observed, i.e., IAF power did not significantly differ from pre-stimulation levels neither in the sham nor the stim group. Contrary to the results in the eyes closed experiment, an effect on the oscillatory power, limited to the alpha range, was found in the eyes open experiment. The power increase from the pre- to the post stimulation period was significant in the stimulated group, but not in the sham group. This effect lasted for the complete duration of the 30 min post-stimulation recording period.

Via the application of tACS, we intended to modulate alpha oscillations; however, under conditions of high endogenous alpha power, tACS fails to influence alpha power. One possible explanation to account for this finding is that with eyes closed, endogenous alpha power has reached a maximum (Nunez et al., 2001) and cannot be further enhanced by tACS, due to ceiling effects. This hypothesis cannot be rejected with respect to our results. A second, more mechanistic, explanation would suggest that the low oscillating currents introduced to the brain by tACS are not strong enough to modulate high endogenous oscillations, but only low endogenous oscillations. From a recent simulation study, we know that 1 mA of tDCS/tACS results in an electric field of 417 μV/mm in occipital areas (Neuling et al., 2012b). Intracranial recordings taken from the visual cortex of wake behaving monkeys performing a task revealed alpha powers in the range of 400 μV/mm (Bollimunta et al., 2008), which is almost identical to the maximum voltage gradient resulting from tACS in occipital cortex. Since monkeys had their eyes open during the experiment, we expect that these values represent the case of low endogenous alpha power. With closed eyes, the power of endogenous alpha oscillations are increased by a factor of 2.27 ± 0.93 compared to the power with open eyes (Könönen and Partanen, 1993). This suggests stimulation intensities more than twice as high as used by us are required to enhance alpha powers in the eyes closed condition. Although this mechanistic explanation is intriguing, further studies with variable stimulation power are required to rule out the ceiling-effect explanation. Our results demonstrate that endogenous oscillations exhibiting lower power before tACS are more prone to the effects of tACS and are enhanced over a long period of time. It might be speculated that the enhancement effect would last even longer than 30 min.

It is interesting to compare electrical stimulation with repetitive sensory stimulation. It has been demonstrated repeatedly that flickering light is able to entrain brain oscillations in form of so called visually steady state evoked potentials (SSEP; Regan, 1989). Systematic variation of the driving frequency has revealed a resonance peak in the SSEP at subject's IAF (Herrmann, 2001). Intriguingly, this resonance effect occurs particularly in subjects with high alpha power (Pigeau and Frame, 1992). In contrast to their study, we were only able to achieve entrainment with eyes open, i.e., at low alpha power. At first glance, this seems like a contradiction; however, high and low alpha power between subjects due to eye opening is not comparable to inter-individual variations of alpha power. Even subjects with low alpha power will show variations due to eye opening. Nevertheless, the study by Pigeau and Frame (1992) demonstrates that visual stimulation has a stronger effect on visual cortex than our electrical stimulation, since even high alpha subjects could be entrained.

It may be argued that the observed effects of increased IAF power in the eyes open experiment do not result from tACS, but instead result from sensory deprivation and the monotonous task. This possibility can be ruled out by our data, because the IAF power of the *sham* group was not significantly enhanced in the post stimulation block. It is also unlikely that tACS increases tiredness and had resulted in increased alpha power, because ratings on the questionnaire items *tiredness* and *trouble concentrating* did not differ between groups, neither in the eyes open, nor in the eyes closed experiment.

A further concern about tACS effects in the visual cortex is whether they are of cortical or retinal origin (e.g., Schwiedrzik, 2009). We used the same electrode montage as Kanai et al. (2008). The authors reported phosphenes thresholds in a dark room at 500 μA stimulation intensity at alpha frequency; however, Kanai et al. (2008) used a smaller electrode over the occipital cortex compared to the current study (3 × 4 cm vs. 5 × 7 cm) leading to a higher current density under the stimulation electrode. Their current density was 42 $\mu A/cm^2$, which exceeds our highest density of 29 $\mu A/cm^2$ that was reached at a stimulation intensity of 1000 μA. This means, with our stimulation intensity, we were below the phosphene threshold, which was additionally confirmed by our questionnaire results. Furthermore, Kar and Krekelberg (2012) demonstrated that even with occipital electrode montage, perceived phosphenes are of retinal origin. Nevertheless, as no phosphenes were reported in the current study, we assume that the long lasting after-effects are due to direct cortical modulation.

The current results further support existing evidence for successful entrainment of oscillatory brain activity (Thut et al., 2011a). We applied tACS at a frequency that was predominant in the spontaneous brain activity of the individual subjects and our results demonstrate that we successfully enhanced the spontaneous activity in a frequency-dependent manner. Furthermore, topographies demonstrate that tACS effects on alpha power are local and enhance alpha oscillations that could be observed before stimulation (cf. **Figure 5**). One of the main questions is, how tACS of the intensity used in our study is able to modulate the neuronal network activity at all. The electrode configuration used in this study targeted the occipito-parietal alpha rhythm (Nunez et al., 2001). A modeling approach by Neuling et al. (2012a) demonstrated that this electrode layout is well suited to affect the occipital cortex (cf. **Figure 1**). The authors report that TES with an intensity of 1 mA, similar to the intensities used in the current study, results in currents of 420 μV/mm in gray matter, which is of sufficient strength to modulate neuronal network activity in the ferret visual cortex (Fröhlich and McCormick, 2010).

Sinusoidal electric fields generate periodic states of depolarization and hyperpolarization relative to the resting membrane potential of individual neurons, thereby generating periods of higher and lower firing probability of the neuron and consequently guiding the entire neuronal population (Fröhlich and McCormick, 2010). The authors demonstrated that although this effect is small on individual neurons it has a strong effect on network dynamics. During continuous stimulation with an oscillating current, spontaneous activity of an increasing number of individual neurons starts to synchronize[1] with the external oscillation, which in turn results in a power increase of the whole network (**Figure 7**). These findings are congruent with the current study, where elevated power levels have been reported.

A population of simple oscillators with similar intrinsic frequencies can be entrained by a single external oscillator (Winfree, 1980). This also applies for neuronal oscillators. An ideal condition for entrainment is a frequency match between the periodic external force and the intrinsic oscillation (Hutcheon and Yarom, 2000; Pikovsky et al., 2003). This means that neurons oscillating in the range of the external stimulation frequency will be entrained but neurons with intrinsic frequencies outside the stimulation frequency will not be affected (Fröhlich and McCormick, 2010). This is confirmed by the result that only IAF power is increased, whereas, surrounding frequency bands remain unaffected.

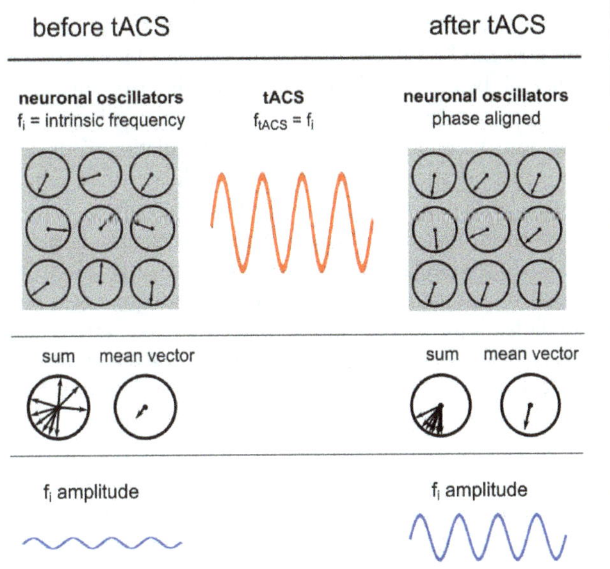

FIGURE 7 | Power increase by synchronization. Illustration of the proposed underlying neuronal mechanism of the power effect. **Upper row:** Single neuronal oscillators, depicted as vectors on a unit circle, with a specific intrinsic frequency synchronize to an external sinusoidal force with the same frequency. **Middle row:** The mean resultant vector of the single oscillating elements represents the amplitude of the oscillation. Due to phase alignment of each single oscillator to the external oscillation, the length of this mean vector increases and likewise the amplitude. **Lower row:** Schematic illustration of the amplitude recorded via EEG.

[1]Note that an oscillator can be phase-locked and/or frequency-locked to an external driving force. Frequency-locking can occur without phase-locking, but phase-locking implies also frequency-locking (Izhikevich, 2007, p. 460); however, our data cannot differentiate between these two states of synchronization.

Unfortunately it is not yet possible to record EEG online during tACS due to the artefact induced by the electric stimulation current. This would yield important insights into the mechanism of action of tACS and its immediate effect on the EEG and the dynamics of brain functions (Miniussi et al., 2012).

Sustained entrainment after the end of oscillatory TES in the alpha range has been reported by Zaehle et al. (2010) and Neuling et al. (2012a). However, these studies only analyzed 3 min directly after the stimulation. The current study demonstrates that these after-effects can outlast the stimulation for at least 30 min. Compared to Zaehle et al. (2010), who also targeted the occipital cortex with tACS at IAF, the current study found a stronger increase of individual IAF power (mean increase: 14% vs. 48%). This difference could be explained by two important parameters: Zaehle et al. (2010) stimulated for 10 min while we applied 20 min of tACS. Furthermore, we used a medial electrode configuration compared to the bilateral configuration used by Zaehle et al. (2010). A medial configuration might be beneficial to synchronize both hemispheres at 0° which might lead to the more pronounced power effect, while bilateral stimulation will lead to a phase difference of 180° between hemispheres.

We found a significant difference in the increase of alpha coherence between groups in the eyes closed condition. This difference was not found in the eyes open condition. One explanation for this effect might be a ceiling effect: if the coherence is already high before stimulation, it does not increase further. We found a negative correlation between the coherence before stimulation and the relative coherence after stimulation. This result suggests that pre stimulation coherence modulates the effect, but the correlation did not reach statistical significance. Although our hypothesis that the coherence before stimulation affects the increase after stimulation cannot be confirmed by our results, the negative correlation encourages further experiments to reveal the underlying mechanism of the coherence effect. Interestingly, results of another recent study of ours are in line with the data of the eyes closed condition (Strüber et al., under revision). We were only able to influence to coherence, but not the amplitude of EEG oscillations.

So far, after-effects of tACS up to an hour post-stimulation have only been reported regarding excitability, measured via motor evoked potentials (MEP) evoked with transcranial magnetic stimulation (Moliadze et al., 2010; Wach et al., 2012). However, EEG was not recorded in these studies, thus no statements can be given regarding effects on EEG power. After-effects lasting up to 90 min have been reported after tDCS (Nitsche and Paulus, 2001). After 13 min of stimulation with 1 mA, cerebral excitability enhancement up to 90 min has been detected via TMS evoked MEPs. Even though EEG was not recorded, these findings are in line with the duration of our effect.

A possible neurophysiological mechanism accounting for the long term after-effects in our study is based on synaptic plasticity (Zaehle et al., 2010). By means of spike-timing-dependent-plasticity (Markram et al., 1997), synapses can be strengthened, a mechanism known as long term potentiation or weakened, referred to as long term depression. During stimulation, synapses in neuronal circuits with an intrinsic frequency (Hutcheon and Yarom, 2000) of the external oscillation (tACS) are strengthened and are thought to persist after stimulation. This assumption was supported by network simulations (Zaehle et al., 2010), which resulted in enhanced synaptic weights of those synapses that were incorporated into neural loops whose frequency was close to that of tACS.

The duration of the after-effects presented here is a prerequisite for clinical applications of tACS for diseases correlated with altered oscillatory brain activity. For example, in schizophrenia, a dysregulation of oscillatory gamma activity may correlate with distinct schizophrenic symptoms (Lee et al., 2003). In Parkinson's disease, abnormal beta activity can lead to motor slowing (Hammond et al., 2007). Furthermore, evoked gamma-band activity is altered in children with attention deficit hyperactivity disorder (Lenz et al., 2010).

One can conclude that tACS has the potential to regulate brain dysfunctions that are related to EEG frequencies. Long lasting changes of endogenous brain oscillations could be used to balance modified brain oscillations. Furthermore, the knowledge that endogenous power has effects on tACS efficacy can be employed to improve attempts of task-related modulations of brain rhythms to modify behavior and improve learning.

ACKNOWLEDGMENTS

We thank Kim Möhrke for assistance with data acquisition and Christina Lavallee for proofreading the manuscript and improving the English style. This work was supported by grants of the German Research foundation to Christoph S. Herrmann (DFG, SFB/TRR 31) and to Stefan Rach (DFG, RA2357/1-1).

REFERENCES

Antal, A., Boros, K., Poreisz, C., Chaieb, L., Terney, D., and Paulus, W. (2008). Comparatively weak after-effects of transcranial alternating current stimulation (tACS) on cortical excitability in humans. *Brain Stimulat.* 1, 97–105.

Başar, E., Başar-Eroğlu, C., Karakas, S., and Schuermann, M. (2001). Gamma, alpha, delta, and theta oscillations govern cognitive processes. *Int. J. Psychophysiol.* 39, 241–248.

Berger, H. (1929). Über das Elektrenkephalogramm des Menschen. *Archiv für Psychiatrie und Nervenkrankheiten* 87, 527–570.

Bergmann, T., Groppa, S., Seeger, M., Mölle, M., Marshall, L., and Siebner, H. (2009). Acute changes in motor cortical excitability during slow oscillatory and constant anodal transcranial direct current stimulation. *J. Neurophysiol.* 102, 2303–2311.

Bollimunta, A., Chen, Y., Schroeder, C., and Ding, M. (2008). Neuronal mechanisms of cortical alpha oscillations in awake-behaving macaques. *J. Neurosci.* 28, 9976–9988.

Brignani, D., Ruzzoli, M., Mauri, P., and Miniussi, C. (2013). Is transcranial alternating current stimulation effective in modulating brain oscillations? *PLoS ONE* 8:e56589. doi: 10.1371/journal.pone.0056589

Brunoni, A. R., Amadera, J., Berbel, B., Volz, M., Rizzerio, B., and Fregni, F. (2011). A systematic review on reporting and assessment of adverse effects associated with transcranial direct current stimulation. *Int. J. Neuropsychopharmacol.* 14, 1133–1145.

Buzsáki, G. (2006). *Rhythms of the Brain.* Oxford: Oxford University Press.

Buzsáki, G., and Draguhn, A. (2004). Neuronal oscillations in cortical networks. *Science* 304, 1926–1929.

Delorme, A., and Makeig, S. (2004). EEGLAB: an open source toolbox for analysis of single-trial EEG dynamics including independent component analysis. *J. Neurosci. Meth.*134, 9–21.

Feurra, M., Paulus, W., Walsh, V., and Kanai, R. (2011). Frequency specific modulation of human somatosensory cortex. *Front. Psychol.* 2:13. doi: 10.3389/fpsyg.2011.00013

Fröhlich, F., and McCormick, D. A. (2010). Endogenous electric fields may guide neocortical network activity. *Neuron* 67, 129–143.

Hammond, C., Bergman, H., and Brown, P. (2007). Pathological synchronization in parkinson's disease: networks, models and treatments. *Trends Neurosci.* 30, 357–364.

Herrmann, C. S. (2001). Human EEG responses to 1–100.Hz flicker: resonance phenomena in visual cortex and their potential correlation to cognitive phenomena. *Exp. Brain Res.* 137, 346–353.

Herrmann, C. S., and Demiralp, T. (2005). Human EEG gamma oscillations in neuropsychiatric disorders. *Clin. Neurophysiol.* 116, 2719–2733.

Herrmann, C. S., Grigutsch, M., and Busch, N. (2004). "EEG oscillations and wavelet analysis," in *Event-Related Potentials: A Methods Handbook*, ed T. Handy (Cambridge: Bradford Books), 229–259.

Hutcheon, B., and Yarom, Y. (2000). Resonance, oscillation and the intrinsic frequency preferences of neurons. *Trends Neurosci.* 23, 216–222.

Izhikevich, E. M. (2007). *Dynamical Systems in Neuroscience: The Geometry of Excitability and Bursting*. Cambridge: The MIT Press.

Kanai, R., Chaieb, L., Antal, A., Walsh, V., and Paulus, W. (2008). Frequency-dependent electrical stimulation of the visual cortex. *Curr. Biol.* 18, 1839–1843.

Kar, K., and Krekelberg, B. (2012). Transcranial electrical stimulation over visual cortex evokes phosphenes with a retinal origin. *J. Neurophysiol.* 108, 2173–2178.

Könönen, M., and Partanen, J. V. (1993). Blocking of EEG alpha activity during visual performance in healthy adults. a quantitative study. *Electroencephalogr. Clin. Neurophysiol.* 87, 164–166.

Kuo, M.-F., and Nitsche, M. A. (2012). Effects of transcranial electrical stimulation on cognition. *Clin. EEG Neurosci.* 43, 192–199.

Lee, K., Williams, L., Breakspear, M., and Gordon, E. (2003). Synchronous gamma activity: a review and contribution to an integrative neuroscience model of schizophrenia. *Brain Res. Rev.* 41, 57–78.

Lenz, D., Krauel, K., Flechtner, H. H., Schadow, J., Hinrichs, H., and Herrmann, C. S. (2010). Altered evoked gamma-band responses reveal impaired early visual processing in ADHD children. *Neuropsychologia* 48, 1985–1993.

Markram, H., Lübke, J., Frotscher, M., and Sakmann, B. (1997). Regulation of synaptic efficacy by coincidence of postsynaptic APs and EPSPs. *Science* 275, 213–215.

Marshall, L., Helgadottir, H., Molle, M., and Born, J. (2006). Boosting slow oscillations during sleep potentiates memory. *Nature* 444, 610–613.

Miniussi, C., Brignani, D., and Pellicciari, M. C. (2012). Combining transcranial electrical stimulation with electroencephalography: a multimodal approach. *Clin. EEG Neurosci.* 43, 184–191.

Moliadze, V., Antal, A., and Paulus, W. (2010). Boosting brain excitability by transcranial high frequency stimulation in the ripple range. *J. Physiol.* 588, 4891–4904.

Neuling, T., Rach, S., and Herrmann, C. S. (2012a). Good vibrations: oscillatory phase shapes perception. *Neuroimage* 63, 771–778.

Neuling, T., Wagner, S., Wolters, C. H., Zaehle, T., and Herrmann, C. S. (2012b). Finite-element model predicts current density distribution for clinical applications of tDCS and tACS. *Front. Psychiatry* 3:83. doi: 10.3389/fpsyt.2012.00083

Nitsche, M. A., and Paulus, W. (2001). Sustained excitability elevations induced by transcranial DC motor cortex stimulation in humans. *Neurology* 57, 1899–1901.

Nunez, P. L., Wingeier, B. M., and Silberstein, R. B. (2001). Spatial-temporal structures of human alpha rhythms: theory, microcurrent sources, multiscale measurements, and global binding of local networks. *Hum. Brain Mapp.*13, 125–164.

Oldfield, R. C. (1971). The assessment and analysis of handedness: the Edinburgh inventory. *Neuropsychologia* 9, 97–113.

Osipov, G. V., Kurths, J., and Zhou, C. (2007). *Synchronization in Oscillatory Networks*. Berlin; Heidelberg; New York: Springer.

Pigeau, R. A., and Frame, A. M. (1992). Steady-state visual evoked responses in high and low alpha subjects. *Electroencephalogr. Clin. Neurophysiol.* 84, 101–109.

Pikovsky, A., Rosenblom, M., and Kurths, J. (2003). *Synchronization*. New York, NY: Cambridge University Press.

Pogosyan, A., Gaynor, L. D., Eusebio, A., and Brown, P. (2009). Boosting cortical activity at beta-band frequencies slows movement in humans. *Curr. Biol.*19, 1637–1641.

Polania, R., Nitsche, M. A., Korman, C., Batsikadze, G., and Paulus, W. (2012). The importance of timing in segregated theta phase-coupling for cognitive performance. *Curr. Biol.* 22, 1314–1318.

Regan, D. (1989). *Human Brain Electrophysiology: Evoked Potentials and Evoked Magnetic Fields in Science and Medicine*. New York, NY: Elsevier.

Romei, V., Gross, J., and Thut, G. (2010). On the role of prestimulus alpha rhythms over occipito-parietal areas in visual input regulation: correlation or causation? *J. Neurosci.* 30, 8692–8697.

Schroeder, C. E., and Lakatos, P. (2009). Low-frequency neuronal oscillations as instruments of sensory selection. *Trends Neurosci.* 32, 9–18.

Schwiedrzik, C. M. (2009). Retina or visual cortex? The site of phosphene induction by transcranial alternating current stimulation. *Front. Integr. Neurosci.* 3:6. doi: 10.3389/neuro.07.006.2009

Thut, G., Schyns, P., and Gross, J. (2011a). Entrainment of perceptually relevant brain oscillations by non-invasive rhythmic stimulation of the human brain. *Front. Psychol.* 2:170. doi: 10.3389/fpsyg.2011.00170

Thut, G., Veniero, D., Romei, V., Miniussi, C., Schyns, P., and Gross, J. (2011b). Rhythmic TMS causes local entrainment of natural oscillatory signatures. *Curr. Biol.* 21, 1176–1185.

Uhlhaas, P. J., Haenschel, C., Nikolić, D., and Singer, W. (2008). The role of oscillations and synchrony in cortical networks and their putative relevance for the pathophysiology of schizophrenia. *Schizophr. Bull.* 34, 927–943.

Wach, C., Krause, V., Moliadze, V., Paulus, W., Schnitzler, A., and Pollok, B. (2012). Effects of 10 Hz and 20 Hz transcranial alternating current stimulation (tACS) on motor functions and motor cortical excitability. *Behav. Brain Res.* 241, 1–6.

Wickens, T. (2001). *Elementary Signal Detection Theory*. New York, NY: Oxford University Press.

Winfree, A. (1980). *The Geometry of Biological Time*. New York; Heidelberg; Berlin: Springer.

Zaehle, T., Rach, S., and Herrmann, C. (2010). Transcranial alternating current stimulation enhances individual alpha activity in human EEG. *PLoS ONE* 5:e13766. doi: 10.1371/journal.pone.0013766

19

tDCS over the left inferior frontal cortex improves speech production in aphasia

***Paola Marangolo*[1,2]*, *Valentina Fiori*[2], *Maria A. Calpagnano*[2], *Serena Campana*[2], *Carmelina Razzano*[2], *Carlo Caltagirone*[2,3] and *Andrea Marini*[2,4]**

[1] *Facoltà di Medicina, Università Politecnica Marche, Ancona, Italy*
[2] *Department of Clinical and Behavioural Neurology, Istituto di Ricovero a Carattere Scientifico Fondazione Santa Lucia, Roma, Italy*
[3] *Department of Neurology, Universitá di Tor Vergata, Roma, Italy*
[4] *Dipartimento di Scienze Umane, Università di Udine, Udine, Italy*

Correspondence:
Paola Marangolo, Faculty of Medicine, Università Politecnica delle Marche, Via Tronto 10/A, 60020 Ancona, Italy
e-mail: p.marangolo@univpm.it

In this study, we investigated the combined effect of transcranial direct current stimulation (tDCS) and an intensive Conversational therapy treatment on discourse skills in 12 persons with chronic aphasia. Six short video clips depicting everyday life contexts were prepared. Three videoclips were used to elicit spontaneous conversation during treatment. The remaining three were presented only before and after the therapy. Participants were prompted to talk about the contents of each videoclip while stimulated with tDCS (20 min 1 mA) over the left hemisphere in three conditions: anodic tDCS over the Broca's area, anodic tDCS over the Wernicke's area, and a sham condition. Each experimental condition was performed for 10 consecutive daily sessions with 14 days of intersession interval. After stimulation over Broca's area, the participants produced more Content Units, verbs and sentences than in the remaining two conditions. Importantly, this improvement was still detectable 1 month after the end of treatment and its effects were generalized also to the three videoclips that had been administered at the beginning and at the end of the therapy sessions. In conclusion, anodic tDCS applied over the left Broca's area together with an intensive "Conversational Therapy" treatment improves informative speech in persons with chronic aphasia. We believe that positive tDCS effects may be further extended to other language domains, such as the recovery of speech production.

Keywords: tDCS, speech production, aphasia recovery, stroke, language rehabilitation

INTRODUCTION

Failure to spontaneously produce fluent and informative speech is the most persistent disabling consequence after stroke, particularly in persons with aphasia with left anterior hemispheric lesions (SPREAD, 2012). Traditional linguistic-based therapies have proved reasonably effective (Jensen, 2000; Kemmerer and Tranel, 2000; Raymer and Ellsworth, 2002; Wambaugh et al., 2002; Marangolo, 2012). However, in many cases a severe reduction of the ability to produce informative speech does persist (Basso, 2010; Marangolo, 2010; Andreetta et al., 2012). For this reason, several efforts have been devoted to the development of new approaches aimed at enhancing the use of language in daily-life communicative situations (e.g., Ulatowska et al., 1983; Saffran et al., 1989; Glosser and Deser, 1990; Nicholas and Brookshire, 1993). Among these, "Conversational therapy" is probably one of the most used (Holland, 1991; Lai, 1993; Basso, 2010; Marini and Carlomagno, 2004; Vigorelli, 2007; Marangolo, 2010; Wilkinson and Wielaert, 2012). Within the conversational therapy approach the therapist and the person with aphasia are engaged in a natural conversation and the latter is encouraged to use all of his/her communicative means to convey informative speech (Grice, 1975; Basso, 2010; Marangolo, 2010).

Parallel to this growing interest in the way language is processed in daily communicative interactions, the traditional views of how to assess language deficits in persons with aphasia have been challenged. Several studies have shown that traditional standardized aphasia tests may not be sensitive enough to adequately assess linguistic deficits and recovery patterns in persons with aphasia (Larfeuil and Le Dorze, 1997). As a result, both functional and structural methods for the analysis of connected language samples from people with aphasia have been proposed (see Armstrong, 2000; Prins and Bastiaanse, 2004; Marini et al., 2011). One procedure for quantifying information content was originally developed by Yorkston and Beukelman (1980). They administered the Cookie Theft Picture description task (Goodglass and Kaplan, 1972) to a group of participants with aphasia. The levels of informativeness of these language samples were quantified in terms of Content Units (C-Units), clusters of elements and/or isolated phrases not always accompanied by a verb, but with high communicative value (Loban, 1966).

Over the last few years, converging evidence has suggested the usefulness of therapies associating intensive language treatment with brain stimulation. Indeed, persons with aphasia exhibit greater recovery of lexical-retrieval deficits when the language treatment is coupled with repeated transcranial magnetic stimulation (rTMS; Naeser et al., 2005, 2010, 2011; Martin et al., 2009; Cotelli et al., 2011) or transcranial direct current stimulation (tDCS; Baker et al., 2010; Fiori et al., 2011; Fridriksson et al., 2011; Kang et al., 2011; Marangolo et al., 2013; see Elsner et al., 2013 and Monti et al., 2013 for reviews). However, these studies did not demonstrate whether the improvements found in the naming tasks would enhance the individuals' ability to use language in daily life interactions (see Brady et al., 2012 for a review).

To the best of our knowledge, only four studies have reported spontaneous speech production in individuals receiving rTMS stimulation (Naeser et al., 2005; Martin et al., 2009; Barwood et al., 2011; Medina et al., 2012). However, even in these investigations the TMS was not coupled with concomitant language training and discourse productivity was merely quantified in terms of phrase length (Naeser et al., 2005; Martin et al., 2009; Barwood et al., 2011) and production of narrative words (Medina et al., 2012).

Considering the benefical effects of tDCS on lexical recovery (Monti et al., 2008; Baker et al., 2010; Fiori et al., 2011; Fridriksson et al., 2011; Marangolo et al., 2013), we hypothesize that a Conversational therapy coupled with repeated stimulation might induce significant linguistic improvements also on other aspects of language processing. Recent evidence suggests a potential role for Broca's area and the adjacent cortex in the processes of lexical selection and unification, that is the combination of word information into larger units that span multi-word utterances (e.g., Hagoort, 2005; Indefrey and Cutler, 2005; Marini and Urgesi, 2012). As such, the left Inferior Frontal Gyrus (LIFG) might play a pivotal role in the recovery of units with a high communicative value (i.e., Content Units). Then, it might be an ideal candidate for the stimulation during conversational therapy.

The present study was aimed to investigate linguistic and functional aspects of language recovery in 12 chronic participants with non-fluent aphasia whose linguistic production showed reduced information content and poor syntactic organization. Three different stimulation conditions were employed: the target condition included anodic stimulation of the Broca's area (i.e., LIFG); a control condition with anodic stimulation of the Wernicke's area (i.e., posterior portiong of the left superior temporal gyrus, LSTC) allowed us to control for the specificity of the effects obtained within the target condition; a further control condition included sham stimulation. We hypothesized that if the Broca's area is indeed involved in the recovery of informative words, we would find a greater improvement only in this condition. The linguistic skills were assessed using different approaches, namely standard aphasia testing and the analysis of speech samples obtained through the administration of a series of videoclips reproducing common everyday situations. In order to assess the extent of any potential recovery, the videoclips were also administered to a group of healthy individuals. This allowed us to further control for significant improvements in the group of aphasic participants with respect to normality.

Overall, this study aimed to determine the efficacy of tDCS coupled with Conversational therapy in improving the informative skills of the aphasic group and their ability to produce adequate content in terms of production of C-Units. We also hypothesized that the potential lexical improvement would be particularly evident for verbs, a category of content words that are particularly impaired in these patients and that are thought to play a crucial role in the structural formulation of sentences (see also Wambaugh et al., 2002).

MATERIALS AND METHODS

PARTICIPANTS

Control group

Twenty healthy individuals (10 males and 10 females) matched for age (40–75 years) and education level (13–17 years) with the aphasic group were enrolled in the experiment. All of them were native Italian speakers with no history of neurological or psychiatric illness.

Aphasic group

Twelve participants (8 males and 4 female) who had sustained a single left hemisphere stroke were included in the study. Inclusion criteria were native Italian proficiency, pre-morbid right handedness, a single left hemispheric stroke at least 6 months prior to the investigation, and no acute or chronic neurological symptoms requiring medication. The data analyzed in the current study were collected in accordance with the Helsinky Declaration and the Institutional Review Board of the IRCCS Fondazione Santa Lucia, Rome, Italy. Prior to participation, all participants signed informed consent forms.

NEUROPSYCHOLOGICAL ASSESMENT

The aphasic disorders were assessed using standardized language testing [the Battery for the analysis of aphasic disorders, BADA test (Miceli et al., 1994)] and the Token test (De Renzi and Vignolo, 1962). Participants were also administered different tasks to investigate the principal attentional functions [selective, divided and sustained attention tests (Zimmermann and Fimm, 1994)] and a visual memory test [the Ray Figure test (Orsini et al., 1987)] to exclude the presence of attention and memory deficits that might have biased their performance.

CLINICAL DATA

All participants had an ischemic lesion involving the left hemisphere. The lesion mapping analysis indicated that the areas of maximal lesion overlap were localized in the capsula estrema, the claustrum, part of the capsula esterna and the putamen (see **Figure 1**). The 12 participants were diagnosed with non-fluent aphasia as they had reduced verbal output in spontaneous speech. Their utterances were short and characterized by omissions of verbs and function words as well as errors in verb inflection. Patients with severe articulatory impairments were excluded, in order to avoid a possible confound in data analysis. Their basic comprehension skills were preserved and indeed they were able to engage in verbal exchanges with the therapist. All patients had some difficulties in word reading and writing and in comprehending complex verbal materials (Token test). In the noun and verb naming tasks, severe word-finding difficulties were present (see **Table 1**).

MATERIALS

Six short videoclips (15 min each) reproducing common everyday life situations were prepared for the therapy. Three of them were employed to elicit spontaneous speech during the treatment (T[reatment]-videoclips: two persons eating at the restaurant, people leaving at the station, a woman attending to household chores). The remaining three videoclips were presented to the participants only before and after the therapy to control for generalization effects (G[eneralization]-videoclips: a girl making a coffee at home, a woman shopping at the supermarket, the housekeepers cleaning inside a hotel).

PROCEDURE

Prior to the experiment, all six videoclips (T- and G-videoclips) were shown to the control group. Each participant was asked to freely describe each video accurately, with no interference from the examiner.

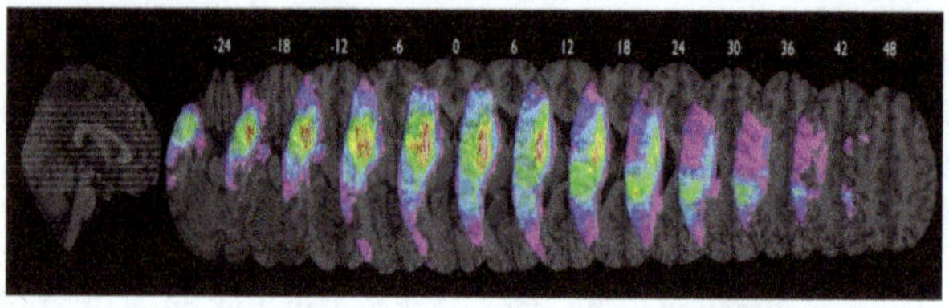

FIGURE 1 | Axial views of color coded probability map of lesion overlap (range 1% purple to 91% white). Individual volume lesions were drawn manually on the re-oriented brain volume transformed into MNI standardized stereotaxic coordinate system using a computational semi-automatic procedure of REGISTER software provided by Brain Imaging Center, Montreal Neurological Institute, McGill University. Averaging the labeled voxels of the individual lesion volumes re-aligned in MNI space generated the probability map revealing the localization of areas of percentage of lesion overlap. Maximal overlap includes the capsula estrema, the claustrum, part of the capsula esterna and the putamen. The inferior frontal gyrus (including the Broca's area) and the superior temporal gyrus (including the Wernicke's area) were similary damaged both having about 45% of lesion overlap.

TRANSCRANIAL DIRECT CURRENT STIMULATION (tDCS)

tDCS was applied using a battery driven Eldith (neuroConn GmbH) Programmable Direct Current Stimulator with a pair of surface-soaked sponge electrodes (5 × 7 cm). A constant current of 1 mA intensity was applied on the skin for 20 min. If applied according to safety guidelines, tDCS is considered to be a safe brain stimulation technique with minor adverse effects (Poreisz et al., 2007). Two different electrode stimulation positions were used: the F5 of the extended International 10–20 system for EEG electrode placement, which correspond best to the Broca's area (Nishitani et al., 2005; Naeser et al., 2010) and the CP5 of the extended International 10–20 system for EEG electrode placement, which has been found to correspond best to the Wernicke's area (Oliveri et al., 1999; Fiori et al., 2011). In both conditions the reference electrode was placed over the contralateral frontopolar cortex (Nitsche and Paulus, 2000; Sparing et al., 2008).

The persons with aphasia underwent two different stimulation conditions: (1) anodic (F5-A) stimulation over the Broca's area; (2) anodic (CP5-A) stimulation over the Wernicke's area; a sham condition was also included (F5/CP5 S). The sham condition was performed exactly like anodic stimulation. To better simulate the two stimulation conditions in half of the participants the electrode was applied over the Broca's area, whereas in the remaining half over the Wernicke's area. In both conditions, the stimulator was turned off after 30 s. It has been shown that this procedure

Table 1 | Sociodemographic and Clinical data of the 12 non-fluent aphasic participants.

Subjects	Sex	Age	Educational level	Time post-onset	Type of aphasia	Noun naming	Verb naming	Noun compreh	Verb compreh	Token test
B.C.	Female	63	8	3 year, 5 months	Non-fluent	5/30	2/28	40/40	20/20	16/36
F.S.	Female	71	5	1 year, 8 months	Non-fluent	3/30	3/28	40/40	20/20	22/36
P.C.	Male	65	9	1 year, 7 months	Non-fluent	6/30	6/28	40/40	20/20	9/36
P.F.	Male	44	13	7 years	Non-fluent	3/30	8/28	40/40	20/20	17/36
A.C	Male	64	13	4 years, 5 months	Non-fluent	4/30	2/28	40/40	20/20	19/36
N.M.	Female	65	13	3 years, 7 months	Non-fluent	5/30	3/28	40/40	20/20	18/36
P.M.	Male	52	13	1 year, 2 months	Non-fluent	6/30	4/28	40/40	20/20	12/36
R.L.	Male	61	11	4 years, 7 months	Non-fluent	3/30	4/28	40/40	20/20	10/36
R.F.	Male	53	13	7 months	Non-fluent	4/30	2/28	40/40	20/20	9/36
R.A.	Female	59	18	3 years, 3 months	Non fluent	6/30	3/28	40/40	20/20	16/36
P.E.	Male	68	18	1 year, 8 months	Non-fluent	5/30	4/28	40/40	20/20	11/36
M.A.	Male	50	18	4 years, 4 months	Non-fluent	8/30	6/28	40/40	20/20	13/36

Legend. Compreh, Comprehension.

For each language task, the number of correct responses are reported.

makes it possible to blind subjects as to the respective stimulation condition (Gandiga et al., 2006). Each stimulation condition was performed with concurrent speech therapy (the Conversational therapy approach). Although tDCS stimulation was delivered from the beginning of the therapy sessions up to 20 min, the language treatment lasted 2 h per day, in 10 consecutive daily sessions (Monday–Friday, weekend off, Monday–Friday). There was a 14-day intersession interval between each condition (see **Figure 2**).

During the language treatment, each T-videoclip was assigned to a different stimulation condition. The order of presentation of the T-videoclips and of stimulation conditions was randomized across subjects. The randomization procedure was delivered through allocation concealment. A clinician not involved in the rest of the study assigned each participant to the stimulation's condition. The random sequence was generated using sequentially numbered, opaque, sealed envelopes. Each language sample was tape-recorded and transcribed verbatim by a clinician. Both the person with aphasia and the clinician were blind with respect to the administration of tDCS. At the end of each condition, subjects were asked if they were aware of which condition (real or sham) they had been exposed to. None of the subjects was able to ascertain differences in intensity of sensation between the two conditions. To measure baseline performance, at the beginning of each experimental condition, all participants were asked to describe the T-videoclip without the therapist's help. The same was done at the end of each experimental condition.

LANGUAGE TREATMENT

According to the Conversational Therapy approach, the main goal of the clinician is to set up a natural conversation with the person with aphasia in which both interlocutors participate using their available communicative resources. Both the aphasic and the therapist were left free to use any communicative means (e.g., gestures, drawings, orthographic or phonological cues) to exchange salient information about the videoclip. The therapist was instructed to accept all the information provided by the patient and tried to relate it to the topic of conversation in order to improve its content and informative level. The goal of the therapy was to make the person with aphasia as much informative as possible on a daily basis and to bring him/her to talk about the video without the therapist's support.

In order to measure generalization of treatment effects, at the beginning and at the end of each experimental condition, all participants were re-administered the language tests and asked to describe the three G-videoclips without the therapist's support. Each language sample was tape-recorded and transcribed verbatim by two independent transcribers. The transcriptions were then compared so to obtain highly-reliable discourse samples that we could segment and analyze. The scoring procedure was performed independently by two raters and then compared. Reproducibility of the scoring procedures resulted in substantial agreement among the coders. The few discrepancies were resolved through discussion.

FOLLOW-UP

At 1 month after the end of each experimental condition, all subjects were again shown the corresponding T-video and asked to describe it without help. Also in this case, each language sample was tape-recorded and transcribed verbatim.

DATA ANALYSIS

Data were analyzed with SPSS 13.0 software. For the healthy and aphasic group, the mean number of C-Units, verbs and sentences produced for each T and G videoclip is reported in **Table 2**. Since during the treatment the videoclips were randomized across subjects and conditions, for the T-videoclips the data are reported only for the pre-and-post treatment sessions.

Before and after each treatment session, the mean number (and standard deviation) of correct C-Units, verbs and sentences produced by each aphasic in the T-and-G videoclips was divided by the mean number collected in the healthy control group for the same linguistic variables and videoclips. The final result was converted into a mean percentage of correct responses and then analyzed.

In the aphasic group, two different analyses were run: the former focused on the results achieved before and after therapy using the videoclips as treatment materials (T-videoclips); the latter focused on the generalization effects obtained on the videoclips presented only before and after the therapy (G-videoclips). For each analysis, a 2 × 3 repeated-measures ANOVA ($ANOVA_{rm}$) with two within-subject factors: *Time* [baseline (T1) vs. end of treatment (T10)] and *Condition* (anodic Broca's area vs. anodic Wernicke's area vs. Sham) was run separately for C-Units, verbs and sentences. The Interaction was explored by using the Scheffè post-hoc test.

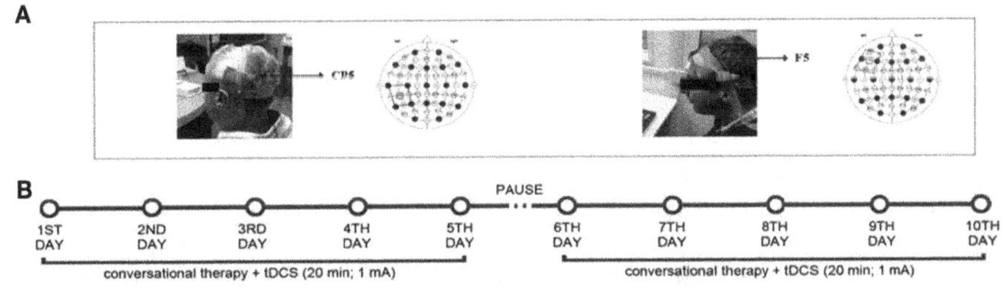

FIGURE 2 | Localization of the tDCS area (A) and overview of study design (B): one video-clip was used for the anodic Broca's stimulation, one for the anodic Wernicke's stimulation and a third one for the sham Broca's or Wernicke's condition. Each condition was performed in 10 consecutive daily sessions over 3 months, with 14 days of intersession interval, while the subjects underwent the "Conversational Therapy" treatment.

Table 2 | Mean number (± Standard Deviation) of C Units, Verbs, Sentences for the control and aphasic group collected in each T- and G-Videoclips.

	Control group	Aphasic group PRE-POST treatment		Control group	Aphasic group PRE/POST treatment		Control group	Aphasic group PRE- POST treatment	
	C-Units	C-Units	C-Units	Verbs	Verbs	Verbs	Sentences	Sentences	Sentences
T-VIDEOCLIPS									
Eating at the restaurant	38 (±9)	7** (±6)	14*/** (±11)	45 (±10)	14** (±9)	21*/** (±13)	35 (±8)	6** (±6)	14*/** (±11)
At the station	35 (±9)	9** (±6)	16*/** (±8)	44 (±10)	24** (±11)	31*/** (±12)	31 (±9)	8** (±5)	13*/** (±7)
At home	40 (±9)	9** (±5)	17*/** (±10)	47 (±11)	18** (±9)	27*/** (±12)	37 (±8)	9/** (±5)	16*/** (±9)
G-VIDEOCLIPS									
Making a coffee									
Broca	15 (±5)	5 (±5)**	10 (±6)*/**	13 (±4)	9 (±8)	12 (±8)*	13 (±3)	4 (±4)**	5 (±6)**
Wernicke		6 (±5)**	6 (±4)**		9 (±6)	9 (±6)		3 (±2)**	3(±3)**
Sham		5 (±5)**	5 (±5)**		9 (±7)	8 (±7)		3 (±3)**	3(±2)**
Shopping at the supermarket									
Broca	14 (±4)	2 (±2)**	6 (±5)*/**	14 (±4)	5 (±4)**	6 (±6)**	14 (±3)	2 (±2)**	6 (±4)*/**
Wernicke		2 (±3)**	3 (±3)**		5 (±4)**	5 (±3)**		1 (±1)**	2 (±2)**
Sham		3 (±3)**	2 (±2)**		5(±5)**	5 (±4)**		2(±2)**	1 (±1)**
The housekeepers									
Broca	14 (±2)	3 (±3)**	4 (±6)**	15 (±4)	7 (±6)**	9 (±6)	12 (±4)	2 (±2)**	6 (±5)*/**
Wernicke		4 (±3)**	5 (±3)**		8 (±4)**	7 (±5)**		3 (±2)**	4 (±3)**
Sham		3 (±3)**	3 (±3)**		7 (±6)**	7 (±5)**		3 (±3)**	3 (±2)**

*Since during the treatment the videoclips were randomized across subjects and conditions, for the T-videoclips data are reported only for the pre-post treatment sessions (pre/post treatment sessions in the aphasic group all paired t-test *p < 0.05; across groups **p < 0.01).*

In addition, to measure long-lasting beneficial effect of the treatment a 2 × 3× 3 repeated-measures ANOVA ($ANOVA_{rm}$) with three within-subject factors: *Time* [end of treatment (T10) vs. follow up (F1)], *Condition* (anodic Broca's area vs. anodic Wernicke's area vs. Sham) and *Category* (Verbs vs. C-Units vs. Sentences) was run. The Interaction was explored by using the Scheffè *post-hoc* test.

Finally, before and after each treatment session, the aphasic's responses to the different re-administration of the standardized language tests were analyzed. Since no significant differences were found in each language task (chi square tests, all *ps* = n.s.), the data were not further investigated.

RESULTS

TREATMENT

C-units

The analysis showed a significant effect of *Time* [baseline (T1) vs. end of treatment (T10), $F_{(1, 11)} = 51.50$; $p = 0.000$] and of *Condition* [anodic Broca's area vs. anodic Wernicke's area vs. Sham, $F_{(2, 22)} = 5.22$; $p = 0.014$]. Subjects' performance significantly improved at the end of training with respect to baseline [mean = 48%, SEM = 6 (T10) vs. mean = 28%, SEM = 4 (T1) $p = 0.000$]. Moreover, the mean percentage of C-Units in the anodic Broca's condition was significantly greater than in the other two conditions (mean = 48%, SEM = 7 (anodic Broca's) vs. mean = 35%, SEM = 4 (anodic Wernicke's) vs. mean = 31%, SEM = 6 (Sham) $p = 0.014$). The interaction of *Time* × *Condition* [$F_{(2, 22)} = 24.18$; $p = 0.000$] was also significant. While no significant differences emerged in the mean percentage of C-Units between the three conditions at baseline (differences between Broca vs. Wernicke = 1%, $p = 0.768$; differences between Broca vs. Sham = 2%, $p = 0.509$; differences between Wernicke vs. Sham = 1%, $p = 0.713$), at the end of training, the mean percentage of C-Units was significantly greater in the anodic Broca's condition with respect to the other two conditions, which did not differ from each other (differences between Broca vs. Wernicke = 27%; $p = 0.000$; differences between Broca vs. Sham = 34%; $p = 0.000$; differences between Sham vs. Wernicke = −7%; $p = 0.064$) (see **Figure 3** and **Table 3**).

Verbs

The analysis showed a significant effect of *Time* [baseline (T1) vs. end of treatment (T10), $F_{(1, 11)} = 34.53$; $p = 0.000$] but not of *Condition* [anodic Broca's area vs. anodic Wernicke's area vs. Sham, $F_{(2, 22)} = 1.54$; $p = 0.235$]. Subjects' performance significantly improved at the end of training with respect to baseline [mean = 47%, SEM = 3 (T10) vs. mean = 29%, SEM = 4 (T1) $p = 0.000$]. The interaction of *Time* × *Condition* [$F_{(2, 22)} = 7.38$; $p = 0.004$] was also significant. While no significant differences emerged in the mean percentage of verbs between the three conditions at baseline (differences between Broca vs. Wernicke = −3%, $p = 0.588$; differences between Broca vs. Sham = 1%,

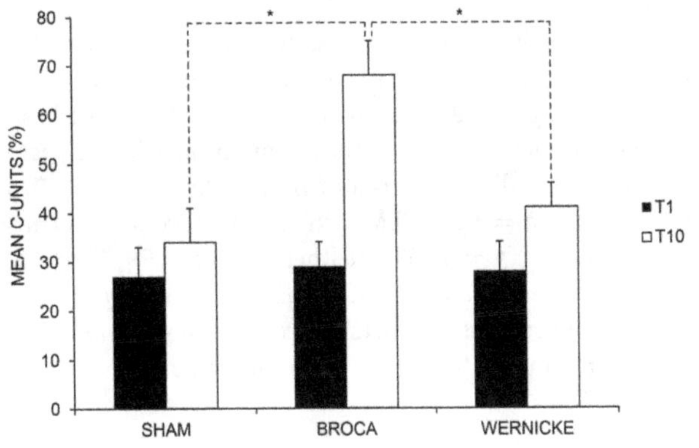

FIGURE 3 | Mean percentage of correct "C-Units" at baseline (T1) and at the end of treatment (T10) for the left anodic Wernicke's, Broca's and sham conditions (* < 0.01), respectively. Error bars represent standard error of the mean.

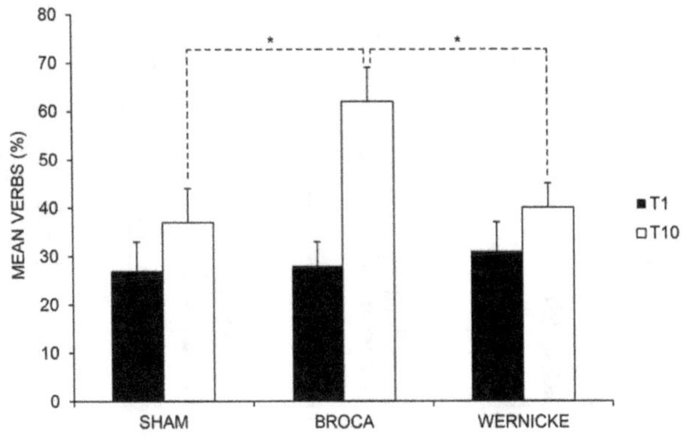

FIGURE 4 | Mean percentage of correct verbs at baseline (T1) and at the end of treatment (T10) for the left anodic Wernicke's, Broca's and sham conditions (* < 0.01), respectively. Error bars represent standard error of the mean.

Table 3 | Mean percentage of correct C-Units, Verbs and Sentences (±SEM) for the 12 aphasic participants at the baseline (T1), at the end of treatment (T10) and at follow-up (1 month after the end of treatment) for the Broca's, Wernicke's and sham condition, respectively (SEM = error standard of the mean).

	BROCA	WERNICKE	SHAM	Total mean
C-UNITS				
T1	29 (±6)	28 (±4)	27 (±6)	28 (±4)
T10	68 (±9)	41 (±5)	34 (±7)	48 (±6)
FOLLOW UP	64 (±9)	43 (±6)	36 (±7)	48 (±6)
Total mean	53(± 8)	37 (± 5)	32 (±7)	
VERBS				
T1	28 (±5)	31 (±6)	27 (±6)	29 (±4)
T10	62 (±7)	40 (±5)	37 (±7)	47 (±3)
FOLLOW UP	60 (±6)	41 (±5)	38 (±6)	47 (±3)
Total mean	50 (±5)	37 (±5)	34 (±6)	
SENTENCES				
T1	32 (±7)	28 (±4)	28 (±7)	30 (±5)
T10	67 (±9)	40 (±6)	36 (±7)	48 (±6)
FOLLOW UP	65 (±9)	40 (±6)	35 (±7)	47 (±6)
Total mean	55 (±8)	36 (±5)	33 (±7)	

$p = 0.950$; differences between Wernicke vs. Sham = −4%, $p = 0.546$), at the end of training, the mean percentage of verbs was significantly greater in the anodic Broca's condition with respect to the other two conditions, which did not differ from each other (differences between Broca vs. Wernicke = 22%; $p = 0.000$; differences between Broca vs. Sham = 25%; $p = 0.000$; differences between Sham vs. Wernicke = −3%; $p = 0.642$) (see **Figure 4** and **Table 3**).

Sentences

The analysis showed a significant effect of *Time* [baseline (T1) vs. end of treatment (T10), $F_{(1, 11)} = 44.77$; $p = 0.000$] and of *Condition* [anodic Broca's area vs. anodic Wernicke's area vs. Sham, $F_{(2, 22)} = 6.29$; $p = 0.007$]. Subjects' performance significantly improved at the end of training with respect to baseline [mean = 48%, SEM = 6 (T10) vs. mean = 30%, SEM = 5 (T1) $p = 0.000$]. Moreover, the mean percentage of sentences in the anodic Broca's condition was significantly greater than in the other two conditions (mean = 50%, SEM = 8 (anodic Broca's) vs. mean = 34%, SEM = 5 (anodic Wernicke's) vs. mean = 32%, SEM = 6 (Sham) $p = 0.007$). The interaction of *Time* × *Condition* [$F_{(2, 22)} = 76.62$; $p = 0.000$] was also significant. While no significant differences emerged in the mean percentage of sentences between the three conditions at baseline (differences between Broca vs. Wernicke = 4%, $p = 0.238$; differences between Broca vs. Sham = 4 %, $p = 0.275$; differences between Wernicke vs. Sham = 0%, $p = 0.927$), at the end of training, the mean percentage of sentences was significantly greater in the anodic Broca's condition with respect to the other two conditions, which did not differ from each other (differences between Broca vs. Wernicke = 27%; $p = 0.000$; differences between Broca vs. Sham = 31%; $p = 0.000$; differences between Sham vs. Wernicke = −4%; $p = 0.190$) (see **Figure 5** and **Table 3**).

GENERALIZATION OF THE TREATMENT

For the "Making a Coffee" video, we found a greater improvement in the Broca's condition with respect to the other two conditions in the mean number of verbs (differences between Broca vs. Wernicke = 26%; $p = 0.000$; differences between Broca vs. Sham = 29%; $p = 0.000$; differences between Sham vs. Wernicke = −3%; $p = 0.604$) and C-Units (differences between Broca vs. Wernicke = 30%; $p = 0.000$; differences between Broca vs. Sham = 34%; $p = 0.000$; differences between Sham vs. Wernicke = −4%; $p = 0.559$). An improvement in C-Units was also found for the "The supermarket" video, which was significantly greater in the Broca's condition with respect to the other two conditions (differences between Broca vs. Wernicke = 23%; $p = 0.000$; differences between Broca vs. Sham = 24%; $p = 0.000$; differences between Sham vs. Wernicke = −1%; $p = 0.829$). For the same video and again for the Broca's condition, we also observed a significant greater change in the mean number of correct sentences with respect to the other two conditions (differences between Broca vs. Wernicke = 18%; $p = 0.000$; differences between

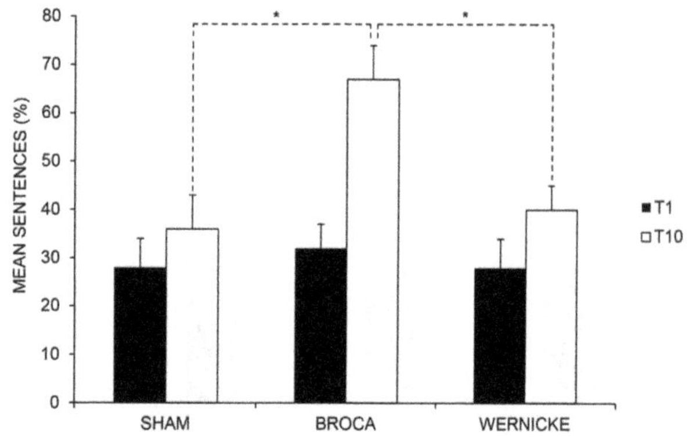

FIGURE 5 | Mean percentage of correct sentences at baseline (T1) and at the end of treatment (T10) for the left anodic Wernicke's, Broca's and sham conditions (* < 0.01), respectively. Error bars represent standard error of the mean.

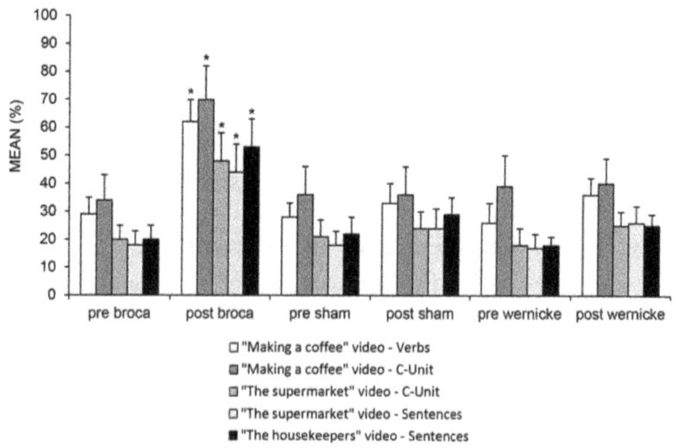

FIGURE 6 | Mean percentage of correct "C-Units", verbs and sentences during the presentation of the three videos ("Making a coffee", "The Supermarket" and "The Housekeepers") presented only at baseline and at the end of treatment in the pre-and post-anodic Broca's, sham and Wernicke's conditions (* < 0.01), respectively.

Broca vs. Sham = 20%; $p = 0.002$; differences between Sham vs. Wernicke = −2%; $p = 0.705$). This last result significantly changed in the same condition also for "The housekeepers" video (differences between Broca vs. Wernicke = 28%; p=0.000; differences between Broca vs. Sham = 24%; $p = 0.000$; differences between Sham vs. Wernicke = 4%; $p = 0.455$) (see **Figure 6**).

The relationship between C-Units, Verbs and Sentences after stimulation of Broca's area was further investigated using Pearson product-moment correlation coefficient. Preliminary analyses were performed to ensure no violation of the assumptions of normality, linearity, and homoscedasticity. There was a strong positive correlation between C-Units and Verbs [$r = 0.75$; $p = 0.005$] and between verbs and sentences [$r = 0.75$; $p = 0.005$]. This suggests that the stimulation of Broca's area increased the production of informative units and that such increase boosted the production of verbs. Furthermore, the increased ability to have access to the morphosyntactic information contained in these verbs allowed them to produce more accurate sentences.

FOLLOW-UP

Overall, the analysis showed a significant effect of *Condition* [Broca's vs. Wernicke's vs. Sham conditions, $F_{(2, 22)} = 11.43$; $p = 0.000$] indicating a greater improvement for C-Units, Verbs and Sentences production in the Broca's condition with respect to the other two conditions [Broca's (mean = 64%, SEM = 7) vs. Wernicke's (mean = 41%, SEM = 5) vs. Sham condition (mean = 36%, SEM = 6) $p = 0.000$]. Neither the *Time* [$F_{(1, 11)} = 0.21$; $p = 0.654$] nor the *Category* effect [$F_{(2, 22)} = 0.04$; $p = 0.963$] were significant suggesting a persistence of the results obtained at the end of treatment after 1 month for all categories (see **Table 3** and **Figure 7**).

DISCUSSION

The aim of this study was to determine if tDCS delivered over the Broca's area coupled with an intensive treatment based on Conversational therapy improves informative speech in persons with chronic non-fluent aphasia. To keep high ecological validity and, therefore, to analyze communication in natural contexts, our materials included six videoclips depicting common everyday situations.

Overall, three major findings will be discussed: (1) after Broca's stimulation, the ability of the persons with aphasia to produce informative speech showed the greatest improvement as they produced descriptions with more C-Units; (2) changes in informativeness during therapy corresponded to relevant changes in the production of verb that, in turn, boosted the participants' ability to use relevant morphosyntactic information and increased the number of sentences produced; (3) significant changes after therapy persisted after 1 month and were observed not only on the videoclips used during the treatment but also in the three videoclips presented to the participants only at the beginning and at the end of the therapy sessions, while no changes were found on the standard aphasia assessment.

The production of informative messages is an effortful endeavor that relies on the interaction between microlinguistic (i.e., lexical and grammatical) and macrolinguistic (i.e., pragmatic and discourse) levels of processing. The goal of the therapy used in the present study was to encourage the use of informative speech even if not always formally correct. Therefore, the approach was mainly focused onto the pragmatic aspects of language. Indeed, patients were required to select the lexical representations that were appropriate to the given context and to organize them within a communicative interaction. To date, although the neural correlates of microlinguistic processing have been extensively studied (Vigneau et al., 2006), the investigation of the ability to organize the macrolinguistic aspects of message production have been much less explored. Recent neuropsychological, neuroimaging and fMRI studies have suggested that Broca's area and the adjacent portion of the left inferior frontal cortex may play a major role for the top-down controlled selection and/or retrieval of contextually adequate words from the mental lexicon (Loban, 1966; Wagner et al., 2001; Hagoort, 2005; Koechlin and Jubault, 2006; Lau et al., 2008; Kim et al., 2011; Whitney et al., 2011; Marini and Urgesi, 2012; Schuhmann et al., 2012). Once retrieved, this lexical information is unified into an overall representations that spans multi-word utterances

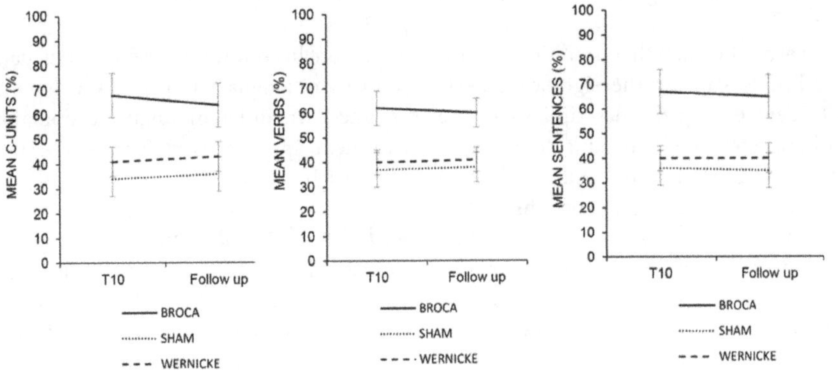

FIGURE 7 | Mean percentage of correct C-Units, Verbs and Sentences at the end of treatment (T10) and at the follow-up for the left anodic Wernicke's, Broca's and sham condition. Error bars represent standard error of the mean.

(Indefrey and Cutler, 2005). As a result, by faciliting the process of lexical selection and retrieval, the stimulation of this region likely elicits the integration of word meanings into an unfolding discourse representation of the context (Hagoort, 2005). Our results are coherent with this interpretation. Indeed, after Broca's stimulation, the patients who were initially unable to communicate verbally could sustain a conversation and produce more content units (i.e., informative chunks). Recently, Marini and Urgesi (2012) reached similar conclusions. In their study, rTMS applied over the dorsal portion of the anterior left, but not right, inferior frontal gyrus (LIFG) reduced the levels of lexical informativeness of narratives produced by a group of healthy individuals. In the authors' interpretation, since the LIFG is involved in the selection of specific lexical concepts, the inhibition of this area through rTMS hampered this process forcing the speakers to change the flow of discourse so to occasionally produce utterances conceptually incongruent with the story.

However, since verbs carry critical meaning in the communicative process, after the treatment we also found a significant increase in verb production. This result is in line with recent reports which showed that excitatory stimulation applied over the left Broca's area or over the surrounding frontal region (left dorsolateral frontal cortex, LDLFC), together with simultaneous intensive language training, led to the greatest amount of verb naming improvement (Cotelli et al., 2012; Marangolo et al., 2013).

It is widely acknowledged that verb representation constrains the assignment of retrieved lexical items to positions within the syntactic frame, and, therefore, plays a crucial role in the structural formulation of sentences (Zingeser and Berndt, 1990; Wambaugh et al., 2002). Accordingly, the speech samples of our participants after the treatment included more grammatically correct sentences. Again, this improvement was greatest after the anodic stimulation over Broca's area. This result is in agreement with recent findings from fMRI studies on spontaneous production in healthy participants, which showed a significant association between syntactic skills and activation of the left inferior frontal gyrus (Grande et al., 2012; see also Menenti et al., 2012).

Taken together, these results suggest that Broca's area is a cortical epicenter subserving the selection of contextually appropriate semantic representations. This conceptual information triggers the generation of appropriate propositions that must be organized at the macrolinguistic level by means of coherent links and increases discourse informativeness.

One important finding of our study was that the enhanced recovery in the participants' ability to communicate, as measured in terms of C-Units, Verbs and Sentences, still persisted at 1 month after the end of treatment. Furthermore, this recovery was generalized also to other contexts which were presented to the participants only before and after each treatment condition.

It has been suggested that long-lasting functional changes in the cortex as the result of electrical stimulation are the consequence of modulation of the strength of synaptic connections (i.e., synaptic plasticity, Nitsche and Paulus, 2000). In our study, the choice to stimulate the left-language hemisphere regions was related to previous results indicating that the stimulation of these sites in persons with chronic aphasia might enhance functional improvement inducing the reactivation of left-hemispheric perilesional structures (Baker et al., 2010; Fiori et al., 2011; Fridriksson et al., 2011; Marangolo et al., 2011, 2013). These results agree with the hypothesis that, in individuals with chronic aphasia, language recovery mostly involved the left unaffected cortical areas (Saur et al., 2006; Warburton et al., 1999; Winhuisen et al., 2007). Although it is often assumed that the right homologue of Broca's area takes over the function of the left if it is infarcted, the evidence for this is slender. Recent studies have stressed the importance of left Broca's area or adjacent tissue in the natural recovery from post-stroke aphasia (Saur et al., 2006, 2008) and there is some evidence that the right homologue of Broca's area inhibits recovery (Naeser et al., 2005, 2010, 2011).

In our aphasic group, the lesion mapping analysis over the two stimulated areas allowed us to exclude that the better recovery observed after Broca's stimulation was due to a greater sparing of this region to cerebral damage compared to Wernicke's area. Indeed, the same percentage of damage was present into the two stimulated areas (45%) (see **Figure 1**) However, in those subjects in which Broca's area was partly or completely damaged, it might be speculated that tDCS has influenced the activity of the brain centers close to the stimulated site producing a rearrangement of synaptic efficiency within the underlying network which in turn led to an improvement of the cognitive language ability (Miniussi et al., 2008; Cotelli et al., 2011).

One final comment regards the fact that traditional standardized language tests failed to capture the significant post-therapy effect that was evident during the descriptions of the videoclips. Likely, this discrepancy might be due to the specific nature of these different tasks. Indeed, while traditional language tests require to produce words under the administration of static pictures, the dynamic therapeutic setting devised for this study employed videoclips representing highly realistic contexts that exerted a positive influence on lexical retrieval. Overall, these considerations are in line with the hypothesis that a multi-level approach to language analysis is more adequate than standardized language tests to quantify communicative improvement in persons with aphasia (Larfeuil and Le Dorze, 1997; Marini et al., 2007, 2011; Andreetta et al., 2012).

In conclusion, we believe that our data clearly show that the recovery of language in persons with aphasia can be successfully enhanced in different linguistic domains by coupling specific treatment approaches with relatively simple stimulation procedures such as tDCS.

AUTHOR CONTRIBUTIONS

Conceived and designed the experiments: Paola Marangolo, Valentina Fiori. Performed the experiments: Valentina Fiori, Carmelina Razzano. Analyzed the data: Valentina Fiori, Maria Antonietta Calpagnanot. Analyzed neuroimaging data Serena Campana. Wrote the paper: Paola Marangolo. Editing and critical revision of the manuscript: Andrea Marini, Carlo Caltagirone.

REFERENCES

Andreetta, S., Cantagallo, A., and Marini, A. (2012). Narrative discourse in anomic aphasia. *Neuropsychologia* 50, 1787–1793. doi: 10.1016/j.neuropsychologia.2012.04.003

Armstrong, E. (2000). Aphasic discourse analysis: the story so far. *Aphasiology* 14, 875–892. doi: 10.1080/02687030050127685

Baker, J. M., Rorden, C., and Fridriksson, J. (2010). Using transcranial direct-current stimulation to treat stroke patients with aphasia. *Stroke* 41, 1229–1236. doi: 10.1161/STROKEAHA.109.576785

Barwood, C. H., Murdoch, B. E., Whelan, B. M., Lloyd, D., Riek, S., O'Sullivan, J. D., et al. (2011). Improved language performance subsequent to low-frequency rTMS in patients with chronic non-fluent aphasia post-stroke. *Eur. J. Neurol.* 18, 935–943. doi: 10.1111/j.1468-1331.2010.03284.x

Basso, A. (2010). "Natural" conversation: a treatment for severe aphasia. *Aphasiology* 24, 466–479. doi: 10.1080/02687030802714165

Brady, M. C., Kelly, H., Godwin, J., and Enderby, P. (2012). Speech and language therapy for aphasia folowing stroke (Review). *Cochrane Library* 5, 1–229.

Cotelli, M., Fertonani, A., Miozzo, A., Rosini, S., Manenti, R., Padovani, A., et al. (2011). Anomia training and brain stimulation in chronic aphasia. *Neuropsychol. Rehabil.* 21, 717–741. doi: 10.1080/09602011.2011.621275

Cotelli, M., Manenti, R., Alberici, A., Brambilla, M., Cosseddu, M., Zanetti, O., et al. (2012). Prefrontalcortex rTMS enhances action naming in progressive non-fluent aphasia. *Eur. J. Neurol.* 19, 1404–1412. doi: 10.1111/j.1468-1331.2012.03699.x

De Renzi, E., and Vignolo, L. A. (1962). The token test: a sensitive test to detect receptive disturbances in aphasia. *Brain* 85, 665–678. doi: 10.1093/brain/85.4.665

Elsner, B., Kugler, J., and Mehrholz, J. (2013). Transcranial direct current stimulation (tDCS) for improving aphasia in patients after stroke (Review). *Cochrane Library.* 6, 1–45.

Fiori, V., Coccia, M., Marinelli, C. V., Vecchi, V., Bonifazi, S., Ceravolo, M. G., et al. (2011). Transcranial direct current stimulation improves word retrieval in healthy and nonfluent aphasic subjects. *J. Cogn. Neurosci.* 23, 2309–2323. doi: 10.1162/jocn.2010.21579

Fridriksson, J., Richardson, J. D., Baker, J. M., and Rorden, C. (2011). Transcranial direct current stimulation improves naming reaction time in fluent aphasia: a double-blind, sham-controlled study. *Stroke* 42, 819–821. doi: 10.1161/STROKEAHA.110.600288

Gandiga, P. C., Hummel, F. C., and Cohen, L. G. (2006). Transcranial DC stimulation (tDCS): a tool for double-blind sham-controlled clinical studies in brain stimulation. *Clin. Neurophysiol.* 117, 845–850. doi: 10.1016/j.clinph.2005.12.003

Glosser, G., and Deser, T. (1990). Patterns of discourse production among neurological patients with fluent language disorders. *Brain Lang.* 40, 67–88. doi: 10.1016/0093-934X(91)90117-J

Goodglass, H., and Kaplan, E. (1972). *The Boston Diagnostic Aphasia Examination.* Philadelphia, PA: Lea and Febiger.

Grande, M., Meffert, E., Schoenberger, E., Jung, S., Frauenrath, T., Huber, W., et al. (2012). From a concept to a word in a syntactically complete sentence: An fMRI study on spontaneous language production in an overt picture description task. *Neuroimage* 61, 702–714. doi: 10.1016/j.neuroimage.2012.03.087

Grice, P. (1975). "Logic and conversation," in *Syntax and Semantics. 3 Speech Acts,* eds P. Cole and J. Morgan (New York, NY: Academic Press), 183–198.

Hagoort, P. (2005). On Broca, brain, and binding: a new framework. *Trends Cogn. Sci.* 9, 416–423. doi: 10.1016/j.tics.2005.07.004

Holland, A. L. (1991). Pragmatic aspects of intervention in aphasia. *J. Neurolinguist.* 6, 197–211. doi: 10.1016/0911-6044(91)90007-6

Jensen, L. R. (2000). Canonical structure without access to verbs? *Aphasiology* 14, 827–850.

Indefrey, P., and Cutler, A. (2005). "Prelexical and lexical processing in listening," in *The Cognitive Neurosciences,* ed M. S. Gazzaniga (New York, NY: MIT Press), 759–774.

Kang, E. K., Kim, Y. K., Sohn, H. M., Cohen, L. G., and Paik, N. J. (2011). Improved picture naming in aphasia patients treated with cathodal tDCS to inhibit the right Broca's homologue area. *Restor. Neurol. Neurosci.* 29, 141–152.

Kemmerer, D., and Tranel, D. (2000). Verb retrieval in brain-damaged subjects: 1. analysis of stimulus, lexical, and conceptual factors. *Brain Lang.* 73, 347–392. doi: 10.1006/brln.2000.2311

Kim, K. K., Karunanayaka, P., Privitera, M. D., Holland, S. K., and Szaflarski, J. P. (2011). Semantic association investigated with functional MRI and independent component analysis. *Epilepsy Behav.* 20, 613–622. doi: 10.1016/j.yebeh.2010.11.010

Koechlin, E., and Jubault, T. (2006). Broca's area and the hierarchical organization of human behavior. *Neuron* 50, 963–974. doi: 10.1016/j.neuron.2006.05.017

Lai, G. (1993). "Conversazionalismo," Torino: Bollati Boringhieri.

Larfeuil, C., and Le Dorze, G. (1997). An analysis of the word-finding difficulties and of the content of the discourse of recent and chronic aphasic speakers. *Aphasiology* 11, 783–811. doi: 10.1080/02687039708250456

Lau, E. F., Phillips, C., and Poeppel, D. (2008). A cortical network for semantics: (De)constructing the N400. *Nat. Rev. Neurosci.* 9, 920–933. doi: 10.1038/nrn2532

Loban, W. (1966). *Language Ability: Grades Seven, Eight, and Nine.* Washington, DC: Government Printing Office.

Marangolo, P. (2010). Riabilitazione nella fase degli esiti. *Acta Phoniatrica Latina* 32, 289–300.

Marangolo, P., Marinelli, C. V., Bonifazi, S., Fiori, V., Ceravolo, M. G., Provinciali, L., et al. (2011). Electrical stimulation over the left inferior frontal gyrus (IFG) determines long-term effects in the recovery of speech apraxia in three chronic aphasics. *Behav. Brain Res.* 225, 498–504. doi: 10.1016/j.bbr.2011.08.008

Marangolo, P. (2012). "La Riabilitazione dei deficit semantico-lessicali," in *La Riabilitazione Neuropsicologica,* ed A. Mazzucchi (Il Mulino, OR: Masson), 44–60.

Marangolo, P., Fiori, V., Di Paola, M., Cipollari, S., Razzano, C., Oliveri, M., et al. (2013). Differential processing of the left frontal and temporal regions in verb naming: a tDCS treatment study. *Restor. Neurol. Neurosci.* 31, 63–72.

Marini, A., and Carlomagno, S. (2004). *Analisi Del Discorso e Patologia Del Linguaggio.* Milan: Springer Verlag Italia.

Marini, A., Caltagirone, C., Pasqualetti, P., and Carlomagno, S. (2007). Patterns of language improvement in adults with non-chronic non-fluent aphasia after specific therapies. *Aphasiology* 21, 164–186. doi: 10.1080/02687030600633799

Marini, A., Andreetta, S., Del Tin, S., and Carlomagno, S. (2011). A multi-level approach to the analysis of narrative language in aphasia. *Aphasiology* 25, 1372–1392. doi: 10.1080/02687038.2011.584690

Marini, A., and Urgesi, C. (2012). Please get to the point! A cortical correlate of linguistic informativeness. *J. Cogn. Neurosci.* 24, 2211–2222. doi: 10.1162/jocn_a_00283

Martin, P. I., Naeser, M. A., Ho, M., Doron, K. W., Kurland, J., Kaplan, J., et al. (2009). Overt naming fMRI pre- and post-TMS: two nonfluent aphasia patients, with and without improved naming post-TMS. *Brain Lang.* 111, 20–35. doi: 10.1016/j.bandl.2009.07.007

Medina, J., Norise, C., Faseyitan, O., Coslett, H. B., Turkeltaub, P. E., and Hamilton, R. H. (2012). Finding the right words: transcranial magnetic stimulation improves discourse productivity in non-fluent aphasia after stroke. *Aphasiology* 26, 1153–1168. doi: 10.1080/02687038.2012.710316

Menenti, L., Segaert, K., and Hagoort, P. (2012). The neuronal infrastructure of speaking. *Brain Lang.* 122, 71–80. doi: 10.1016/j.bandl.2012.04.012

Miceli, G., Laudanna, A., Burani, C., and Capasso, R. (1994). *Batteria per L'analisi dei deficit afasici BADA*. Roma: CEPSAG, Policlinico Gemelli, Università Cattolica del Sacro Cuore.

Miniussi, C., Cappa, S. F., Cohen, L. G., Floel, A., Fregni, F., Nitsche, M. A., et al. (2008). Efficacy of repetitive transcranial magnetic stimulation/transcranial direct current stimulation in cognitive neurorehabilitation. *Brain Stimul.* 1, 326–336. doi: 10.1016/j.brs.2008.07.002

Monti, A., Cogiamanian, F., Marceglia, S., Ferrucci, F., Mameli, F., Mrakic-Sposta, S., et al. (2008). Improved naming after transcranial direct current stimulation in aphasia. *J. Neurol. Neurosurg. Psychiatry* 79, 451–453. doi: 10.1136/jnnp.2007.135277

Monti, A., Ferrucci, F., Fumagalli, M., Mameli, F., Cogiamanian, F., Ardolino, G., et al. (2013). Transcranial direct current stimulation (tDCS) and language. *J. Neurol. Neurosurg. Psychiatry* 84, 832–842. doi: 10.1136/jnnp-2012-302825

Naeser, M. A., Martin, P. I., Nicholas, M., Baker, E. H., Seekins, H., Kobayashi, M., et al. (2005). Improved picture naming in chronic aphasia after TMS to part of right Broca's area: an open-protocol study. *Brain Lang.* 93, 95–105. doi: 10.1016/j.bandl.2004.08.004

Naeser, M. A., Martin, P. I., Treglia, E., Ho, M., Kaplan, E., Bashir, S., et al. (2010). Research with rTMS in the treatment of aphasia. *Restor. Neurol. Neurosci.* 28, 511–529.

Naeser, M. A., Martin, P. I., Theoret, H., Kobayashi, M., Fregni, F., Nicholas, M., et al. (2011). TMS suppression of right pars triangularis, but not pars opercularis, improves naming in aphasia. *Brain Lang.* 119, 206–213. doi: 10.1016/j.bandl.2011.07.005

Nicholas, L., and Brookshire, R. (1993). A system for quantifying the informativeness and efficiency of the connected speech of adults with aphasia. *J. Speech Hear. Res.* 36, 338–350.

Nishitani, N., Schürmann, M., Amunts, K., and Hari, R. (2005). Broca's region: from action to language. *Physiology* 20, 60–69. doi: 10.1152/physiol.00043.2004

Nitsche, M. A., and Paulus, W. (2000). Excitability changes induced in the human motor cortex by weak transcranial direct current stimulation. *J. Physiol.* 527, 633–639. doi: 10.1111/j.1469-7793.2000.t01-1-00633.x

Oliveri, M., Rossini, P. M., Traversa, R., Cicinelli, P., Filippi, M. M., Pasqualetti, P., et al. (1999). Left frontal transcranial magnetic stimulation reduces contralesional extinction in patients with unilateral right brain damage. *Brain* 122, 1731–1739. doi: 10.1093/brain/122.9.1731

Orsini, A., Grossi, D., Capitani, E., Laiacona, M., Papagno, C., and Vallar, G. (1987). Verbal and spatial immediate memory span: normative data from 1355 adults and 1112 children. *Ital. J. Neurol. Sci.* 8, 537–548. doi: 10.1007/BF02333660

Poreisz, C., Boros, K., Antal, A., and Paulus, W. (2007). Safety aspects of transcranial direct current stimulation concerning healthy subjects and patients. *Brain Res. Bull.* 72, 208–214. doi: 10.1016/j.brainresbull.2007.01.004

Prins, R., and Bastiaanse, R. (2004). Analysing the spontaneous speech of aphasic patients. *Aphasiology* 18, 1075–1091. doi: 10.1080/02687030444000534

Raymer, A. M., and Ellsworth, T. A. (2002). Response to contrasting verb retrieval treatments: a case study. *Aphasiology* 16, 1031–1045. doi: 10.1080/026870401430000609

Saffran, E. M., Berndt, R. S., and Schwartz, M. F. (1989). The quantitative analysis of agrammatic production: procedure and data. *Brain Lang.* 37, 440–479. doi: 10.1016/0093-934X(89)90030-8

Saur, D., Lange, R., Baumgaertner, A., Schraknepper, V., Willmes, K., Rijntjes, M., et al. (2006). Dynamics of language reorganization after stroke. *Brain* 129, 1371–1384. doi: 10.1093/brain/awl090

Saur, D., Kreher, B. W., Schnell, S., Kümmerer, D., Kellmeyer, P., Vry, M. S., et al. (2008). Ventral and dorsal pathways for language. *Proc. Natl. Acad. Sci. U.S.A.* 105, 18035–18040. doi: 10.1073/pnas.0805234105

Schuhmann, T., Schiller, N. O., Goebel, R., and Sack, A. T. (2012). Speaking of which: Dissecting the neurocognitive network of language production in picture naming. *Cereb. Cortex* 22, 701–709. doi: 10.1093/cercor/bhr155

Sparing, R., Dafotakis, M., Meister, I. G., Thirugnanasambandam, N., and Fink, G. R. (2008). Enhancing language performance with non-invasive brain stimulation-a transcranial direct current stimulation study in healthy humans. *Neuropsychologia* 46, 261–268. doi: 10.1016/j.neuropsychologia.2007.07.009

Ulatowska, H. K., Freedman-Stern, R., Doyel, A. W., Macaluso-Haynes, S., and North, A. J. (1983). Production of narrative discourse in aphasia. *Brain Lang.* 19, 317–334. doi: 10.1016/0093-934X(83)90074-3

Vigorelli, P. (2007). *L'Approccio conversazionale nella cura del malato di Alzheimer: I principi generali*, Vol. 1, Milano: J Medical Bools Edizioni.

Vigneau, M., Beaucousin, V., Hervé, P. Y., Duffau, H., Crivello, F., Houdé, O., et al. (2006). Meta-analyzing left hemisphere language areas: phonology, semantics, and sentence processing. *Neuroimage* 30, 1414–1432. doi: 10.1016/j.neuroimage.2005.11.002

Wagner, A. D., Pare-Blagoev, E. J., Clark, J., and Poldrack, R. A. (2001). Recovering meaning: Left prefrontal cortex guides controlled semantic retrieval. *Neuron* 31, 329–338. doi: 10.1016/S0896-6273(01)00359-2

Wambaugh, J. L., Doyle, P. J., Martinez, A. L., and Kalinyak-Fliszar, M. (2002). Effects of two lexical retrieval cueing treatments on action naming in aphasia. *J. Rehabil. Res. Dev.* 39, 455–466.

Warburton, E., Price, C. J., Swinburn, K., and Wise, R. J. (1999). Mechanisms of recovery from aphasia: evidence from positron emission tomography studies. *J. Neurol. Neurosurg. Psychiatry* 66, 155–161. doi: 10.1136/jnnp.66.2.155

Whitney, C., Kirk, M., O'Sullivan, J., Lambon Ralph, M. A., and Jefferies, E. (2011). The neural organization of semantic control: TMS evidence for a distributed network in left inferior frontal and posterior middle temporal gyrus. *Cereb. Cortex* 21, 1066–1075. doi: 10.1093/cercor/bhq180

Wilkinson, R., and Wielaert, S. (2012). Rehabilitation targeted at everyday communication: can we change the talk of people with aphasia and their significant others within conversation? *Arch. Phys. Med. Rehabil.* 93, 70–76. doi: 10.1016/j.apmr.2011.07.206

Winhuisen, L., Thiel, A., Schumacher, B., Kessler, J., Rudolf, J., Haupt, W. F., et al. (2007). The right inferior frontal gyrus and post-stroke aphasia: a follow up investigation. *Stroke* 38, 1286–1292. doi: 10.1161/01.STR.0000259632.04324.6c

Yorkston, K. M., and Beukelman, D. R. (1980). An analysis of connected speech samples of aphasic and normal speakers. *J. Speech Hear. Disor.* 45, 27–36.

Zimmermann, P., and Fimm, B. (1994). *Tests d'evaluation de l'attention* (TEA). IRCCS Fondazione Santa Lucia, Rome: Psytest.

Zingeser, L. B., and Berndt, R. S. (1990). Retrieval of nouns and verbs in agrammatism and anomia. *Brain Lang.* 39, 14–32. doi: 10.1016/0093-934X(90)90002-X

Permissions

All chapters in this book were first published in MAHBD, by Frontiers; hereby published with permission under the Creative Commons Attribution License or equivalent. Every chapter published in this book has been scrutinized by our experts. Their significance has been extensively debated. The topics covered herein carry significant findings which will fuel the growth of the discipline. They may even be implemented as practical applications or may be referred to as a beginning point for another development.

The contributors of this book come from diverse backgrounds, making this book a truly international effort. This book will bring forth new frontiers with its revolutionizing research information and detailed analysis of the nascent developments around the world.

We would like to thank all the contributing authors for lending their expertise to make the book truly unique. They have played a crucial role in the development of this book. Without their invaluable contributions this book wouldn't have been possible. They have made vital efforts to compile up to date information on the varied aspects of this subject to make this book a valuable addition to the collection of many professionals and students.

This book was conceptualized with the vision of imparting up-to-date information and advanced data in this field. To ensure the same, a matchless editorial board was set up. Every individual on the board went through rigorous rounds of assessment to prove their worth. After which they invested a large part of their time researching and compiling the most relevant data for our readers.

The editorial board has been involved in producing this book since its inception. They have spent rigorous hours researching and exploring the diverse topics which have resulted in the successful publishing of this book. They have passed on their knowledge of decades through this book. To expedite this challenging task, the publisher supported the team at every step. A small team of assistant editors was also appointed to further simplify the editing procedure and attain best results for the readers.

Apart from the editorial board, the designing team has also invested a significant amount of their time in understanding the subject and creating the most relevant covers. They scrutinized every image to scout for the most suitable representation of the subject and create an appropriate cover for the book.

The publishing team has been an ardent support to the editorial, designing and production team. Their endless efforts to recruit the best for this project, has resulted in the accomplishment of this book. They are a veteran in the field of academics and their pool of knowledge is as vast as their experience in printing. Their expertise and guidance has proved useful at every step. Their uncompromising quality standards have made this book an exceptional effort. Their encouragement from time to time has been an inspiration for everyone.

The publisher and the editorial board hope that this book will prove to be a valuable piece of knowledge for researchers, students, practitioners and scholars across the globe.

List of Contributors

Marco Zanon
Cognitive Neuroscience Sector, International School for Advanced Studies, SISSA, Trieste, Italy

Piero P. Battaglini, Joanna Jarmolowska and Pierpaolo Busan
Department of Life Sciences, BRAIN Center for Neuroscience, University of Trieste, Trieste, Italy

Gilberto Pizzolato
Department of Medical, Surgical and Health Sciences, University of Trieste, Trieste, Italy

Maria Concetta Pellicciari, Stefano Bignotti and Anna Gazzoli
Cognitive Neuroscience Section, IRCCS Centro San Giovanni di Dio Fatebenefratelli, Brescia, Italy

Susanna Cordone, Cristina Marzano and Luigi De Gennaro
Department of Psychology, University of Rome Sapienza, Rome, Italy

Carlo Miniussi
Cognitive Neuroscience Section, IRCCS Centro San Giovanni di Dio Fatebenefratelli, Brescia, Italy
Department of Clinical and Experimental Sciences, National Institute of Neuroscience, University of Brescia, Brescia, Italy
Neuroscience Section, Department of Clinical and Experimental Sciences, University of Brescia, Brescia, Italy

KentaroYamanaka
Graduate School of Human Life Sciences, Showa Women's University, Tokyo, Japan

Daichi Nozaki
Graduate School of Education, The University of Tokyo, Tokyo, Japan

Hiroshi Kadota
Graduate School of Education, The University of Tokyo, Tokyo, Japan
Research Institute, Kochi University of Technology, Kochi, Japan

Naoko Uedaand Katsuyuki Sakai
Department of Cognitive Neuroscience, Graduate School of Medicine, The University of Tokyo, Tokyo, Japan

Rei Akaishi
Department of Cognitive Neuroscience, Graduate School of Medicine, The University of Tokyo, Tokyo, Japan
Department of Experimental Psychology, University of Oxford, Oxford, UK

Tuomas Mutanen, Jaakko O. Nieminen and Risto J. Ilmoniemi
Department of Biomedical Engineering and Computational Science, Aalto University School of Science, Espoo, Finland
BioMag Laboratory, HUSLAB, Helsinki University Central Hospital, Helsinki, Finland

Masahiro Kawasaki
Department of Intelligent Interaction Technology, Graduate School of Systems and Information Engineering, University of Tsukuba, Tsukuba, Japan
Rhythm-based Brain Information Processing Unit, RIKEN BSI-TOYOTA Collaboration Center, Wako, Japan
Laboratory for Advanced Brain Signal Processing, RIKEN Brain Science Institute, Wako, Japan

Yutaka Uno
Rhythm-based Brain Information Processing Unit, RIKEN BSI-TOYOTA Collaboration Center, Wako, Japan

Keiichi Kitajo
Rhythm-based Brain Information Processing Unit, RIKEN BSI-TOYOTA Collaboration Center, Wako, Japan
Laboratory for Advanced Brain Signal Processing, RIKEN Brain Science Institute, Wako, Japan

Jumpei Mori and Kenji Kobata
Rhythm-based Brain Information Processing Unit, RIKEN BSI-TOYOTA Collaboration Center, Wako, Japan
School of Fundamental Science and Technology, Graduate School of Science and Technology, Keio University, Yokohama, Japan

M. Honda
Department of Functional Brain Research, National Center of Neurology and Psychiatry, National Institute of Neuroscience, Kodaira, Japan

H. Shitara
Department of Functional Brain Research, National Center of Neurology and Psychiatry, National Institute of Neuroscience, Kodaira, Japan
Department of Orthopedic Surgery, Gunma University Graduate School of Medicine, Maebashi, Japan

K. Takagishi
Department of Orthopedic Surgery, Gunma University Graduate School of Medicine, Maebashi, Japan

T. Shinozaki
Department of Orthopedic Surgery, Maki Hospital, Takasaki, Japan

T. Hanakawa
Department of Functional Brain Research, National Center of Neurology and Psychiatry, National Institute of Neuroscience, Kodaira, Japan
Department of Advanced Neuroimaging, Integrative Brain Imaging Center, National Center of Neurology and Psychiatry, Kodaira, Japan
PRESTO, Japan Science and Technology Agency, Kawaguchi, Japan

Domenica Veniero
Neuroscience Section, Department of Clinical and Experimental Sciences, University of Brescia, Brescia, Italy
Cognitive Neuroscience Section, IRCCS Centro San Giovanni di Dio Fatebenefratelli, Brescia, Italy

Marta Bortoletto
Cognitive Neuroscience Section, IRCCS Centro San Giovanni di Dio Fatebenefratelli, Brescia, Italy

Luca Falciati, Tiziana Gianesini and Claudio Maioli
Department of Clinical and Experimental Sciences and National Institute of Neuroscience, University of Brescia, Brescia, Italy

Alessandra Del Felice and Silvia F. Storti
Clinical Neurophysiology and Functional Neuroimaging Unit, Section of Neurology, Department of Neurological and Movement Sciences, University of Verona, Verona, Italy

Paolo Manganotti and Antonio Fiaschi
Clinical Neurophysiology and Functional Neuroimaging Unit, Section of Neurology, Department of Neurological and Movement Sciences, University of Verona, Verona, Italy
Department of Neurophysiology, Foundation IRCCS San Camillo Hospital, Venice, Italy

Emanuela Formaggio
Department of Neurophysiology, Foundation IRCCS San Camillo Hospital, Venice, Italy

Alessandro Zamboni, Alessandra Bertoldo and Gianna M.Toffolo
Department of Information Engineering, University of Padova, Padova, Italy

Richard G. Carson
Trinity College Institute of Neuroscience and School of Psychology, Trinity College Dublin, Dublin, Ireland
School of Psychology, Queen's University Belfast, Belfast, UK

Niamh C. Kennedy
School of Psychology, Queen's University Belfast, Belfast, UK
School of Rehabilitation Sciences University of East Anglia, Norwich, UK

Jui-Yang Chang and Barry D. Van Veen
Department of Electrical and Computer Engineering, University of Wisconsin, Madison, WI, USA

Andrea Pigorini and Marcello Massimini
Department of Clinical Sciences, University of Milan, Milan, Italy

Giulio Tononi
Department of Psychiatry, University of Wisconsin, Madison, WI, USA

Lino Nobili
Centre of Epilepsy Surgery "C. Munari," Niguarda Hospital, Milan, Italy

Olivia M. Lapenta and Paulo S. Boggio
Social and Cognitive Neuroscience Laboratory, Center for Healthy and Biological Sciences, Mackenzie Presbyterian University, Sao Paulo, Brazil

Ludovico Minati
U.O. Direzione Scientifica, Fondazione IRCCS Istituto Neurologico "Carlo Besta", Milano, Italy

Felipe Fregni
Laboratory of Neuromodulation, Harvard Medical School, Spaulding Rehabilitation Hospital, Massachusetts General Hospital, Boston, MA, USA

Susanna Cipollari
Istituto Di Ricovero e Cura a Carattere Scientifico Fondazione Santa Lucia, Roma, Italy

Margherita Di Paola
Istituto Di Ricovero e Cura a Carattere Scientifico Fondazione Santa Lucia, Roma, Italy
Dipartimento di Medicina Interna e Sanità Pubblica, Università de L'Aquila, L'Aquila-Coppito, Italy

Nathan A. Parks
Department of Psychological Science, University of Arkansas, Fayetteville, AR, USA

Catarina Saiote, Zsolt Turi, Walter Paulus and Andrea Antal
Clinic for Clinical Neurophysiology, Universitätsmedizin, Georg-August-Universität, Göttingen, Germany

Toralf Neuling
Experimental Psychology Lab, Center of excellence Hearing4all, Department for Psychology, Faculty for Medicine and Health Sciences, Carl von Ossietzky, Universität, Ammerländer Heerstr, Oldenburg, Germany

Christoph S. Herrmann, Stefan Rach and Daniel Strüber
Experimental Psychology Lab, Center of excellence Hearing4all, Department for Psychology, Faculty for Medicine and Health Sciences, Carl von Ossietzky, Universität, Ammerländer Heerstr, Oldenburg, Germany
Research Center Neurosensory Science, Carl von Ossietzky Universität, Oldenburg, Germany

Toralf Neuling
Experimental Psychology Lab, University of Oldenburg, Oldenburg, Germany

Stefan Rach and Christoph S. Herrmann
Experimental Psychology Lab, University of Oldenburg, Oldenburg, Germany
Research Center Neurosensory Science, University of Oldenburg, Oldenburg, Germany

Paola Marangolo
Facoltà di Medicina, Università Politecnica Marche, Ancona, Italy
Department of Clinical and Behavioural Neurology, Istituto di Ricovero a Carattere Scientifico Fondazione Santa Lucia, Roma, Italy

Valentina Fiori, Maria A. Calpagnano, Serena Campana and Carmelina Razzano
Department of Clinical and Behavioural Neurology, Istituto di Ricovero a Carattere Scientifico Fondazione Santa Lucia, Roma, Italy

Carlo Caltagirone
Department of Clinical and Behavioural Neurology, Istituto di Ricovero a Carattere Scientifico Fondazione Santa Lucia, Roma, Italy
Department of Neurology, Universitá di Tor Vergata, Roma, Italy

Andrea Marini
Department of Clinical and Behavioural Neurology, Istituto di Ricovero a Carattere Scientifico Fondazione Santa Lucia, Roma, Italy
Dipartimento di Scienze Umane, Università di Udine, Udine, Italy

Index

www.ingramcontent.com/pod-product-compliance
Lightning Source LLC
LaVergne TN
LVHW082205200926
848484LV00008B/2213